Perspectives in Medicine

New Trends in Neurosonology and Cerebral Hemodynamics – an Update

Eva Bartels, Susanne Bartels and Holger Poppert, Editors

Volume 1 · 2012

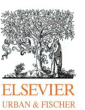
ELSEVIER
URBAN & FISCHER

Amsterdam · Boston · London · New York · Oxford · Paris · Philadelphia · San Diego · St. Louis

© 2012 Elsevier GmbH. All rights reserved.
This journal and the individual contributions contained in it are protected under copyright by Elsevier GmbH, and the following terms and conditions apply to their use:

Photocopying
Single photocopies of single articles may be made for personal use as allowed by national copyright laws. Permission of the Publisher and payment of a fee is required for all other photocopying, including multiple or systematic copying, copying for advertising or promotional purposes, resale, and all forms of document delivery. Special rates are available for educational institutions that wish to make photocopies for non-profit educational classroom use.
For information on how to seek permission visit www.elsevier.com/permissions or call: (+44) 1865 843830 (UK) / (+1) 215 239 3804 (USA).

Derivative Works
Subscribers may reproduce tables of contents or prepare lists of articles including abstracts for internal circulation within their institutions. Permission of the Publisher is required for resale or distribution outside the institution. Permission of the Publisher is required for all other derivative works, including compilations and translations (please consult www.elsevier.com/permissions).

Electronic Storage or Usage
Permission of the Publisher is required to store or use electronically any material contained in this journal, including any article or part of an article (please consult www.elsevier.com/permissions).
Except as outlined above, no part of this publication may be reproduced, stored in a retrieval system or transmitted in any form or by any means, electronic, mechanical, photocopying, recording or otherwise, without prior written permission of the Publisher.

Notice
No responsibility is assumed by the Publisher for any injury and/or damage to persons or property as a matter of products liability, negligence or otherwise, or from any use or operation of any methods, products, instructions or ideas contained in the material herein. Because of rapid advances in the medical sciences, in particular, independent verification of diagnoses and drug dosages should be made.
Although all advertising material is expected to conform to ethical (medical) standards, inclusion in this publication does not constitute a guarantee or endorsement of the quality or value of such product or of the claims made of it by its manufacturer.

Publisher: Elsevier GmbH, Hackerbrücke 6, 80335 Munich, Germany
Phone: (+49) (89) 53830, Fax: (+49) (89) 5383939
e-mail: info@elsevier.de

Perspectives in Medicine is Elsevier's new open access journal serial for the publication of concise and well-defined medical topics, each delivered as a distinct topical issue, serving as a platform for content that usually falls somewhere in between traditional journal articles and more expansive books or textbooks.

This journal is published **"open access"**. There are no fees for accessing the publication.

For detailed journal information see our homepage **www.elsevier.com/locate/permed**

As of vol. 1, number 1 (2012) the paper used in this publication meets the requirements of ANSI/NISO Z39.48-1992 (Permanence of Paper).

Typesetting: Thomson Digital, B/10-12, Noida Special Economic Zone, Noida 201 305, India
Printing and binding: Stürtz GmbH, Alfred-Nobel-Straße 33, 97080 Würzburg, Germany
Coverdesign: Studio eljott, Lothar Jähnichen, Dornburg, Germany

ISSN 2211-968X
ISBN 978-3-437-41034-5

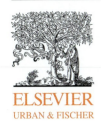
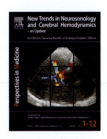

Bartels E, Bartels S, Poppert H (Editors):
New Trends in Neurosonology and Cerebral Hemodynamics — an Update.
Perspectives in Medicine (2012) 1, 1—12

journal homepage: www.elsevier.com/locate/permed

Contents

Prefaces
The European Society of Neurosonology and Cerebral Hemodynamics (ESNCH)
    D. Russell, E.B. Ringelstein, K. Niederkorn 1
Foreword
    L. Csiba 3
Foreword
    E. Bartels, S. Bartels, H. Poppert 4

1 Advances in Neurosonology - Brain Perfusion, Sonothrombolysis, Plaque Perfusion
Advances in neurosonology – Brain perfusion, sonothrombolysis and CNS drug delivery
    S. Meairs 5
Sonothrombolysis: Current status
    P.D. Schellinger, C.A. Molina 11
Sonothrombolysis for treatment of acute ischemic stroke: Current evidence and new developments
    J. Eggers 14
Current trends in sonothrombolysis for acute ischemic stroke
    A.V. Alexandrov 21
Safety evaluation of superheated perfluorocarbon nanodroplets for novel phase change type neurological therapeutic agents
    J. Shimizu, R. Endoh, T. Fukuda, T. Inagaki, H. Hano, R. Asami, K.-i. Kawabata, M. Yokoyama,
    H. Furuhata 25
Update on ultrasound brain perfusion imaging
    G. Seidel 30
Brain tissue perfusion monitoring using Sonopod for transcranial color duplex sonography
    T. Shiogai, M. Koyama, M. Yamamoto, K. Yoshikawa, T. Mizuno, M. Nakagawa 34
Relationship between refill-kinetics of ultrasound perfusion imaging and vascular obstruction in acute middle cerebral artery stroke
    M. Bolognese, D. Artemis, A. Alonso, M.G. Hennerici, S. Meairs, R.R. Kern 39
Imaging of plaque perfusion using contrast-enhanced ultrasound – Clinical significance
    E. Vicenzini, M.F. Giannoni, G. Sirimarco, M.C. Ricciardi, M. Toscano, G.L. Lenzi, V. Di Piero 44
Plaque angiogenesis identification with Contrast Enhanced Carotid Ultrasonography: Statement of the Consensus after the 16th ESNCH Meeting - Munich, 20-23 May 2011
    H. Poppert, E. Vicenzini, K. Stock, E. Bartels 51

2 Novel Technologies
Mechanical recanalization in acute stroke treatment
    P. Mordasini, G. Schroth, J. Gralla 54
Functional guidance in intracranial tumor surgery
    S.M. Krieg, F. Ringel, B. Meyer 59
Endovascular sono-lysis using EKOS system in acute stroke patients with a main cerebral artery occlusion – A pilot study
    M. Kuliha, M. Roubec, T. Fadrná, D. Šaňák, R. Herzig, T. Jonszta, D. Czerný, J. Krajča, V. Procházka,
    D. Školoudík 65

Act on Stroke – Optimization of clinical processes and workflow for stroke diagnosis and treatment
    B.M. Hofmann, U. Zikeli, E.B. Ringelstein 73
Telestroke – How does that work?
    S. Boy 77
Ultrasound fusion imaging
    J. Stoll 80
Threedimensional imaging of carotid arteries: Advantages and pitfalls of ultrasound investigations
    E. Vicenzini, S. Pro, G. Sirimarco, P. Pulitano, O. Mecarelli, G.L. Lenzi, V. Di Piero 82
Four-dimensional ultrasound imaging in neuro-ophthalmology
    E. Titianova, S. Cherninkova, S. Karakaneva, B. Stamenov 86
Clinical application of laser Doppler flowmetry in neurology
    Z. Stoyneva 89

3 Stroke Prevention, Diagnostics and Therapy

The role of extracranial ultrasound in the prevention of stroke based on the new guidelines
    B. Léránt, L. Csiba 94
Optimized prevention of stroke: What is the role of ultrasound?
    D. Sander 100
Measuring the degree of internal carotid artery stenosis
    G.-M. von Reutern 104
Early ultrasound imaging of carotid arteries in the acute ischemic cerebrovascular patients
    M.F. Giannoni, E. Vicenzini, E. Sbarigia, V. Di Piero, G.L. Lenzi, F. Speziale 108
How to treat an asymptomatic carotid stenosis? The view of the neurologist
    D. Sander, M. Valet 112
Medical management of asymptomatic carotid stenosis
    M. Jauss 116
When to perform transcranial Doppler to predict cerebral hyperperfusion after carotid endarterectomy?
    C.W. Pennekamp, S.C. Tromp, R.G. Ackerstaff, M.L. Bots, R.V. Immink, W. Spiering, J.-P.P. de Vries,
    J. Kappelle, F.L. Moll, W.F. Buhre, G.J. de Borst 119
Predictors of carotid artery in-stent restenosis
    K. Wasser, S. Gröschel, J. Wohlfahrt, K. Gröschel 122
Post-carotid stent ultrasound provides critical data to avoid rare but serious complications
    J.J. Volpi, Z. Garami, R. Kabir, O. Diaz-Daza, R. Klucznik 129

4 Atherosclerotic Plaque, Intima-Media Thickness

How local hemodynamics at the carotid bifurcation influence the development of carotid plaques
    D. Liepsch, A. Balasso, H. Berger, H.-H. Eckstein 132
In vivo wall shear stress patterns in carotid bifurcations assessed by 4D MRI
    A. Harloff, M. Markl 137
Carotid intima-media thickness (cIMT) and plaque from risk assessment and clinical use to genetic discoveries
    S. Bartels, A.R. Franco, T. Rundek 139
Arterial wall dynamics
    G. Baltgaile 146
Morphological, hemodynamic and stiffness changes in arteries of young smokers
    B. Léránt, C. Straesser, R.K. Kovács, L. Oláh, L. Kardos, L. Csiba 152
Breath holding index and arterial stiffness in evaluation of stroke risk in diabetic patients
    I. Zavoreo, V. Bašić Kes, L. Ćorić, V. Demarin 156
Intima-media thickness of the carotid artery in OSAS patients
    S. Andonova, D. Petkova, Y. Bocheva 160
The association of carotid intima-media thickness (cIMT) and stroke: A cross sectional study
    S. Harris 164
Carotid atherosclerosis: Socio-demographic issues, the hidden dimensions
    F. Abd-Allah, N. Abo-Krysha, E. Baligh 167
Comparative *in vivo* and *in vitro* postmortem ultrasound assessment of intima-media thickness with additional histological analysis in human carotid arteries
    S. Farkas, S. Molnár, K. Nagy, T. Hortobágyi, L. Csiba 170

5 Cerebral Hemodynamics in Ischemic Stroke

Hemodynamic causes of deterioration in acute ischemic stroke
G. Tsivgoulis, N. Apostolidou, S. Giannopoulos, V.K. Sharma 177

Transcranial Doppler in acute stroke management – A "real-time" bed-side guide to reperfusion and collateral flow
C. Levi, H. Zareie, M. Parsons 185

Cerebral autoregulation in acute ischemic stroke
M. Reinhard, S. Rutsch, A. Hetzel 194

Vertebral artery hypoplasia and the posterior circulation stroke
A.S. Szárazová, E. Bartels, P. Turčáni 198

Volume flow rate
D. Ratanakorn, J. Keandaoungchan 203

Intra- and extracranial stenoses in TIA – Findings from the Aarhus TIA-study: A prospective population-based study
P. von Weitzel-Mudersbach, S.P. Johnsen, G. Andersen 207

Symptomatic intracranial stenosis: A university hospital-based ultrasound study
F. Viaro, F.M. Farina, A. Onofri, G. Meneghetti, C. Baracchini 211

6 Detection of Microembolic Signals, Right-to-Left Shunt (Patent Foramen Ovale)

The contribution of microembolic signals (MES) detection in cardioembolic stroke
M.A. Ritter 214

Exploration of a zero-tolerance regime on cerebral embolism in symptomatic carotid artery disease
R.W.M. Keunen, A. van Sonderen, M. Hunfeld, M. Remmers, D.L. Tavy, S.F.T.M. de Bruijn, A. Mosch 218

Late septic encephalopathy and septic shock are not associated with ongoing cerebral embolism
M. Hunfeld, M. Remmers, R. Hoogenboezem, M. Frank, M. van der Mee, H.S.M. Hazra, S.C. Tromp, E.H. Boezeman, D.L. Tavy, R.W. Keunen 224

Patent foramen ovale
S. Horner, K. Niederkorn, F. Fazekas 228

Microbubble signal properties from PFO tests using transcranial Doppler ultrasound
C. Banahan, R. Patel, V. Jeyagopal, A. Mistri, J.P. Hague, D.H. Evans, E.M.L. Chung 232

Italian patent foramen ovale survey (I.P.O.S.): Early results
L. Caputi, G. Butera, E. Parati, G. Sangiorgi, E. Onorato, G.P. Anzola, M. Chessa, M. Carminati, G.P. Ussia, I. Spadoni, G. Santoro, on behalf of IPOS investigators 236

An increased frequency of right-to-left shunt in patients with chronic hyperventilation syndrome
J. Staszewski, K. Tomczykiewicz, B. Brodacki, R.A. Piusińska-Macoch, A. Stępień, Z. Podgajny, P. Smużyński, M. Zarębiński 241

7 Non Atherosclerotic Stroke Etiology

Diagnosis of non-atherosclerotic carotid disease
A. Lovrencic-Huzjan 244

Ultrasound in spontaneous cervical artery dissection
R. Dittrich, M.A. Ritter, E.B. Ringelstein 250

Diagnosis and management of Takayasu arteritis
N. Venketasubramanian 255

Moyamoya like arteriopathy: Neurosonological suspicion and prognosis in adult asymptomatic patients
G. Malferrari, M. Zedde, G. De Berti, M. Maggi, N. Marcello 257

Posttraumatic vasospasm and intracranial hypertension after wartime traumatic brain injury
R.A. Armonda, T.A. Tigno, S.M. Hochheimer, F.L. Stephens, R.S. Bell, A.H. Vo, M.A. Severson, S.A. Marshall, S.M. Oppenheimer, R. Ecker, A. Razumovsky 261

Role of TCD in sickle cell disease: A review
V.F. Zétola 265

Transcranial Doppler sonography in children with sickle cell disease and silent ischemic lesions
F.M. Farina, P. Rampazzo, L. Sainati, R. Manara, A. Onofri, R. Colombatti, C. Baracchini, G. Meneghetti 269

Intellectual impairment and TCD evaluation in children with sickle cell disease and silent stroke
A. Onofri, M. Montanaro, P. Rampazzo, R. Colombatti, F.M. Farina, R. Manara, L. Sainati, M. Ermani, C. Baracchini, G. Meneghetti 272

8 Cerebral Autoregulation and Functional Testing

Cerebral blood flow velocity in sleep
J. Klingelhöfer 275

Asymmetry of cerebral autoregulation does not correspond to asymmetry of cerebrovascular pressure reactivity
B. Schmidt, M. Czosnyka, J. Klingelhöfer 285

Adaptation of cerebral pressure-velocity hemodynamic changes of neurovascular coupling to orthostatic challenge
P. Castro, R. Santos, J. Freitas, B. Rosengarten, R. Panerai, E. Azevedo 290

Are impaired endothelial function in the posterior cerebral circulation and intact endothelial function in the anterior cerebral and systemic circulation associated with migraine: A post hoc study
D. Perko, J. Pretnar-Oblak, B. Žvan, M. Zaletel 297

Effect of helium on cerebral blood flow: A $n = 1$ trial in a healthy young person
S.M. Zinkstok, D. Bertens, J.R. de Kruijk, S.C. Tromp 301

Cerebral blood flow in the chronic heart failure patients
T. Lepic, G. Loncar, B. Bozic, D. Veljancic, B. Labovic, Z. Krsmanovic, M. Lepic, R. Raicevic 304

Withdraw of statin improves cerebrovascular reserve in radiation vasculopathy
J.J. Volpi, R. Kabir, Z. Garami, P. New 309

Informativity of pulsatility index and cerebral autoregulation in hydrocephalus
V. Semenyutin, V. Aliev, V. Bersnev, A. Patzak, L. Rozhchenko, A. Kozlov, S. Ramazanov 311

The long-term effects of hypobaric and hyperbaric conditions on brain hemodynamic: A transcranial Doppler ultrasonography of blood flow velocity of middle cerebral and basilar arteries in pilots and divers
S.-M. Fereshtehnejad, M. Mehrpour, S.M.H. Mahmoodi, P. Bassir, B. Dormanesh, M.R. Motamed . . . 316

Oscillating transcranial Doppler patterns of brain death associated with therapeutic maneuvers
P. Cardona, H. Quesada, L. Cano, J. Campelacreu, A. Escrig, P. Mora, F. Rubio 321

9 Transcranial Duplex Ultrasonography

Transcranial color-coded duplex ultrasonography in routine cerebrovascular diagnostics
E. Bartels 325

Evaluation of very early recanalization after tPA administration monitoring by transcranial color-coded sonography
H. Mitsumura, M. Yogo, R. Sengoku, H. Furuhata, S. Mochio 331

Transcranial sonography of the cerebral parenchyma: Update on clinically relevant applications
U. Walter 334

Intra- and post-operative monitoring of deep brain implants using transcranial ultrasound
U. Walter 344

Transcranial ultrasound in adults and children with movement disorders
J. Liman, M. Bähr, P. Kermer 349

Possibilities of transcranial color-coded sonography in pathology of deep brain veins in children
M. Abramova, I. Stepanova, S. Shayunova 353

Transcranial sonography in psychiatric diseases
M.D. Mijajlovic 357

The role of color duplex sonography in the brain death diagnostics
I.D. Stulin, D.S. Solonskiy, M.V. Sinkin, R.S. Musin, A.O. Mnushkin, A.V. Kascheev, L.A. Savin, M.A. Bolotnov 362

10 Cerebral and Cervical Venous Ultrasonography

Ultrasound examination techniques of extra- and intracranial veins
E. Stolz 366

Fact or fiction: Chronic cerebro-spinal insufficiency
C. Baracchini, P. Gallo 371

Chronic cerebrospinal venous insufficiency in patients with multiple sclerosis: A case-control study from Iran
M. Mehrpour, N. Najimi, S.-M. Fereshtehnejad, F.N. Safa, S. Mirzaeizadeh, M.R. Motamed, M. Nabavi, M.A. Sahraeian 375

Ultrasound findings of the optic nerve and its arterial venous system in multiple sclerosis patients with and without optic neuritis vs. healthy controls
N. Carraro, G. Servillo, V.M. Sarra, A. Bignamini, G. Pizzolato, M. Zorzon 381

Contents

Virtual Navigator study: Subset of preliminary data about cerebral venous circulation
  M. Zedde, G. Malferrari, G. De Berti, M. Maggi, L. Lodigiani 385
Ipsilateral evaluation of the transverse sinus: Transcranial color-coded sonography approach in comparison with magnetic resonance venography
  M. Zedde, G. Malferrari, G. De Berti, M. Maggi 390
Intraoperative color-coded duplex sonography of the superior sagittal sinus in parasagittal meningiomas
  V.B. Semenyutin, D.A. Pechiborsch, V.E. Olyushin, V.A. Aliev, V.Y. Chirkin, A.V. Kozlov,
  G.K. Panuntsev. 395
Italian multicenter study on venous hemodynamics in multiple sclerosis: Advanced Sonological Protocol
  G. Malferrari, M. Del Sette, M. Zedde, S. Sanguigni, N. Carraro, C. Baracchini, M. Mancini,
  E. Stolz 399

11 Nonvascular Neurosonography – Muscle, Nerve and Eye
B-mode sonography of the optic nerve in neurological disorders with altered intracranial pressure
  J. Bäuerle, M. Nedelmann. 404
The retrobulbar spot sign in sudden blindness – Sufficient to rule out vasculitis?
  M. Ertl, M. Altmann, E. Torka, H. Helbig, U. Bogdahn, A. Gamulescu, F. Schlachetzki 408
Ultrasonography of the optic nerve sheath in brain death
  A. Lovrencic-Huzjan, D.S. Simicevic, I.M. Popovic, M.B. Puretic, V.V. Cvetkovic, A. Gopcevic, M. Vucic,
  B. Rode, V. Demarin 414
Ultrasonography of the peripheral nervous system
  H. Kele 417
Ultrasonography of peripheral nerves – Clinical significance
  U. Schminke. 422
An overview of musculoskeletal ultrasound – A thirteen years experience in Pakistan
  S.A. Gilani 427
Four-dimensional ultrasound calf muscle imaging in patients with genetic types of distal myopathy
  E. Titianova, T. Chamova, V. Guergueltcheva, I. Tournev. 431

12 Case Reports
"A horse, a horse, my kingdom for a horse" – Saddle thrombosis of carotid bifurcation in acute stroke
  E.B. Vicenzini, M.F. Giannoni, M.C. Ricciardi, G. Sirimarco, M. Toscano, G.L. Lenzi, V. Di Piero . . . 435
Intravascular papillary endothelial hyperplasia at the origin of internal carotid artery: A rare cause of stroke
  N. Carraro, V.M. Sarra, A. Gorian, F. Pancrazio, S. Bucconi, P. Martingano, G. Pizzolato, F.C. Grandi . . . 440
Reversible cerebral vasoconstriction syndrome after preeclampsia
  R. Müller, O. Meier, R.L. Haberl. 443
Transcranial and cervical duplex: A feasible approach to the diagnosis of pulsatile tinnitus
  P. Cardona, H. Quesada, L. Cano, J. Campdelacreu, A. Escrig, P. Mora, F. Rubio 446
Pitfall of vertebral artery insonation: Bidirectional flow without subclavian artery pathology
  S. Johnsen, S.J. Schreiber, F. Connolly, K. Schepelmann, J.M. Valdueza. 449
Migraine-like presentation of vertebral artery dissection after cervical manipulative therapy
  D. Jatuzis, J. Valaikiene 452
The impact of recanalization on ischemic stroke outcome: A clinical case presentation
  S. Andonova, F. Kirov, C. Bachvarov. 455
Semantic aphasia in a sonothrombolysed patient. A treatment without use of rt-PA
  M. Klissurski, E. Vavrek, N. Nicheva-Vavrek 459
My worst case with sonothrombolysis
  E.V. Vavrek 462
Transient brainstem ischemia and dural arteriovenous malformation
  J. Valaikiene, J. Dementaviciene, D. Jatuzis, L. Cimbalistiene 465

List of Contributors III

Subject index IX

Acknowledgments XVIII

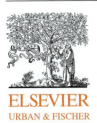

Bartels E, Bartels S, Poppert H (Editors):
New Trends in Neurosonology and Cerebral Hemodynamics — an Update.
Perspectives in Medicine (2012) 1, 1—2

journal homepage: www.elsevier.com/locate/permed

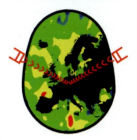

Foreword
The European Society of Neurosonology and Cerebral Hemodynamics (ESNCH)

The formation of the European Society of Neurosonology and Cerebral Hemodynamics (ESNCH) was proposed by Professor David Russell in a letter to leading European Scientists in this field in December 1993. In August 1994 Professor Russell sent a more general invitation to European scientists inviting them to attend an inaugural meeting during the 8th International Cerebral Hemodynamics Symposium from 25th to 27th September 1994 which was chaired by Professor E.Bernd Ringelstein in Münster, Germany, from 25th to 27th September 1994. The inaugural meeting of the ESNCH was held on 26th September 1994. The first meeting of the ESNCH was chaired by Professor Jürgen Klingelhöfer and Professor Eva Bartels in Munich, Germany, from 29th August to 1st September 1996. The statutes of the Society were accepted by a General Assembly on 27th May 1997 during the 2nd meeting of the ESNCH in Zeist/Utrecht, Netherlands, which was chaired by Professor Rob G. A. Ackerstaff.

The first Executive Committee consisted of Professor David Russell (President), Professor Jürgen Klingelhöfer (secretary), Professor Eva Bartels (treasurer), Professor Rob G. A. Ackerstaff, Professor Donald Grosset, Professor Kurt Niederkorn, Professor E. Bernd Ringelstein and Professor Elietta Zanette.

The ESNCH has grown in the last 18 years to become one of the most important societies in the world in the field of neurosonology and cerebral hemodynamics. We pride ourselves by being a society of the highest academic discipline while always maintaining a welcoming family atmosphere at all of our meetings. We also follow strict financial discipline in order to keep our membership and meeting fees at a level which enables younger colleagues from all countries to become a member and attend our meetings. The number of members continues to grow and we now are a truly international society with members from 29 different countries.

The backbone of a society is dependent on the contributions of its members and we would like to thank all of our colleagues who have contributed to the ESNCH especially on the executive board and different scientific committees. The main reason for our success has been the scientific contributions at our yearly meetings which have made significant contributions in the field of neurosonology and cerebral hemodynamics. It is with sincere thanks and pride that we recall the 16 very successful yearly meetings which the ESNCH has had. The success of these meetings is also without doubt due to the hard work done by the organizing chairpersons and their committees.

We would therefore like you to take a walk down memory lane and to look back and remember the wonderful science and social activities that we had in many different European countries: the 1st meeting of the ESNCH in Munich, Germany, from 29th August 1996, chaired by Professor Jürgen Klingelhöfer and Professor Eva Bartels, the 2nd meeting of the ESNCH in Zeist/Utrecht, Netherlands, May 1997, chaired by Professor Rob G. A. Ackerstaff, the 3rd meeting of the ESNCH in Glasgow, Scotland, May 1998, chaired by Professor Donald G. Grosset, the 4th meeting of the ESNCH in Venice, Italy, April 1999, chaired by Professor Elietta Zanette, the 5th meeting of the ESNCH in Graz, Austria, May 2000, chaired by Professor Kurt Niederkorn, the 6th meeting of the ESNCH in Lisbon, Portugal, May 2001, chaired by Professor Victor Oliveira, the 7th meeting of the ESNCH in Bern, Switzerland, from May 2002, chaired by Professor Matthias Sturzenegger, the 8th meeting of the ESNCH in Alicante, Spain, from May 2003, chaired by Dr. José-Manuel Moltó-Jorda, the 9th meeting of the ESNCH in Wetzlar, Germany, May 2004, chaired by Professor Manfred Kaps, the 10th meeting of the ESNCH in Abano Terme, Padova, Italy, May 2005, chaired by Professor Giorgio Meneghetti, the 11th meeting of the ESNCH took place in Düsseldorf, Germany, from May 2006, chaired by Professor Mario Siebler, the 12th meeting of the ESNCH took place in Budapest, Hungary, May 2007, chaired by Professor László Csiba, the 13th meeting of the ESNCH in Geneva, Italy, May 2008, chaired by Professor Massimo Del Sette, the 14th meeting of ESNCH took place in Riga, Latvia, May 2009, chaired by Dr. Galina Baltgaile, the 15th meeting of the

2211-968X/$ — see front matter © 2012 Elsevier GmbH. All rights reserved.
http://dx.doi.org/10.1016/j.permed.2012.05.001

ESNCH took place in Madrid, Spain, May 2010, chaired by Dr. Joaquin Carneado-Ruiz and the 16th meeting of the ESNCH in Munich, May 2011, chaired by Professor Eva Bartels.

We are now looking forward to our 17th meeting which will be held in Venice from 17th to 20th of May 2012, and will be chaired by Dr. Claudio Baracchini and Professor Giorgio Meneghetti.

The society has also had its very sad moments and we still feel the loss of three very dear friends who were pioneers in the field of neurosonology and cerebral hemodynamics: William Markley McKinney, Elietta Maria Zanette and Merrill P. Spencer (honorary member).

The society has the pleasure and privilege of having three esteemed honorary members: Professor Rune Aaslid, Professor Hiroshi Furuhata and Professor Karl-Fredrik Lindegaard.

The ESNCH has had three past presidents: Professor David Russell (Founding President), Professor E. Bernd Ringelstein and Professor Kurt Niederkorn. The serving president of the ESNCH is Professor László Csiba.

We would lastly like to thank Professor Eva Bartels for her contributions to the ESNCH since its beginning and congratulate her on the publication of New Trends in Neurosonology and Cerebral Hemodynamics — an Update which is based on scientific contributions made by ESNCH members at the 16th meeting of the ESNCH in Munich, May 2011. There is no doubt that this book will promote the goals of the ESNCH with regard to the clinical use of neurosonology and our understanding of cerebral hemodynamics.

Founding President of ESNCH
David Russell[*]
Department of Neurology, Oslo University Hospital,
Norway
Past President of ESNCH
E. Bernd Ringelstein
Department of Neurology, University Hospital of Münster,
Münster, Germany
Past President of ESNCH
Kurt Niederkorn
Department of Neurology, Medical University of Graz,
Austria

[*] Corresponding author.
E-mail address: david.russell@medisin.uio.no (D. Russell)

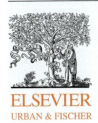
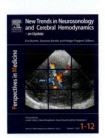

Bartels E, Bartels S, Poppert H (Editors):
New Trends in Neurosonology and Cerebral Hemodynamics — an Update.
Perspectives in Medicine (2012) 1, 3

journal homepage: www.elsevier.com/locate/permed

Foreword

Stroke is an increasing health care problem and social burden in our societies. The neurosonological methods play an important role in CNS research and prevention, diagnostics and therapy of vascular and non-vascular neurological diseases (e.g. neuromuscular, degenerative, peripheral nervous system diseases).

It is pleasing to see the increasing number of sonographic equipment in the departments of neurology and intensive care units (ICU) for monitoring vascular and heart surgery, as well as in studying the effects of new drugs in clinical trials.

Thanks to the development over the past few years, the ultrasonographic methods proved their power not only in prevention and diagnostics of vascular diseases but also in ICU monitoring and in therapeutic intervention (e.g. thrombolysis and gene therapy) and in monitoring regeneration processes in the CNS.

These widely used methods enable the investigation and follow the early impairment of endothelial function and changes of cerebral hemodynamics before and after pharmacological interventions.

Written by international experts this book reviews present knowledge and summarizes the recent results of diagnostic and therapeutic neurosonology.

Updated results of arterial wall imaging, endothelial dysfunction testing, cerebral blood flow measurement, enhancing of thrombolysis are detailed.

This book describes the diagnostic and therapeutic advances of extra- and transcranial ultrasonography, possible research, clinical and pharmacological applications, and besides "the state of the art" the future perspectives are also presented.

To make an annual survey on the growing utilization of ultrasonic methods is justified by the fast improvement in the field of diagnostics and therapy of vascular and other diseases.

I hope that this book will be useful in the daily work and will stimulate our sonologists to use these non-invasive techniques more intensively for the benefit of our patients and for clinical research.

Debrecen, February, 2012

President of ESNCH
László Csiba
University of Debrecen Medical and Health Science Center, Department of Neurology, Móricz Zsigmond str. 22, 4032 Debrecen, Hungary
E-mail address: csiba@dote.hu

2211-968X/$ — see front matter © 2012 Elsevier GmbH. All rights reserved.
http://dx.doi.org/10.1016/j.permed.2012.05.002

Foreword

During the past three decades, the diagnosis and treatment of patients with cerebrovascular diseases have advanced rapidly, whereby especially the field of neuroimaging has made a huge progress. In comparison to other imaging techniques, neurosonology encompasses different ultrasonographic methods which offer excellent time resolution, a bedside approach and noninvasiveness.

In 1996, the first meeting of the European Society of Neurosonology and Cerebral Hemodynamics (ESNCH) in Munich became the cornerstone for further successful cooperation in developing new ultrasound diagnostics and even for new therapeutic techniques in neurosonology. In 1997, selected contributions to the aforementioned symposium were published in the book "New Trends in Cerebral Hemodynamics and Neurosonology". The subsequent annual European meetings have become a popular platform for scientific exchange among all who are interested in neurosonology — not only in Europe, but also worldwide. This successful tradition continued in 2011, when the 16th ESNCH Meeting again took place in Munich.

Because of the large number of high-quality scientific contributions at the 2011 Munich Meeting, we decided to build on our first 1997 book success and to follow with a new book, "New Trends in Neurosonology and Cerebral Hemodynamics — an Update", which features lectures and some of the best-rated posters presented at the meeting, and which highlights the most interesting current topics in the field of neurosonology and cerebral hemodynamics. The concept of this book is very modern due to its additional online access. It enables the reader to view ultrasound images and videos that were included in the scientific contributions.

This new book reflects the development in the field of neurosonology during the past 16 years. In addition to covering the current state of the art in traditional neurosonographic topics, such as extra- and transcranial Doppler- and duplex ultrasonography, emboli detection, cerebral autoregulation, functional testing, etc., we also included articles presenting the newest imaging and therapeutic technologies, such as imaging of plaque perfusion, cerebral perfusion techniques, or sonothrombolysis. We are grateful that not only neurologists but also authors from other disciplines have contributed with their articles — among others — about mechanical recanalization in acute stroke treatment, about neuro-navigation and functional guidance in intracranial tumor surgery, and about ultrasound fusion imaging as well, so that readers will find a comprehensive overview of the latest discoveries and knowledge in neuroimaging and of therapeutic strategies in this field.

Scientists from 51 countries all over the world participated at the Munich meeting. It is a great pleasure for us to also present the contributions of colleagues from those countries where neuroimaging techniques were not established until recent years. Despite the starting difficulties in implementing ultrasonography and introducing it into clinical routine, these colleagues are playing an important role in transferring neurosonographic methods worldwide.

This book would not have been possible without the generous support of Boehringer Ingelheim GmbH, Bracco Imaging Deutschland GmbH, Compumedics Germany GmbH, Esaote Biomedica Deutschland GmbH, Philips GmbH and Toshiba Medical Systems. We would like to express our special gratitude to Dr. Alrun Albrecht, and to Mrs. Rabea Osterloh from Elsevier Publisher for their assistance throughout the planning and preparation of this book. Furthermore, we would like to thank Kashif Kanak and his team for their help during the production process. Finally, we would like to thank all authors for their scientific contributions and for their cooperation.

Eva Bartels*
Center for Neurological Vascular Diagnostics, München, Germany
Susanne Bartels
Albert-Ludwigs-University Freiburg, Department of Psychiatry and Psychotherapy, Freiburg, Germany
Holger Poppert
Klinikum rechts der Isar, Universität München, Department of Neurology, München, Germany

* Corresponding author.
E-mail address: bartels.eva@t-online.de (E. Bartels)

1. Advances in Neurosonology – Brain Perfusion, Sonothrombolysis, Plaque Perfusion

Advances in neurosonology — Brain perfusion, sonothrombolysis and CNS drug delivery

Stephen Meairs*

Department of Neurology, Universitätsklinikum Mannheim, University of Heidelberg, Germany

KEYWORDS
Microbubbles;
Ultrasound;
Stroke;
Therapy;
Sonothrombolysis;
Perfusion;
Drug delivery;
BBB

Summary Advances in microbubble pharmacology together with novel ultrasound technologies are leading to new emerging applications for both assessment and treatment of stroke patients. Ultrasound perfusion imaging, for example, has added new perspectives for diagnosis and monitoring of both ischemic and hemorrhagic stroke. Real-time brain perfusion imaging of cerebral infarctions is now possible and quantitative algorithms for evaluation of regional cerebral blood flow are being applied for the first time in humans. There is growing interest in therapeutic applications of ultrasound, particularly in the field of sonothrombolysis. Recent results indicate that ultrasound and microbubbles may be effective in clot lysis of ischemic stroke even without additional thrombolytic drugs. Moreover, this combination may be effective in treating the microcirculation, which will give new dimensions to the application of sonothrombolysis in stroke patients. Further therapeutic avenues include opening of the blood–brain barrier (BBB) with ultrasound and microbubbles to enable novel drug delivery to the brain.
© 2012 Elsevier GmbH. All rights reserved.

Brain perfusion imaging — towards new clinical applications

The most important advance in brain perfusion imaging during the last several years has been low-mechanical index (MI) real time perfusion scanning. This technique allows the detection of ultrasound contrast agent (UCA) in the cerebral microcirculation with little or no bubble destruction as compared to the high MI-imaging. Because of minimal contrast agent bubble destruction, a high frame rate can be applied, which leads to a better time resolution of bolus kinetics (Fig. 1). Low-MI imaging of contrast agent also avoids the shadowing effect, a significant problem associated with high mechanical index imaging. Because of the high acoustic intensities that are emitted by bursting bubbles, bubbles that are "behind" the emitting bubbles (further away from the ultrasound transducer) are "shadowed" by this effect and thus obscured from data analysis. Thus, areas of tissue that are shadowed may not be available for analysis of tissue perfusion. The problem of shadowing is basically eliminated with low mechanical index imaging, since bubbles are not destroyed with such low acoustic pressures. Moreover, the technique can obtain multi-planar real-time images of brain perfusion [1]. This is a significant breakthrough for ultrasound perfusion imaging, since previous approaches were confined to a single image plane and therefore limited in their assessment of the extents of brain infarction and low perfusion states. The disadvantage of this new low-MI technique, however, is the limited investigation depth due to the low MI used. Recent technological advances suggest, however, that perfusion imaging of the contralateral hemisphere through the temporal bone window will be possible.

* Correspondence address: Department of Neurology, Universitätsklinikum Mannheim, University of Heidelberg, 68167 Mannheim, Germany. Tel.: +49 621 383 3550/3953; fax: +49 621 383 3807.
E-mail address: meairs@neuro.ma.uni-heidelberg.de

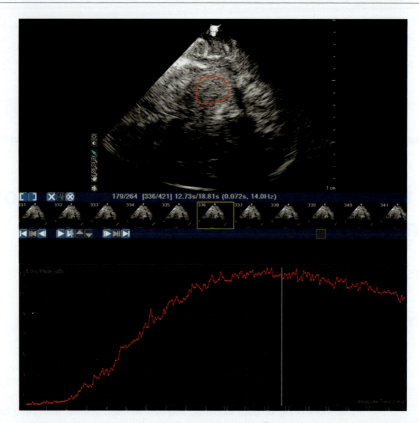

Figure 1 Real-time acoustic intensity curve of the contrast agent SonoVue™ after bolus injection on a Philips IU22 platform using a 1–5 MHz dynamic pulsed array transducer. A very low mechanical index of 0.017 is used, which is then attenuated about 90% by the skull bone before entering the brain. A region of interest has been drawn in the upper image to determine where mean acoustic intensity will be measured. The smaller images in the middle of the figure are the individual image frames at 14 Hz. The red curve displays the mean acoustic intensity of contrast bolus arrival from the region of interest for a total of 264 frames during 18.81 s.

If a constant concentration of contrast agent is delivered to brain tissue using a constant UCA infusion rate, then after destruction with high MI ultrasound, new microbubbles will enter this field with a certain velocity, will travel a determined distance and fill a certain tissue volume depending on blood velocity. The intensity of the echo response signal is directly related to the contrast agent concentration in the tissue; therefore, the blood flow assessment is based on monitoring the intensity of the echo response signal of the insonated volume after bubbles destruction. Low-MI ultrasound imaging can be used to monitor microbubble replenishment in real time (Fig. 2) following the application of destruction pulses at high MI. The behavior of the refill kinetics can be assessed with an exponential curve fit [2]. The parameters of this exponential curve are related to cerebral blood flow: blood flow velocity is directly related to the rate constant β, the fractional vascular volume is related to the plateau echo enhancement (A), and the product of both ($A \cdot \beta$) is associated with blood flow [3]. More sophisticated algorithms for characterization of microbubble refill have been recently introduced [4,5], which should increase reproducibility and improve the quantification of cerebral blood flow with ultrasound perfusion imaging.

Since individual microbubbles can be depicted flowing through small vessels in the brain with low MI imaging, it is possible to track these bubbles and map perfusion over time. Dynamic microvascular microbubble maps provide excellent demarcation of MCA infarctions (Fig. 3) and provide impressive displays of low velocity tissue microbubble refill following destruction with high mechanical index imaging. In brain regions showing delayed contrast bolus arrival on perfusion-weighted MRI, ultrasound shows decreased or absent microbubble refill kinetics. This new technique has been applied for diagnosis of acute ischemic stroke. Recent results demonstrate that real-time ultrasound perfusion imaging with analysis of microbubble replenishment correctly identifies ischemic brain tissue in acute MCA stroke [6]. Pulse compression methods are being combined with the nonlinear bubble imaging techniques discussed above for highly sensitive contrast imaging with very low noise. These advances will lead to further improvements of microbubble imaging of the brain microcirculation, making ultrasound perfusion imaging a viable application for bedside assessment of acute stroke patients.

Therapeutic applications of ultrasound — sonothrombolysis

Ultrasound applied as an adjunct to thrombolytic therapy improves recanalization of occluded intracerebral vessels and microbubbles can amplify this effect. New data suggest that ultrasound and microbubbles alone may be as

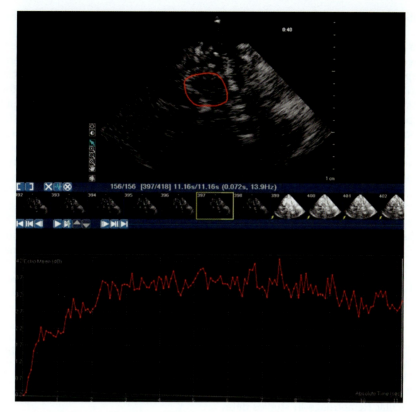

Figure 2 Real-time acoustic intensity curve of the contrast agent SonoVue™ demonstrating refill following bubble destruction with transient high mechanical index imaging. Mean acoustic intensity is measured in the region of interest in the upper image. The smaller images in the middle of the figure are the individual image frames at 14 Hz. The yellow arrow shows the first of a series of high mechanical index images for microbubble destruction.

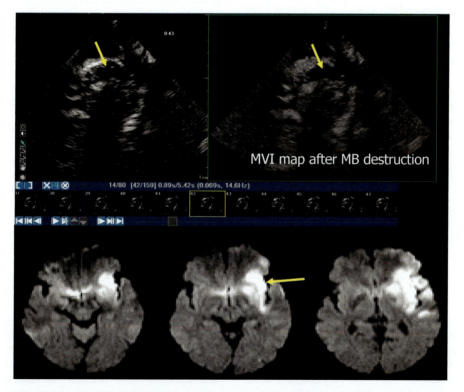

Figure 3 Microvascular map of left MCA infarction (arrows) characterized by absent or diminished contrast agent. The excellent infarction demarcation compares well with MRI diffusion-weighted imaging (bottom images).

effective as t-PA thrombolysis and also safer with less risk of hemorrhage [7,8].

Ultrasound-sensitive thrombolytic drug delivery combined with specific targeting is highly attractive. Targeting of clot-dissolving therapeutics can potentially decrease the frequency of complications while simultaneously increasing treatment effectiveness by concentrating the available drug at the desired site and permitting a lower systemic dose [9].

Clinical studies support the use of ultrasound for therapy of ischemic stroke, and first trials of enhancing sonothrombolysis with microbubbles have been encouraging. A recent meta-analysis of all published clinical sonothrombolysis studies confirmed that ultrasound and tPA (with or without microbubbles) increases recanalization compared to tPA alone [10]. These observations have led to design of CLOTBUSTER, a phase III controlled clinical trial of sonothrombolysis.

Sonothrombolysis of spontaneous intracranial hemorrhages

One emerging clinical application is sonothrombolysis of intracranial hemorrhages for clot evacuation using catheter-mounted transducers. As compared with MISTIE (Minimally Invasive Surgery plus T-PA for Intracerebral Hemorrhage Evacuation) and CLEAR (Clot Lysis Evaluating Accelerated Resolution of Intraventricular Hemorrhage II) studies data, the rate of lysis during treatment for IVH and ICH was faster in patients treated with sonothrombolysis plus rt-PA *versus* rt-PA alone [11]. Thus, lysis and drainage of spontaneous ICH and IVH with a reduction in mass effect can be accomplished rapidly and safely through sonothrombolysis using stereotactically delivered drainage and ultrasound catheters *via* a bur hole.

MRI-guided focused ultrasound for clot lysis

Histotripsy is a process which fractionates soft tissue through controlled cavitation using focused, short, high-intensity ultrasound pulses. Histotripsy can be used to achieve effective thrombolysis with ultrasound energy alone at peak negative acoustic pressures >6 MPa, breaking down blood clots in about 1.5–5 min into small fragments less than 5 μm diameter [12]. Recent developments in using MR-guided focused ultrasound therapy through the intact skull suggest that this technology could be useful for clot lysis in humans. Experimental studies are currently being undertaken to test this possibility, both in ischemic and hemorrhagic stroke.

Ultrasound and microbubbles for treatment of the microcirculation

Ultrasound and microbubbles may improve flow to the microcirculation irrespective of recanalization, thus opening new opportunities for application of sonothrombolysis in acute ischemic stroke. This was suggested by results of a study on possible adverse bioeffects [13] of 2 MHz ultrasound and microbubbles (Sonovue™) in a middle cerebral artery permanent occlusion model in rats at different steps in the cascade of tissue destruction after ischemic stroke [14]. While deleterious effects were not observed, infarctions were unexpectedly smaller in the treatment group, despite the fact that in all animals recanalization of the MCA did not occur. This suggested a beneficial effect of ultrasound and microbubbles in the microcirculation. A similar tissue protective effect has been found in an *in vivo* animal study using intravenous microbubbles and transthoracic ultrasound to treat acute coronary thromboses. Pigs treated with ultrasound and intravenous perfluorocarbon microbubbles (PESDA) had significantly greater improvements in ST segments over a 30-minute treatment period when compared with pigs treated with ultrasound alone or with control animals. Moreover, there was a significantly smaller myocardial contrast defect size after treatment with ultrasound and PESDA [15]. Recently, nano-CT was used to demonstrate complete reversal of microcirculatory impairment in a rodent reperfusion model following treatment with rt-PA, ultrasound and microbubbles [16]. The mechanism of the microcirculatory effect of ultrasound and microbubbles may involve improvement of blood flow to risk tissue *via* collaterals and changes in the microenvironment of damaged tissue, like decreased cell damaging factors, *e.g.* glutamate or enhanced enzyme activity of endothelial nitric oxide [17]. Further work is necessary to elucidate the exact mechanisms of salvaging of tissue-at-risk by ultrasound-mediated microbubble thrombolysis.

Opening the blood–brain barrier with focused ultrasound and microbubbles

The blood–brain barrier is a significant obstacle for delivery of both small molecules and macromolecular agents. Indeed, potential therapeutic substances, which cannot be applied in the presence of an intact BBB are neuropeptides, proteins and chemotherapeutic agents. Likewise, large-molecules such as monoclonal antibodies, recombinant proteins, antisense, or gene therapeutics do not cross the BBB.

There is a good deal of evidence showing that ultrasound can be used to permeate blood-tissue barriers. Large molecules and genes can cross the plasma membrane of cultured cells after application of acoustic energy [18]. Indeed, electron microscopy has revealed ultrasound-induced membrane porosity in both *in vitro* and *in vivo* experiments [19]. High-intensity focused ultrasound has been shown to allow selective and non-destructive disruption of the BBB in rats [20]. If microbubbles are introduced to the blood stream prior to focused US exposure, the BBB can be transiently opened at the ultrasound focus without acute neuronal damage [21]. Thus, the introduction of cavitation nuclei into the blood stream can confine the ultrasound effects to the vasculature and reduce the intensity needed to produce BBB opening (Fig. 4). This can diminish the risk of tissue damage and make the technique more easily applied through the intact skull. In most studies, the confirmation of BBB disruption has been obtained with MR contrast imaging at targeted locations [21–23] or with post mortem histology [20,24].

Targeted delivery of antibodies to the brain has been accomplished with focused ultrasound. Dopamine D(4) receptor-targeting antibody was injected intravenously and shown to recognize antigen in the murine brain following disruption of the BBB with ultrasound [22]. Likewise,

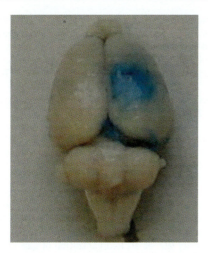

Figure 4 Example of blood—brain disruption by ultrasound and microbubbles in a rat brain. Extravasation of Evans blue marks BBB disruption. Exposure time was 20 s with a 1 MHz sector transducer at a pressure amplitude of 2.5 MPa through the rat skull with about 50% attenuation.

doxorubicin, a chemotherapeutic drug that does not cross the BBB, has been administered to the brain using ultrasound and microbubbles [25]. Different levels of doxorubicin in the brain were accomplished through alteration of the microbubble concentration. These results are encouraging and provide an important framework for future studies aimed at local disruption of the BBB for delivery of macromolecular agents to the brain.

Several avenues of transcapillary passage after ultrasound sonication have been identified. These include transcytosis, passage through endothelial cell cytoplasmic openings, opening of tight junctions and free passage through injured endothelium [26]. One study investigated the integrity of the tight junctions (TJs) in rat brain microvessels after BBB disruption by ultrasound bursts (1.5-MHz) in combination with Optison [27]. BBB disruption, as evidenced by leakage of i.v. administered horseradish peroxidase (HRP) and lanthanum chloride, was paralleled by the apparent disintegration of the TJ complexes, the redistribution and loss of the immunosignals for occludin, claudin-5 and ZO-1. At 6 and 24 h after sonication, no HRP or lanthanum leakage was observed and the barrier function of the TJs, as indicated by the localization and density of immunosignals, appeared to be completely restored. The results of these studies demonstrate that the effect of ultrasound upon TJs is very transient, lasting less than 4 h.

Although much effort has been undertaken to demonstrate the safety of BBB opening with ultrasound and microbubbles, further work is needed to elucidate the molecular effects of this application. Recent data demonstrate that at the upper thresholds of acoustic pressure for safe BBB opening a reorganization of gap-junctional plaques in both neurons and astrocytes may occur [28]. This is important because gap junctions allow transfer of information between adjacent cells and are responsible for tissue homeostasis. Likewise, there is evidence that focused ultrasound-induced opening of the BBB in the presence of ultrasound contrast agents can lead to increased ubiquitinylation of proteins in neuronal cells [29], indicating that brain molecular stress pathways are affected by this treatment. Nevertheless, this new technology for delivering drugs across the BBB will offer exciting opportunities for treatment of a variety of brain diseases in the future.

References

[1] Kern R, Perren F, Kreisel S, Szabo K, Hennerici M, Meairs S. Multi-planar transcranial ultrasound imaging—standards, landmarks and correlation with magnetic resonance imaging. Ultrasound Med Biol 2005;31:311—5.

[2] Meairs S. Contrast-enhanced ultrasound perfusion imaging in acute stroke patients. Eur Neurol 2008;59(Suppl. 1):17—26.

[3] Wei K, Jayaweera AR, Firoozan S, Linka A, Skyba DM, Kaul S. Quantification of myocardial blood flow with ultrasound-induced destruction of microbubbles administered as a constant venous infusion. Circulation 1998;97:473—83.

[4] Hudson JM, Karshafian R, Burns PN. Quantification of flow using ultrasound and microbubbles: a disruption replenishment model based on physical principles. Ultrasound Med Biol 2009;35:2007—20.

[5] Arditi M, Frinking PJ, Zhou X, Rognin NG. A new formalism for the quantification of tissue perfusion by the destruction-replenishment method in contrast ultrasound imaging. IEEE Trans Ultrason Ferroelectr Freq Control 2006;53:1118—29.

[6] Kern R, Diels A, Pettenpohl J, Kablau M, Brade J, Hennerici MG, et al. Real-time ultrasound brain perfusion imaging with analysis of microbubble replenishment in acute MCA stroke. J Cereb Blood Flow Metab 2011;31:1716—24.

[7] Culp WC, Flores R, Brown AT, Lowery JD, Roberson PK, Hennings LJ, et al. Successful microbubble sonothrombolysis without tissue-type plasminogen activator in a rabbit model of acute ischemic stroke. Stroke 2011;42:2280—5.

[8] Flores R, Hennings LJ, Lowery JD, Brown AT, Culp WC. Microbubble-augmented ultrasound sonothrombolysis decreases intracranial hemorrhage in a rabbit model of acute ischemic stroke. Invest Radiol 2011;46:419—24.

[9] Marsh JN, Senpan A, Hu G, Scott MJ, Gaffney PJ, Wickline SA, et al. Fibrin-targeted perfluorocarbon nanoparticles for targeted thrombolysis. Nanomedicine 2007;2:533—43.

[10] Tsivgoulis G, Eggers J, Ribo M, Perren F, Saqqur M, Rubiera M, et al. Safety and efficacy of ultrasound-enhanced thrombolysis: a comprehensive review and meta-analysis of randomized and nonrandomized studies. Stroke 2010;41:280—7.

[11] Newell DW, Shah MM, Wilcox R, Hansmann DR, Melnychuk E, Muschelli J, et al. Minimally invasive evacuation of spontaneous intracerebral hemorrhage using sonothrombolysis. J Neurosurg 2011;115:592—601.

[12] Maxwell AD, Cain CA, Duryea AP, Yuan L, Gurm HS, Xu Z. Noninvasive thrombolysis using pulsed ultrasound cavitation therapy—histotripsy. Ultrasound Med Biol 2009;35:1982—94.

[13] Fatar M, Stroick M, Griebe M, Alonso A, Kreisel S, Kern R, et al. Effect of combined ultrasound and microbubbles treatment in an experimental model of cerebral ischemia. Ultrasound Med Biol 2008;34:1414—20.

[14] Dirnagl U, Iadecola C, Moskowitz MA. Pathobiology of ischaemic stroke: an integrated view. Trends Neurosci 1999;22:391—7.

[15] Xie F, Slikkerveer J, Gao S, Lof J, Kamp O, Unger E, et al. Coronary and microvascular thrombolysis with guided diagnostic ultrasound and microbubbles in acute ST segment elevation myocardial infarction. J Am Soc Echocardiogr 2011;24:1400—8.

[16] Nedelmann M, Ritschel N, Doenges S, Langheinrich AC, Acker T, Reuter P, et al. Combined contrast-enhanced ultrasound and rt-PA treatment is safe and improves impaired microcirculation after reperfusion of middle cerebral artery occlusion. J Cereb Blood Flow Metab 2010;30:1712—20.

[17] Altland OD, Dalecki D, Suchkova VN, Francis CW. Low-intensity ultrasound increases endothelial cell nitric oxide synthase activity and nitric oxide synthesis. J Thromb Haemost 2004;2:637—43.

[18] Taniyama Y, Tachibana K, Hiraoka K, Namba T, Yamasaki K, Hashiya N, et al. Local delivery of plasmid DNA into rat carotid artery using ultrasound. Circulation 2002;105:1233—9.

[19] Ogawa K, Tachibana K, Uchida T, Tai T, Yamashita N, Tsujita N, et al. High-resolution scanning electron microscopic evaluation of cell-membrane porosity by ultrasound. Med Electron Microsc 2001;34:249—53.

[20] Mesiwala AH, Farrell L, Wenzel HJ, Silbergeld DL, Crum LA, Winn HR, et al. High-intensity focused ultrasound selectively disrupts the blood—brain barrier in vivo. Ultrasound Med Biol 2002;28:389—400.

[21] Hynynen K, McDannold N, Vykhodtseva N, Jolesz FA, Noninvasive MR. imaging-guided focal opening of the blood—brain barrier in rabbits. Radiology 2001;220:640—6.

[22] Kinoshita M, McDannold N, Jolesz FA, Hynynen K. Targeted delivery of antibodies through the blood—brain barrier by MRI-guided focused ultrasound. Biochem Biophys Res Commun 2006;340:1085—90.

[23] McDannold N, Vykhodtseva N, Hynynen K. Targeted disruption of the blood—brain barrier with focused ultrasound: association with cavitation activity. Phys Med Biol 2006;51:793—807.

[24] McDannold N, Vykhodtseva N, Raymond S, Jolesz FA, Hynynen K. MRI-guided targeted blood—brain barrier disruption with focused ultrasound: histological findings in rabbits. Ultrasound Med Biol 2005;31:1527—37.

[25] Treat LH, McDannold N, Vykhodtseva N, Zhang Y, Tam K, Hynynen K. Targeted delivery of doxorubicin to the rat brain at therapeutic levels using MRI-guided focused ultrasound. Int J Cancer 2007;121:901—7.

[26] Sheikov N, McDannold N, Vykhodtseva N, Jolesz F, Hynynen K. Cellular mechanisms of the blood—brain barrier opening induced by ultrasound in presence of microbubbles. Ultrasound Med Biol 2004;30:979—89.

[27] Sheikov N, McDannold N, Sharma S, Hynynen K. Effect of focused ultrasound applied with an ultrasound contrast agent on the tight junctional integrity of the brain microvascular endothelium. Ultrasound Med Biol 2008;34:1093—104.

[28] Alonso A, Reinz E, Jenne JW, Fatar M, Schmidt-Glenewinkel H, Hennerici MG, et al. Reorganization of gap junctions after focused ultrasound blood—brain barrier opening in the rat brain. J Cereb Blood Flow Metab 2010;30:1394—402.

[29] Alonso A, Reinz E, Fatar M, Jenne J, Hennerici MG, Meairs S. Neurons but not glial cells overexpress ubiquitin in the rat brain following focused ultrasound-induced opening of the blood—brain barrier. Neuroscience 2010;169:116—24.

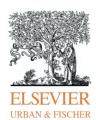

Sonothrombolysis: Current status

Peter D. Schellinger [a,*], Carlos A. Molina [b]

[a] Departments of Neurology and Geriatry, Johannes Wesling Klinikum Minden, Germany
[b] Vall d'Hebron Stroke Unit, Department of Neurosciences, Hospital Universitari Vall d'Hebron, Barcelona, Spain

KEYWORDS
Sonothrombolysis;
rt-PA;
Microbubbles

Summary This contribution summarizes the past and present status of ultrasound-facilitated thrombolysis (sonolysis) with and without the use of microspheres. Different ultrasound techniques are addressed and advantages as well as pitfalls are discussed.
© 2012 Elsevier GmbH. All rights reserved.

Introduction

Intravenous thrombolysis with rt-PA is the only approved therapy for treating acute ischemic stroke and needs to be administered within the first 4.5 h after symptom onset [1]. Among other factors, the speed and completeness of recanalization, and successive reperfusion of ischemic brain tissue is associated with final infarct size, restoration of function, and finally clinical outcome. With i.v. rt-PA only, there is a rather low percentage of patients achieving early (30—40%) and complete (18%) recanalization [2]. Therefore, various ways to improve speed and completeness of recanalization have been studied, among others the therapeutic use of ultrasound, alone or in combination with thrombolytics. The following brief overview reflects the current clinical status of sonothrombolysis. For an extensive recent review (and the basis for this chapter) including the experimental background of sonothrombolysis the reader is referred to Amaral-Silva et al. [3].

Delivery of tPA to the thrombus is dependent on the residual flow to and around the arterial obstruction, and better residual flow signals detected by Transcranial Doppler (TCD) are associated with higher recanalization rates and consequently better clinical courser in stroke patients treated with i.v. tPA [3,4]. Proximal arterial occlusions are a marker of clot burden and poorer response to thrombolysis in terms of recanalization [5,6]. Therefore, proximal intracranial occlusion is a target for more advanced reperfusion strategies, among them ultrasound-enhanced thrombolysis. While several ultrasound techniques have been applied, the focus of this contribution shall remain on the techniques that are also used in standard diagnostic ultrasound, i.e. transcranial color coded duplex (TCCD) and TCD.

TCD is a non-invasive technique that uses ultrasound to access regional blood flow by determining flow velocities of intracranial arteries. TCD is a fast and reliable method of obtaining real-time information on the presence and location of arterial occlusion and recanalization during or shortly after thrombolysis [3]. The patterns of intracranial arterial occlusion and recanalization on TCD have been validated against angiography with high sensitivity and specificity values resulting in the now widely used derived *thrombolysis in brain ischemia* (TIBI) grading system [7].

Clinical studies

High frequencies lead to greater attenuation of ultrasound, lower frequencies may be harmful due to tissue heating. There are only very limited data on the effect of ultrasound alone (without thrombolytic drugs) to facilitate clot lysis in acute stroke.

The TRUMBI study, a phase II clinical trial testing the use of low frequency ultrasound insonation in acute stroke patients treated with i.v. t-PA, showed a significant increase in hemorrhage, both symptomatic and asymptomatic [8]. The trial included i.v. rt-PA patients within 6h of symptom onset but was closed early because of signs of ICH in 13/14 patients compared with 5/12 patients on rt-PA only albeit identical recanalization rates. Since then, clinical trials restricted the use of ultrasound for therapeutical purposes to the settings usually used for diagnostic purposes (1–2 MHz), which have proved their safety and efficacy in several experimental and clinical trials.

Alexandrov et al. reported one of the first clinical reports on the use of sonothrombolysis in acute stroke patients [9] and showed with 2 MHz TCD a higher response rate to i.v. t-PA at 24h than previously documented (40% of patients versus 27% in the NINDS trial showed a >10 points improvement in NIHSSS or complete recovery). This pilot trial was followed by a phase II randomized controlled trial CLOTBUST (Combined Lysis of Thrombus in Brain Ischemia using Transcranial Ultrasound and Systemic TPA), which demonstrated that enhancement of the thrombolytic activity of tPA could be safely achieved by using higher frequency (2 MHz) and low intensity (<700 mW/cm^2) single element pulsed-wave ultrasound [2]. In 126 patients randomized in a 1:1 fashion acute rt-PA treated stroke patients were either insonated within a 3-h time window for 2h or not. rt-PA induced arterial recanalization was increased by ultrasound (sustained complete recanalization rates at 2h: 38% versus 13%, $p = 0.002$) with a non-significant trend toward an increased rate of clinical recovery from stroke, as compared with placebo and at no increased cost of bleeding complications (4.8% in both arms). A phase III trial has been planned for quite some time and protocols have been published [10]. The problem, however, is still the lack of an investigator independent device, although this may be solved in the close future (Andrei Alexandrov, personal communication).

Transcranial color coded duplex ultrasound (TCCD) has been used in four smaller trials of ultrasound enhanced thrombolysis [3]. In general, the results were somewhat better than control rt-PA patients with regard to recanalization and trends for outcome, but again at the cost of higher bleeding rates fortunately not in the same range as in the TRUMBI trial.

Microbubble-enhanced sonothrombolysis

Microbubbles (MBs, microspheres), originally developed as ultrasound contrast agents, have been utilized for increasing ultrasound performance in neurovascular imaging and sonolysis by enhanced cavitation and microstreaming [11,12]. Derived from experimental studies in the 90s [13], the approach was consecutively applied to the clinical setting [12,14]. In a first study Molina and colleagues used levovist® given at 3 time points in 38 patients compared to 73 patients treated with either 2 MHz TCD and rt-PA or rt-PA alone [12]. Complete recanalization rate 2h after t-PA bolus was significantly higher in the tPA/US/MB group (54.5%) compared with tPA/US (40.8%) and tPA (23.9%) groups ($p = 0.038$). No systemic symptoms deriving from MBs use were documented. Symptomatic ICH rates did not differ. A French TCCD (plus rt-PA plus MB versus rt-PA alone) study was terminated prematurely because of safety concerns [15]. Other MBs have been tested but none have emerged so far as superior to others.

Newer submicron lipid coated perflutren MBs ("nanobubbles") were tested in a pilot trial and a phase IIa study [14,16]. Preliminary data compared to historic controls from the CLOTBUST trial showed a higher rate of complete recanalization (50% versus 18%, $p = 0.028$) and sustained complete recanalization at 2h (42% versus 13%, $p = 0.003$). Interestingly, in a majority of patients MBs were detected in areas with no pretreatment flow, indicating permeation beyond intracranial occlusions [17]. The phase IIa TUCSON study [14] aimed to determine the safety, tolerability, and activity of perflutren-lipid MBs MRX-801 plus TCD insonation in sonothrombolysis. Thirty-five patients with pretreatment proximal intracranial occlusions on TCD were randomized (2:1 ratio) to increasing doses of MRx-801 MBs infusion over 90 min. The study was terminated prematurely by the sponsor because of bleeding events in the 2nd dose tier, although all the 3 bleedings could have been attributed to very severe strokes and high blood pressures during treatment. Despite that, a trend toward higher sustained complete recanalization rates in both MBs dose tiers compared to control was observed (67% for Cohort 1, 46% for Cohort 2, and 33% for controls, $p = 0.255$). To date this was the last sonothrombolysis study also using MBs, and the concept remains to be rechallenged in the authors' opinion.

Conclusions

Early and effective reperfusion is the key for early ischemic tissue rescue and further good clinical outcomes. However, i.v. tPA alone can only accomplish this goal in less than 50% of the patients. Ultrasound may be a tool to enhance clot lysis, albeit the final verdict has to be spoken. At the current stage a phase III trial with an investigator blinded 2 MHz device using the settings of the original CLOTBUST study is underway, and the protocol has been finalized. Future research should be dedicated to optimizing the technical setting of ultrasound, the development of untargeted and targeted MBs and optimizing the feasibility of this not so novel therapeutic approach to acute stroke.

Financial disclosures

Peter D Schellinger is Honoraria, Advisory Board, Travel grants, Speaker Board for Boehringer Ingelheim, Coaxia Inc., Photothera, Cerevast, ImARX, Sanofi, Ferrer, ev3/covidien, GSK, Haemonetics, Bayer.

Carlos A Molina is Honoraria, Advisory Board, Travel grants, Speaker Board for Boehringer Ingelheim, Coaxia Inc., Cerevast, ImARX, Sanofi, Ferrer, Haemonetics.

References

[1] Hacke W, Kaste M, Bluhmki E, Brozman M, Davalos A, Guidetti D, et al. Thrombolysis with alteplase 3 to 4.5 hours after acute ischemic stroke. N Engl J Med 2008;359(13):1317−29.

[2] Alexandrov AV, Molina CA, Grotta JC, Garami Z, Ford SR, Alvarez-Sabin J, et al. Ultrasound-enhanced systemic thrombolysis for acute stroke. N Engl J Med 2004;351(21):2170−8.

[3] Amaral-Silva A, Pineiro S, Molina CA. Sonothrombolysis for the treatment of acute stroke: current concepts and future directions. Expert Rev Neurother 2011;11(2):265−73.

[4] Alexandrov AV, Burgin WS, Demchuk AM, El-Mitwalli A, Grotta JC. Speed of intracranial clot lysis with intravenous tissue plasminogen activator therapy: sonographic classification and short-term improvement. Circulation 2001;103(24):2897−902.

[5] Riedel CH, Jensen U, Rohr A, Tietke M, Alfke K, Ulmer S, et al. Assessment of thrombus in acute middle cerebral artery occlusion using thin-slice nonenhanced computed tomography reconstructions. Stroke 2010;41.

[6] Riedel CH, Zimmermann P, Jensen-Kondering U, Stingele R, Deuschl G, Jansen O. The importance of size: successful recanalization by intravenous thrombolysis in acute anterior stroke depends on thrombus length. Stroke 2011;42(6):1775−7.

[7] Demchuk AM, Burgin WS, Christou I, Felberg RA, Barber PA, Hill MD, et al. Thrombolysis in brain ischemia (TIBI) transcranial Doppler flow grades predict clinical severity, early recovery, and mortality in patients treated with intravenous tissue plasminogen activator. Stroke 2001;32(1):89−93.

[8] Daffertshofer M, Gass A, Ringleb P, Sitzer M, Sliwka U, Els T, et al. Transcranial low-frequency ultrasound-mediated thrombolysis in brain ischemia: increased risk of hemorrhage with combined ultrasound and tissue plasminogen activator results of a phase II clinical trial. Stroke 2005;36(7):1441−6.

[9] Alexandrov AV, Demchuk AM, Felberg RA, Christou I, Barber PA, Burgin WS, et al. High rate of complete recanalization and dramatic clinical recovery during tPA infusion when continuously monitored with 2-MHz transcranial Doppler monitoring. Stroke 2000;31(3):610−4.

[10] Saqqur M, Tsivgoulis G, Molina CA, Demchuk AM, Garami Z, Barreto A, et al. Design of a PROspective multi-national CLOTBUST collaboration on reperfusion therapies for stroke (CLOTBUST-PRO). Int J Stroke 2008;3(1):66−72.

[11] Bogdahn U, Becker G, Schlief R, Reddig J, Hassel W. Contrast-enhanced transcranial color-coded real-time sonography. Results of a phase-two study. Stroke 1993;24(5):676−84.

[12] Molina CA, Ribo M, Rubiera M, Montaner J, Santamarina E, Delgado-Mederos R, et al. Microbubble administration accelerates clot lysis during continuous 2-MHz ultrasound monitoring in stroke patients treated with intravenous tissue plasminogen activator. Stroke 2006;37(2):425−9.

[13] Tachibana K, Tachibana S. Albumin microbubble echo-contrast material as an enhancer for ultrasound accelerated thrombolysis. Circulation 1995;92(5):1148−50.

[14] Molina CA, Barreto AD, Tsivgoulis G, Sierzenski P, Malkoff MD, Rubiera M, et al. Transcranial ultrasound in clinical sonothrombolysis (TUCSON) trial. Ann Neurol 2009;66(1):28−38.

[15] Tsivgoulis G, Eggers J, Ribo M, Perren F, Saqqur M, Rubiera M, et al. Safety and efficacy of ultrasound-enhanced thrombolysis: a comprehensive review and meta-analysis of randomized and nonrandomized studies. Stroke 2010;41(2):280−7.

[16] Barreto AD, Sharma VK, Lao AY, Schellinger PD, Amarenco P, Sierzenski P, et al. Safety and dose-escalation study design of Transcranial Ultrasound in Clinical SONolysis for acute ischemic stroke: the TUCSON Trial. Int J Stroke 2009;4(1):42−8.

[17] Alexandrov AV, Mikulik R, Ribo M, Sharma VK, Lao AY, Tsivgoulis G, et al. A pilot randomized clinical safety study of sonothrombolysis augmentation with ultrasound-activated perflutren-lipid microspheres for acute ischemic stroke. Stroke 2008;39(5):1464−9.

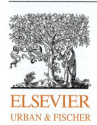
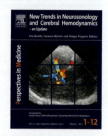

Bartels E, Bartels S, Poppert H (Editors):
New Trends in Neurosonology and Cerebral Hemodynamics — an Update.
Perspectives in Medicine (2012) 1, 14—20

journal homepage: www.elsevier.com/locate/permed

Sonothrombolysis for treatment of acute ischemic stroke: Current evidence and new developments

Jürgen Eggers*

Neurology, University Hospital Schleswig-Holstein, Campus Lübeck, Ratzeburger Allee 160, 23538 Lübeck, Germany

KEYWORDS
Acute ischemic stroke;
Therapy;
Transcranial ultrasound;
Thrombolysis;
Sonothrombolysis

Summary Sonothrombolysis is a novel therapy for recanalization of acute intracranial arterial occlusion. So far, safety and efficacy has been shown for transcranial ultrasound with diagnostic probes in combination with standard thrombolysis treatment. However, there are several new developments including special designed ultrasound probes, microspheres for enhancement of the thrombolytic effect of ultrasound and other new approaches. This review provides an overview of current evidence from randomized controlled trials and perspectives on this topic.
© 2012 Elsevier GmbH. All rights reserved.

Introduction

Sonothrombolysis has been introduced for treatment of acute intracranial occlusions during the first years of the last decade. Improved recanalization has been demonstrated with ''diagnostic'' transcranial ultrasound (US) in combination with standard intravenous (IV) thrombolysis with recombinant tissue-plasminogen activator (rtPA) in two randomized trials [1,2]. A study with limited sample size on middle cerebral artery (MCA) main stem occlusion has indicated that this method might be a possible alternative to interventional therapy [2]. The occurrence of an increased rate of symptomatic hemorrhagic transformation of brain infarction after sonothrombolysis with diagnostic US has not been confirmed thus far [3]. In the absence of other therapies (e.g., in cases of contraindication to thrombolytic drugs or thrombus extraction), this method may serve as an alternative treatment, as indicated by the findings of a small randomized study using transcranial color-coded sonography (TCCS)-guided pulsed-wave (PW) US [4]. Novel developments include microspheres-enhanced thrombolysis for improved drug delivery and enhancement of microcirculation [5,6]. A recent pilot study has tested the feasibility of using an intra-arterial high-energy US catheter for recanalization [7]. Although many promising advances have been made in the field of sonothrombolysis, ''diagnostic'' transcranial US remains the only method that has been shown to be effective and safe. The aim of this review is to provide an overview of confirmed evidence and perspectives on sonothrombolysis for the treatment of acute ischemic stroke (AIS).

Clinical evidence

From random observation to therapy

The thrombolytic effect of ''diagnostic'' transcranial US in acute intracranial occlusion was discovered more than 10 years ago at 3 stroke therapy centers, independently of each other. At the Center for Noninvasive Brain Perfusion Studies at the University of Texas-Houston Medical School, physicians noticed that patients receiving continuous transcranial US monitoring for determination of rtPA-associated

* Tel.: +49 451 500 3334; fax: +49 451 500 5457.
E-mail addresses: juergen.eggers@neuro.uni-luebeck.de, juergeneggers@gmx.net

2211-968X/$ — see front matter © 2012 Elsevier GmbH. All rights reserved.
doi:10.1016/j.permed.2012.02.022

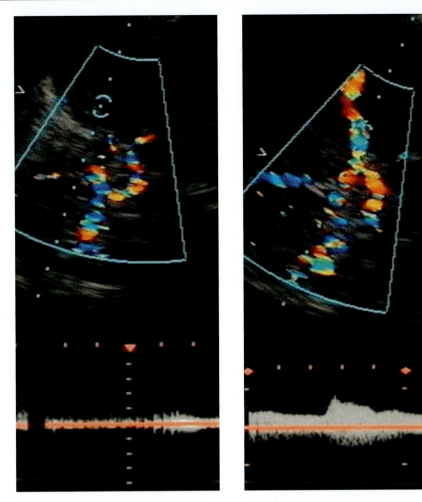

Figure 1 Transcranial image in color-coded mode of transcranial color-coded sonography (TCCS). Proximal middle cerebral artery (MCA) main stem occlusion (left) with complete recanalization at 1 h after intravenous (IV) recombinant tissue-type plasminogen activator (rtPA) plus sonothrombolysis (right).

recanalization more frequently exhibited a favorable clinical course in comparison to patients without monitoring [8]. Based on these results, a randomized, multicenter clinical trial, known as the Combined Lysis of Thrombus in Brain Ischemia Using Transcranial Ultrasound and Systemic tPA (CLOTBUST) trial, was performed to study this effect. A similar effect was observed with TCCS in the stroke unit at the University of Lübeck, Germany [9] (Fig. 1). In contrast to the multicenter CLOTBUST trial, this monocenter, randomized study also included patients with contraindications to rtPA. In addition, neurologists at the University Hospital Ostrava, Czech Republic, observed a similar effect in patients with acute cerebral artery occlusion during examination with TCCS [10].

Results of randomized studies

The CLOTBUST trial included a total of 126 patients with occlusion of the main segment of the stem or branches of the MCA. All subjects were treated with standard IV rtPA and were additionally randomized for a 2-h insonation with transcranial Doppler (TCD). The primary endpoint (complete recanalization or substantial clinical improvement) was more frequently reached in the sonothrombolysis group (40%) than in the standard therapy group (30%). No significant differences were found in the clinical results obtained after 24 h and after 3 months. However, a clear tendency for functional independence after 3 months was detected in the sonothrombolysis group. The rate of symptomatic intracranial hemorrhage (sICH) was the same for each group (4.8%) [1]. Some limitations of the CLOTBUST trial were the inclusion of an inhomogeneous patient sample (MCA main stem and branch occlusions) and the definition of the primary endpoint. The US imaging of the thrombus, carried out with blind TCD sonography by means of a probe attached to the head, may also have been inadequate, particularly in branch occlusions or occlusions of the main stem without residual flow. Despite these limitations, this multicenter trial can be considered a proof of principle study.

In the Lübeck study, patients were randomly selected to receive TCCS-guided PW mode US for 1 h. The color duplex mode was used to improve the accuracy of focusing the US on the thrombus. Patients with exclusively proximal MCA main stem occlusions without residual flow who underwent simultaneously insonation and rtPA standard treatment were included in the study. The homogeneity of the sample was not only a major strength of the study but also its weakness (i.e., only a relatively low number of patients [n = 37] were included in this monocenter study). Similar to the findings of the CLOTBUST trial, continuous insonation for 1 h (instead of 2 h like in the CLOTBUST trial) resulted in significantly improved recanalization (partial or complete recanalization: 58% in the continuous insonation group vs. 22% in the control group). Additionally, an improvement in neurological deficits after 4 days, and a clear trend toward better functional outcome after 3 months in patients was shown. Tendencies for increased symptomatic cerebral bleeding (3 patients in the sonothrombolysis group vs. 1 patient in the control group) and increased hemorrhagic transformation of infarcts were also found in patients who underwent continuous insonation [2]. A total of 15 patients were randomized in the arm of the trial for patients with contraindications to rtPA. Recanalization (all of them were partial recanalizations) after 1 h occurred only in the sonothrombolysis group (62.5% in the sonothrombolysis group vs. 0% in the control group). Significant improvements in clinical course after 4 days and functional independence after 3 months were found in 2 of 8 patients in the sonothrombolysis group (compared with none of the 7 patients in the control group) [4]. No sICHs occurred in the sonothrombolysis group. At the end of the randomized trial, this treatment principle was continued in the context of a clinical register. Currently available data (obtained from a total of 116 patients with MCA main stem occlusions, with or without rtPA treatment) confirm these results (unpublished data).

Sonothrombolysis with TCCS in combination with rtPA: an alternative to interventional treatment?

For occlusions of the main intracranial arteries, IV thrombolysis alone is probably not adequate to achieve early recanalization, which explains why interventional therapy, either intra-arterial thrombolysis or thrombus extraction, is often regarded as an alternative. However, in addition to the yet unsatisfactory evidence attained from randomized clinical trials for these interventional therapies, there are two important limitations: the time delay to the start of the intra-arterial intervention and the lack of availability of these types of interventional treatment in nonspecialized centers. Sonothrombolysis as a tool to improve the effectiveness of IV thrombolysis may be a promising alternative option. A comparison of the published randomized data and those from the randomized study of intra-arterial thrombolysis, known as Prolyse in Acute Cerebral Thromboembolism II (PROACT II) [11], revealed very similar recanalization rates, although more severe occlusions were treated in the sonothrombolysis study (proximal MCA-M1 occlusions in contrast to M1 and M2 branch occlusions in PROACT II). As shown in Fig. 2, rates of recanalization in the PROACT II study were quite similar to those obtained in the sonothrombolysis with TCCS and rtPA study. The PROACT II study randomized patients with MCA main stem or M2 branch occlusions within a 6-h time window for intra-arterial thrombolysis with pro-urokinase. The sonothrombolysis with TCCS and IV rtPA study randomized patients with proximal MCA main stem occlusions without residual flow (including patients with additional ipsilateral internal carotid artery occlusion) within a 3-h time window for 1 h of continuous insonation. As

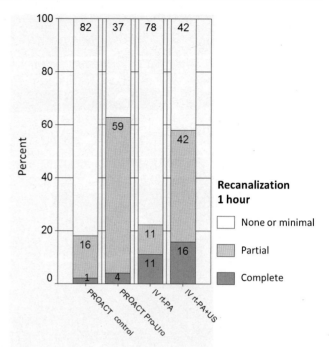

Figure 2 Recanalization rates after 1 h from the Prolyse in Acute Cerebral Thromboembolism II (PROACT II) study compared with those from the sonothrombolysis with TCCS and rtPA study. Partial/complete recanalization was defined as follows: Thrombolysis in Myocardial Infarction (TIMI) 2/3 in PROACT II, and Thrombolysis in Brain Ischemia (TIBI) Doppler score [40] 2—3/4—5 in the sonothrombolysis with TCCS and rtPA study. For the PROACT II study, 162 patients were 2:1 randomized for therapy vs. control, for the sonothrombolysis study 37 patients were randomized 1:1 for rtPA plus 1 h insonation (US) vs. rtPA alone.

shown in Fig. 3, comparable outcome results after 3 months (3—4 months in PROACT II) were obtained for the sonothrombolysis with TCCS and IV rtPA group and the pro-urokinase treatment group. The strong tendency toward a worse outcome for patients in the IV rtPA group without sonothrombolysis compared with those in the PROACT II control group may indicate that patients in the Lübeck randomized study may have been more severely affected than those in the PROACT II study.

Limitations of sonothrombolysis

The lack of a temporal bone window is one main limitation of sonothrombolysis. Research studies have revealed that the frequency of an insufficient temporal sound window for TCCS can vary from 8% [12] to 27% [13]. On the other hand, also the interventional therapy may not be applicable for all patients. A common limitation of interventional therapy is the lack of patency of the proximal carotid artery. Data from the own register of MCA-M1 occlusions have revealed the presence of an additional proximal occlusion of the internal carotid artery in 23% of patients (unpublished data).

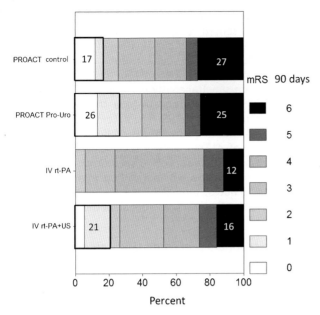

Figure 3 Functional results after 90 days (in the Prolyse in Acute Cerebral Thromboembolism II [PROACT II] collective, 90—120 days) as measured on the modified Rankin scale (mRS). Median National Institutes of Health Stroke Scale (NIHSS) scores on inclusion: PROACT II, 17 for control group and 17 for pro-urokinase group; sonothrombolysis with transcranial color-coded sonography (TCCS) and recombinant tissue-type plasminogen activator (rtPA) study, 18 for IV rtPA and 18 for IV rtPA plus ultrasound (US). The percentages in the bars give the rate of mRS scores (0—1) or the mortality at 90 days (90—120 days in PROACT II). Number of randomized patients in PROACT II, 162; in the sonothrombolysis study, 37. Rate of symptomatic intracranial hemorrhage (sICH): 10% in the pro-urokinase group, 15% in the sonothrombolysis group. Differences were not statistically significant.

Meta-analysis of clinical results of sonothrombolysis

A meta-analysis conducted by Tsivgoulis et al. [3] on sonothrombolysis with transcranial US (TCCS or TCD) included over 400 patients. They found that in comparison to patients with rtPA treatment alone, patients who underwent sonothrombolysis had a 3 times higher chance for complete recanalization and a 2 times higher chance for non-disability after 3 months. There was no evidence for increased risk of cerebral bleeding with US treatment.

From bedside to bench: experimental evidence

When the thrombolytic effect of ''diagnostic'' transcranial US was clinically observed for the first time, no experimental data on the effect of high-frequency, low-energy PW US on thrombolysis were available at the time. However, during the 1990s (after much time had passed since the first description of the thrombolytic effect of US in the late 1970s [14]), in vitro studies using high-frequency (1 MHz) and high-energy (spatial peak temporal average intensity [I_{SPTA}] of 2 W/cm^2) US demonstrated improved US-mediated binding of rtPA to fibrin, as well as reversible disintegration of fibrin without thrombolytics [15]. By contrast, in the Lübeck study, the transducers for ''diagnostic'' transcranial use employed frequencies between 1.8 and 2.5 MHz and had a I_{SPTA} of 179/cm^2, and most of the energy was absorbed by the skull. For neurological disorders, only two in vitro studies on the transcranial use of US for acceleration of thrombolysis were available at this time: These studies showed the effect of low-frequency US in combination with a thrombolytic on fibrin-rich thrombi [16,17]. However, the US used in these two studies differed substantially from the diagnostic US of a probe for TCCS: The frequencies used in the in vitro studies were in the range of 33—211 kHz, leading to good penetration of emitted US energy through the skull (e.g., by 40% in the Akiyama et al. [16] study). In comparison, up to 90% of energy from a high-frequency (1.8—2.5 MHz) ''diagnostic'' transcranial US probe was absorbed by the skull [18,19]. To obtain more information about the thrombolytic effect of ''diagnostic'' transcranial US, corresponding in vitro studies were done. In addition to the effect on the thrombolysis of whole venous blood clots, the effect on platelet-rich clots (PRCs) was investigated. The effect of US in combination with abciximab, the glycoprotein IIb/IIIa receptor inhibitor, was also examined and compared with the effect of rtPA. One main finding was that sonothrombolysis in combination with rtPA had a greater effect on whole venous blood clots and PRCs than sonothrombolysis in combination with abciximab. Because sonothrombolysis in combination with abciximab produced very disappointing results, including a weak effect on PRCs, this combination could not be recommended [20,21]. A study by Pfaffenberger et al. [19], which compared the impact of duplex-Doppler, continuous wave-Doppler, and PW-Doppler on rtPA-mediated thrombolysis, found that only the PW mode significantly accelerated rtPA-mediated thrombolysis.

Perspectives for sonothrombolysis

Operator-independent device for sonothrombolysis

A multicenter, randomized clinical trial will be launched to evaluate the safety and applicability of a novel operator-independent device for sonothrombolysis. A total of 900 patients who receive standard IV rtPA treatment will be randomized for 2-MHz PW US vs. sham treatment. The primary outcome endpoint will be functional independence after 3 months, and sICH will be assessed as the primary safety endpoint [22]. The introduction of a semi-automatic novel device for sonothrombolysis may overcome the disadvantages of conventional diagnostic US probes, which are considered time-consuming and operator intensive.

Other types of US

The results of previously conducted randomized clinical trials were based on the randomly observed effects of transcranial imaging generated by commercial diagnostic US devices. An early attempt to enhance thrombolysis by using US probes dedicated for optimized sonothrombolysis did not yield promising results. A multicenter, randomized clinical trial investigating the effectiveness of a specially developed "sonothrombolysis probe" with a higher energy and lower frequency for improved penetration of the skull (Transcranial Low-frequency Ultrasound-mediated Thrombolysis in Brain Ischemia [TRUMBI] study) unfortunately resulted in a higher rate of sICH [23]. Cerebral bleeding after treatment also occurred on the opposite side of the brain infarction, suggesting a causal link to the substantially higher energy and lower frequency of the "sonothrombolysis probe" compared with the energy of diagnostic US probes. In vivo experiments evaluating the therapeutic efficacy and safety of using highly energetic, low-frequency (20 kHz) US in treating rats with an embolic MCA occlusion showed an increased incidence of cerebral edema [24,25], thus indicating the unsuitability of this kind of US for clinical use. So far, "diagnostic" transcranial US remains the only form of US appropriate for sonothrombolysis.

Endovascular sonothrombolysis: results from a pilot study

Skoloudik et al. [7] performed a pilot study on 9 patients who had suffered an AIS with acute MCA or basilar artery occlusion and undergone endovascular sonothrombolysis within an 8-h time window from symptom onset. For this purpose, a 3F microcatheter with a US probe of 2.05—2.35 MHz was used. Complete recanalization at the end of treatment was achieved in one third of patients, and partial recanalization occurred in an additional 44% of patients at the end of the procedure. At admission, the National Institutes of Health Stroke Scale (NIHSS) scores were in the range of 10—33 (median, 19.0). At 3 months, 4 (44%) patients were functionally independent (modified Rankin Scale [mRS] score, 0—3; median mRS score, 4). No sICHs occurred for 24 h after endovascular sonothrombolysis until a control computed tomography (CT) scan at 24 h. These researchers concluded that this endovascular system might serve as a new treatment option for patients suffering from acute stroke.

US can control embolus growth—can transcranial US prevent early reocclusion?

The thrombolytic effect of US has generally been regarded as a tool for improving recanalization. However, as several US follow-up studies have shown, reocclusion of a vessel after recanalization can occur in 20% or more (up to 29%) of patients after rtPA treatment [1,26]. Sawaguchi et al. [27] recently reported interesting results from a novel use of US treatment in AIS. They found that continuous US (500 kHz, 0.72—0.28 W/cm^2) significantly suppressed thrombus growth in vitro. Based on their findings, these researchers suggested low-intensity, low-energy US as a possible simple and safe tool to prevent reocclusion of intracranial vessels after rtPA treatment.

What is the most effective US for sonothrombolysis? Systemic evaluation using standardized experimental settings

Determining the most efficient US settings for sonothrombolysis is complicated by the fact that there is a tremendous number of possible combinations of its parameters. Wang et al. [28] presented results from an in vitro experiment for the systematic and rapid evaluation of the thrombolytic effect of 500-kHz US as the ultrasonic spatial intensity increased from 0.1 to 0.7 mW/cm^2. For this purpose, flat discoid clots were simultaneously made in specially designed wells with a thin polycarbonate base that is transparent to light and reflects little US. The extent of clot lysis was automatically measured by means of light absorbance at a wavelength of 412 nm using a spectrometer before and after thrombolytic treatment. This method allowed the researchers to measure automatically a total of 200 positions within minutes, representing a throughput about 100 times as large as that of conventional methods.

Magnetic resonance imaging (MRI)-guided US for sonothrombolysis

Magnetic resonance-guided focused ultrasound (MRgFUS) is a novel method for optimizing US treatment. In general, magnetic resonance imaging (MRI) enables the adjustment of the US beam, based on differences in temperature measurements in the targeted parenchyma. For the purpose of sonothrombolysis, preliminary steps have involved using in vitro models with human skull and porcine brain. In future, it may be possible to detect the thrombus within the vessel, to focus the US beam on this target, and make corrections to the US beam so as to avoid side effects of US caused by distortion and shifting of the human skull [29,30].

Microspheres for enhancement of sonothrombolysis: current state and new developments

Another way of enhancing the effect of sonothrombolysis involves the use of microspheres. Commercially manufactured ultrasonic contrast amplifiers have been used in several studies: SonoVue®, which consists of sulfur hexafluoride-filled microbubbles of phospholipids, and Levovist®, a granulate of galactose and palmitic acid, which binds to micrometer-sized air bubbles. Following IV injection, they take energy on under influence of US, and by oscillation or rupture, this energy is released again, which reinforces the US effectiveness. Various experiments have shown the effectiveness of this method without an increase in the intracranial bleeding rate, which has been demonstrated in vivo. Molina et al. [31] showed an improvement by intermittent bolus injection of Levovist® in addition to tPA treatment plus 2-h insonation with TCD monitoring. A similar study was conducted by Perren et al. [32] in which patients who had suffered from an MCA stroke underwent IV rtPA thrombolysis and 2-MHz TCCS monitoring for 1 h with SonoVue®, resulting in clinical improvement in these patients. No additional intracranial bleedings were noted in these studies. In the transcranial ultrasound in clinical sonothrombolysis (TUCSON) randomized clinical trial, intravenously applied microspheres, which had been developed for the purpose of strengthening the effect of sonothrombolysis, were clinically tested [5]. This dose-escalation study of microspheres showed increased bleeding in the second dose tier, prompting the sponsor of the study to discontinue this approach.

Microspheres with abciximab for better thrombus binding and identification and improved sonothrombolysis

In vivo molecular imaging of the human thrombus can be carried out with microspheres conjugated with abciximab, a glycoprotein IIb/IIIa receptor inhibitor that is involved in ligand targeting of the thrombus. In vitro experiments have shown that improved binding of microspheres to the clot enhances sonothrombolysis [33,34].

Nanodroplet-enhanced sonothrombolysis

In their 2011 study, Shimizu et al. [35] reported preliminary results from an in vivo animal safety evaluation in vivo experiment with superheated perfluorocarbon nanodroplets (SPNs). When triggered by US, these nanodroplets turn into microbubbles. During this in vivo experiment, rabbits received either an IV injection of SPNs or a placebo without additional insonation. Within an hour after administration of SPNs, 4 cases showed a reversible change in respiration; 1 animal showed transient horizontal nystagmus about 20 min after administration of SPNs. Following euthanasia, no neuropathological damage or histological damage could be shown in any organ sample from any of the animals included in the study. The biochemical blood examination revealed no significant differences between the SPN-treated group and the placebo group. These researchers plan to conduct a study investigating the SPN-assisted sonothrombolytic effect of 500-kHz US exposure.

US-targeted drug delivery to the brain

In addition to enhancing sonothrombolysis, the combination of transcranial US and microspheres may have another purpose—that is, facilitating the delivery of drugs across the blood—brain barrier (BBB). Substances or drugs (e.g., large-molecule agents such as monoclonal antibodies, recombinant proteins, and gene therapeutics) that would be potentially useful for treatment of a variety of central nervous system disorders cannot penetrate the BBB. New developments have shown that noninvasive, targeted, US-induced disruption of the BBB could facilitate drug delivery. Transcranial-focused US penetrates the skull, thus preventing the need for trepanation. Targeting of the US beam can also be optimized by MRI [36—38].

Improvement of microcirculation

In addition to recanalization, microcirculation of ischemic brain parenchyma can be a target for transcranial US treatment of AIS. This possible effect of US was first described by Suchkova et al. [39]; this effect may also be achieved with US combined with microspheres [6].

Conclusion

Several clinical studies have shown that sonothrombolysis using ''diagnostic'' transcranial US in combination with rtPA improves recanalization of an acute intracranial artery occlusion. The chance of a favorable functional outcome after 3 months is doubled with this method of treatment when compared with rtPA treatment alone. TCCS has several advantages (e.g., visualization of an occlusion in a shorter insonation time) over TCD; thus, it is considered a more advanced tool. Although results of sonothrombolysis with TCCS have thus far been based on limited sample size, this method seems to provide a degree of effectiveness in achieving early recanalization of proximal MCA main stem occlusion that is similar to that provided by intra-arterial thrombolysis. For this reason, sonothrombolysis using TCCS should be considered an alternative treatment to intra-arterial recanalization procedures. A tendency toward increased cerebral infarction bleeding in patients treated with sonothrombolysis in combination with IV rtPA has not been confirmed thus far. Sonothrombolysis with TCCS alone in cases of contraindication for rtPA administration should be considered as a treatment option. Several studies have shown that microspheres may have a dual role: They may be used to enhance the effect of sonothrombolysis and assist in targeted drug delivery. To date, transcranial US has mainly been developed for diagnostic purposes. Several experimental studies have been conducted or are being undertaken to optimize US settings for sonothrombolysis. A need still exists to determine the optimal US frequency and energy so as to achieve the safest and most effective form of US for sonothrombolysis.

References

[1] Alexandrov AV, Molina CA, Grotta JC, Garami Z, Ford SR, Alvarez-Sabin J, et al. CLOTBUST Investigators. Ultrasound-enhanced systemic thrombolysis for acute ischemic stroke. N Engl J Med 2004;351:2170—8.

[2] Eggers J, König IR, Koch B, Händler G, Seidel G. Sonothrombolysis with transcranial color-coded sonography and recombinant tissue-type plasminogen activator in acute middle cerebral artery main stem occlusion: results from a randomized study. Stroke 2008;39:1470—5.

[3] Tsivgoulis G, Eggers J, Ribo M, Perren F, Saqqur M, Rubiera M, et al. Safety and efficacy of ultrasound-enhanced thrombolysis: a comprehensive review and meta-analysis of randomized and nonrandomized studies. Stroke 2010;41:280—7.

[4] Eggers J, Seidel G, Koch B, König IR. Sonothrombolysis in acute ischemic stroke for patients ineligible for rt-PA. Neurology 2005;64:1052—4.

[5] Molina CA, Barreto AD, Tsivgoulis G, Sierzenski P, Malkoff MD, Rubiera M, et al. Transcranial ultrasound in clinical sonothrombolysis (TUCSON) trial. Ann Neurol 2009;66:28—38.

[6] Nedelmann M, Ritschel N, Doenges S, Langheinrich AC, Acker T, Reuter P, et al. Combined contrast-enhanced ultrasound and rt-PA treatment is safe and improves impaired microcirculation after reperfusion of middle cerebral artery occlusion. J Cereb Blood Flow Metab 2010;30:1712—20.

[7] Skoloudik D, Fadrna T, Roubec M, Kuliha M, Prochazka V, Jonszta T, et al. Intravascular sonothrombolysis using Ekos system in acute stroke patients — a pilot study. Cerebrovasc Dis 2011;31(Suppl. 1):19.

[8] Alexandrov AV, Demchuk AM, Felberg RA, Christou I, Barber PA, Burgin WS, et al. High rate of complete recanalization and dramatic clinical recovery during tPA infusion when continuously monitored with 2-MHz transcranialdoppler monitoring. Stroke 2000;31:610–4.

[9] Eggers J, Koch B, Meyer K, König I, Seidel G. Effect of ultrasound on thrombolysis of middle cerebral artery occlusion. Ann Neurol 2003;53:797–800.

[10] Skoloudik D, Bar M, Skoda O, Vaclavik D, Hradilek P, Allendoerfer J, et al. Safety and efficacy of the sonographic acceleration of the middle cerebral artery recanalization: results of the pilot thrombotripsy study. Ultrasound Med Biol 2008;34:1775–82.

[11] Furlan A, Higashida R, Wechsler L, Gent M, Rowley H, Kase C, et al. Intra-arterial prourokinase for acute ischemic stroke. The PROACT II study: a randomized controlled trial. Prolyse in Acute Cerebral Thromboembolism. JAMA 1999;282:2003–11.

[12] Krejza J, Swiat M, Pawlak MA, Oszkinis G, Weigele J, Hurst RW, et al. Suitability of temporal bone acoustic window: conventional TCD versus transcranial color-coded duplex sonography. J Neuroimaging 2007;17:311–4.

[13] Nolte CH, Doepp F, Schreiber SJ, Gerischer LM, Audebert HJ. Quantification of target population for ultrasound enhanced thrombolysis in acute ischemic stroke. J Neuroimaging 2011, doi:10.1111/j.1552-6569.2011.00632.x [Epub ahead of print].

[14] Trubestein G, Engel C, Etzel F, Sobbe A, Cremer H, Stumpff U. Thrombolysis by ultrasound. Clin Sci Mol Med 1976;(Suppl. 3):697–8.

[15] Siddiqi F, Odrljin TM, Fay PJ, Cox C, Francis CW. Binding of tissue-plasminogen activator to fibrin: effect of ultrasound. Blood 1998;91:2019–25.

[16] Akiyama M, Ishibashi T, Yamada T, Furuhata H. Low-frequency ultrasound penetrates the cranium and enhances thrombolysis in vitro. Neurosurgery 1998;43:828–32.

[17] Behrens S, Daffertshofer M, Spiegel D, Hennerici M. Low-frequency, low-intensity ultrasound accelerates thrombolysis through the skull. Ultrasound Med Biol 1999;25:269–73.

[18] Grolimund P. Transmission of ultrasound through the temporal bone. In: Aaslid R, editor. Transcranial Doppler sonography. New York: Springer-Verlag Wien; 1986.

[19] Pfaffenberger S, Devcic-Kuhar B, Kollmann C, Kastl SP, Kaun C, Speidl WS, et al. Can a commercial diagnostic ultrasound device accelerate thrombolysis? An in vitro skull model. Stroke 2005;36:124–8.

[20] Eggers J, Ossadnik S, Seidel G. Enhanced clot dissolution in vitro by 1.8-MHz pulsed ultrasound. Ultrasound Med Biol 2009;35:523–6.

[21] Eggers J, Ossadnik S, Hütten H, Seidel G. Sonothrombolysis is effective with recombinant tissue-type plasminogen activator, but not with Abciximab. Results from an in vitro study with whole blood clots and platelet-rich clots. Thromb Haemost 2009;102:1274–347.

[22] Alexandrov AV, Brandt G, Barreto A, Schellinger PD, Kohrmann M, Barlinn K, et al. Planning a multi-center efficacy trial of sonothrombolysis. Cerebrovasc Dis 2011;31(Suppl. 1):27.

[23] Daffertshofer M, Gass A, Ringleb P, Sitzer M, Sliwka U, Els T, et al. Transcranial low-frequency ultrasound-mediated thrombolysis in brain ischemia: increased risk of hemorrhage with combined ultrasound and tissue plasminogen activator: results of a phase II clinical trial. Stroke 2005;36:1441–6.

[24] Nedelmann M, Reuter P, Walberer M, Sommer C, Alessandri B, Schiel D, et al. Detrimental effects of 60 kHz sonothrombolysis in rats with middle cerebral artery occlusion. Ultrasound Med Biol 2008;34:2019–27.

[25] Wilhelm-Schwenkmezger T, Pittermann P, Zajonz K, Kempski O, Dieterich M, Nedelmann M. Therapeutic application of 20-kHz transcranial ultrasound in an embolic middle cerebral artery occlusion model in rats: safety concerns. Stroke 2007;38:1031–5.

[26] Saqqur M, Molina CA, Salam A, Siddiqui M, Ribo M, Uchino K, et al. CLOTBUST Investigators. Clinical deterioration after intravenous recombinant tissue plasminogen activator treatment: a multicenter transcranial Doppler study. Stroke 2007;38:69–74.

[27] Sawaguchi Y, Wang Z, Furuhata H. Ultrasound can control embolus growth. Cerebrovasc Dis 2011;31(Suppl. 1):19.

[28] Wang Z, Fukuda T, Furuhata H. High efficient evaluation method for sonothrombolysis. Cerebrovasc Dis 2011;31(Suppl. 1):18–9.

[29] Hertzberg Y, Volovick A, Zur Y, Medan Y, Vitek S, Navon G. Ultrasound focusing using magnetic resonance acoustic radiation force imaging: application to ultrasound transcranial therapy. Med Phys 2010;37:2934–42.

[30] Durst C, Monteith S, Sheehan J, Moldovan K, Snell J, Eames M, et al. Optimal imaging of in vitro clot sonothrombolysis by MR-guided focused ultrasound. J Neuroimaging 2011, doi:10.1111/j.1552-6569.2011.00662.x [Epub ahead of print].

[31] Molina CA, Ribo M, Rubiera M, Montaner J, Santamarina E, Delgado-Mederos R, et al. Microbubble administration accelerates clot lysis during continuous 2-MHz ultrasound monitoring in stroke patients treated with intravenous tissue plasminogen activator. Stroke 2006;37:425–9.

[32] Perren F, Loulidi J, Poglia D, Landis T, Sztajzel R. Microbubble potentiated transcranial duplex ultrasound enhances IV thrombolysis in acute stroke. J Thromb Thrombolysis 2008;25:219–23.

[33] Alonso A, Della Martina A, Stroick M, Fatar M, Griebe M, Pochon S, et al. Molecular imaging of human thrombus with novel abciximab immunobubbles and ultrasound. Stroke 2007;38:1508–14.

[34] Alonso A, Dempfle CE, Della Martina A, Stroick M, Fatar M, Zohsel K, et al. In vivo clot lysis of human thrombus with intravenous abciximab immunobubbles and ultrasound. Thromb Res 2009;124:70–4.

[35] Shimizu J, Endoh R, Fukuda T, Inagaki T, Hano H, Asami R, et al. Safety evaluation of superheated perfluorocarbon nanodroplets for novel neurological therapy. Cerebrovasc Dis 2011;31(Suppl. 1):23–4.

[36] Meairs S, Alonso A. Ultrasound, microbubbles and the blood–brain barrier. Prog Biophys Mol Biol 2007;93:354–62.

[37] Hynynen K. Focused ultrasound for blood–brain disruption and delivery of therapeutic molecules into the brain. Expert Opin Drug Deliv 2007;4:7–35.

[38] Vykhodtseva N, McDannold N, Hynynen K. Progress and problems in the application of focused ultrasound for blood–brain barrier disruption. Ultrasonics 2008;48:279–96.

[39] Suchkova VN, Baggs RB, Francis CW. Effect of 40-kHz ultrasound on acute thrombotic ischemia in a rabbit femoral artery thrombosis model: enhancement of thrombolysis and improvement in capillary muscle perfusion. Circulation 2000;101:2296–301.

[40] Demchuk AM, Burgin WS, Christou I, Felberg RA, Barber PA, Hill MD, et al. Thrombolysis in brain ischemia (TIBI) transcranial Doppler flow grades predict clinical severity, early recovery, and mortality in patients treated with intravenous tissue plasminogen activator. Stroke 2001;32:89–93.

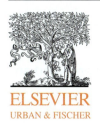

Current trends in sonothrombolysis for acute ischemic stroke

Andrei V. Alexandrov*

Comprehensive Stroke Center, University of Alabama Hospital, Birmingham, USA

KEYWORDS
Thrombolysis;
Recanalization;
Stroke;
Outcome

Summary Intravenous tissue plasminogen activator (tPA) remains the only approved, fastest and widely feasible treatment of acute ischemic stroke. Systemic tPA induces recanalization of an occluded vessel, the process thought to lead to neurological recovery. Augmentation of this fibrinolytic activity can be safely achieved with diagnostic ultrasound frequencies and intensities. Ultrasound delivers mechanical pressure waves to thrombi exposing more thrombus surface to circulating drug. International multi-center CLOTBUST trial showed that patients with acute stroke treated with sonothrombolysis (tPA+2 MHz TCD) had more dramatic clinical recovery coupled with arterial recanalization (25% vs 8%) at no increase in the risk of symptomatic intracerebral hemorrhage (sICH). Based on this trial and subsequent phase I—II studies of a novel operator-independent device for delivery of the CLOBUST levels of ultrasound energy, a phase III efficacy trial of sonothrombolysis (named CLOTBUSTER) is being launched in Europe and North America.
© 2012 Elsevier GmbH. All rights reserved.

Introduction

Intravenous tissue plasminogen activator (tPA) remains the only approved therapy for acute ischemic stroke [1] that can be administered fast and at any level emergency room equipped with a non-contrast CT scanner. Even though patients with severe strokes and proximal arterial occlusions are less likely to respond to tPA, they still do better than placebo-treated patients [1]. The presence of a proximal arterial occlusion should not be viewed as an insurmountable predictor of tPA failure since nutritious recanalization can occur even with large middle cerebral (MCA) or internal carotid artery (ICA) thrombi [2,3]. Even if intra-arterial interventions are approved in the future for stroke treatment, it is unrealistic to expect that all patients with MCA occlusions either will reach comprehensive stroke centers in time or their risk factor profile would always make catheter intervention feasible. With bridging intravenous—intra-arterial protocols being tested, there is even further need to amplify the systemic part of reperfusion therapy so that more patients could benefit from early treatment initiation [4].

Arterial recanalization and reversibility of stroke

Early clinical improvement after stroke usually occurs after arterial recanalization [5—8]. The so-called ''recanalization hypothesis'' links the occurrence of recanalization with increase of good functional outcome and reduction of death

* Corresponding author at: Department of Neurology, Comprehensive Stroke Center, The University of Alabama at Birmingham, RWUH M226, 619 19th Street South, Birmingham, AL 35249-3280, USA. Tel.: +1 205 975 8508; fax: +1 205 975 6785.
E-mail address: avalexandrov@att.net

[9], however this hypothesis has not been confirmed in a prospective clinical trial, subject of an ongoing CLOTBUST-PRO multi-center study [10]. In the CLOTBUST trial [11], early recanalization coupled with early dramatic recovery was more common among tPA treated patients who were exposed to continuous vs intermittent monitoring with pulsed wave 2 MHz TCD (25% vs 8%). This, in turn, produced a trend towards more patients recovering at 3 months to modified Ranking score 0–1 (42% vs 29%) [11].

Diagnosis of an acute intracranial occlusion, recanalization and re-occlusion in the CLOTBUST trial was based on the thrombolysis in brain ischemia (TIBI) residual flow grading system [12]. It describes typical waveforms that identify residual flow around an arterial occlusion, and their detailed definitions were published elsewhere [13].

Delivery of tPA to and through the thrombus is dependent on minuscule residual blood cell flow around the thrombus and plasma flow through the thrombus and the need for ultrasound exposure to facilitate drug delivery, enzymatic and mechanical thrombus dissolution has been emphasized by many research groups [14–22]. Acute stroke provided the clinical setting to test the effect of continuous exposure to ultrasound energy in human subjects, goal less attainable in acute coronary syndromes. The CLOTBUST trial demonstrated the positive biological effect of low intensity 2 MHz pulsed wave transcranial Doppler on enhancement of tPA-induced early recanalization. It paved the road for subsequent studies that included combination of ultrasound with gaseous microspheres [23–29] (Table 1). Detailed analysis of microspheres data is beyond the scope of this update since at the moment the clinical developments in the field of sonothrombolysis are focused on the ultrasound device, i.e. drug–device combination. Testing tPA combination with such a device alone is necessary in the first place before more complex combination products (drug–drug–device or drug–device–device) can be tested in clinical trials of microspheres activated with ultrasound in the presence of tPA.

CLOTBUST levels of ultrasound energy and an operator independent device

The main limitation of TCD technology used in the CLOTBUST trial is its extreme operator dependency and the need for a qualified sonographer to be present at bedside to find, aim and deliver ultrasound beam to the thrombus residual flow interface. Our collaborative group first measured outputs of all devices used in the CLOTBUST trial [30], then designed multi-transducer assembly to cover conventional windows used for TCD examinations [31], and prospectively evaluated its safety in human volunteers [35] and ischemic stroke patients treated with intravenous tPA [36]. In these phase I–II clinical studies, the novel operator-independent device showed no safety concerns, caused no disruption of the blood–brain barrier on sequential MRI imaging and yielded recanalization rates comparable to the CLOTBUST trial.

Since this operator-independent device can be quickly mounted by medical personnel with no prior experience in ultrasound, the device enables us to conduct large scale sonothrombolysis trials at all levels of emergency rooms capable of administering tPA as the standard of care. Thus, sonothrombolysis for acute ischemic stroke enters testing in the pivotal efficacy multi-national trial called CLOTBUSTER (Combined Lysis of ThromBus using 2 MHz pulsed wave Ultrasound and Systemic TPA for Emergent Revascularization, NCT01098981). Briefly, all patients will receive 0.9 mg/kg intravenous tPA therapy (10% bolus, 90% continuous infusion over 1 h, maximum dose 90 mg) as standard of care according to national labels (i.e. within 3 or 4.5 h from symptom onset). All patients with National Institutes of

Table 1 Clinical trials of microsphere-potentiated sonothrombolysis for acute ischemic stroke using trancranial ultrasonography (modified from Ref. [34]).

Trial	F	Microspheres	Design	Recanalization	Asymptomatic ICH	Symptomatic ICH	Outcome
Molina et al. [23]	2 MHz	Galactose-based	tPA/TCD/μS vs tPA/TCD vs tPA	55%	23%	3%	56% (mRS 0–2)
Alexandrov et al. [24]	2 MHz	Perflutren-lipid	tPA/TCD/μS vs tPA/TCD	42%	25%	0%	40% (mRS 0–1)
TUCSON [25]	2 MHz	Perflutren-lipid	tPA/TCD/μS 2 doses vs tPA	67%	17%	0%, 27%	75% (mRS 0–1)
Larrue et al. [28]	2 MHz	Galactose-based	tPA/TCCD/μS vs tPA	48%	78%	0%	N/A
Perren et al. [26]	2 MHz	Phospholipid encapsulated sulphur hexafluoride	tPA/TCCD/μS vs tPA	63%	N/A	9%	N/A
Nicoli et al. [29]	2 MHz	Phospholipid encapsulated sulphur hexafluoride	tPA/TCD/μS vs tPA/TCD	86%	N/A	5.7%	N/A

F — frequency of ultrasound; ICH — intracerebral hemorrhage; tPA — tissue plasminogen activator; TCD — transcranial Doppler; μS — microspheres; mRS — modified Rankin scale; TCCD — transcranial color-coded duplex; N/A — not available.

Health Stroke Scale (NIHSS) scores ≥ 10 points are eligible and after signing a written informed consent they will wear an operator-independent ultrasound emitting device for 2 h. The proprietary device (Cerevast Therapeutics, Redmond, WA) exposes traditional transcranial Doppler bone windows for sequential insonation of the 12 proximal intracranial segments that most commonly contain thrombo-embolic occlusions causing disabling strokes. Patients will be randomized 1:1 to continuous exposure to 2 MHz PW ultrasound versus sham exposure. No pre-treatment proof of a proximal arterial occlusion would be required since angiography is not a standard of care for evaluation of tPA-eligible patients at most institutions. Furthermore, NIHSS ≥ 10 points identify severe cerebral ischemia caused by proximal occlusions in >80% of patients [32,33].

Safety will be determined by the incidence of sICH within 24 h of treatment. Functional recovery will be determined by modified Ranking scores (primary end-point mRS 0—1) at 3 months. CLOTBUSTER is a large simple efficacy clinical trial, the first of its kind for sonothrombolysis.

Once CLOTBUSTER establishes safety and efficacy of an operator-independent 2 MHz PW ultrasound device, the next phase clinical trials can commence combining experimental microspheres with regulatory-approved tPA therapy and safe ultrasound exposure. This exposure is needed to activate microspheres, however a proof of safety and efficacy of ultrasound is required before a complex combinatory treatment with or without tPA can be tested any further in the clinical setting.

References

[1] The National Institutes of Neurological Disorders and Stroke rt-PA Stroke Study Group. Tissue plasminogen activator for acute ischemic stroke. N Engl J Med 1995;333:1581—7.

[2] Saqqur M, Uchino K, Demchuk AM, Molina CA, Garami Z, Calleja S, et al. Site of arterial occlusion identified by transcranial Doppler (TCD) predicts the response to intravenous thrombolysis for stroke. Stroke 2007;38:948—54.

[3] Christou I, Felberg RA, Demchuk AM, Burgin WS, Grotta JC, Malkoff M, et al. Intravenous tissue plasminogen activator and flow improvement in acute ischemic stroke patients with internal carotid artery occlusion. J Neuroimaging 2002;12:119—23.

[4] The IMS II Study Investigators. The interventional management of stroke (IMS II) study. Stroke 2007;38:2127—35.

[5] Demchuk AM, Felberg RA, Alexandrov AV. Clinical recovery from acute ischemic stroke after early reperfusion of the brain with intravenous thrombolysis. N Engl J Med 1999;340:894—5.

[6] Grotta JC, Alexandrov AV. TPA-associated reperfusion in acute ischemic stroke demonstrated by SPECT. Stroke 1998;29:429—32.

[7] Heiss W-D, Grond M, Thiel A, von Stockhausen H-M, Rudolf J, Ghaemi M, et al. Tissue at risk of infarction rescued by early reperfusion: a positron emission tomography study in systemic recombinant tissue plasminogen activator thrombolysis of acute stroke. J Cereb Blood Flow Metab 1998;18:1298—307.

[8] Ringelstein EB, Biniek R, Weiller C, Ammeling B, Nolte PN, Thron A. Type and extent of hemispheric brain infarctions and clinical outcome in early and delayed middle cerebral artery recanalization. Neurology 1992;42:289—98.

[9] Rha JH, Saver JL. The impact of recanalization on ischemic stroke outcome: a meta-analysis. Stroke 2007;38:967—73.

[10] Saqqur M, Tsivgoulis G, Molina CA, Demchuk AM, Garami Z, Barreto A, et al. Design of a PROspective multi-national collaboration on reperfusion therapies for stroke (CLOTBUST-PRO). Intl J Stroke 2008;3:66—72.

[11] Alexandrov AV, Molina CA, Grotta JC, Garami Z, Ford SR, Alvarez-Sabin J, et al. Ultrasound-enhanced systemic thrombolysis for acute ischemic stroke. N Engl J Med 2004;351:2170—8.

[12] Demchuk AM, Burgin WS, Christou I, Felberg RA, Barber PA, Hill MD, et al. Thrombolysis in brain ischemia (TIBI) transcranial Doppler flow grades predict clinical severity, early recovery, and mortality in patients treated with intravenous tissue plasminogen activator. Stroke 2001;32(1):89—93.

[13] Alexandrov AV. Ultrasound-enhanced thrombolysis for stroke: clinical significance. Eur J Ultrasound 2002;16:131—40.

[14] Trubestein R, Bernard HR, Etzel F, et al. Thrombolysis by ultrasound. Clin Sci Mol Med 1976;51:697—8.

[15] Tachibana K, Tachibana S. Ultrasonic vibration for boosting fibrinolytic effects of urokinase in vivo. Thromb Haemost 1981;46:211.

[16] Lauer CG, Burge R, Tang DB, Bass BG, Gomez ER, Alving BM. Effect of ultrasound on tissue-type plasminogen activator-induced thrombolysis. Circulation 1992;86:1257—64.

[17] Kimura M, Iijima S, Kobayashi K, Furuhata H. Evaluation of the thrombolytic effect of tissue-type plasminogen activator with ultrasound irradiation: in vitro experiment involving assay of the fibrin degradation products from the clot. Biol Pharm Bull 1994;17:126—30.

[18] Francis CW, Blinc A, Lee S, Cox C. Ultrasound accelerates transport of recombinant tissue plasminogen activator into clots. Ultrasound Med Biol 1995;21:419—24.

[19] Suchkova V, Siddiqi FN, Carstensen EL, Dalecki D, Child S, Francis CW. Enhancement of fibrinolysis with 40-kHz ultrasound. Circulation 1998;98:1030—5.

[20] Behrens S, Daffertshoffer M, Spiegel D, Hennerici M. Low frequency, low-intensity ultrasound accelerates thrombolysis through the skull. Ultrasound Med Biol 1999;25:269—73.

[21] Saguchi T, Onoue H, Urashima M, Ishibashi T, Abe T, Furuhata H. Effective and safe conditions of low-frequency transcranial ultrasound thrombolysis for acute ischemic stroke. Neurologic and histologic evaluation in a rat middle cerebral artery stroke model. Stroke 2008;39:1007—11.

[22] Shaw GJ, Meunier JM, Huang SL, Lindsell CJ, McPherson DD, Holland CK. Ultrasound-enhanced thrombolysis with tPA-loaded echogenic liposomes. Thromb Res 2009;124:306—10.

[23] Molina CA, Ribo M, Rubiera M, Montaner J, Santamarina E, Delgado-Mederos R, et al. Microbubble administration accelerates clot lysis during continuous 2-MHz ultrasound monitoring in stroke patients treated with intravenous tissue plasminogen activator. Stroke 2006;37:425—9.

[24] Alexandrov AV, Mikulik R, Ribo M, Sharma VK, Lao AY, Tsivgoulis G, et al. A pilot randomized clinical safety study of sonothrombolysis augmentation with ultrasound-activated perflutren-lipid microspheres for acute ischemic stroke. Stroke 2008;39:1464—9.

[25] Molina CA, Barreto AD, Tsivgoulis G, Sierzenski P, Malkoff MD, Rubiera M, et al. Transcranial ultrasound in clinical sonothrombolysis (TUCSON) trial. Ann Neurol 2009;66:28—38.

[26] Perren F, Loulidi J, Poglia D, Landis T, Sztajzel R. Microbubble potentiated transcranial duplex ultrasound enhances IV thrombolysis in acute stroke. J Thromb Thrombolysis 2008;25:219—23.

[27] Dinia L, Rubiera M, Ribo M, Maisterra O, Ortega G, del Sette M, et al. Reperfusion after stroke sonothrombolysis with microbubbles may predict intracranial bleeding. Neurology 2009;73:775—80.

[28] Larrue V, Viguier A, Arnaud C, Cognard C, Petit R, Rigal M, et al. Transcranial ultrasound combined with intravenous microbubbles and tissue plasminogen activator for acute ischemic stroke: a randomized controlled study. Stroke 2007;38:472.

[29] Nicoli FJL, Squarcioni C, Grimaud L, Barberet M, Girard N. Microbubble administration during prolonged 2 MHz TCD improves recanalization and long-term functional outcome in acute stroke patients treated with IV thrombolysis for isolated MCA M1 occlusion. Cerebrovasc Dis 2010;29(Suppl 2):Q39.

[30] Ramaswami R, Zhou Y, Schafer M, Zutshi R, Alexandrov AV. Ultrasound energy levels in the CLOTBUST trial: a step towards optimization of clinical sonothrombolysis. Stroke 2008;39:610.

[31] Alexandrov A, Schafer M. Operator-independent device for sonothrombolysis. Cerebrovasc Dis 2008;26(Suppl. 1):6.

[32] Fischer U, Arnold M, Nedeltchev K, Brekenfeld C, Ballinari P, Remonda L, et al. NIHSS score and arteriographic findings in acute ischemic stroke. Stroke 2005;36:2121—5.

[33] Lewandowski CA, Frankel M, Tomsick TA, Broderick J, Frey J, Clark W, et al. Combined intravenous and intra-arterial r-TPA versus intra-arterial therapy of acute ischemic stroke: Emergency Management of Stroke (EMS) Bridging Trial. Stroke 1999;30:2598—605.

[34] Zivanovic Z, Barlinn K, Balucani C, Alexandrov AV. What is the role of ultrasound in systemic thrombolysis? Curr Top Neurol Psychiatr Relat Discip 2010;18:33—41.

[35] Barlinn K. Late-Breaking Science presentation at the International Stroke Conference. 2011.

[36] Barreto AD. Late-Breaking Science presentation at the International Stroke Conference. 2012.

Safety evaluation of superheated perfluorocarbon nanodroplets for novel phase change type neurological therapeutic agents

Jun Shimizu [a,*], Reiko Endoh [a], Takahiro Fukuda [b], Takuya Inagaki [c], Hiroshi Hano [c], Rei Asami [d], Ken-ichi Kawabata [d], Masayuki Yokoyama [a,e], Hiroshi Furuhata [a]

[a] *Medical Engineering Laboratory, Research Center for Medical Sciences, Jikei University School of Medicine, 3-25-8, Nishi-shinbashi, Minato-ku, Tokyo 105-8461, Japan*
[b] *Division of Neuropathology, Department of Neuroscience, Research Center for Medical Sciences, Jikei University School of Medicine, 3-25-8, Nishi-shinbashi, Minato-ku, Tokyo 105-8461, Japan*
[c] *Department of Pathology, Jikei University School of Medicine, 3-25-8, Nishi-shinbashi, Minato-ku, Tokyo 105-8461, Japan*
[d] *Life Science Research Center, Central Research Laboratory, Hitachi Ltd, 1-280, Higasi-koigakubo, Kokubunju-shi, Tokyo 185-8601, Japan*
[e] *Kanagawa Academy of Science and Technology, 3-2-1, Sakato, Takatsu-ku, Kawasaki-shi, Kanagaga 213-0012, Japan*

KEYWORDS
Perfluorocarbon;
Nanodroplets;
Microbubble;
Sonothrombolysis;
Safety

Summary

Background and purpose: Sonothrombolysis using diagnostic ultrasound (US) in combination with microbubble (MB) contrast agents is an attractive trial. Superheated perfluorocarbon nanodroplet (SPN), which can turn into MBs upon US trigger, may have advantages in sonothrombolysis. As a preliminary investigation of SPN-assisted sonothrombolysis, we performed a safety evaluation *in vivo*.

Method: Twenty male rabbits (2.59 ± 0.14 kg) were assigned to three groups: the Control group ($n=6$), 2.2 mL/kg of physiological saline intravascular (i.v.) injection into auricular vein; the PL group ($n=8$), 25 mg/kg of phospholipid-coated SPN i.v.; and the AA group ($n=6$), 25 mg/kg of SPN coated with poly aspartic acid derivative i.v. Rectal temperatures were maintained at $39.08 \pm 0.98\,°C$. Neurological evaluation and biochemical blood examinations were performed at pre-injection, 1, 4, and 7 days after injection. Organ samples including heart, lungs, liver, spleen and kidneys were harvested after euthanasia.

Abbreviations: US, ultrasound; MB, microbubble; SPN, superheated perfluorocarbon nanodroplets; PFC, perfluorocarbon; rt-PA, recombinant tissue-type plasminogen activator; PL, phospholipid-coated; SPN-AA, poly aspartic acid derivative-coated SPN.
 * Corresponding author. Tel.: +81 33433 1111; fax: +81 33459 6005.
   E-mail address: jun-sh@jikei.ac.jp (J. Shimizu).

Results: Within an hour after administration of SPNs, both the PL and AA groups showed a reversible change in respiration. One animal in the AA showed transient nystagmus about 20 min after administration; however, there was no pathological damage. One animal in the PL died 2 days after. No histological damage was found in any organ sample from any of the animals. Moreover, no significant differences were found in the biochemical blood examination between the PL, AA, and Control groups.

Conclusions: No neurological damage or histological change was found with two SPNs. We will further investigate the SPN-assisted sonothrombolysis based on the 500-kHz US exposure with bubble liposome acceleration of rt-PA efficacy.

© 2012 Elsevier GmbH. All rights reserved.

Introduction

Sonothrombolysis using diagnostic ultrasound (US) in combination with microbubble (MB) contrast agents is a potentially productive means to improve the efficiency of rt-PA thrombolysis [1]. Meanwhile, 500 kHz US exposure with liposome MBs can accelerate rt-PA thrombolysis efficacy *in vitro* [2]. Superheated perfluorocarbon nanodroplet (SPN) which can turn into MB upon US trigger, have been studied as a next-generation US contrast agent and therapeutic enhancer [3]. Based on these reports, SPNs may have advantages in sonothrombolysis. However, perfluorocarbon (PFC) is currently approved for diagnostic use only because of the adverse effects including cerebrovascular damage [4,5]. As a preliminary investigation of SPN-assisted sonothrombolysis, we investigated the possible pharmacological toxicity of newly developed SPNs in rabbits as a means of evaluating the safety of PFCs.

Materials and methods

Character of SPN

SPNs are small in size, typically 200—400 nm in diameter, and have compromised sensitivity to US and stability in the body [3,6].

We used two types of SPNs for investigation in animals: a phospholipid-coated SPN, 400 nm in size, that was developed at the Central Research Laboratory, Hitachi [3,6]; and a SPN coated with poly aspartic acid derivative, 200 nm in diameter, that was developed at the Kanagawa Academy of Science and Technology (KAST) [7]. According to previous experiments in rat liver, the SPN dose used in the present study was assumed to be high enough to generate MBs *in vivo* by 1 or 3 MHz US [8]. Before this investigation, we had already confirmed that these two SPNs turn into MBs *in vitro* (Fig. 1) and *in vivo* (Fig. 2).

Experimental animal groups

We selected rabbits as the subject animals for testing the safety of PFCs because they are known to have high sensitivity to the effects of i.v. injection of PFCs [9]. The experimental animal protocol was approved by the animal research committees of Jikei University School of Medicine (Tokyo, Japan).

Twenty male Japanese white rabbits (2.59 ± 0.14 kg) were divided into three groups: the Control group (n = 6), 2.2 mL/kg of physiological saline i.v. into the auricular vein; the PL group (n = 8), 25 mg/kg of phospholipid-coated SPNs i.v.; and the AA group (n = 6), 25 mg/kg of SPNs coated with poly aspartic acid derivative i.v. The administered dosage was determined in a previous investigation of rabbit VX tumors in which 30 mg/kg of phospholipid-coated SPNs was injected i.v., revealing severe respiratory side effects in three of seven rabbits, including two animals that did not survive. In the present study, saline and SPNs were injected i.v. via a 22-G catheter (Angiocath, BD Japan, Fukushima, Japan).

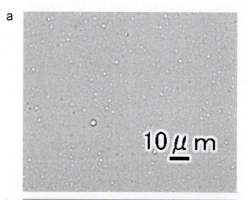
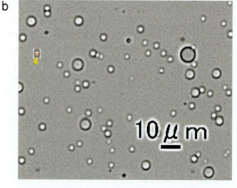

Figure 1 Images of conversion of SPNs into MBs *in vitro*. SPNs turn into MBs in acrylamide gel with exposure to 15 repetition of 7 MHz flash echo. Mechanical index (MI) 0.86, pulse repetition frequency (PRF) 2 Hz, pulse duration (PD) 5 min (Aplio XG, Toshiba, Tokyo, Japan). (a) Phospholipid-coated SPN (Hitachi); (b) SPN coated with poly aspartic acid derivative (KAST).

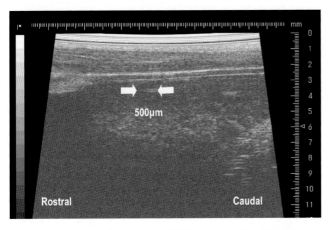

Figure 2 Ultrasonic image of SPNs converted to MB *in vivo*. Intravenously injected SPNs turn into MBs in rat liver with 3 MHz flash echo. 2 kW/cm^2 of spatial peak-temporal peak (SPTP), PRF 50 Hz, 100 waves (Vevo 770, Visualsonics, Toronto, Canada).

Animal set-up and maintenance

Anesthesia was maintained by i.m. injection of midazolam (0.04 mg/kg) and medetomidine (0.08 mg/kg). In a clinical study, Krafft et al. reported that flu-like symptoms with light fever and myalgia had occurred when PFC was excreted from the respiratory system into the air [10]. In our study, animals were placed on a temperature-controlled plate and their homeostatic thermal condition was maintained by measuring rectal temperature (mean ± standard deviation = 39.08 ± 0.98 °C) with a rectal digital thermometer (AW-601H and AW-650H; Nihon Koden, Tokyo, Japan). Animals were supplied pure oxygen via a face mask (1 L/min). Measured parameters included arterial blood pressure (ABP) by cuff and SpO$_2$ with pulse rate (PR) by pulse oximeter (BSM-2301; Nihon Koden). Animals awakened spontaneously and were returned to their cages with free access to water and food on a 12-h light—dark cycle in the animal research facility at Jikei University School of Medicine.

Neurological evaluation

Neurological evaluation was performed according to a previous experimental report in which rabbits were injected with PFC, the neurological check points were the occurrence of paresis, convulsion, anisocoria, and nystagmus [9].

Blood plasma evaluation

Biochemical blood plasma examination including hepatobiliary and renal functions, blood lipid were performed at pre-injection, and 1, 4, and 7 days after injection of SPN. Blood samples were taken from the auricular marginal vein. Biochemically estimated items were as follows: total protein (TP) [g/L], albumin (Alb) [g/L], lactate dehydrogenase (LDH) [U/L], alanine amino transferase (ALT) [U/L], aspartate amino transferase (AST) [U/L], γ-glutanyl transpeptidase (γ-GTP) [U/L], alkaline phosphatase (ALP) [U/L], total bilirubin (T-bil) [mg/dL] for hepatobiliary estimation, blood urea nitrogen (BUN) [mg/dL], creatinine (Cr) [mg/dL] for renal estimation, and total cholesterol (Tch) [mg/dL], triglyceride (TG) [mg/dL], and phospholipid (PL) [mg/dL] for plasma lipid estimation. Statistical analysis was performed with using Dunnett's test.

Histological evaluation

All animals were euthanized with i.v. injection of pentobarbital (20 mg/kg) after blood sampling in 7 days. Organ samples including heart, lungs, liver, spleen and kidneys were harvested after euthanasia. The brain of neurologically positive animal was obtained after perfusion with 10% buffered formalin via the right common carotid artery. Paraffin sections were cut at a thickness of 6 μm. Sections were stained with hematoxylin and eosin (HE), and Masson trichrome.

Results

Change of SpO$_2$ after SPN injection

Within 10 min after administration of SPN, animals in both PL and AA group showed a statistically significant decrease in SpO$_2$ with rapid breathing (Fig. 3). However, in all cases, SpO$_2$ recovered within 1 h. During this investigation, no animals showed an elevated rectal core temperature.

Neurological findings after SPN injection

No animals showed signs of paresis, convulsion or anisocoria. One animal in the AA group showed transient horizontal nystagmus about 20 min after SPN administration, and the duration of nystagmus was 20 min (Table 1).

Neuropathological finding of a nystagmus case in AA group

There was no neuropathological damage, such as hemorrhage, ischemia or any degeneration in brain tissue including the cerebellum and brain stem (Fig. 4).

Pathological findings of each organ

One animal in the PL group died 2 days after injection of SPN. The following description of pathological findings in this paragraph and biochemical plasma results from the PL group includes results from the seven surviving animals.

No histological damage or leukocyte aggregation was found in any organ sample including the heart, lungs, liver, kidneys and spleen in any of the animals. No macrophage hypertrophy or vacuolation was found in the lung, liver or spleen of any animals (Fig. 5).

Table 1 Neurological findings after SPN injection.

	n	Paresis	Convulsion	Anisocoria	Nystagmus
Control	6	0	0	0	0
PL	8	0	0	0	0
AA	6	0	0	0	1

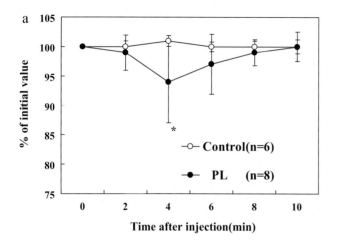

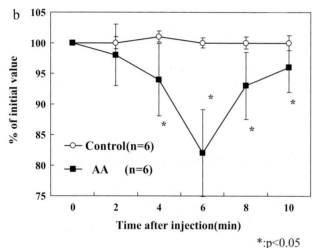

Figure 3 Changes of SpO_2 after SPN injection. Data are percentages of the pre-injection value. (a) Phospholipid-coated SPN (Hitachi); (b) SPN coated with poly aspartic acid derivative (KAST). * $p < 0.05$, versus Control group, Mann—Whitney test.

Biochemical plasma statistical analysis

On biochemical blood examination, including hepatobiliary, renal function and plasma lipid, no significant differences were found between PL, AA, and Control groups ($p > 0.05$).

Autopsy of a dead animal in PL group

In necropsy of the one dead animal in the PL group, diffuse alveolar damage with deposition of fibrin was apparent. Hyaline membrane formation and migration of macrophages were clear, suggesting a state of shock. However, a direct relationship between SPN injection and the histopathological findings could not be detected (Fig. 6).

Discussion

Canaud initially reported the ''perfluorocarbon syndrome'' as a previously unrecognized hazard of a dialysis-related clinical pathologic event in 2002. He also pointed out that PFC foam was identified in blood mainly in the right ventricle in autopsied patients, leading to speculation that death was caused by gas embolism. Oxygen transport characteristic

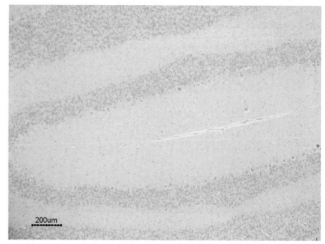

a. cerebellum

b. brain stem (pons)

Figure 4 Photomicrographs of animal with nystagmus in the AA group.

of PFC emulsions are fundamentally different from those of blood [11]. Nieuwoudt et al. reported that PFC is not metabolized, but rather is excreted from the respiratory system into the air. In the first 24 h, the PFC is cleared from the circulation by the mononuclear phagocyte system accumulating in the liver, spleen, and bone marrow [12]. Using macroscopic histology, they also demonstrated leukocyte aggregation and alveolar macrophage hypertrophy in several PFC-injected rats 2 and 4 days after administration.

Canaud et al. (2005) investigated the pharmacological toxicity of PF-5070 in rabbits [9]. Rabbits were given the low (4 μL/kg) or intermediate dose (40 μL/kg) exhibited generalized malacia of the cerebrum and cerebellum. Notably, one animal showed horizontal nystagmus and pulmonary infarcts were detected in some rabbits given the intermediate dose. Neurologically positive animal in the intermediate and high dose (160 μL/kg) groups showed hemorrhagic or ischemic damage in the cerebrum and cerebellum. The necrosis was sharply demarcated from adjacent viable tissue, a characteristic morphologic sign of ischemic infarct. Histopathologic findings from other organs in their study were extensive pulmonary edema,

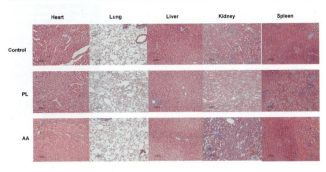

Figure 5 Photomicrographs of each organ in the Control, PL and AA groups.

hemorrhages and infarction, and disseminated patchy necrosis of kidney, liver and spleen.

In our study, SpO_2 was remarkably decreased in both the PL and AA groups without histological damage. There was no macrophage phagocytosis of MBs or necrosis in the lungs, liver, spleen or kidneys. These phenomena may have been due to transient pulmonary alveolar occlusion while intravascular SPNs were present before they were excreted to the air. This speculation could be extended to the animal with transient nystagmus in the AA group without cerebellum and brain stem damage. According to the study by Canaud et al. and our study, i.v. administration of PFC in rabbits might have the potential to cause occlusion within the vertebrobasilar system [9]. Moreover, one animal in the PL group that died after injection did not appear to have leukocyte aggregation or macrophage hypertrophy in the lungs [12]. However, the causes may also be attributable to delayed allergic reaction or some other unknown factor related to SPN injection.

In summary, the side effects of our newly developed SPNs are reversible respiratory disturbance and transient horizontal nystagmus without permanent neurological deficits, and biochemical changes in the plasma. One animal in the PL group died apparently of delayed shock. The most noteworthy point in this study is that no pathological damage due to gas embolism was found in any organs, including the brain tissue of case that developed temporary nystagmus.

Our next challenges for novel neurological US therapies including sonothrombolysis are further evaluation of the safety administration dosages, other kinds of SPNs, and research into transcranial US trigger conditions which can convert SPNs into MBs in the cerebrovascular system.

Conclusions

No permanent neurological deficit, biochemical changes in plasma, or histological damage were observed after injection of the two SPNs in surviving animals.

One animal in the PL group died of delayed shock 2 days after injection.

Acknowledgments

This study was supported, in part, by the New Energy and Industrial Technology Development Organization, Japan. The authors thank Shiho Sasanuki for her help in performing the experiments.

References

[1] Molina CA, Ribo M, Rubiera M, Montaner J, Santamarina E, Delgado-Mederos R, et al. Microbubble administration accelerates clot lysis during continuous 2-MHz ultrasound monitoring in stroke patients treated with intravenous tissue plasminogen activator. Stroke 2006;37:425—9.

[2] Zenitani T, Suzuki R, Maruyama K, Furuhata H. Accelerating effects of ultrasonic thrombolysis with bubble liposome. J Med Ultrasonics 2008;35:5—10.

[3] Asami R, Ikeda T, Azuma T, Kawabata K, Umemura S. Acoustic signal characterization of phase change nanodroplets in tissue mimicking phantom gels. Jpn J Appl Phys 2010;49:07HF16.

[4] Canaud B. Performance liquid test as a cause for sudden deaths of dialysis patients: perfluorocarbon, a previously unrecognized hazard for dialysis patients. Nephrol Dial Transplant 2002;17:545—8.

[5] Castro CI, Briceno CJ. Perfluorocarbon-based oxygen carriers: review of products and trials. Artif Organs 2010:622—34.

[6] Kawabata K, Sugita N, Yoshikawa H, Azuma T, Umemura S. Nanoparticles with multiple perfluorocarbon for controllable ultrasonically induced phase shifting. Jpn J Appl Phys 2005;44:4548—52.

[7] Shiraishi K, Endoh R, Furuhata H, Nishihara M, Suzuki R, Maruyama K, et al. A facile preparation method of a PFC-containing nano-sized emulsion for theranotics of solid tumor. Int J Pharma 2011;421:379—87.

[8] Asami R, Azuma T, Kawabata K. Fluorocarbon droplets as next generation contrast agents—their behavior under 1—3 MHz ultrasound. In: IEEE Proc Int Ultrasonnic Symp. 2009. p. 1294—7.

[9] Canaud B, Aljama P, Tielemans C, Gasparovic V, Gutierrez A, Locatelli F. Pathochemical toxicity of perfluorocarbon-5070, a liquid test performance fluid previously used in dialyzer manufacturing, confirmed in animal experiment. J Am Soc Nephrol 2005;16:1819—23.

[10] Krafft MP, Riess JG. Perfluorocarbons: life sciences and biomedical uses. J Polym Sci A 2007;45:1185—98.

[11] Barrione P, Mastrone A, Salvo RA, Spaccaminlio A, Grasso L, Angeli A. Oxygen delivery enhancer: past, present, and future. J Endcrinol Invest 2008;31:185—92.

[12] Nieuwoudt M, Engelbrecht GH, Sentle L, Auer R, Kahn D, van der Merwe SW. Non-toxicity of IV injected perfluorocarbon oxygen carrier in animal model of liver regeneration following surgical injury. Artifi Cells Blood Substit Immobil Biotechnol 2009;37:117—24.

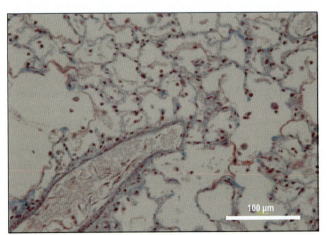

Figure 6 Photomicrograph of lung from one animal in the PL group that died after injection.

Update on ultrasound brain perfusion imaging

Günter Seidel*

Department of Neurology, Asklepios Klinik Hamburg Nord — Heidberg, Tangstedter Landstrasse 400, D-22417 Hamburg, Germany

KEYWORDS
Ultrasound contrast;
Brain perfusion;
Ischemic stroke

Summary Several studies have demonstrated the value of ultrasound perfusion imaging to visualize the area of perfusion deficit in patients with acute ischemic stroke.
Triggered high mechanical index (MI) imaging, which uses contrast microbubble destruction to analyze bolus contrast kinetics in the brain parenchyma, was used in these studies. Recently high sensitive, low MI imaging was introduced. With this new technology real-time bolus kinetics as well as refill kinetics could be analyzed without triggering. In the early phase of ischemic stroke, ultrasound perfusion imaging is useful in detecting the area of perfusion deficit and to assess outcome prognosis of the patient. This bedside technology is available for use in the stroke unit when patients with acute ischemic stroke undergo a color-coded duplex work-up to evaluate their vascular status.
© 2012 Elsevier GmbH. All rights reserved.

Technical background

Several studies using trigger high mechanical index (MI) techniques for visualization of cerebral perfusion after ultrasound contrast agent (UCA) injection have been published in the last 13 years [1—6]. The studies were mostly performed with triggered harmonic gray scale imaging techniques (conventional, power modulation or pulse-inversion) analyzing

Abbreviations: A, fractional vascular volume related to the plateau echo enhancement (refill kinetics); AUC, area under the curve; β, rate constant (slope of the wash in curve of refill kinetics); FWHM, full width at half the maximum intensity; IU, intensity units (linear scale); MI, mechanical index; MTT, mean transit time; PG, positive gradient; PI, peak intensity; PPI, pixelwise peak intensity; PSI, peak signal increase; PW, peak width; ROI, region of interest; TPI, time to peak intensity; TTP, time between start of contrast signal and peak intensity; UCA, ultrasound contrast agent.
 * Tel.: +49 040 18 18 87 3076; fax: +49 040 18 18 87 3069.
 E-mail address: g.seidel@asklepios.com

the bolus kinetics in healthy subjects to find out the best way for the detection of UCA in the cerebral microcirculation.

Recently low mechanical index gray scale imaging was introduced. With this new real-time technology bolus kinetics as well as refill kinetics could be analyzed. Refill kinetics is based on the reappearance of echo contrast in tissue after complete microbubble destruction using a high MI pulse. After destruction of the contrast agent within the scanning plane new microbubbles enter the volume with a certain velocity, thus allowing calculation of regional blood flow (Fig. 1). Refill kinetics to measure regional cerebral blood flow was first studied in dogs after craniectomy [7]. Recent technological advances in ultrasound equipment with improved sensitivity for detection of microbubbles in the cerebral microcirculation through the acoustic bone window in humans now enable real-time ultrasound perfusion imaging [8,9]. This new real-time refill technology has several advantages over the triggered high MI techniques. First refill kinetics could be recorded and analyzed within seconds (Fig. 2); therefore, several insonation planes could be evaluated with one contrast bolus injection. Second software tools like microvascular imaging (display of the

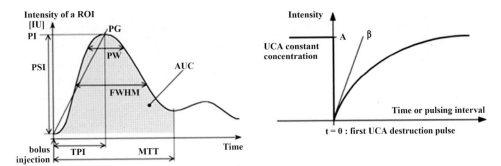

Figure 1 Schematic representation of different parameters of the time—intensity curve available from bolus kinetics (left) and refill kinetics (right). (a) Bolus kinetics: ROI = region of interest, IU = intensity units (linear scale), PI = peak intensity, PG = positive gradient, PSI = peak signal increase, PW = peak width, FWHM = full width at half the maximum intensity, AUC = area under the curve, TPI = time to peak intensity, TTP = time between start of contrast signal and peak intensity, MTT = mean transit time. (b) Refill kinetics: β = rate constant (slope of the wash in curve), A = fractional vascular volume related to the plateau echo enhancement. Adapted from [11].

amount of contrast signals over time [8]) help in visualization and documentation of perfusion deficits. On the other hand there are some disadvantages like the limited maximal insonation depth and the high rate of insonation artifacts.

As of yet, it is not evident which method is superior for the analysis of brain perfusion, because studies with a direct comparison are missing.

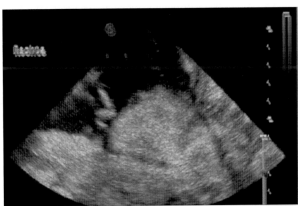

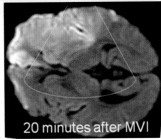

Figure 2 Microvascular imaging: captured contrast signals over 8 s after destruction pulse using low MI real time contrast imaging (iU22 ultrasound system) in a 41-year-old female patient suffering from middle and anterior cerebral artery infarction 11.5 h after symptom onset. We used 2.4 ml SonoVue™ as a bolus. MRI scan (DWI, below) was performed 20 min after the ultrasound perfusion study. Notice the insonation plane within the yellow margins. The area of diffusion disturbance in the MRI (white area) showed no contrast signal in the ultrasound perfusion study (dark area).

The commercially available ultrasound contrast agents Levovist™ (Schering), Optison™ (Amersham Health), and SonoVue™ (Bracco) proved to have contrast enhancing properties in human brain perfusion imaging. No severe adverse events were documented in numerous volunteer studies published on brain perfusion analysis using these contrast agents including more than 200 subjects.

Various curve parameters have been described for the analysis of the different contrast kinetics (bolus and refill). To date (12/2011), it is not evident which kinetics or which parameter is the most valuable for the analysis of brain perfusion in healthy subjects. Theoretically, time-dependent parameters like time to peak intensity (bolus kinetics) or the β-value (refill kinetics) should be more useful than amplitude-dependent parameters, because the latter depend also on insonation depth. Parametric images of certain properties of the time—intensity curves have been generated, which facilitate the evaluation of regional brain perfusion (Fig. 3) [6].

Several studies were reported on ultrasound perfusion imaging in healthy volunteers using perfusion weighted MRI as reference for ultrasound perfusion imaging (Contrast Burst and Time Variance Imaging as well as high MI harmonic imaging) [5,10]. In these studies the time to peak intensity and in one study [5] the area under the time—intensity curve of ultrasound perfusion imaging showed a good correlation to the time to peak intensity as measured in perfusion weighted MRI.

Stroke studies

In most clinical studies on ischemic stroke patients contrast bolus kinetics was analyzed using different high MI harmonic imaging modalities (harmonic imaging, power modulation, and pulse inversion imaging). Levovist™, Optison™, and SonoVue™ were used as contrast agents [12—16]. With new, more sensitive multi-pulse ultrasound technologies it is possible to analyze brain perfusion not only in the ipsilateral but also in the contralateral hemisphere within one investigation improving the geometry of the insonation plane and overcoming near-field artifacts [16]. When using this approach, additional artifacts (calcification of pineal gland

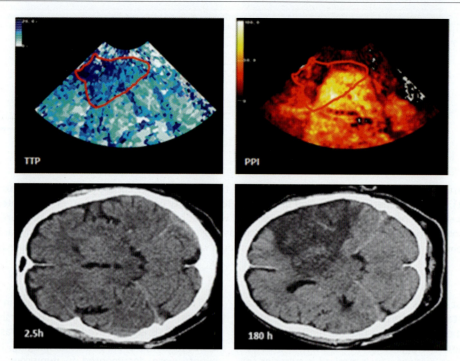

Figure 3 Ultrasound perfusion study using parametric imaging (high-MI imaging, 2.4 ml SonoVue™ bolus kinetics). Ultrasound (SONOS 5500, Philips) was performed 6 h after symptom onset in a 70-year-old male patient suffering from MCA occlusion (M1-segment). Upper row: Time-to-peak image (TTP) and peak signal increase image (PPI—pixelwise peak intensity). Notice the area of delayed contrast arrival in the TTP image (within the red line), which showed in the anterior section a decrease of contrast amplitude in the PPI image. CCT follow-up in the same imaging plane as investigated by ultrasound is shown in the lower row. In the follow-up 180 h after symptom onset a complete middle cerebral artery infarction was displayed, which fits with the initial delay of contrast arrival in the TTP image.

and choroid plexus of lateral ventricles causing shadowing artifacts) have to be considered.

In recent low MI real time refill kinetics studies [17,18] perfusion deficits in acute ischemic stroke patients could be visualized qualitatively with high sensitivity in the ipsilateral hemisphere. The maximal area without detectable contrast signal correlates with the severity of stroke symptoms [17]. Besides this, quantitative thresholds for the occurrence of ischemia were calculated ($\beta < 0.76$ and $A \times \beta < 1.91$ [18]).

Different parameters of the bolus kinetics curve acquired from ischemic brain regions in the acute phase of stroke were compared with follow-up CT to visualize the infarction. A combination of the peak intensity increase (PI) and time-to-peak (TTP) proved to be most helpful in detecting the area of infarction, with a sensitivity between 75% and 86% as well as a specificity between 96% and 100% [13,15].

In more recent studies color-coded parametric images were evaluated [12,19]. They provide information on the time—intensity data in all pixels under evaluation, thus facilitating the visualization of the perfusion state [19]. Although the supplying artery was found patent by color-coded duplex, in 13—14% of acute ischemic stroke patients a perfusion deficit in the middle cerebral artery territory could be identified with parametric perfusion imaging [13,19]. The areas of disturbed perfusion in the parametric images (especially the PPI image) correlate with the area of infarction in follow-up CT and the severity of stroke symptoms in the early phase as well as after four months [16].

Some more investigations based on contrast bolus kinetics were performed on smaller populations using Xenon-CT [20] and MRI [14] as reference methods. These case reports demonstrate the potential of different contrast-specific modalities for the assessment of pathologic brain perfusion using contrast ultrasound imaging. In a small study analyzing local correlations of ultrasound perfusion parameters of bolus kinetics with the occurrence of a perfusion-diffusion mismatch on Stroke MRI (penumbra) thresholds were calculated. Penumbra could be assumed if the relative time delay exceeded 4 s and the relative signal amplitude exceeded 1/3 [21]. These preliminary data should be verified by a prospective study.

Besides the high potential of ultrasound perfusion imaging as a fast, semi-invasive bedside method to evaluate supratentorial brain perfusion in acute ischemic stroke patients, there are some drawbacks like the insonation artifacts, which occur in most of the patients and the inability to scan the whole brain. Besides these technical limitations there are potential side effects of the new contrast agents, which restrict the employment of these substances in severe cardiac or pulmonary disease.

Disclosure statement

Prof. Seidel is employed by Asklepios Kliniken Hamburg GmbH and is professor of Neurology at the University of

Luebeck, Germany. He has previously received unrestricted educational grants from Schering, Bracco Imaging SpA, Philips Medical Systems, Boehringer Ingelheim, Solvay, Bayer HealthCare, Biogen idec, Desitin, Merck Serono, Meda, MSD, Novartis Neuroscience, Talecris, UCB, Grunenthal, Lundbeck, Merz, Teva and Sanofi Aventis. He has worked together with Bracco Imaging SpA and Philips Medical Systems in research projects funded by the European Union.

References

[1] Seidel G, Greis C, Sonne J, Kaps M. Harmonic grey scale imaging of the human brain. J Neuroimaging 1999;9:171—4.

[2] Postert T, Hoppe P, Federlein J, Helbeck S, Ermert H, Przuntek H, et al. Contrast agent specific imaging modes for the ultrasonic assessment of parenchymal cerebral echo contrast enhancement. J Cereb Blood Flow Metab 2000;20:1709—16.

[3] Eyding J, Krogias C, Wilkening W, Meves S, Ermert H, Postert T. Parameters of cerebral perfusion in phase-inversion harmonic imaging (PIHI) ultrasound examinations. Ultrasound Med Biol 2003;29:1379—85.

[4] Harrer JU, Klötzsch C. Second harmonic imaging of the human brain: the practicability of coronal insonation planes and alternative perfusion parameters. Stroke 2002;33:1530—5.

[5] Harrer J, Klötzsch C, Stracke CP, Möller-Hartmann W. Cerebral perfusion sonography in comparison with perfusion MRT: a study with healthy volunteers. Ultraschall Med 2004;25:263—9.

[6] Wiesmann M, Seidel G. Ultrasound perfusion imaging of the human brain. Stroke 2000;31:2421—5.

[7] Rim SJ, Leong-Poi H, Lindner JR, Couture D, Ellegala D, Mason H, et al. Quantification of cerebral perfusion with ''real-time'' contrast-enhanced ultrasound. Circulation 2001;104:2582—7.

[8] Powers J, Averkiou M, Bruce M. Principles of cerebral ultrasound contrast imaging. Cerebrovasc Dis 2009;27(Suppl. 2):14—24.

[9] Seidel G, Meairs S. Ultrasound contrast agents in ischemic stroke. Cerebrovasc Dis 2009;27(Suppl. 2):25—39.

[10] Meves SH, Wilkening W, Thies T, Eyding J, Hölscher T, Finger M, et al. Comparison between echo contrast agent-specific imaging modes and perfusion-weighted magnetic resonance imaging for the assessment of brain perfusion. Stroke 2002;33:2433—7.

[11] Della Martina A, Meyer-Wiethe K, Allemann E, Seidel G. Ultrasound contrast agents for brain perfusion imaging and ischemic stroke therapy. J Neuroimaging 2005;15:217—32.

[12] Seidel G, Meyer-Wiethe K, Berdien G, Hollstein D, Toth D, Aach T. Ultrasound perfusion imaging in acute middle cerebral artery infarction predicts outcome. Stroke 2004;35:1107—11.

[13] Federlein J, Postert T, Meves SH, Weber S, Przuntek H, Büttner T. Ultrasonic evaluation of pathological brain perfusion in acute stroke using second harmonic imaging. J Neurol Neurosurg Psychiatry 2000;69:616—22.

[14] Meyer K, Wiesmann M, Albers T, Seidel G. Harmonic imaging in acute stroke: detection of a cerebral perfusion deficit with ultrasound and perfusion MRI. J Neuroimaging 2003;13:166—8.

[15] Seidel G, Albers T, Meyer K, Wiesmann M. Perfusion harmonic imaging in acute middle cerebral artery infarction. Ultrasound Med Biol 2003;29:1245—51.

[16] Eyding J, Krogias C, Wilkening W, Postert T. Detection of cerebral perfusion abnormalities in acute stroke using phase inversion harmonic imaging (PIHI): preliminary results. J Neurol Neurosurg Psychiatry 2004;75:926—9.

[17] Kern R, Diels A, Pettenpohl J, Kablau M, Brade J, Hennerici MG, et al. Real-time ultrasound brain perfusion imaging with analysis of microbubble replenishment in acute MCA stroke. J Cereb Blood Flow Metab 2011;31:1716—24.

[18] Seidel G, Roessler F, Al-Khaled M. Microvascular imaging in acute ischemic stroke. J Neuroimaging; in press.

[19] Wiesmann M, Meyer K, Albers T, Seidel G. Parametric perfusion imaging with contrast-enhanced ultrasound in acute ischemic stroke. Stroke 2004;35:508—13.

[20] Meairs S, Daffertshofer M, Neff W, Eschenfelder C, Hennerici M. Pulse-inversion contrast harmonic imaging: ultrasonographic assessment of cerebral perfusion. Lancet 2000;355:550—1.

[21] Meyer-Wiethe K, Cangur H, Schindler A, Koch C, Seidel G. Ultrasound perfusion imaging: determination of thresholds for the identification of critically disturbed perfusion in acute ischemic stroke—a pilot study. Ultrasound Med Biol 2007;33:851—6.

Brain tissue perfusion monitoring using Sonopod for transcranial color duplex sonography

Toshiyuki Shiogai [a,*], Mari Koyama [a], Mayumi Yamamoto [a], Kenji Yoshikawa [b], Toshiki Mizuno [c], Masanori Nakagawa [c]

[a] Department of Clinical Neurosciences, Kyoto Takeda Hospital, Minamikinuta-cho 11, Nishinanajo, Shimogyo-ku, Kyoto 600-8884, Japan
[b] Department of Stroke Medicine, Hoshigaoka Kouseinenkin Hospital, Hoshigaoka 4-8-1, Hirakata City, Osaka 573-8511, Japan
[c] Department of Neurology, Kyoto Prefectural University of Medicine, Kajii-cho 465, Kawaramachi-Hirokoji, Kamigyo-ku, Kyoto 602-8566, Japan

KEYWORDS
Transcranial color duplex sonography;
Transducer holder (Sonopod);
Brain tissue perfusion;
Acetazolamide vasoreactivity;
Second harmonic imaging;
Power modulation imaging

Summary

Objective: We have introduced and improved a transducer holder, named the Sonopod, for transcranial color duplex sonography (TCDS) monitoring via both temporal/foraminal windows (TW/FW). The objective is to clarify clinical usefulness and identify problems in TCDS-Sonopod monitoring during the evaluation of brain tissue perfusion.

Methods: Brain tissue perfusion monitoring was evaluated in 11 patients (ages 31–94, mean 66). After a bolus intravenous Levovist®, power modulation imaging (PMI) in all cases was evaluated in comparison with second harmonic imaging (SHI) in two cases at the diencephalic horizontal plain via the TWs on the basis of time—intensity curves (TICs) in five regions of interest (ROIs); bilateral basal ganglia (BG) and thalamus (Th), and contra-lateral temporal lobe (TL). After a SONOS5500 S3 transducer was installed in the Sonopod, acetazolamide (ACZ) cerebral vasoreactivity utilizing PMI was evaluated in 10 cases via the bilateral (five cases) and unilateral (five cases) TWs. A total of 30 TICs were evaluated before/after ACZ administration.

Results: (1) All patients could be monitored continuously by one examiner. (2) We confirmed that PMI proves superior to SHI in quantitative evaluation of the bilateral hemispheres via the unilateral TWs. (3) Brain tissue perfusion could be precisely quantified before/after ACZ in the same ROIs. (4) TIC base-line drifts during monitoring were observed in 4 (seven TICs) of 10 (30 TICs) patients. However, fixed-probe shifts during monitoring were easily readjustable and the TIC recovered to the base-line in all cases. (5) Due to re-fixation needed for contralateral TW monitoring, it was not possible to evaluate completely in the same ROIs.

Conclusions: TCDS-Sonopod monitoring succeeds in continuously and quantitatively evaluating precise and reproducible intracranial hemodynamics in the brain tissue.
© 2012 Elsevier GmbH. All rights reserved.

* Corresponding author. Tel.: +81 75 312 7001; fax: +81 75 325 2295.
E-mail address: shiogait@pop11.odn.ne.jp (T. Shiogai).

Introduction

Compared to conventional transcranial Doppler sonography (TCD), transcranial color duplex sonography (TCDS) is

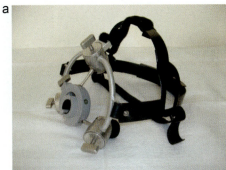
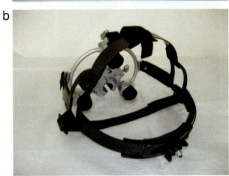

Figure 1 Transducer holder (Sonopod) for transcranial color duplex sonography (TCDS) monitoring. We have developed and improved the transducer holder (Sonopod) for TCDS monitoring (a and b).

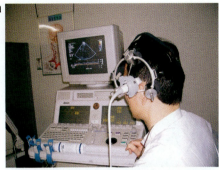
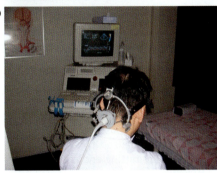

Figure 2 TCDS-Sonopod monitoring in sitting position via both temporal (a) and foraminal (b) windows.

able to measure much more accurately on the basis of angle-collected velocities in the intracranial major vessels. Furthermore, TCDS is able to visualize intracranial lesions in stroke [1], severe head injury [2], and other neurological disorder cases [3]. Utilizing ultrasound contrast agents (UCA), TCDS has been able to evaluate brain tissue perfusion non-invasively, particularly in ischemic stroke patient investigations [4,5]. Possibilities of quantitative measurements have been evaluated in an identical way to neuroradiological perfusion imaging, based on the bolus dye-dilution principle. However, quantitative reliability has not yet been established, due to problems of skull- and depth-dependent ultrasound attenuation, shadowing effects, bubble saturation, and low data reproducibility (the latter due to UCA administration methods, transducer fixation, data analysis, etc.) [4,5].

Transducer holders or probe fixation devices for conventional TCD monitoring have been introduced into clinical settings [6—9]. However, a transducer holder for TCDS has yet to be clinically introduced. We have developed and improved such a transducer holder (Sonopod) (Fig. 1) for TCDS monitoring via both temporal and foraminal windows (TW and FW) (Fig. 2).

To overcome the inherent problems and establish the clinical significance of transcranial ultrasound perfusion imaging, we have clinically introduced the Sonopod for TCDS monitoring [10,11] and evaluated acetazolamide (ACZ) vasoreactivity [12,13]. The objective of this study is to clarify clinical usefulness and identify problems in TCDS-Sonopod monitoring in the evaluation of brain tissue perfusion.

Material and methods

Brain tissue perfusion monitoring was evaluated in 11 patients (ages 31—94, mean 66). Details of patient demographics are shown in Table 1. After a 5 ml-bolus Levovist® injection (2.5 g, 400 mg/ml) via the antecubital vein, power modulation imaging (PMI) in all cases in comparison with

Table 1 Patient demographics.

Total patients: $n = 11$	
Causes of brain injury	
Cerebral infarction (atherothrombotic 5, lacunar 2, embolic 1)	8
Hypertensive putaminal hemorrhage	1
Ruptured anterior communicating aneurysm	1
Chronic subdural hematoma	1
Ages: 31—94 years (mean 66)	
Gender: male 9, female 2	
Monitoring (via temporal window)	
Perfusion imaging	
Power modulation imaging only	9
Second harmonic imaging and Power modulation imaging	2
Acetazolamide vasoreactivity test (bilateral 5, unilateral 5)	10 (30 TIC analyses)
TIC base-line drift during monitoring	4 (7 TIC analyses)

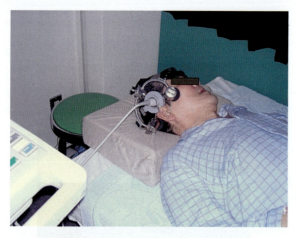

Figure 3 TCDS-Sonopod monitoring in supine position via the temporal window.

second harmonic imaging (SHI) in the initial two cases were evaluated in the supine position via TWs (Fig. 3). Both imaging types were visualized by an integrated backscatter method. The transmitting and receiving frequencies of PMI and SHI were 1.7/1.7 MHz and 1.3/2.6 MHz, respectively. The investigation depth was 16 cm with a focus of 8 cm. Settings were mechanical index 1.6, system gain 75, and compression 70. ACZ cerebral vasoreactivity, before and after 500 mg Diamox® intravenous injection, was evaluated in 10 cases utilizing a SONOS5500 S3 transducer (Philips Electronics Japan, Ltd.) installed in the Sonopod. Time—intensity curves (TICs) on the diencephalic horizontal plain were evaluated before and after ACZ in five regions of interest (ROI); bilateral basal ganglia (BG) and thalamus (Th), and contra-lateral temporal lobe (TL). A total of 30 TICs with a duration of 10 min via the bilateral (five cases) and unilateral (five cases) TWs were analyzed before and after ACZ.

Results

Hand-held monitoring utilizing PMI and SHI

Conventional SHI and PMI utilizing hand-held monitoring were compared in two cases. In the visualization of the contralateral hemispheres via the unilateral TWs, PMI was superior to SHI as shown in the upper panels of Fig. 4a and b. As shown in the lower panels of the quantitative TIC evaluations in both PMI and SHI, peak intensity (PI) in the contralateral hemisphere ROIs was lower than in the ipsilateral hemisphere ROIs. During hand-held monitoring, TICs were not always stable in all cases and drifted from the base-line due to patients' movements as shown in the lower panels of Fig. 4.

Sonopod ACZ monitoring utilizing PMI

All patients could be fitted and monitored continuously by one examiner. Brain tissue perfusion could be precisely quantified before/after ACZ in the same ROI as shown in Fig. 5. Due mainly to patient's movements, drifts from the base-line were observed in the TICs of 4 (seven TIC analyses)

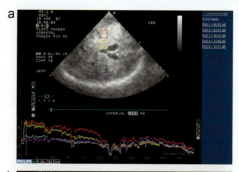
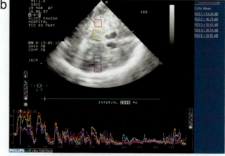

Figure 4 Hand-held monitoring via the left temporal windows utilizing second harmonic imaging (SHI) and power modulation imaging (PMI). Hand-held monitoring of brain tissue perfusion via the left TW utilizing SHI (a) and PMI (b) are depicted in a post-operative patient with an anterior communicating artery aneurysm. TICs derived from the five ROIs, placed in the bilateral BG and Th, and contra-lateral TL, are shown in the lower panels. TICs have drifted from the base-line and are unstable due to patient's movements.

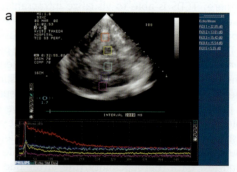
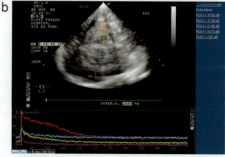

Figure 5 Sonopod acetazolamide (ACZ) vasoreactivity test utilizing PMI. Sonopod monitoring of brain tissue perfusion via the right TW utilizing PMI before (a) and after (b) ACZ administration, demonstrated in a postoperative patient with chronic subdural hematoma. TICs are completely stable during 10 min of monitoring.

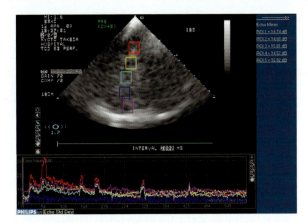

Figure 6 Sonopod PMI monitoring before ACZ administration. Sonopod PMI monitoring of brain tissue perfusion via the left TW before ACZ administration is shown in a patient with right putaminal hemorrhage. TICs have drifted from the baseline due to patients' movements, but have been returned to the baseline easily through readjustment of fixed-probe positions during monitoring.

out of 10 (30 TIC analyses) patients. However, fixed-probe shifts due to patients' movements during monitoring were easily re-adjustable and the TICs could be returned to the baseline in all patients as shown in Fig. 6. Regarding contralateral TW monitoring in the five bilaterally ACZ examined patients, it was not possible to evaluate precisely in the same ROI locations due to Sonopod re-fixation.

Discussion

Transducer holder for TCD and TCDS

Transducer holders or probe fixation devices for conventional TCD monitoring have been introduced into clinical settings. Previously, for the examination of neonates, a hood-like probe fixation device via the transfontanellar window has been investigated [14]. Trials in adult patients have focused not only on the middle cerebral artery (MCA) via the TWs [7,15], but also in the vertebrobasilar arteries via the FW for high intensity transient signals (HITS) monitoring [16]. More recently, a commercially available head-frame (Marc 600, Spencer Technologies) for monitoring via the TWs has been used for detection of recanalization in the MCA during tissue plasminogen activator studies [6]. Furthermore, a long-term ambulatory TCD monitoring device placed on a spectacle frame has been introduced for HITS detection in the MCAs via the TWs [9]. A modified head-frame combining two Spencer Technologies' head-frames for both the TWs and FW has been tried for vasoreactivity tests [8].

Our TCDS transducer fixation device, the Sonopod, is able to monitor not only via the TWs, but also via the FW (Fig. 2). A further important advantage is long-duration stable TCDS monitoring that implies accurate quantitative measurements in the major cerebral arteries and brain tissue. Proposed criteria for probe-holding systems include ease of application, stability during patient movement, low-cost, compatibility with multiple probes, comfort and durability [7]. The durability of a prototype of this transducer, the Sonopod, has been proven, with no problems in our four-year experience. However, it is still so heavy that long-time TW monitoring in the sitting position will probably result in discomfort caused by fatigue of the neck muscles. This problem will be improved in changing materials from heavy stainless steel to light weight aluminum, titanium, or similar. For FW monitoring, the Sonopod is unable to be applied in a supine position, therefore patients should be instructed to lie down semi-laterally. It is necessary to tighten four screws during setup of the Sonopod and this may prove a slight time-consuming drawback while searching for appropriate location of vessels or anatomical places. In our experience however, we were usually ready for monitoring in around 5—10 min. Improvements of the Sonopod have been planned for the SONOS 5500 S3 transducer (Philips), compatibility with multiple probes and costs of marketing the products should be confirmed in the near future.

Comparison of SHI and PMI

Since the clinical introduction of transcranial ultrasound perfusion imaging of brain tissue, depth dependant ultrasound attenuation has been the most challenging problem for qualitative and quantitative evaluation [17,18]. In our study, significant depth dependant PI attenuation on the TICs was observed in both image types, particularly in the contralateral hemisphere. In the pioneering work utilizing SHI with Levovist® by Postert et al. [17], not only PI but also the area under the TIC was shown to be significantly higher in the BG and white matter ROIs than in the Th ROI. Furthermore, SHI utilizing an alternative UCA (Optison) showed significantly higher Th ROI in the ipsilateral hemisphere than in the contralateral hemisphere [18]. More recent studies utilizing phase-inversion harmonic imaging (PIHI) utilizing Optison and SonoVue [19] showed typical depth dependant PI attenuation in the contralateral hemisphere rather than the ipsilateral hemisphere in bilateral or unilateral (ipsilateral) approaches. A bilateral approach utilizing PIHI [19,20] has been suggested for evaluating contralateral hemispheres. Our previous study of ultrasound perfusion imaging also showed that PMI utilizing transient response high power images is superior to conventional SHI in evaluation of the contra-lateral cerebral hemisphere [21]. This study reconfirmed that result. However, limitations of the contralateral approach, e.g. shadowing [19], have been pointed out [5].

ACZ vasoreactivity utilizing PMI

In order to overcome the problems in quantifying brain tissue perfusion, e.g. depth dependant ultrasound attenuation, we have applied transcranial ultrasound perfusion imaging to the ACZ vasoreactivity test [10,13]. In ACZ vasoreactivity tests, the same ROI placements before and after ACZ are very important for accurate quantification. From this point of view, the Sonopod is very useful for precise quantification of brain tissue perfusion.

Conclusions

TCDS-Sonopod monitoring succeeds in continuously and quantitatively evaluating precise and reproducible intracranial hemodynamics in the major cerebral arteries and brain tissue.

References

[1] Seidel G, Kaps M, Dorndorf W. Transcranial color-coded duplex sonography of intracerebral hematomas in adults. Stroke 1993;24:1519—27.
[2] Shiogai T, Nagayama K, Damrinjap G, Saruta K, Hara M, Saito I. Morphological and hemodynamic evaluations by means of transcranial power Doppler imaging in patients with severe head injury. Acta Neurochir Suppl 1998;71:94—100.
[3] Tsai CF, Wu RM, Huang YW, Chen LL, Yip PK, Jeng JS. Transcranial color-coded sonography helps differentiation between idiopathic Parkinson's disease and vascular parkinsonism. J Neurol 2007;254:501—7.
[4] Martina AD, Meyer-Wiethe K, Allemann E, Seidel G. Ultrasound contrast agents for brain perfusion imaging and ischemic stroke therapy. J Neuroimaging 2005;15:217—32.
[5] Seidel G, Meyer-Wiethe K. Acute stroke: perfusion imaging. Front Neurol Neurosci 2006;21:127—39.
[6] Alexandrov AV, Demchuk AM, Felberg RA, Christou I, Barber PA, Burgin WS, et al. High rate of complete recanalization and dramatic clinical recovery during tPA infusion when continuously monitored with 2 MHz transcranial Doppler monitoring. Stroke 2000;31:610—4.
[7] Giller CA, Giller AM. A new method for fixation of probes for transcranial Doppler ultrasound. J Neuroimaging 1997;7:103—5.
[8] Hong JM, Joo IS, Huh K, Sheen SS. Simultaneous vasomotor reactivity testing in the middle cerebral and basilar artery with suboccipital probe fixation device. J Neuroimaging 2010;20:83—6.
[9] Mackinnon AD, Aaslid R, Markus HS. Long-term ambulatory monitoring for cerebral emboli using transcranial Doppler ultrasound. Stroke 2004;35:73—8.
[10] Shiogai T, Ikeda K, Morisaka A, Nagakane Y, Mizuno T, Nakagawa M, et al. Acetazolamide vasoreactivity evaluated by transcranial power harmonic imaging and Doppler sonography. Acta Neurochir Suppl 2008;102:177—83.
[11] Shiogai T, Koyama M, Yamamoto M, Yoshikawa K, Mizuno T, Nakagawa M. Monitoring of brain tissue perfusion utilizing Sonopod for transcranial color duplex sonography. Cerebrovasc Dis 2011;31(Suppl. 1):18 [abstract].
[12] Shiogai T, Matsumoto M, Ikeda K, Morisaka A, Yoshikawa K, Nagakane Y, et al. Continuous monitoring in the vertebrobasilar artery utilizing a newly developed transducer holder (Sonopod) for transcranial color duplex sonography. Cerebrovasc Dis 2008;25(Suppl 1):36 [abstract].
[13] Shiogai T, Koyama M, Mizuno T, Nakagawa M, Furuhata H. Cerebral vasoreactivity in the brain tissue and the major cerebral arteries evaluated by transcranial power modulation imaging and color duplex sonography. Cerebrovasc Dis 2010;29(Suppl. 1):23—4 [abstract].
[14] Michel E, Zernikow B, Rabe H, Jorch G. Adaptive multipurpose probe fixation device for use on newborns. Ultrasound Med Biol 1993;19:581—6.
[15] Gehring H, Meyer zu Westrup L, Berndt S, Joubert-Hübner E, Eleftheriadis S, Schmucker P. A new probe holding device for continuous bilateral measurements of blood flow velocity in basal brain vessels. Anasthesiol Intensivmed Notfallmed Schmerzther 1997;32:355—9.
[16] Woodtli M, Müller HR. A head and transducer holding technique for TCD monitoring of the vertebrobasilar circulation. Ultraschall Med 1994;15:293—5.
[17] Postert T, Muhs A, Meves S, Federlein J, Przuntek H, Buttner T. Transient response harmonic imaging: an ultrasound technique related to brain perfusion. Stroke 1998;29:1901—7.
[18] Seidel G, Algermissen C, Christoph A, Claassen L, Vidal-Langwasser M, Katzer T. Harmonic imaging of the human brain. Visualization of brain perfusion with ultrasound. Stroke 2000;31:151—4.
[19] Eyding J, Krogias C, Wilkening W, Meves S, Ermert H, Postert T. Parameters of cerebral perfusion in phase-inversion harmonic imaging (PIHI) ultrasound examinations. Ultrasound Med Biol 2003;29:1379—85.
[20] Eyding J, Krogias C, Wilkening W, Postert T. Detection of cerebral perfusion abnormalities in acute stroke using phase inversion harmonic imaging (PIHI): preliminary results. J Neurol Neurosurg Psychiatry 2004;75:926—9.
[21] Shiogai T, Ikeda K, Matsumoto M, Morisaka A, Mizuno T, Nakagawa M, et al. Comparison of quantitative parameters in transcranial brain tissue perfusion images between power modulation imaging and second harmonic imaging. Cerebrovasc Dis 2009;27(Suppl. 5):20 [abstract].

Relationship between refill-kinetics of ultrasound perfusion imaging and vascular obstruction in acute middle cerebral artery stroke

Manuel Bolognese*, Dimitrios Artemis, Angelika Alonso, Michael G. Hennerici, Stephan Meairs, R. Rolf Kern

Department of Neurology, UniversitätsMedizin Mannheim, University of Heidelberg, Mannheim, Germany

KEYWORDS
Ultrasound perfusion imaging;
Refill kinetics;
Ischemic stroke;
Microbubbles

Summary

Background: Ultrasound perfusion imaging (UPI) with bolus kinetic has been shown to be feasible at bedside for evaluation of perfusion deficits in stroke patients. Recent technical advances allow perfusion imaging with refill kinetics using a low mechanical index.

Methods: We examined 31 acute middle cerebral artery (MCA) stroke patients with transcranial color-coded duplex ultrasound (TCCD) and UPI. The refill of microbubbles was calculated from regions of interest in the ischemic area and the contralateral MCA territory by using the exponential function $y = A(1 - e^{\beta t})$; A = acoustic intensity of the plateau (dB), β = slope (1/s).

Results: We found significantly lower values of β in the ischemic area compared with the contralateral MCA territory (0.75 vs. 1.05 1/s, $p < 0.05$); particularly in patients with a pathological MCA flow pattern on TCCD (0.61 vs. 1.01, $p < 0.01$). There was a high interindividual variance without significant difference of the plateau of acoustic intensity (A) in any subgroup of patients.

Discussion: The slope parameter β of refill kinetics is useful for assessing brain perfusion in patients with acute stroke and pathological flow pattern of the ipsilateral MCA. The parameter A, however, seems more dependent from the quality of the temporal bone window.
© 2012 Elsevier GmbH. All rights reserved.

Introduction

Assessment of cerebral perfusion is highly relevant for the immediate diagnostic work-up of acute ischemic stroke. MRI and CT perfusion are routinely used to identify patients who may benefit from recanalizing therapy beyond the standard time window, identifying salvageable tissue at risk of infarction by the MR diffusion-perfusion-based mismatch concept [1]. Other perfusion imaging methods like PET-CT and SPECT are not feasible in acute stroke patients because of logistic limitations.

Ultrasound perfusion imaging (UPI) has been shown to be able to likewise identify perfusion deficits of the brain parenchyma [2–4]. The advantages of UPI are the possibility to perform and repeat the examination at patient's bedside, allowing a non-invasive, cheap and quickly applicable assessment of cerebral perfusion on an intensive care unit or a stroke unit.

* Corresponding author at: UniversitätsMedizin Mannheim, University of Heidelberg, Department of Neurology, Theodor-Kutzer-Ufer 1-3, 68167 Mannheim, Germany. Tel.: +49 621 383 2885.
E-mail addresses: bolognese@neuro.ma.uni-heidelberg.de, manuel.bolognese@gmx.de (M. Bolognese).

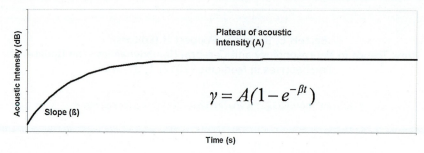

Figure 1 Exponential function of microbubbles replenishment after destruction of microbubbles. γ is the acoustic intensity measured at pulse interval t, A represents the plateau of acoustic intensity during refill kinetic and β is the slope of the acoustic intensity over time.

The main limitations of this method are the attenuation of ultrasound by the human skull and the interindividual variance of skull thickness [5]. In order to guarantee a sufficient penetration of ultrasound, a high ultrasound energy (high mechanical index = MI) was necessary in earlier UPI protocols. This led, however, to an early destruction of the echo-contrast agent microbubbles, which made it necessary to trigger the ultrasound impulses with a frequency of 1—2/s. This resulted in a relevant decrease of the temporal resolution of UPI and thus of the sensitivity of this method to detect small differences of cerebral perfusion between different regions of interest (ROI) [6].

Recent advances in ultrasound technology now allow to perform UPI using low ultrasound energy (i.e. low MI), which enables perfusion studies in real time (rt-UPI) without the need of triggering the impulses, leading to improved temporal resolution [7]. Bolus kinetics, where the time after application of the ultrasound contrast agent until the maximum of acoustic intensity (=time to peak) is measured, has been already established as a valid method to assess human brain perfusion with ultrasound [4]. Another interesting method to measure tissue perfusion with UPI is refill kinetics, which has been first used by Wei and coworkers in myocardial tissue [8]. After injection of echo-contrast agents, the circulating microbubbles in the ultrasound plane are destroyed by a repetitive ultrasound pulse with high MI, followed by registration of the replenishment of microbubbles in the cerebral microvasculature with low MI. The replenishment can be demonstrated by an exponential equitation $y = A(1 - e^{\beta t})$, where A represents the plateau of the acoustic intensity and β the slope factor of the exponential curve (Fig. 1).

Refill kinetics has been also employed successfully to measure cerebral perfusion in an animal model of trepanated dogs, showing a good correlation with cerebral blood flow [9]. We have recently reported that refill kinetics is also feasible for assessing cerebral perfusion in acute middle cerebral artery (MCA) stroke patients [10]. In the present study, we investigated the relationship between the rt-UPI parameters of refill kinetics and the degree of underlying arterial obstruction of the MCA as assessed by transcranial color-coded duplex ultrasound (TCCD).

Methods

We used a Philips IU 22 system and a 1—5 MHz sector transducer for rt-UPI and TCCD studies. Inclusion criteria were sufficient transtemporal bone windows bilaterally and a territorial acute MCA stroke as shown by either CT or MRI. Exclusion criteria were any contraindication against SonoVue®, a second-generation ultrasound contrast agent based on sulfurhexafluoride microbubbles [11].

TCCD and rt-UPI studies were performed within the first 24 h after onset of stroke. TCCD was used to evaluate the quality of the temporal bone window. The maximum systolic flow velocity of the MCA was measured in different depths bilaterally (Fig. 2). The severity of vascular obstruction was expressed by the COGIF grades [12] indicating different degrees of persistent arterial obstruction (COGIF grades 0—3) or residual stenosis/reperfusion (COGIF grade

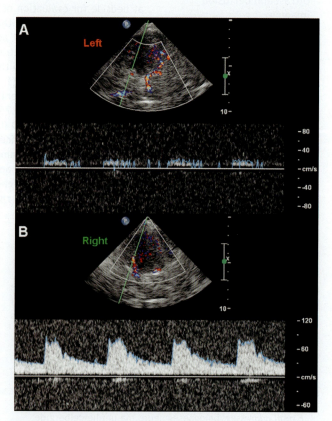

Figure 2 Example of patient with left middle cerebral artery (MCA) stroke: TCCD of the left (A) and right hemisphere (B) showing an occlusion of the proximal left MCA (COGIF-Score 2) and a normal flow pattern of the right MCA.

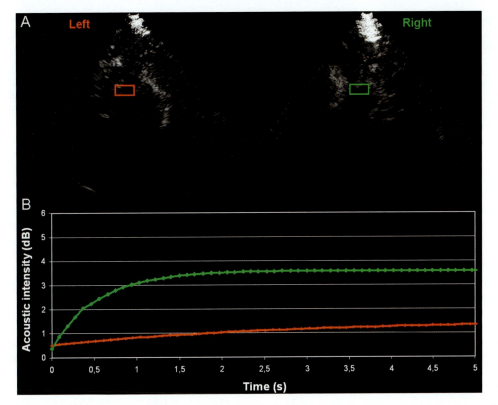

Figure 3 Real time ultrasound perfusion imaging (rt-UPI) of both hemispheres (A) with corresponding regions of interest in the ischemic area of the left (red) and the contralateral MCA territory (green). Refill kinetics (B) show a flattened curve with low slope of the exponential function in ischemic tissue (red), and a normal replenishment of microbubbles in the contralateral hemisphere (green).

4). For rt-UPI the ultrasound plane was tilted 20° cranially from the mesencephalic plane, displaying lateral and third ventricle and the thalamus. A bolus of 2.5 ml Sonovue® was injected and parameters of refill kinetics were calculated from selected ROIs in the ischemic area under avoidance of large vessels. After 10 min, we examined the contralateral hemisphere with the same protocol. We selected ROIs in the contralateral MCA territory, which corresponded in size, shape and localization to the ischemic ROIs (Fig. 3). Parameters of refill kinetics (A, β and the product $A \times \beta$) were extracted from each ROI for statistical analysis. To analyze the potential relationship between MCA flow velocity and the parameters of refill kinetics, we subdivided patients in two groups: patients with persisting MCA pathology defined by COGIF grades of 3 or lower, and patients with symmetrical or increased MCA flow (COGIF grade 4).

Results

We examined 31 patients (17 male, 14 female, mean age 68.3 ± 13.4) who were admitted to our stroke unit with acute ischemic stroke in the MCA territory (Table 1). 58% of patients were treated with intravenous thrombolysis. At the time point of examination, TCCD showed a persistent pathological flow pattern of the ipsilateral MCA (COGIF grades 0—3) in 21/31 (67.7%) patients. Pathological flow patterns were more frequent among patients who were not treated with tPA (11/13 vs. 10/18, $p = 0.08$). Rt-UPI showed significantly lower values of the refill parameter β in the ischemic area compared to the contralateral MCA territory (β (1/s): 0.75 ± 0.41 vs. 1.05 ± 0.51, $p < 0.05$). The difference between ischemic and contralateral ROIs was more prominent in patients with persisting MCA obstruction ($n = 21$; β (1/s): 0.61 ± 0.31 vs. 1.01 ± 0.53, $p = 0.005$). Correspondingly, in patients with symmetrical or increased ipsilateral MCA flow, β values were not significantly different between both hemispheres ($n = 10$; β (1/s): 1.04 ± 0.47 vs. 1.14 ± 0.49, $p = $ n.s.). There was no significant difference between β values of the ischemic tissue of patients treated with tPA and those who did not receive systemic thrombolysis (β (1/s): 0.72 ± 0.32 vs. 0.78 ± 0.53, $p = $ n.s.). For the plateau of acoustic intensity (A) and the product of A and β ($A \times \beta$), there was a high interindividual variance of the values, resulting in no significant difference between ischemic or contralateral healthy tissue in any group of patients (Table 2).

Discussion

This study investigated the feasibility of rt-UPI with refill kinetics to assess perfusion deficits related to persistent or already recanalized arterial obstruction in acute MCA stroke patients. The parameter β, which represents the slope factor of the exponential function of refill kinetics, shows overall significant differences between ischemic and healthy tissue. This finding was more pronounced in patients

Table 1 rt-UPI parameters and COGIF grades of the ipsilateral MCA as assessed by TCCD.

	COGIF grade (ipsilateral MCA)	Ischemic tissue			Normal tissue		
		A	β	A × β	A	β	A × β
1	4	2.78	1.83	5.09	9.33	1.05	9.80
2	3	1.66	0.92	1.53	4.24	0.67	2.84
3	4	0.35	0.61	0.21	0.17	0.69	0.12
4	3	1.13	0.33	0.37	1.64	0.61	1.00
5	3	1.8	0.82	1.48	1.9	2.2	4.18
6	4	1.08	0.81	0.87	1.97	0.67	1.32
7	4	2.57	1.17	3.01	2.36	1.36	3.21
8	1	7.58	0.04	0.30	6.06	1.47	8.91
9	3	1.79	0.63	1.13	0.5	0.96	0.48
10	3	0.99	0.68	0.67	0.86	1.17	1.01
11	1	3.92	0.3	1.18	3.89	0.86	3.35
12	4	0.51	0.67	0.34	2.29	2.24	5.13
13	3	4.26	0.5	2.13	2.58	1.22	3.15
14	3	1.13	0.87	0.98	0.93	0.89	0.83
15	4	2.66	0.63	1.68	3.99	0.88	3.51
16	4	2.98	1.66	4.95	0.76	1.45	1.10
17	4	3.15	1.51	4.76	1.23	0.88	1.08
18	3	0.77	0.82	0.63	1.42	0.63	0.89
19	3	6.18	0.63	3.89	13.37	0.41	5.48
20	4	10.22	0.75	7.67	13.17	1.43	18.83
21	3	2.37	0.39	0.92	3.4	0.48	1.63
22	4	3.81	0.74	2.82	5.53	0.78	4.31
23	3	2.86	1.31	3.75	0.89	1.26	1.12
24	1	20.2	1.11	22.42	3.88	0.95	3.69
25	3	1.46	0.44	0.64	20.75	0.66	13.70
26	2	20.3	0.58	11.77	1.95	1.23	2.40
27	3	24.83	0.28	6.95	12.43	1.94	24.11
28	2	0.97	0.39	0.38	3.22	1.85	5.96
29	3	2.42	0.78	1.89	0.59	1.08	0.64
30	3	0.78	0.29	0.23	0.72	0.28	0.20
31	1	0.01	0.62	0.01	0.4	0.33	0.13

Table 2 Mean values of rt-UPI parameters and subgroup analysis according to the degree of vascular obstruction.

	All patients			COGIF 0–3			COGIF 4		
	Ischemic tissue	Normal tissue	p-Value	Ischemic tissue	Normal tissue	p-Value	Ischemic tissue	Normal tissue	p-Value
A	4.44 ± 6.20	4.08 ± 4.84	n.s.	5.11 ± 7.26	4.08 ± 5.22	n.s.	3.01 ± 2.79	4.08 ± 4.18	n.s.
β	0.75 ± 0.41	1.05 ± 0.51	<0.05	0.61 ± 0.31	1.01 ± 0.53	0.005	1.04 ± 0.47	1.14 ± 0.49	n.s.
A × β	3.05 ± 4.48	4.33 ± 5.67	n.s.	3.01 ± 5.23	4.08 ± 5.65	n.s.	3.14 ± 2.45	4.84 ± 5.66	n.s.

with COGIF grades 0–3 and was absent in COGIF grade 4. The parameters A and the product $A \times \beta$ showed high standard deviations in our study, which resulted in a lack of significance between ischemic and non-ischemic tissue for these parameters. The most likely reason for the failure of establishing the plateau of acoustic intensity as a reliable parameter of rt-UPI is the strong relationship between the acoustic intensity and the individually varying level of acoustic attenuation by the temporal skull bone. Reliable mathematical algorithms developed to estimate the level of attenuation of ultrasound by the human skull may improve the diagnostic confidence of these parameters in future.

Conclusion

The slope parameter β of refill kinetics is useful for the assessment perfusion deficits in the acute phase of MCA stroke. According to our data, the severity of the perfusion deficit as measured with β is strongly related to the underlying vascular pathology of the ipsilateral MCA.

References

[1] Schellinger PD, Thomalla G, Fiehler J, Kohrmann M, Molina CA, Neumann-Haefelin T, et al. MRI-based and CT-based thrombolytic therapy in acute stroke within and beyond established time windows: an analysis of 1210 patients. Stroke 2007;38:2640–5.

[2] Kern R, Perren F, Schoeneberger K, Gass A, Hennerici M, Meairs S. Ultrasound microbubble destruction imaging in acute middle cerebral artery stroke. Stroke 2004;35:1665–70.

[3] Seidel G, Albers T, Meyer K, Wiesmann M. Perfusion harmonic imaging in acute middle cerebral artery infarction. Ultrasound Med Biol 2003;29:1245–51.

[4] Seidel G, Meyer-Wiethe K, Berdien G, Hollstein D, Toth D, Aach T. Ultrasound perfusion imaging in acute middle cerebral artery infarction predicts outcome. Stroke 2004;35:1107–11.

[5] Deverson S, Evans DH, Bouch DC. The effects of temporal bone on transcranial Doppler ultrasound beam shape. Ultrasound Med Biol 2000;26:239–44.

[6] Della Martina A, Meyer-Wiethe K, Allemann E, Seidel G. Ultrasound contrast agents for brain perfusion imaging and ischemic stroke therapy. J Neuroimaging 2005;15:217–32.

[7] Seidel G, Meairs S. Ultrasound contrast agents in ischemic stroke. Cerebrovasc Dis 2009;27(Suppl. 2):25–39.

[8] Wei K, Jayaweera AR, Firoozan S, Linka A, Skyba DM, Kaul S. Quantification of myocardial blood flow with ultrasound-induced destruction of microbubbles administered as a constant venous infusion. Circulation 1998;97:473–83.

[9] Rim SJ, Leong-Poi H, Lindner JR, Couture D, Ellegala D, Mason H, et al. Quantification of cerebral perfusion with "Real-Time" contrast-enhanced ultrasound. Circulation 2001;104:2582–7.

[10] Kern R, Diels A, Pettenpohl J, Kablau M, Brade J, Hennerici MG, et al. Real-time ultrasound brain perfusion imaging with analysis of microbubble replenishment in acute MCA stroke. J Cereb Blood Flow Metab 2011;31:1716–24.

[11] Bokor D, Chambers JB, Rees PJ, Mant TG, Luzzani F, Spinazzi A. Clinical safety of SonoVue, a new contrast agent for ultrasound imaging, in healthy volunteers and in patients with chronic obstructive pulmonary disease. Invest Radiol 2001;36:104–9.

[12] Nedelmann M, Stolz E, Gerriets T, Baumgartner RW, Malferrari G, Seidel G, et al. Consensus recommendations for transcranial color-coded duplex sonography for the assessment of intracranial arteries in clinical trials on acute stroke. Stroke 2009;40:3238–44.

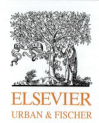
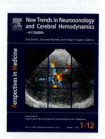

Bartels E, Bartels S, Poppert H (Editors):
New Trends in Neurosonology and Cerebral Hemodynamics — an Update.
Perspectives in Medicine (2012) 1, 44—50

journal homepage: www.elsevier.com/locate/permed

Imaging of plaque perfusion using contrast-enhanced ultrasound — Clinical significance

Edoardo Vicenzini [a,*], Maria Fabrizia Giannoni [a,b], Gaia Sirimarco [a], Maria Chiara Ricciardi [a], Massimiliano Toscano [a], Gian Luigi Lenzi [a], Vittorio Di Piero [a]

[a] Stroke Unit — Neurosonology, Department of Neurology and Psychiatry, Sapienza University of Rome, Italy
[b] Vascular Ultrasound Investigation, Department ''Paride Stefanini'', Sapienza University of Rome, Italy

KEYWORDS
Carotid stenosis;
Unstable plaque;
Angiogenesis;
Acute stroke;
Contrast carotid ultrasound

Summary   The identification of vulnerable and unstable carotid atherosclerotic lesions is up-to-date an important topic of research, in order to adopt the adequate strategy for preventing cerebrovascular events. Plaque inflammation, presence of adventitial vasa vasorum, intimal angiogenesis and plaque neovascularization have been identified in histological studies as indicators of the instability of the atheroma of carotid arteries in cerebrovascular patients and of coronary arteries in cardiovascular patents. Consequently, the identification ''in vivo'' of these pathophysiological aspects has been objective for the development of new imaging techniques. Ultrasound of carotid arteries, with ultrasound contrast agents, is not only able to provide an enhanced visualization of the arterial lumen and plaque morphology, but also allows to directly visualize adventitial vasa-vasorum and carotid plaque neovascularization. This technique and its clinical implications in the unstable plaque identification are discussed in the present paper.
© 2012 Elsevier GmbH. All rights reserved.

Introduction

The degree of internal carotid stenosis is nowadays no more considered the only parameter to be evaluated when identifying the ''plaque at risk'' to be addressed to carotid endarterectomy [1—3]. Since the 1980s the characterization of the morphology of the carotid plaque has become standard for stroke risk definition and, hence, the efforts for the definition of the ''unstable plaque'' [1,4]. In these regards, carotid ultrasound imaging has represented the cornerstone to describe the plaque characteristics that reflect a higher risk of vulnerability [4—7]. Plaques of moderate echogenicity and with hyperechoic spots are composed of ''hard'' fibrous tissue and calcifications; these plaques are less harmful than heterogeneous plaques with hypoechoic areas that correspond to ''soft'' atheromatous material consisting of cholesterol, lipid deposits, cell debris and necrotic residuals. Intraplaque hemorrhage, another cause of the sudden increase of plaque volume and rupture, is also of low echogenicity. Summarizing, the lower the degree of the echogenicity of a plaque, the higher the risk of the cap thinning and the surface endothelium rupture with subsequent ulceration, distal embolization and stroke. To reduce the biases of the subjective image interpretation, the computerized analysis of ultrasound images has also proved a reliable objective tool for identifying plaques

* Corresponding author at: Department of Neurology and Psychiatry, Sapienza University of Rome, Viale dell'Università 30, 00185 Rome, Italy. Tel.: +39 06 49914705; fax: +39 06 49914194.
  E-mail address: edoardo.vicenzini@uniroma1.it (E. Vicenzini).

with low Gray Scale Median scores, at a "major risk" of developing future cerebrovascular events [8,9].

A turning point in the history of atherosclerosis pathophysiological mechanisms comprehension has been the concept that "inflammation" may be linked with the disease development and progression. From histology, indeed, it was already known that while stable atheromatic lesions are characterized by a chronic inflammatory infiltrate, in vulnerable and ruptured plaques an active and acute inflammatory process regarding the surface and the plaque core takes place [10]. Consequently, adventitial vasa vasorum, intimal angiogenesis and plaque neovascularization have been considered, and confirmed by histological studies, as important predictors of instability in atheromasic lesions of cerebro and cardiovascular patients [11–19]. Angiogenesis occurs indeed regularly within atherosclerotic plaques and atheroma vulnerability and symptomatic carotid disease have been associated with an increased number of microvessels [16] that may also be responsible of the intra-plaque hemorrhage, when the rupture of these small newly generated and vulnerable vessels within the plaque occurs.

The possibility that inflammation could represent an index of plaque vulnerability has brought the scientific interest to concentrate on imaging "in vivo" the pathophysiological "functional" status of the atheroma with the goal to identify, as early as possible, the more vulnerable ones, to adopt the adequate preventive strategy. For this reason, several conventional radiological imaging, such as Computerized Tomography Angiography, Magnetic Resonance Angiography and also 18-FDG Positron Emission Tomography have focused on the evaluation of the "plaque metabolic activity", but — up to date — this is an evolving methodology requiring further consensus [20]. Contrast carotid ultrasound (CCU) is nowadays a well-established tool for angiogenesis detection in several fields with the principal advantage of being a simple, low cost and minimally invasive technique. Since the first data of 2006, several papers have now described the possibility to identify adventitial vasa vasorum and neovascularization also in carotid plaques [22–40], with a specific pattern of vascularization in acute symptomatic lesions [41].

Aim of this paper is to describe the methodology and the efficacy of contrast carotid ultrasound to identify plaque vascularization and to discuss the related clinical implications.

Contrast ultrasound investigation methodology and findings

Our experience is based on patients with carotid stenosis electively referred to our ultrasound laboratory for contrast ultrasound investigation [23,27,28,41] and from still ongoing data. The population consists of both asymptomatic patients, referred for vascular screening, as well as by symptomatic stroke patients. Plaques of different morphologies and various degree of stenosis have been investigated. According to the specific indications and guidelines for carotid endarterectomy, symptomatic and asymptomatic patients with a severe degree of stenosis were operated and histological/samples confronted with the ultrasonographic findings.

Apparatus, plaque morphology and technique of ultrasound contrast investigation

Ultrasound carotid duplex scanning were performed with Acuson/Siemens Sequoia 512 and Siemens S2000 systems, with standard vascular presets, and equipped with contrast multi-pulse non-harmonic imaging software "Cadence contrast Pulse Sequencing" (CPS) technology. Linear phased array probes (6, 8 and 15 MHz for the Sequoia, 9L4 for S2000) with standard presettings were used. The same machine presets were maintained constant. The technique of investigation is also reported in other published papers on this topic from our group [23,27,28,41].

Plaque echographic morphology was categorized according to criteria already well established in literature [4,7]. Plaque structure according to the echogenicity, and considered as hyperechoic with acoustic shadow, hyperechoic, isoechoic, hypoechoic, and consequently as calcific, fibrous, fibro-calcific, fibro-fatty and hemorrhagic. Plaque surface was defined as regular, irregular and ulcerated, when an excavation ≥2 mm was observed. Echogenicity was also quantified with the Gray Scale Median (GSM) computerized analysis [8], in order to better define the plaque risk. The degree of stenosis was evaluated according to European Carotid Surgery Trial (ECST) criteria [42], as percentage of the difference between the original vessel lumen diameter/area and the residual lumen diameter/area at the maximum site of stenosis, and according to blood flow velocities [4,43].

After the standard basal investigation of the plaque, contrast ultrasound investigations were performed with repeated short (0.5–1 ml) bolus injections in an antecubital vein (20 Gauge Venflon) of Sonovue (Bracco Altana Pharma, Konstanz, Germany), for a total contrast administration of up to 2.5 ml, each bolus being promptly followed by a saline flush. The 15 MHz linear array probe for the Sequoia (MI 0.4–1.1) and the 9L4 MHz for the S2000 (MI 0.10) were used for the CPS continuous real-time imaging. The "Contrast Agent only" software feature, in which the image is derived only from the signals of the microbubbles, has been used. All the investigations were digitally stored and DICOM files transferred to an external PC equipped with Showcase (v 5.1, Trillium Technology) for the off-line analysis.

Angiogenesis and neovascularization detection

After the bolus injection, few seconds are required for the contrast to be carried through the venous system to the pulmonary filter, heart and to the carotid arterial lumen. After the contrast is detected in the carotid axis, few seconds later, mainly during the diastolic cardiac phase, probably because of the reduced local pressure on the atherosclerotic lesion, the dynamic distribution of the contrast agent inside the plaque allows the visualization of the plaque vascularization. As previously already reported elsewhere [23,27,28], vascularization was detected at the shoulder of the plaque at the adventitial layers, and in the iso-hyperechoic fibrous and fibro-fatty tissue. It is represented by little echogenic spots rapidly moving within the texture of the atheromasic lesion, easily identifiable in the real time motion, and depicting the small microvessels (Fig. 1, Clip 1). In

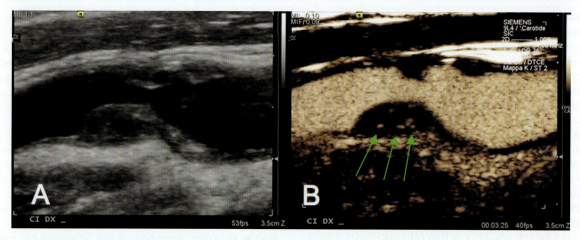

Figure 1 B-Mode high-resolution ultrasound (A) and contrast CPS imaging (B) of an isohypoechoic plaque with a central hypoechoic core, moderate internal carotid stenosis. Note the microbubbles in the fibrous tissue in image B (green arrows).

ulcerated plaques small vessels are constantly observed under the ulceration (Fig. 2, Clip 2). The diffusion of the contrast agent appears to be in an ''outside-in'' direction, namely from the external adventitial layers toward the inside of the plaque and vessel lumen [Fig. S1, online supplementary file]. Only in plaques in which the surface was fissurated or ulcerated the contrast agent appeared to have an ''inside-out'' direction, namely ''filling'' the void signal of the ulceration from the vessel lumen and better depicting the plaque surface rupture [Fig. S2, online supplementary file]. In recent atherotrombotic occlusion, vascularization, expression of the highly active remodeling process, was also observed [Fig. S3, online supplementary file]. Vascularization was not detected in the hyperechoic with acoustic shadow calcific tissue, nor in the hypoechoic necrotic and hemorrhagic areas. Moreover, plaque vascularization is present in almost every plaque, regardless the degree of stenosis.

In acute symptomatic patients a completely different pattern of vascularization was detected with ultrasound and validated by post-operative histology in a first paper published from our group [41]. In the first seconds after contrast agent administration, no vascularization seemed to be identified in the hypoechoic areas. Few seconds later, vascularization presented as a major diffuse area of contrast enhancement at the base of the plaques, due to an agglomerate of many small microvessels, difficult to differentiate from each other, while the residual hypoechoic part of the plaque, corresponding to the necrotic or hemorrhagic contents, remained avascularized. In operated patients, carotid endoarterectomies were carefully performed in order to obtain the whole plaque with minimal trauma. The pathologist evaluated the removed plaques after formalin fixation: the pathologist and the sonographers discussed the regions of interest previously observed at ultrasound imaging. The intra-operative macroscopic findings confirmed the presence of the unstable plaques observed at contrast ultrasound. The microscopic findings confirmed the presence of plaque vascularization in the ultrasound contrast-enhanced areas. Symptomatic carotid plaques showed a relevant increased number of small (diameter 20–30 μm), immature microvessels in respect to asymptomatic ones, consisting with a strong neoangiogenetic activity. Angiogenesis was less represented in asymptomatic plaques that underwent surgery, with microvessels of a higher caliber (80–100 μm). Immunostaining with VEGF, MMP3, CD 31 and CD 34 depicted

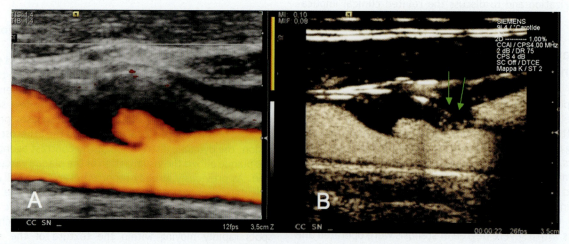

Figure 2 Power duplex (A) and contrast CPS imaging (B) of an ulcerated plaque. Contrast microbubbles diffuse at the base of ulceration (green arrows in B).

a different distribution pattern between asymptomatic and symptomatic lesions: while in the former antigenic activity was of a lesser degree and localized mainly along the microvessels course, in symptomatic plaques a high antigenic fixation was observed also in the external part of the plaque, closer to the adventitial layers. In the same areas, an inflammatory infiltrate constituted by macrophagic foam cells and T lymphocytes, indicative of high plaque activity was detected, with small areas of hemorrhage expression of microvessels rupture.

From the evaluation of subsequent acute stroke patients, it has also been observed that the entity of the internal carotid stenosis may not be directly correlated with clinical symptoms: patients with smaller plaques, even without hemodyamic effect, may present plaque "harmful" characteristics and local areas of vascularization expression of intense "plaque activity", responsible of the distal embolization. In Fig. 3 two examples are shown: in the former case, figure top, a relative small plaque with a distal ulceration is characterized by predominant vascularization in the distal part nearby the ulceration and in the second case, figure bottom, of a more complex lesion vascularization is highly expressed at the base of the plaque. All these features may then be considered expression of intense plaque remodeling — plaque "activity" that may be consequent to local acute inflammation and plaque vulnerability.

Discussion

Pathophysiological mechanisms responsible of plaque progression and developing of clinical symptoms are not yet completely understood. The role of inflammation has been hypothesized as a fundamental factor involved in the progression of the atherosclerotic plaque and the association between inflammation, atherosclerosis progression and cardiovascular events have been well established for coronary and carotid artery diseases.

The presence of newly generated blood vessels within atherosclerotic lesions has been well recognized since many decades [44], but the "in vivo" evaluation of angiogenesis has received attention, for its possible role in understanding the vulnerability of the atheroma only recently. Histological studies have indeed shown that microvessels are not usually present in the normal human intimal layers and that intima becomes vascularized only with the developing of the atherosclerotic process and when its layer growths in thickness [45]. In nearly half of the patients with a non hemodynamic carotid stenosis addressed to medical therapy, if — and when — cerebral ischemic symptoms — be it a TIA or other — will occur, these will be without any warning [46]. Therefore, even in those patients who have a non-severe carotid stenosis, some unknown or undetected mechanisms at the level of the arterial wall produces the rupture of the plaque, with consequent embolism and

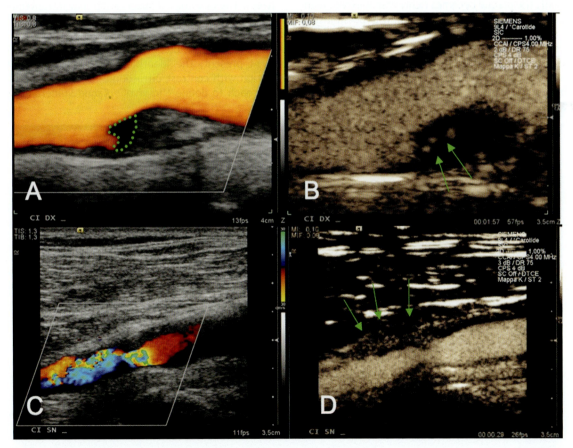

Figure 3 Top: power duplex (A) and contrast CPS imaging (B) of a small ulcerated plaque in an acute stroke patients. Contrast agents diffuse in the distal part of the plaque nearby ulceration (green arrows in B), corresponding to an area of lower echogenicity (dotted green lines in A). Bottom: color duplex (C) and contrast CPS imaging (D) of an ulcerated plaque in an acute stroke patients. Contrast agents are diffusely visualized at the base of the plaque (green arrows in D).

stroke. Nonetheless, the causes for the modifications of a "hard and stable" into a "softer and unstable" plaque are still not yet completely understood. In these regards, the role of angiogenesis and of intimal vasa vasorum may be of particular relevance. Angiogenesis has indeed also been documented in carotid atherosclerosis and in stable atherosclerotic lesions studied after carotid endarterectomy. It is believed that the absence of pericytes in some new angiogenic vessels causes these immature vessels to "leak" potentially noxious and inflammatory plasma components (hemoglobin, oxidized low-density lipoprotein cholesterol, lipoprotein, glucose, advanced glycation end products, and inflammatory cells) into the extracellular matrix of the media/intima, thus increasing the plaque volume. The ongoing deposit of plasma components appears to further reduce vessel wall oxygen diffusion, enhancing further angiogenesis, plaque inflammation. In the final phase, the plaque is enveloped in adventitial vasa vasorum and intraplaque neovascularization, a hallmark of symptomatic atherosclerosis [47]. The histological observation of a higher number of microvessels within operated symptomatic carotid artery plaques further supports this hypothesis [10,15,16]. All these data follow the observation in the cardiology field, where, angiogenesis and microvessels detected in the coronary atheromas in histological studies have proven to be strongly associated with unstable angina and myocardial infarction. Thus, the observation that, in a late phase of development, the plaque becomes richly vascularized, leading to the atheroma vulnerability increase with possibility of coronary artery occlusion and/or distal embolization, with consequent myocardial ischemic damage [9,10,13,15].

Standard ultrasound carotid duplex is one of the most diffuse and available techniques in clinical routine to assess plaque morphology and to identify the "plaque at risk". The recent application of ultrasound contrast agents to carotid plaque imaging lead to the possibility of directly visualizing adventitial vasa vasorum and plaque neovascularization "in vivo" [21—41], with the advantage of ultrasound being a simple, low cost and minimally invasive technique.

From our experience [23,27,28,41], we observed that microbubbles are visualized easily in the fibrous tissue of carotid plaques and that they correspond to the newly generated vessels, so confirming that plaques have angiogenesis that could be related to the progression and remodeling. The processes that lead to intramural hemorrhage and plaque ulcerations are other important issues that have been extensively studied. Some theories claim the hypothesis that atherosclerosis progression is due to an "outside-in" process and, effectively, intimal vessels originating from the adventitial layers have been observed much more frequently than those originating from the luminal side, resembling the microvessels than grow within tumors. This datum was also confirmed in our patients, in which the microbubbles diffusion seems to be oriented from the external adventitial layers toward the internal intimal lumen and, constantly, through a little vessel present under the plaque ulcerations. This latter observation further supports the theory that intraplaque hemorrhage and ulcerations can be related to the rupture of newly formed intraplaque microvessels, that, being immature and with a thin wall, are submitted to local triggering factors such as mechanical forces and shear stress. The histological observation that intraplaque hemorrhages are common in every atherosclerotic lesion, usually deep and not connected with the vessel lumen, is another indicator that the bleeding originates locally [48,49].

At present, the identification of the plaque vascularization with contrast ultrasound may be considered a new approach to define "in vivo" plaque vulnerability. Future

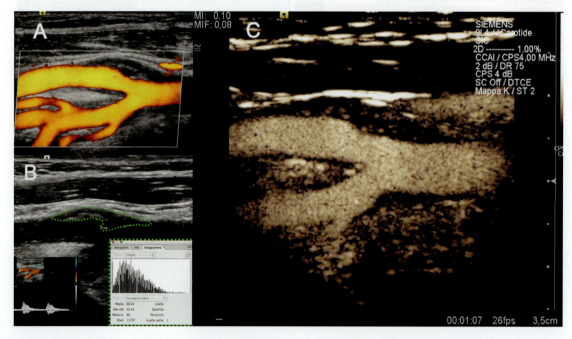

Figure 4 Power duplex (A) of a moderate internal carotid stenosis in an asymptomatic patient. B-Mode imaging (B) with pulsed wave Doppler (small box, bottom left) shows no hemodynamic effect and GSM calculation (small box, bottom right, green dotted line) echogenicity characteristics of low stroke risk (GSM = 60). Contrast CPS imaging (C) shows a high, diffuse vascularization in the whole plaque texture.

development may be represented by the sonographic follow-up of the plaque vascularization, to evaluate the potential benefit or specific effect of medical therapy on plaque remodeling, as regression of plaque vascularization may occur [22]. It is also our experience that vascularization is detectable not only in unstable plaques with a high grade stenosis that are addressed to carotid endoarterectomy, but even in light to moderate stenosis and in asymptomatic patients [23,27,28]. The observation of apparently "stable" plaques in asymptomatic patients, determining internal carotid stenosis without indications for surgery, but with evidence of intense vascularization with contrast ultrasound, may open the discussion for further reconsidering mild, non hemodynamic carotid stenosis, in order to better evaluate stroke risk in these cases (Fig. 4). In this view, further large-scale studies are mandatory for a complete understanding of the natural history of these vascularized lesions, to eventually adopt the adequate preventive strategy.

One limit of this approach of this technique regards the modality for the evaluation of the vascularization: at present, a method of a real numerical objective quantification of the global "plaque perfusion" is indeed not available for carotid plaques. Differently from the evaluation of the heart, in which myocardial tissue perfusion is the expression of a normal condition, and differently from small coronary plaques, in which there is a different ratio due to the size of the vessel, in carotid atherosclerosis this pattern may interest only limited regions of the plaque and therefore quantitative analysis of the mean signal enhancement derived from the whole plaque may not be expressive of the real perfusion. The finding of a "harmful" pattern of plaque vascularization may indeed be limited to a small area of the plaque, but its identification is, in our experience, highly representative of the "plaque activity". This was confirmed in our histologial and immunohistochemical specimen finding of a high angiogenesis with high density of microvessels and with a strong fixation in these areas of endothelial growth factors and inflammatory markers [41]. Moreover, the semi-quantitative evaluation of ultrasound images with time intensity curves, being arbitrary selected areas, may not be considered as really representative of plaque vascularization, also because it is evaluated in bidimensional images. The identification of these patterns then requires a very careful visual and morphological observation, by sonographers trained in this field.

Conclusions

Contrast carotid ultrasound is an emerging technique, easily available and quick to perform, that adds important clinical and research information of the "in vivo" pathophysiological status, with low costs and invasiveness. In symptomatic stroke patients with carotid plaques addressed toward surgery, contrast carotid examinations could help to better analyze plaque morphology and to identify and quantify the presence and degree of neovascularization, allowing a further assessment of the cerebrovascular risk. Larger studies are though needed to clarify the prognostic value of plaque vascularization detection in asymptomatic patients with non-severe carotid stenosis that are not candidated for surgery.

Moreover, the identification and evaluation of plaque angiogenesis may be in the future useful to evaluate the possible effects of therapies aimed to plaque remodeling.

Appendix A. Supplementary data

Supplementary data associated with this article can be found, in the online version, at http://dx.doi.org/10.1016/j.permed.2012.03.017.

References

[1] Hennerici MG. The unstable plaque. Cerebrovasc Dis 2004;17(Suppl 3):17—22.
[2] Rothwell PM, Eliasziw M, Gutnikov SA, Fox AJ, Taylor DW, Mayberg MR, Warlow CP, Barnett HJ. Carotid Endarterectomy Trialists' Collaboration. Analysis of pooled data from the randomised controlled trials of endarterectomy for symptomatic carotid stenosis. Lancet 2003;361:107—16.
[3] Lenzi GL, Vicenzini E. The ruler is dead. An analysis of carotid plaque motion. Cerebrovasc Dis 2007;23:121—5.
[4] Bartels E, editor. Color-Coded Duplex Ultrasound of the cerebral vessels. Atlas and manual. Stuttgart, Germany/New York: Schattauer F.K. Verlagsgesellschaft mBH. 1999.
[5] Ratliff DA, Gallagher PJ, Hames TK, Humphries KN, Webster JH, Chant AD. Characterisation of carotid artery disease: comparison of duplex scanning with histology. Ultrasound Med Biol 1985;11:835—40.
[6] Gray-Weale AC, Graham JC, Burnett JR, Byrne K, Lusby RJ. Carotid artery atheroma: comparison of preoperative B-mode ultrasound appearance with carotid endarterectomy specimen pathology. J Cardiovasc Surg 1988;29:676—81.
[7] Widder B, Paulat K, Hackspacher J, Hamann H, Hutschenreiter S, Kreutzer C, Ott F, Vollmar J. Morphological characterization of carotid artery stenoses by ultrasound duplex scanning. Ultrasound Med Biol 1990;16:349—54.
[8] Biasi GM, Sampaolo A, Mingazzini P, De Amicis P, El-Barghouty N, Nicolaides AN. Computer analysis of ultrasonic plaque echolucency in identifying high risk carotid bifurcation lesions. Eur J Vasc Endovasc Surg 1999;17:476—9.
[9] El-Barghouty N, Gerulakos G, Nicolaides AN, Androulakos A, Bahn V. Computer assisted carotid plaque characterization. Eur J Vasc Endovasc Surg 1995;9:389—93.
[10] Spagnoli LG, Mauriello A, Sangiorgi G. Extracranial thrombotically active carotid plaque as a risk factor of ischemic stroke. JAMA 2004;292:1845—52.
[11] Beeuwkes R, Barger C, Silverman K, Lainery LL. Cinemicrographic studies of the vasa vasorum of the human coronary arteries. In: Glagov S, Newman WP, Schaffer S, editors. Pathobiology of the human atherosclerotic plaque. New York, NY: Springer-Verlag; 1990. p. 425—32.
[12] Clagett GP, Robinowitz M, Youkey JR, Fisher Jr DF, Fry RE, Myers SI, Lee EL, Collins Jr GJ, Virmani R. Morphogenesis and clinicopathologic characteristics of recurrent carotid disease. J Vasc Surg 1986:10—23.
[13] Fryer JA, Myers PC, Appleberg M. Carotid intraplaque hemorrhage: the significance of neovascularity. J Vasc Surg 1987;6:341—9.
[14] Kumamoto M, Nakashima Y, Sueishi K. Intimal neovascularization in human coronary atherosclerosis: its origin and pathophysiological significance. Hum Pathol 1995;26:450—6.
[15] Mofidi R, Crotty TB, McCarthy P, Sheehan SJ, Mehigan D, Keaveny TV. Association between plaque instability, angiogenesis

and symptomatic carotid occlusive disease. Br J Surg 2001;88:945—50.
[16] Fleiner M, Kummer M, Mirlacher M, Sauter G, Cathomas G, Krapf R, Biedermann BC. Arterial neovascularization and inflammation in vulnerable patients: early and late signs of symptomatic atherosclerosis. Circulation 2004;110: 2843—50.
[17] Moreno PR, Fuster V. New aspects in the pathogenesis of diabetic atherothrombosis. J Am Coll Cardiol 2004;44: 2293—300.
[18] Barger AC, Beeuwkes R, Lainey LL, Silverman KJ. Hypothesis: vasa vasorum and neovascularization of human coronary arteries. A possible role in the pathophysiology of atherosclerosis. NEJM 1984;310:175—7.
[19] Dunmore BJ, McCarthy MJ, Naylor AR, Brindle NP. Carotid plaque instability and ischemic symptoms are linked to immaturity of microvessels within plaques. J Vasc Surg 2007;45:155—9.
[20] Warburton L, Gillard J. Functional imaging of carotid atheromatous plaques. J Neuroimaging 2006;16:293—301.
[21] Feinstein SB. The powerful microbubble: from bench to bedside, from intravascular indicator to therapeutic delivery system, and beyond. Am J Physiol Heart Circ Physiol 2004;287:450—7.
[22] Feinstein SB. Contrast ultrasound imaging of the carotid artery vasa vasorum and atherosclerotic plaque neovascularization. J Am Coll Cardiol 2006;48:236—43.
[23] Vicenzini E, Giannoni MF, Puccinelli F, Ricciardi MC, Altieri M, Di Piero V, Gossetti B, Benedetti-Valentini F, Lenzi GL. Detection of carotid adventitial vasa vasorum and plaque vascularization with ultrasound cadence contrast pulse sequencing technique and echo-contrast agent. Stroke 2007;38:2841—3.
[24] Shah F, Balan P, Weinberg M, Reddy V, Neems R, Feinstein M, Dainauskas J, Meyer P, Goldin M, Feinstein SB. Contrast-enhanced ultrasound imaging of atherosclerotic carotid plaque neovascularization: a new surrogate marker of atherosclerosis? Vasc Med 2007;12:291—7.
[25] Purushothaman KR, Sanz J, Zias E, Fuster V, Moreno PR. Atherosclerosis neovascularization and imaging. Curr Mol Med 2006;6:549—56.
[26] Huang PT, Huang FG, Zou CP, Sun HY, Tian XQ, Yang Y, Tang JF, Yang PL, Wang XT. Contrast-enhanced sonographic characteristics of neovascularization in carotid atherosclerotic plaques. J Clin Ultrasound 2008;36:346—51.
[27] Giannoni MF, Vicenzini E. Focus on the "unstable" carotid plaque: detection of intraplaque angiogenesis with contrast ultrasound. Present state and future perspectives. Curr Vasc Pharmacol 2009;7:180—4.
[28] Vicenzini E, Giannoni MF, Benedetti-Valentini F, Lenzi GL. Imaging of carotid plaque angiogenesis. Cerebrovasc Dis 2009;27(Suppl 2):48—54.
[29] Magnoni M, Coli S, Cianflone D. A surprise behind the dark. Eur J Echocardiogr 2009;10:887—8.
[30] Staub D, Patel MB, Tibrewala A, Ludden D, Johnson M, Espinosa P, Coll B, Jaeger KA, Feinstein SB. Vasa vasorum and plaque neovascularization on contrast-enhanced carotid ultrasound imaging correlates with cardiovascular disease and past cardiovascular events. Stroke 2010;41:41—7.
[31] Shalhoub J, Owen DR, Gauthier T, Monaco C, Leen EL, Davies AH. The use of contrast enhanced ultrasound in carotid arterial disease. Eur J Vasc Endovasc Surg 2010;39: 381—7.
[32] Staub D, Schinkel AF, Coll B, Coli S, van der Steen AF, Reed JD, Krueger C, Thomenius KE, Adam D, Sijbrands EJ, ten Cate FJ, Feinstein SB. Contrast-enhanced ultrasound imaging of the vasa vasorum: from early atherosclerosis to the identification of unstable plaques. JACC Cardiovasc Imaging 2010;3: 761—71.

[33] Coll B, Nambi V, Feinstein SB. New advances in noninvasive imaging of the carotid artery: CIMT, contrast-enhanced ultrasound, and vasa vasorum. Curr Cardiol Rep 2010;12:497—502.
[34] Staub D, Partovi S, Schinkel AF, Coll B, Uthoff H, Aschwanden M, Jaeger KA, Feinstein SB. Correlation of carotid artery atherosclerotic lesion echogenicity and severity at standard US with intraplaque neovascularization detected at contrast-enhanced US. Radiology 2011;258:618—26.
[35] Faggioli GL, Pini R, Mauro R, Pasquinelli G, Fittipaldi S, Freyrie A, Serra C, Stella A. Identification of carotid 'vulnerable plaque' by contrast-enhanced ultrasonography: correlation with plaque histology, symptoms and cerebral computed tomography. Eur J Vasc Endovasc Surg 2011;41: 238—48.
[36] Eyding J, Geier B, Staub D. Current strategies and possible perspectives of ultrasonic risk stratification of ischemic stroke in internal carotid artery disease. Ultraschall Med 2011;32:267—73.
[37] Hoogi A, Adam D, Hoffman A, Kerner H, Reisner S, Gaitini D. Carotid plaque vulnerability: quantification of neovascularization on contrast-enhanced ultrasound with histopathologic correlation. AJR Am J Roentgenol 2011;196:431—6.
[38] Clevert DA, Sommer WH, Zengel P, Helck A, Reiser M. Imaging of carotid arterial diseases with contrast-enhanced ultrasound (CEUS). Eur J Radiol 2011;80:68—76.
[39] Clevert DA, Sommer WH, Helck A, Reiser M. Duplex and contrast enhanced ultrasound (CEUS) in evaluation of in-stent restenosis after carotid stenting. Clin Hemorheol Microcirc 2011;48:199—208.
[40] Shalhoub J, Monaco C, Owen DR, Gauthier T, Thapar A, Leen EL, Davies AH. Late-phase contrast-enhanced ultrasound reflects biological features of instability in human carotid atherosclerosis. Stroke 2011;42:3634—6.
[41] Giannoni MF, Vicenzini E, Citone M, Ricciardi MC, Irace L, Laurito A, Scucchi LF, Di Piero V, Gossetti B, Mauriello A, Spagnoli LG, Lenzi GL, Valentini FB. Contrast carotid ultrasound for the detection of unstable plaques with neoangiogenesis: a pilot study. Eur J Vasc Endovasc Surg 2009;37:722—7.
[42] European Carotid Surgery Trialists' Collaborative Group. Randomised trial of endarterectomy for recently symptomatic carotid stenosis: final results of the MRC European Carotid Surgery Trial (ECST). Lancet 1998;351:1379—87.
[43] Sabeti S, Schillinger M, Mlekusch W, Willfort A, Haumer M, Nachtmann T, Mullner M, Lang W, Ahmadi R, Minar E. Quantification of internal carotid artery stenosis with duplex US: comparative analysis of different flow velocity criteria. Radiology 2004;232:431—9.
[44] Paterson JC. Capillary rupture of with intimal haemorrhage as the causative factor in coronary thrombosis. Arch Pathol 1938;25:474—87.
[45] Geiringer E. Intimal vascularisation and atherosclerosis. Histologic characteristics of carotid atherosclerotid plaque. J Pathol Bacteriol 1951;63:201—11.
[46] Executive Committee for the Asymptomatic Carotid Atherosclerosis Study. Endarterectomy for asymptomatic carotid artery stenosis. JAMA 1995;273:1421—8.
[47] Carlier S, Kakadiaris IA, Dib N, Vavuranakis M, O'Malley SM, Gul K, Hartley CJ, Metcalfe R, Mehran R, Stefanadis C, Falk E, Stone G, Leon M, Naghavi M. Vasa vasorum imaging: a new window to the clinical detection of vulnerable atherosclerotic plaques. Curr Atheroscler Rep 2005;7:164—9.
[48] Milei J, Parodi JC, Alonso GF, Barone A, Grana D, Matturri L. Carotid rupture and intraplaque hemorrhage: immunophenotype and role of cells involved. Am Heart J 1998;136: 1096—105.
[49] Bornstein NM, Krajewski A, Lewis AJ, Norris JW. Clinical significance of carotid plaque hemorrhage. Arch Neurol 1990;47:958—9.

Plaque angiogenesis identification with Contrast Enhanced Carotid Ultrasonography: Statement of the Consensus after the 16th ESNCH Meeting — Munich, 20-23 May 2011

Holger Poppert [a,*], Edoardo Vicenzini [b], Konrad Stock [c], Eva Bartels [d]

[a] Klinikum rechts der Isar, Universität München, Department of Neurology, Ismaninger Str. 22, München, Germany
[b] Stroke Unit — Neurosonology, Department of Neurology and Psychiatry, Sapienza University of Rome, Italy
[c] Klinikum rechts der Isar, Universität München, Department of Nephrology, Ismaninger Str. 22, München, Germany
[d] Center for Neurological Vascular Diagnostics, München, Germany

KEYWORDS
Contrast agents;
Carotid artery stenosis;
Atherosclerotic plaques;
Consensus conference

Summary Contrast Enhanced Carotid Ultrasonography (CCU) is capable of detecting angiogenesis within the carotid plaque as a potential index of plaque vulnerability. However, due to a lack of standard of examination technique and documentation, results are not sufficiently, reliably comparable.

To improve this situation and in order to support wide acceptance of this promising technique, experts in this field met in the Consensus conference in May 22, 2011, held during the 16th ESNCH Meeting (20—23 May 2011) in Munich, Germany, to discuss the limitations and problems and to determine guidelines for its proper use in scientific investigations and clinical practice.

The main results of this conference are presented here. The discussion is still in progress and individual conclusions may not reflect the opinion of all participants. It aims to provide a basis for a later comprehensive consensus statement.

© 2012 Published by Elsevier GmbH.

Introduction

The possibility that inflammation may represent an index of plaque vulnerability has brought the scientific interest to concentrate on the "in vivo" imaging the pathophysiological status of the atheroma, with the goal to identify the more vulnerable ones, to adopt the more adequate preventive strategies as early as possible.

Contrast Enhanced Carotid Ultrasonography (CCU) is nowadays a well-established tool for angiogenesis detection in several fields of application, with the principal advantage of ultrasound being a minimally invasive technique that allows "real-time" imaging. Since the first data of 2006, several papers have now described the possibility to identify adventitial vasa-vasorum and neovascularization in carotid plaques, with a specific pattern of vascularization in acute symptomatic lesions, and thus identifying "plaque activity".

Aim of this work is to describe the state of art of the methodology, to propose practical guidelines for CCU exam

* Corresponding author.
E-mail address: poppert@neurovasc.de (H. Poppert).

2211-968X/$ — see front matter © 2012 Published by Elsevier GmbH.
http://dx.doi.org/10.1016/j.permed.2012.04.001

to obtain comparable data and to discuss the related clinical implications of plaque vascularization detection.

When to use

In moderate-to-severe internal carotid artery stenosis, both neurologically symptomatic and asymptomatic.

(a) Advantages in clinical routine:
- better Intima—Media-Thickness visualization;
- better plaque surface definition, especially in cases of large acoustic shadow calcified plaques;
- more sensible identification of plaque rupture and plaque ulcerations;
- improved sensibility in detecting carotid pseudoocclusion.

(b) Research objectives
- to identify vasa-vasorum and intra-plaque angiogenesis.

Suggested protocol and methods

CCU first requires the standard, basal exam of carotid plaques, to obtain the "best view" images, mandatory to be documented for further analysis. Ultrasound carotid duplex scanning should be performed with up-to-date ultrasound equipment, contrast enhanced ultrasound with machine-specific low-Mechanical-Index-software. The same, user defined "machine presets" have to be maintained constant in different examinations, to allow comparisons.

(a) Plaque basal assessment

Plaque echographic morphology has first to be recognized according to the criteria already established in literature. Plaque structure according to the echogenicity, as hyperechoic with acoustic shadow, hyperechoic, isoechoic, hypoechoic, and consequently as calcified, fibrous, fibro-calcified, fibro-fatty and hemorrhagic. Plaque surface as regular, irregular and ulcerated, when an excavation ≥ 2 mm in depth is observed. For easier data analysis in research studies, echogenicity might also be quantified with the Gray Scale Median (GSM) computerized analysis. The degree of stenosis should be evaluated according to North American Symptomatic Carotid Endarterectomy Trial (NASCET) criteria, as percentage of the difference between the distal diameter/area of the internal carotid artery and the residual lumen diameter/area at the maximum site of stenosis, and according to blood flow velocities.

(b) Contrast imaging

After having obtained the "best view" in basal imaging, contrast ultrasound exams can be performed using a linear transducer (9—4 MHz) with repeated short bolus injections in an antecubital vein (20 Gauge Venflon) of Sonovue (Bracco Altana Pharma, Konstanz, Germany), each bolus being promptly followed by a saline flush of 5 ml. Mechanical index should be kept as low as possible to allow vascularization identification. Real-time imaging — with high frequency transducers and high frame rates — should be used. Side to side imaging with B-mode could also be used to keep the "best view" on the screen. The exam should be digitally stored using clips of the real-time exam. These files can be transferred to an external PC for visual or computer-assisted off-line analysis. If possible, a clip of the whole contrast bolus administration should be obtained, to allow second "crop" of more significative findings. When computerized quantification is performed, similar epochs should be analyzed to compare findings from different patients, starting the analysis at the first appearance of the contrast agent in the carotid lumen. Clip length should not be inferior to 90 s each. The timer should be displayed on screen starting at the end of the contrast bolus injection.

Vascularization identification and quantification

After the bolus injection, few seconds are required for the contrast to be carried through the venous system to the pulmonary filter, heart and to the carotid arterial lumen. This time may differ from patient to patient, according to heart rate and ventricular ejection fraction. After the contrast is detected in the carotid axis, few seconds later, mainly during the diastolic cardiac phase, contrast agent may be shown inside the plaques allowing plaque vascularization detection. Microbubbles appear as little echogenic spots rapidly moving within the texture of the atheromatic lesion, easily identifiable in the real-time-motion, and depicting the small microvessels. The diffusion of the contrast agent appears to be in an "outside-in" direction, namely from the external adventitial layers toward the inside of the plaque and vessel lumen. Only in plaques in which the surface is fissurated or ulcerated the contrast agent show an "inside-out" direction, namely "filling" the void signal of the ulceration from the vessel lumen, thus better depicting the plaque surface rupture. In the ulcerated plaques small vessels are constantly observed under the ulceration. In recent atherothrombotic occlusion vascularization, expression of the highly active remodeling process, is usually observed. Vascularization is usually not detected in the hyperechoic plaque with calcific tissue acoustic shadow, nor in the hypoechoic necrotic and hemorrhagic areas of a plaque.

In acute symptomatic stroke patients due to carotid disease, a different pattern of vascularization may be observed: vascularization may be present as a major diffuse area of contrast enhancement at the base of the plaques, due to an agglomerate of many small microvessels, difficult to differentiate from each other, while the residual hypoechoic parts of the plaques, corresponding to the necrotic or hemorrhagic contents, usually remain avascularized. Furthermore, it has also been observed that the entity of the internal carotid stenosis may not be directly correlated with clinical symptoms: patients with smaller plaques, even without hemodyamic effect, may present plaque "harmful" characteristics and local areas of vascularization with intense "plaque activity", responsible for the distal embolization. If possible, all these features should be compared with the post-operative histology.

Contrast enhancement may be evaluated "visually" with qualitative scales, as well as "semi-quantitatively" using time-intensity curves. When visually evaluated, one must always take into account the contrast distribution within the plaque texture (no bubbles detectable within the plaque, bubbles emanating from the adventitial side or shoulder of the plaque and moving toward the plaque core: clearly visible bubbles in the plaque) as well as by focal specific regions of contrast enhancement, usually observed even in smaller lesions and in acute symptomatic patients. Up to date, there is no consensus for time-intensity curves quantification method because: (1) region-of-interest is made only in a biplanar images; (2) the global whole plaque region selection may fail to reveal the small areas of high contrast enhancement; (3) the region-of-interest selection is highly operator dependent. Differently from the evaluation of the heart, in which myocardial tissue perfusion is the expression of a normal condition, and differently from small coronary plaques, in which there is a different ratio due to the size of the vessel, in carotid atherosclerosis this pattern may appear in only limited regions of the plaque and therefore quantitative analysis of the mean signal enhancement deriving from the whole plaque may not be expressive of the real perfusion. The finding of a ''harmful'' pattern of plaque vascularization may indeed be limited to a small area of the plaque, but its visual identification is, in our experience, highly representative of the ''plaque activity''. Some methods to obtain a ''ratio'' carotid lumen versus plaque texture has been proposed, with the same limitations related to the already described pitfalls in semiquantitative computerized analysis.

Conclusion and further implications

Contrast carotid ultrasound is an emerging technique, easily available and quick to perform, that adds important clinical and research information of the ''in vivo'' pathophysiological status, with low costs and invasiveness. In symptomatic stroke patients with carotid plaques addressed toward surgery, contrast carotid examinations could help to better analyze plaque morphology and to identify and quantify the presence and degree of neovascularization, allowing a further assessment of the cerebrovascular risk. Larger studies are though needed to clarify the prognostic value of plaque vascularization detection in asymptomatic patients with non-severe carotid stenosis that are not candidated for surgery. Moreover, the identification and evaluation of plaque angiogenesis may be in the future useful to evaluate the possible effects of therapies aimed to plaque remodeling.

2. Novel Technologies

Mechanical recanalization in acute stroke treatment

Pasquale Mordasini, Gerhard Schroth, Jan Gralla*

Institute of Diagnostic and Interventional Neuroradiology, Inselspital, University of Bern, Switzerland

KEYWORDS
Mechanical recanalization;
Mechanical thrombectomy;
Endovascular stroke treatment;
Acute stroke treatment

Summary Endovascular stroke treatment is a rapidly evolving field in neurointerventions. The article reviews the evolution of the different mechanical thrombolysis and stenting techniques and their working principles for endovascular vessel recanalization and reviews the data on the outcome after acute stroke treatment.
© 2012 Elsevier GmbH. All rights reserved.

Introduction

Ischemic stroke is one of the leading causes of disability and mortality in industrialized countries. Patient outcome mainly depends on the time span between onset of symptoms and revascularization, recanalization rate and the occurrence of symptomatic intracranial hemorrhage (sICH) [1]. Therefore, fast and effective reperfusion in combination with a low rate of sICH is the key to successful stroke treatment. Systemic thrombolysis with intravenously administered tissue plasminogen activator (IV rtPA) and local intra-arterial thrombolysis (IAT) have been shown to be effective to improve patient outcome. However, the time window for treatment and the recanalization rate of both methods are limited [2–4]. Furthermore, the application of thrombolytic drugs increases the risk of sICH [5]. Moreover, recanalization rate is dependent on the site of occlusion: proximal occlusions of large brain supplying vessels such as the internal carotid artery have a limited recanalization rate after either IV rtPA or IAT [3,4]. Therefore, the aim of mechanical recanalization approaches is to improve recanalization rates, reduce the time to recanalization and further expand the window of opportunity. Furthermore, the waiving of thrombolytic drugs is considered to reduce the rate of symptomatic intracranial hemorrhage.

Mechanical treatment approaches

Different techniques and approaches have been advocated for mechanical thrombolysis in acute stroke treatment, which can be divided into: immediate flow restoration using self-expandable stents and thrombectomy.

Stent recanalization

Placement of a permanent intracranial stent achieves immediate flow restoration and recanalization by compressing the thrombus against the vessel wall. Stenting allows fast and effective recanalization without the need of repetitive

---

Abbreviations: sICH, symptomatic intracranial hemorrhage; IV rtPA, intravenously administered tissue plasminogen activator; IAT, local intra-arterial thrombolysis; PTA, percutaneous angioplasty; NIHSS, National Institute of Health Stroke Scale; FDA, Food and Drug Administration.

* Corresponding author at: Department of Diagnostic and Interventional Neuroradiology, Inselspital, University of Bern, Freiburgstrasse 4, CH-3010 Bern, Switzerland.
Tel.: +41 031 6322655; fax: +41 031 6324872.
E-mail address: jan.gralla@insel.ch (J. Gralla).

passing of the occlusion site and retrieval attempts. However, this concept has some disadvantages in general and especially in the setting of acute stroke treatment. Thrombus compression may lead to permanent side branch or perforator occlusion. Moreover, permanent stent placement needs double platelet anti-aggregation medication in order to prevent in-stent thrombosis and re-occlusion. This preventive medication may increase the risk of sICH in the setting of acute stroke [6]. Furthermore, an in-stent re-stenosis rate of bare metal stents has been reported in up to 32% in the treatment of intracranial arteriosclerotic stenosis after a follow-up period of 9 months [7]. The use of different stent systems has been reported in case reports and small case series. In general, self-expandable stents are preferentially used over balloon-mounted stents.

Recanalization rates are reported to be between 79% and 92% with moderate clinical outcome in 33—50% [8,9]. The Stent-Assisted Recanalization in Acute Ischemic Stroke (SARIS) trial is the first FDA approved prospective trial investigating stenting in acute stroke treatment. 20 patients (mean NIHSS 14) were included within 6 h after symptom onset. Recanalization rate was 100% with adjuvant therapies such as angioplasty, IV tPA and IAT applied in 63% of patients. Moderate clinical outcome was achieved in 60% of patients [10,11].

Despite the high recanalization rate reported in these studies, the use of intracranial stenting in acute stroke treatment is debatable due to the risks associated with permanent stent deployment and the recent success of thrombectomy. However, stenting has a clear value in selective cases of rescue therapy.

Mechanical thrombectomy

All mechanical thrombectomy devices are delivered by endovascular access proximal to the occlusion site. The various systems can be divided into 3 major groups according to where they apply mechanical force on the thrombus:

(a) Proximal devices apply force to the proximal base of the thrombus. This group includes various aspiration catheters and systems.
(b) Distal devices approach the thrombus proximally but then are advanced by microguidewire and microcatheter across the thrombus to be unsheathed behind it, where force is applied to the distal base of the thrombus. This group includes brush-like, basket-like or coil-like devices.
(c) The most recently developed devices include stent-like devices, which are placed across the thrombus at the occlusion site, deployed within the thrombus and then are retrieved. This group includes various types of self-expandable, retrievable, stent-like devices, so-called stent retrievers.

Proximal thrombectomy using thrombus aspiration

Vascular access is usually gained with a 7—8-F sheath. After placement of the guiding catheter, a large dedicated aspiration catheter (4—5-F) flexible enough to pass the tortuosity of the cranial vessels (e.g. carotid siphon) is navigated to the proximal surface of the thrombus. Aspiration force is applied to the thrombus using a 60-ml syringe. The aspiration catheter is then retrieved under constant negative pressure to avoid loss of thrombus material. This approach omits repetitive passing of the occlusion site and after each retrieval of clot fragments, the procedure can be repeated. The advantages of this approach are that it is mechanically simple, fast to apply and inexpensive. Therefore, it is widely used, especially in proximal occlusions when the target vessel has a large diameter and an anatomy favorable for device navigation such as the distal cervical internal carotid artery and the carotid artery terminus. Although first reports on mechanical thrombectomy included the use of aspiration catheters [12,13], only few systematic data have been published on this approach so far. A recent single-center study reported on 22 patients (mean NIHSS 18) treated with aspiration thrombectomy alone with a recanalization rate of 81.9% and a good clinical outcome in 45.5% [14].

Penumbra System. The Penumbra System (Penumbra, Almeda, USA) is a modification of the proximal aspiration technique. It has been FDA approved for clot removal in acute stroke treatment in 2007. It consists of a reperfusion catheter attached to continuous aspiration via a dedicated pumping system. A microwire with an olive-shaped tip, called separator, is used to fragmentize the thrombus from proximal to distal and to avoid obstruction of the aspiration catheter by cleaning the catheter tip of clot fragments. Both reperfusion catheter and separator are available in various sizes and diameters (0.26—0.51 in.) to adjust the device to different anatomical settings and to allow thrombectomy even in distal branches such as M2 segments.

The Penumbra System has been investigated in several single-center and multicenter trials. The Penumbra Pivotal Stroke Trial [15] prospectively evaluated 125 stroke patients (mean NIHSS 18) within 8 h after onset of symptoms. Successful recanalization of the target vessel was achieved in 81.6%. Despite the relatively high recanalization rate, favorable clinical outcome was achieved in only 25% of all patients and in 29% of patients with successful recanalization. Overall mortality was 32.8% and sICH occurred in 11.2% with serious adverse events in 3.2%. The high recanalization rate in conjunction with the poor clinical outcome in this trial sparked the discussion on the impact of recanalization using mechanical thrombectomy. However, some single-center studies reported more favorable clinical results with the Penumbra System and then the Pivotal Trial with successful recanalization in 93%, good clinical outcome in 48% and reduced mortality of 11% [16].

Distal thrombectomy

Compared to IAT and the use of proximal devices, the use of distal thrombectomy devices is technically more complex. An 8 F sheath and balloon catheter of similar size are used. After placement of the balloon catheter in the internal carotid artery, a microcatheter (0.18—0.27 in.) is navigated across the occlusion site to pass the thrombus. The device is then introduced into the microcatheter and unsheathed behind the thrombus. This approach applies the retrieval force to the distal base of the thrombus. The device and thrombus are then retracted into the guide catheter under balloon occlusion and additional aspiration.

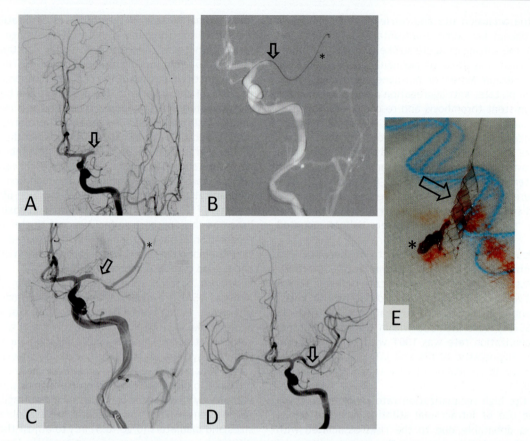

Figure 1 74-year-old male patient 4.5 h after acute onset of right hemiplegia and aphasia, at admission NIHSS 18, bridging therapy. (A) Digital subtraction angiogram of the left internal carotid artery, illustrating proximal occlusion (arrow) of the middle cerebral artery (MCA). (B) Application of a stent-retriever: a microcatheter and microwire are advanced beyond the occlusion side (arrow) and placed into the distal branches of the MCA (*). (C) Angiogram immediately after placement of a stent-retriever (Solitaire FR) covering the occlusion (arrow). The device compresses the thrombus and creates a channel; a temporary bypass to the distal branches of the MCA (*). (D) After retrieval of the device 5 min later complete recanalization of the MCA main trunk (arrow) and the distal braches. (E) The stent-retriever device (arrow) after the successful thrombectomy with the entangled clot from the MCA (*). The patient recovered to NIHSS 5 after 24 h, mRS 1 after 90 days.

Clinical observations have shown that thrombectomy using distal devices has the risk of potentially dislodging thrombotic material during retrieval from the occlusion site into a previously unaffected vascular territory. Such embolic events may worsen the patient's neurological condition. Therefore, distal thrombectomy devices are regularly used in combination with proximal balloon occlusion in the internal carotid artery in conjunction with aspiration from the guiding catheter in order to reduce the risk of thromboembolic events during retrieval. Furthermore, vasospasm and vessel wall damage have been reported more frequently in association with distal thrombectomy devices. Various distal thrombectomy devices with brush-like, basket-like or coil-like designs have been advocated in the past (e.g. Catch, Balt, Montmorency, France; Phenox pCR and CRC, Bochum, Germany), with most of them only available in Europe. The largest clinical experience has been reported on the Merci Retrieval System (Concentric Medical, Mountain View, USA), which is the first device of this group to receive FDA approval in 2004.

Merci Retrieval System. The Merci Retrieval System is somehow the pioneer of intracranial device development for acute stroke treatment. FDA approval was based on the multicenter Mechanical Embolus Removal in Cerebral Ischemia (MERCI) trial [17]. 151 patients (mean NIHSS 20) were evaluated within 8 h after onset of symptoms, who were ineligible for standard IAT. Successful recanalization was achieved in 46% of patients with favorable clinical outcome in 27.7%. Mean procedure time was 2.1 h. Clinically significant procedural complications occurred in 7.1% and rate of sICH was 7.8%. The Multi-MERCI trial [18] was a prospective, multicenter, single-arm registry that included 164 patients (mean NIHSS 19) within 8 h after onset of symptoms. In contrast to the MERCI trial, patients with persistent large vessel occlusion after IV tPA were also included in the study, adjunctive IAT using rtPA and the use of other mechanical recanalization techniques and new generation of Merci devices were allowed. Recanalization success was 57.3% using the Merci device alone and 69.5% in conjunction with other treatment modalities. Favorable clinical outcome was achieved in 36% of patients with clinical significant complications in 5.5% and sICH in 9.8%. Mean time to recanalization was 1.6 h.

The introduction of the Merci device was a landmark of mechanical recanalization in acute stroke treatment. Both MERCI trials demonstrated a significantly better clinical outcome in patients with successful recanalization.

Stent retriever. The most recent developments for mechanical acute stroke treatment are self-expandable, retrievable, stent-like thrombectomy devices. They combine the advantages of intracranial stent placement with immediate flow restoration without the need of permanent device implantation and the advantages of a thrombectomy system with the ability of definitive clot removal. This concept offers a promising new treatment option for acute ischemic stroke with high recanalization rates, marked reduction in procedure time and a marked elevation in the rate of favorable clinical outcome. Stent retrievers are applied in a comparable manner to that of intracranial stents. The occlusion site is passed with a microcatheter (0.21–0.27 in.) and the device is deployed over the entire thrombus. Due to its radial force, the device compresses the thrombus against the contralateral vessel wall leading to immediate partial flow restoration to the distal vessel territory. After an embedding time of 3–10 min the device is retrieved. As for distal thrombectomy devices the use of proximal balloon occlusion and aspiration during retrieval is recommended in order to avoid thromboembolic events.

Several stent retrievers with different designs are currently under development or evaluated in first clinical trials (Trevo, Concentric Medical, Mountain View, USA; PULSE and 3D Separator, Penumbra, Almeda, USA; Revive, Micrus, USA; Aperio, Acandis, Pforzheim, Germany; Bonnet and pREset, Phenox, Bochum, Germany).

The first dedicated combined flow restoration and thrombectomy device for acute stroke treatment was the Solitaire FR (ev3, Irvine, USA). The device is a modification of the Solitaire AB Neurovascular Remodeling Device, originally developed for stent-assisted coil treatment of wide-necked intracranial aneurysms. Within a short period of time several in vivo and clinical studies have reported about the application of the Solitaire FR for acute stroke treatment (Fig. 1).

The first clinical experience was published by Castano et al. [19] in 2010 reporting their initial treatment of 20 patients within 8 h after onset of symptoms. Successful recanalization was achieved in 90% of patients with a favorable clinical outcome in 45%. Mean procedure time was short with 50 min. sICH occurred in 10%. Several other small case series using various stent retrievers have shown similar promising successful recanalization rates (88–91%) and fast procedural times (42–55 min) with comparable rates of favorable clinical outcome (42–54%) [20–22]. Rohde et al. [23] reported their preliminary experience with the Revive system (Micrus Endovascular, San Jose, USA) in the treatment of large vessel occlusion in 10 patients (mean NIHSS 19). The design of the Revive system consists of a closed basket at the distal end of the stent in order to enhance clot removal. Successful recanalization (TICI 2b or 3) was achieved in all patients with favorable outcome in 60% of patients after 30 days. The Solitaire FR with the Intention for Thrombectomy (SWIFT) trial is a randomized trial comparing the efficacy and safety of the Solitaire FR with that of the Merci device. The SWIFT trial was halted by the data monitoring board early in 2011 after inclusion of 126 patients of anticipated 250 patients. The results have not yet been published, but favorable results for the Solitaire FR can be assumed. The Solitaire FR is currently evaluated in the Solitaire FR Thrombectomy for Acute Revascularization (STAR) trial, a prospective, multicenter, single-arm study with an enrolment goal of 200 patients. The study includes patients within 8 h after symptom onset ineligible for or with failed IV rtPA as a bridging therapy or thrombectomy as initial treatment. First results are expected in mid-2012.

Conclusion

Immediate flow restoration is the principle goal of ischemic stroke therapy and is associated with better clinical outcome and reduced mortality. The introduction of mechanical approaches has expanded the time window for stroke treatment and broadened the spectrum of stroke patients for treatment. The latest results of MT using stent-retrievers demonstrate high recanalization rates in conjunction with short recanalization times and a low-risk device-related severe adverse event. Furthermore, recent data show that the increased recanalization rate of MT improves clinical outcome.

The future role of MT in acute stroke treatment is not clear yet. Considering the poor recanalization rate and clinical outcome of patients with proximal vessel occlusions and large thrombus burden (e.g. internal carotid artery occlusion), MT is likely to become a first-line treatment.

References

[1] Rha JH, Saver JL. The impact of recanalization on ischemic stroke outcome: a meta-analysis. Stroke 2007;38(3):967–73.

[2] del Zoppo GJ, Poeck K, Pessin MS, Wolpert SM, Furlan AJ, Ferbert A, et al. Recombinant tissue plasminogen activator in acute thrombotic and embolic stroke. Annals of Neurology 1992;32(1):78–86.

[3] Mori E, Yoneda Y, Tabuchi M, Yoshida T, Ohkawa S, Ohsumi Y, et al. Intravenous recombinant tissue plasminogen activator in acute carotid artery territory stroke. Neurology 1992;42(5):976–82.

[4] Saqqur M, Uchino K, Demchuk AM, Molina CA, Garami Z, Calleja S, et al. Site of arterial occlusion identified by transcranial Doppler predicts the response to intravenous thrombolysis for stroke. Stroke 2007;38(3):948–54.

[5] Brekenfeld C, Remonda L, Nedeltchev K, Arnold M, Mattle HP, Fischer U, et al. Symptomatic intracranial haemorrhage after intra-arterial thrombolysis in acute ischaemic stroke: assessment of 294 patients treated with urokinase. Journal of Neurology, Neurosurgery and Psychiatry 2007;78(3):280–5.

[6] Diener HC, Bogousslavsky J, Brass LM, Cimminiello C, Csiba L, Kaste M, et al. Aspirin and clopidogrel compared with clopidogrel alone after recent ischaemic stroke or transient ischaemic attack in high-risk patients (MATCH): randomised, double-blind, placebo-controlled trial. Lancet 2004;364(9431):331–7.

[7] Stenting of Symptomatic Atherosclerotic Lesions in the Vertebral or Intracranial Arteries (SSYLVIA): study results. Stroke 2004;35(6):1388–92.

[8] Levy EI, Mehta R, Gupta R, Hanel RA, Chamczuk AJ, Fiorella D, et al. Self-expanding stents for recanalization of acute cerebrovascular occlusions. American Journal of Neuroradiology 2007;28(5):816–22.

[9] Brekenfeld C, Schroth G, Mattle HP, Do DD, Remonda L, Mordasini P, et al. Stent placement in acute cerebral artery occlusion: use of a self-expandable intracranial stent for acute stroke treatment. Stroke 2009;40(3):847–52.

[10] Levy EI, Rahman M, Khalessi AA, Beyer PT, Natarajan SK, Hartney ML, et al. Midterm clinical and angiographic follow-up for the first Food and Drug Administration-approved prospective Single-Arm Trial of Primary Stenting for Stroke: SARIS (Stent-Assisted Recanalization for Acute Ischemic Stroke). Neurosurgery 2011;69(4):915–20, discussion 920.

[11] Levy EI, Siddiqui AH, Crumlish A, Snyder KV, Hauck EF, Fiorella DJ, et al. First Food and Drug Administration-approved prospective trial of primary intracranial stenting for acute stroke: SARIS (stent-assisted recanalization in acute ischemic stroke). Stroke 2009;40(11):3552–6.

[12] Chapot R, Houdart E, Rogopoulos A, Mounayer C, Saint-Maurice JP, Merland JJ. Thromboaspiration in the basilar artery: report of two cases. American Journal of Neuroradiology 2002;23(2):282–4.

[13] Lutsep HL, Clark WM, Nesbit GM, Kuether TA, Barnwell SL. Intraarterial suction thrombectomy in acute stroke. American Journal of Neuroradiology 2002;23(5):783–6.

[14] Kang DH, Hwang YH, Kim YS, Park J, Kwon O, Jung C. Direct thrombus retrieval using the reperfusion catheter of the penumbra system: forced-suction thrombectomy in acute ischemic stroke. American Journal of Neuroradiology 2011;32(2):283–7.

[15] The penumbra pivotal stroke trial: safety and effectiveness of a new generation of mechanical devices for clot removal in intracranial large vessel occlusive disease. Stroke 2009;40(8):2761–8.

[16] Kulcsar Z, Bonvin C, Pereira VM, Altrichter S, Yilmaz H, Lovblad KO, et al. Penumbra system: a novel mechanical thrombectomy device for large-vessel occlusions in acute stroke. American Journal of Neuroradiology 2010;31(4):628–33.

[17] Smith WS, Sung G, Starkman S, Saver JL, Kidwell CS, Gobin YP, et al. Safety and efficacy of mechanical embolectomy in acute ischemic stroke: results of the MERCI trial. Stroke 2005;36(7):1432–8.

[18] Smith WS, Sung G, Saver J, Budzik R, Duckwiler G, Liebeskind DS, et al. Mechanical thrombectomy for acute ischemic stroke: final results of the Multi MERCI trial. Stroke 2008;39(4):1205–12.

[19] Castano C, Dorado L, Guerrero C, Millan M, Gomis M, Perez de la Ossa, et al. Mechanical thrombectomy with the Solitaire AB device in large artery occlusions of the anterior circulation: a pilot study. Stroke 2010;41(8):1836–40.

[20] Brekenfeld C, Schroth G, Mordasini P, Fischer U, Mono ML, Weck A, et al. Impact of retrievable stents on acute ischemic stroke treatment. American Journal of Neuroradiology 2011;32(7):1269–73.

[21] Roth C, Papanagiotou P, Behnke S, Walter S, Haass A, Becker C, et al. Stent-assisted mechanical recanalization for treatment of acute intracerebral artery occlusions. Stroke 2010;41(11):2559–67.

[22] Costalat V, Machi P, Lobotesis K, Maldonado I, Vendrell JF, Riquelme C, et al. Rescue, combined, and stand-alone thrombectomy in the management of large vessel occlusion stroke using the solitaire device: a prospective 50-patient single-center study: timing, safety, and efficacy. Stroke 2011;42(7):1929–35.

[23] Rohde S, Haehnel S, Herweh C, Pham M, Stampfl S, Ringleb PA, et al. Mechanical thrombectomy in acute embolic stroke: preliminary results with the revive device. Stroke 2011;42(10):2954–6.

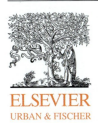
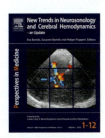

Bartels E, Bartels S, Poppert H (Editors):
New Trends in Neurosonology and Cerebral Hemodynamics — an Update.
Perspectives in Medicine (2012) 1, 59—64

journal homepage: www.elsevier.com/locate/permed

Functional guidance in intracranial tumor surgery

Sandro M. Krieg, Florian Ringel, Bernhard Meyer*

Department of Neurosurgery, Klinikum rechts der Isar, Technische Universität München, Ismaninger Str. 22, 81675 Munich, Germany

KEYWORDS
Preoperative mapping;
Rolandic region;
Tumor;
Transcranial magnetic stimulation;
Navigated brain stimulation

Summary

Objective: Navigated transcranial magnetic stimulation (nTMS) is a newly evolving technique. Despite its supposed purpose of preoperative mapping of the central region, little is known about further applications as well as the accuracy compared to more commonly used modalities like direct cortical stimulation (DCS) and functional MRI (fMRI).

Methods: We examined 30 patients with tumors in or close to the precentral gyrus as well as in the subcortical white matter motor tract using nTMS with the Nexstim eXimia system. Data was sent to the neuronavigation system and correlated with intraoperative direct cortical stimulation.

Results: In the cases of lesions of the precentral gyrus, preoperative motor cortex characterization correlated well with intraoperative DCS with a deviation of 4.5 ± 3.5 mm. When comparing nTMS with fMRI however, deviation was quite larger with 9.6 ± 7.9 mm for upper and 15.0 ± 12.8 mm for lower extremity. In patients with subcortical lesions DTI fiber tracking was performed using nTMS mapping as seed region, which resulted in a subjectively more specific presentation of the corticospinal tract compared to conventional fiber tracking and caused less interobserver variability.

Conclusion: Navigated TMS correlates well with DCS as the best established standard despite many factors, which are supposed to contribute to inaccuracy of the method. Moreover, nTMS-aided DTI fiber tracking is user-independent and, therefore, a method for further standardization of DTI fiber tracking.
© 2012 Elsevier GmbH. All rights reserved.

Abbreviations: BOLD, blood oxygen level dependent; CMAP, compound muscle action potential; CST, corticospinal tract; DCS, direct cortical stimulation; EEG, electroencephalography; EMG, electromyography; fMRI, functional MRI; IOM, intraoperative neuromonitoring; MEG, magneto-encephalography; MEP, motor evoked potential; nTMS, navigated transcranial magnetic stimulation; PET, positron emission tomography; rMT, resting motor threshold; TIVA, total intravenous anesthesia.
* Corresponding author. Tel.: +49 89 4140 2151; fax: +49 89 4140 4889.
E-mail addresses: sandro.krieg@lrz.tum.de (S.M. Krieg), florian.ringel@lrz.tum.de (F. Ringel), bernhard.meyer@lrz.tum.de, sandro.krieg@googlemail.com (B. Meyer).

2211-968X/$ — see front matter © 2012 Elsevier GmbH. All rights reserved.
http://dx.doi.org/10.1016/j.permed.2012.03.014

Introduction

Resection of tumors within or close to motor eloquent areas, particularly the precentral gyrus, is always a compromise between extent of resection and preservation of motor function. Especially in gliomas, surgical tumor reduction has a significant impact on survival and thus has to be as extensive as possible [1,2]. On the other hand, motor function has to be preserved in order to secure quality of life for the patient. To achieve both goals, neurosurgeons use multiple modalities to examine, visualize, and monitor anatomy and motor function presurgically and during resection [3–5]. For preoperative motor cortex mapping, some already established modalities are at hand, such as functional magnetic resonance imaging (fMRI), positron emission tomography (PET), electroencephalography (EEG), and magnetoencephalography (MEG). However, these measures use the distribution of metabolic (fMRI, PET) or electrical (EEG, MEG) activity for detection of activity of neuronal pathways. In theory, metabolic or electrical activity might correlate with neurophysiological pathways but do not have to [6]. In the last two years, we witnessed the increasing use of another modality: navigated transcranial magnetic stimulation (nTMS). It is able to reach cortical neurons by a shortly induced but strong magnetic field, causing α-motoneurons to be excited. However, as a new modality, nTMS is actually capable of giving us specific information where monosynaptic motor evoked potentials (MEP) are elicited in the precentral gyrus as shown in recently published studies [7,8].

Thus, this study was designed to prospectively evaluate the accuracy of nTMS in comparison to DCS as the best known standard and to an already established preoperative mapping method: fMRI. Moreover, we wanted to demonstrate value and feasibility of diffusion tensor imaging fiber tracking (DTI-FT) based on nTMS data as the seed region in patients with tumors within or close to the corticospinal tract (CST).

Materials and methods

Patients

From May to December 2010, 30 patients with tumors within the motor system were mapped by nTMS prior to surgery. Mild preoperative motor deficit occurred in 12 cases (40.0%). There were 15 GBMs, 2 anaplastic astrocytomas, 3 diffuse astrocytomas WHO °II, 1 DNET WHO °I, 1 meningioma °I, 1 AVM, and 7 metastases.

Preoperative magnetic resonance imaging

All patients underwent pre- and postoperative MRI on a clinical 3 Tesla MR scanner (Achieva 3T, Philips Medical Systems, The Netherlands B.V.) with an 8-channel phased array head coil including blood oxygen level dependent (BOLD) functional imaging (fMRI), T2 FLAIR and a contrast-enhanced 3D gradient echo sequence for anatomical coregistration. BOLD data was postprocessed using the IViewBOLD package (Extended MR Workspace, Philips Medical Systems, The Netherlands B.V.). Moreover, 6 orthogonal diffusion directions were used for diffusion tensor imaging (DTI).

Navigated transcranial magnetic stimulation

The used nTMS system (eXimia 3.2 and eXimia 4.3, Nexstim, Helsinki, Finland) was applied the day before surgery as descried earlier [9,10]. In short, while stimulating with nTMS, electromyography (EMG) (eXimia 3.2, Nexstim, Helsinki, Finland) is monitored continuously, with 4 channels for the upper and 2 channels for the lower extremity and site of stimulation and activated muscle are correlated as repeatedly reported earlier [7,8].

Neuronavigation and fiber tracking

Navigated TMS mapping was imported to the neuronavigation planning system (BrainLAB iPlan® Cranial 3.0.1, BrainLAB AG, Feldkirchen, Germany), fused with continuous sagittal images of the T1-weighted 3D gradient echo sequence, T2 FLAIR, and DTI data (Fig. 1). The white matter tracts were computed from the DTI dataset as previously described using BrainLAB iPlan® Cranial 3.0.1 [11] while seeding was performed in two different ways: traditionally outlined according to anatomical landmarks, or generated from the nTMS points of positive eliciting of MEPs as described above. DTI-FT was performed by three different investigators with BrainLAB iPlan® Cranial 3.0.1 (BrainLAB AG, Feldkirchen, Germany) at two different time points.

Intraoperative technique

Total intravenous anesthesia (TIVA) was used in all cases by continuous propofol and remifentanyl application without neuromuscular blocking. For detection of compound muscle action potential (CMAP), subdermal needle electrodes were placed over the same muscles as in nTMS. Immediately after durotomy and determination of motor threshold, mapping of the rolandic region was performed by anodal monopolar navigated DCS (Inomed Medizintechnik, Emmendingen, Germany) with intensities between 5 and 14 mA with the train-of-five technique as described previously [12,13]. After DCS mapping continuous MEP monitoring was performed as also outlined earlier [12,13].

Results

Preoperative nTMS mapping

Preoperative mapping of the primary motor cortex was possible in all patients and required 121–253 stimulation points per patient. In 50.0% of cases, mapping of the lower extremity was possible as well. One patient experienced nTMS mapping as unpleasant, whereas no patient actually stated nTMS mapping was painful.

Correlation of nTMS to DCS and fMRI mapping

Preoperative motor cortex mapping was compared to intraoperative DCS with a navigated DCS electrode. Borders between positive and negative stimulation points of both modalities were then compared on axial slices by recalibrating screenshots and BrainLAB iPlan® Net Cranial 3.0.1. A difference of 4.5 ± 3.5 mm (range 1.9—9.2 mm) between nTMS and intraoperative DCS has been determined for the borders of the mapped primary motor cortex without observing any systematic monodirectional deviation (Figs. 2a and 3). Compared to nTMS data, determination of the primary motor cortex using BOLD data differed strongly between the upper and lower extremities. For the upper extremity, the deviation of nTMS and fMRI was 9.6 ± 7.9 mm (range 5.3—39.7 mm) (Fig. 3). For the lower extremity, this difference was 15.0 ± 12.8 mm (range 8.4—33.5 mm) (Figs. 2b and 3). Again, no monodirectional systematic deviation could be observed.

Differences from standard fiber tracking

When using nTMS as the seed region for DTI-FT, we observed significantly less fibers within the tracked CST (nTMS: 916.0 ± 986.0 fibers; standard: 1297.9 ± 1278.7 fibers; $p < 0.01$; Fig. 4), fewer aberrant tracts (nTMS: 0.33 ± 0.47 aberrant tracts/tracked CST; standard: 0.57 ± 0.5 aberrant tracts/tracked CST; $p < 0.001$; Fig. 5), and less interobserver variability compared to standard tracking. Interobserver variability was evaluated and visualized by a Bland—Altman plot (Fig. 6) [14]. In both modalities, we were not able to show any significant differences between the two measurements of each observer for any examined item (data not shown).

Discussion

Functional MRI vs. nTMS

Today, the only widely used and applicable method for preoperative functional brain mapping is fMRI. But, as repeatedly shown, fMRI is insufficient for reliable delineation of functional motor areas [6,15]. We moreover confirmed the discrepancy between metabolic and electrophysiological (i.e., true functional) mapping (Fig. 3). Especially in cases when tumors with pathologic vasculature compromise the central region, mapping of the primary motor cortex by metabolic measures was demonstrated to be an unreliable method [15—18]. Moreover, metabolically activated brain parenchyma does not have to be essential for

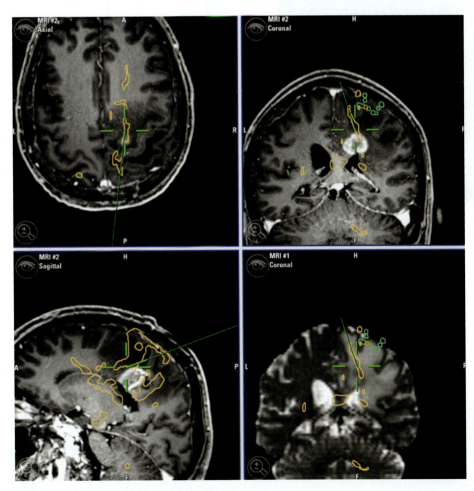

Figure 1 Intraoperative neuronavigation: intraoperative neuronavigation showing preoperative nTMS data (green) as well as nTMS-based DTI-FT (yellow).

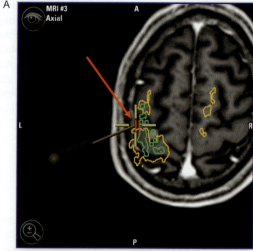

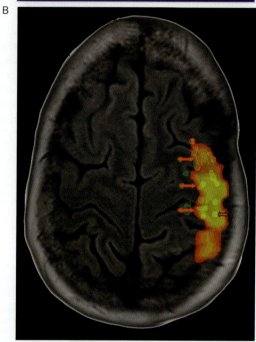

Figure 2 Deviation measurements: (a) intraoperative DCS mapping compared to preoperative nTMS data; (b) preoperative fMRI data vs. nTMS mapping.

motor function. Another disadvantage of fMRI is its frequent affection by the patient's cooperation or claustrophobia as confirmed in our work.

DCS vs. nTMS

Taking standard deviation into account, spatial deviation of DCS and nTMS ranges within the calculated accuracy of the used nTMS system (eXimia 3.2, Nexstim, Helsinki, Finland), which is 5.73 mm [19]. Such precision was already reported in previous reports on nTMS accuracy stating that a spatial resolution of 5 mm is obtainable [20,21].

Furthermore, we recognized that especially for lower extremity mapping, nTMS succeeded more frequently than DCS did, most likely due to the comparatively large stimulated cortical volume, which is calculated to be 1—2 cm^3

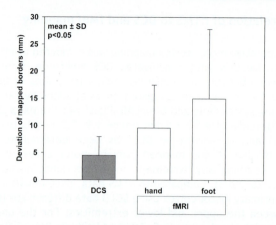

Figure 3 Deviation of nTMS compared to DCS and fMRI: navigated TMS correlates with DCS (4.5 ± 3.5 mm), while the borders of the primary motor cortex as outlined by fMRI differ significantly from nTMS for upper (9.6 ± 7.9 mm) as well as for lower extremity (15.0 ± 12.8 mm).

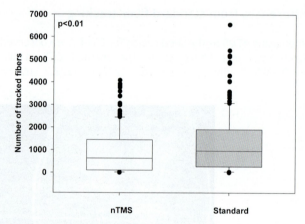

Figure 4 Number of tracked fibers: by using nTMS for defining seed regions for diffusion tensor imaging fiber tracking (DTI-FT), we witness a significantly smaller number of fibers within the tracked corticospinal tract (CST) compared to standard tracking (nTMS: 916.0 ± 986.0 fibers; standard: 1297.9 ± 1278.7 fibers).

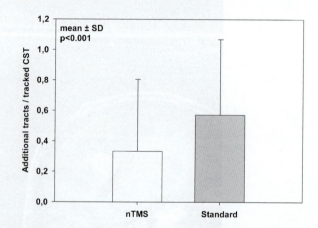

Figure 5 Aberrant tracts: we observe significantly fewer additional tracks differing from the corticospinal tract (CST) when using nTMS data for defining the cortical seed region (nTMS: 0.33 ± 0.47 aberrant tracts per tracked CST; standard: 0.57 ± 0.50 aberrant tracts per tracked CST).

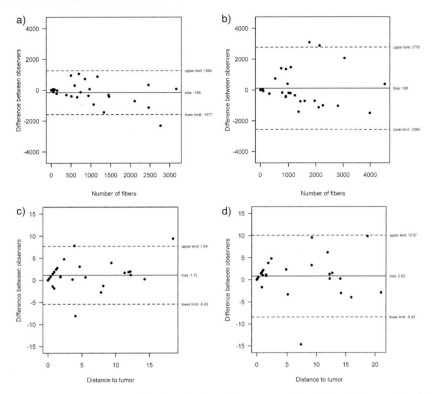

Figure 6 Interobserver variability: variability of both methods as demonstrated by a Bland—Altman plot. The graph shows the difference between standard diffusion tensor imaging fiber tracking (DTI-FT) and nTMS-based DTI-FT between observers in correlation to the number of fibers (a: nTMS; b: standard) and distance to tumor (c: nTMS; d: standard).

for the utilized figure-of-eight coil [22]. Despite the good agreement between nTMS and DCS (Fig. 3), we have to be aware that these results strongly rely on many parameters, such as definition of resting motor threshold (rMT), the voltage at which CMAP is considered significant, registration errors, navigation errors of both systems, and brain shift after durotomy [23,24].

Therefore, it seems to be unlikely that nTMS is capable to completely replace intraoperative neuromonitoring (IOM). Yet, when the rolandic region is compromised by tumor growth, it is highly valuable to have another modality at hand, which confirms the results of DCS mapping.

General results on nTMS

Compared to fMRI, nTMS is also less affected by the patient's cooperation or claustrophobia. Further newly evolved possibilities of nTMS are to decide whether or not DCS is mandatory or not and it enhances IOM by guiding the DCS probe, thus accelerating DCS mapping significantly.

DTI fiber tracking

The adaptation of nTMS motor mapping data for outlining functionally crucial seed regions was simple, and compatibility between the Nexstim eXimia 3.2 and iPlan® Cranial 3.0.1 using iPlan® Net was given by the DICOM standard and remained trouble-free when changing to iPlan® Cranial Unlimited (BrainLAB AG, Feldkirchen, Germany).

Traditional outlining of the primary motor cortex can be quite challenging when tumors affect the rolandic region. Mostly due to mass effects and edema. Such structural alteration with impairment of the anatomy causes an imprecise outlining of the cortical seed region with the manual technique. Thus, even tracts from accidently included non-eloquent regions are incorporated and lead to a broader and therefore less specific definition of the CST. Furthermore, tumors within the CST or the precentral gyrus can cause cerebral plasticity so that functionally important motor areas do not have to coincide anymore with standard anatomical landmarks, which are also regularly hard to identify [17,25—27]. Especially due to this matter, only nTMS data and not anatomical landmarks can reliably identify functionally crucial motor regions prior to surgery. Because our technique, shown in this work, is based on functional and not structural anatomy, it should provide a more accurate white matter fiber reconstruction. Nonetheless, we have to keep in mind that in large volume lesions or largely infiltrating tumors, nTMS might not be able to elicit MEPs in all fibers of the CST due to impairment of these fibers by tumor or edema. Therefore the tract might appear more compact than observed with traditional tractography. In most cases, these missing fibers are located around the tumor in the upper part of the tract in standard tractography, which seem to be missing in the nTMS-designed tracts.

From a neurosurgical point of view, we have to emphasize that DTI-FT can only provide additional information for intraoperative neuromonitoring, e.g., by accelerating subcortical mapping, and, thus, might reduce the duration of surgery, as reported previously [28].

This work demonstrates that accurate and reliable nTMS motor mapping can help us to standardize tractography of the CST to some degree. Combining both techniques seems promising for the preoperative evaluation of functionally essential white matter networks on the one hand but there is also a high potential on the other hand to expand its use to other functional systems within the brain, such as speech or sensory system, but also to investigate brain plasticity or development far beyond neurosurgical purposes.

Conclusions

We were able to show that nTMS is feasible in every patient without major discomfort, and that nTMS highly correlates with intraoperative DCS. In contrast, fMRI differed significantly. Moreover, the use of nTMS data for tractography of the CST was shown to be feasible and leads to higher standardization of DTI-FT.

Yet, more patients have to be enrolled in order to examine the impact of nTMS mapping on extent of resection, patient outcomes, and survival. Thus, the actual value of this method is still unclear.

Disclosure

The authors declare that they have no conflict of interest affecting this work. The presented studies were completely financed by institutional grants of the Department of Neurosurgery.

References

[1] Laws Jr ER, Taylor WF, Clifton MB, Okazaki H. Neurosurgical management of low-grade astrocytoma of the cerebral hemispheres. J Neurosurg 1984;61:665—73.
[2] Stummer W, et al. Extent of resection and survival in glioblastoma multiforme: identification of and adjustment for bias. Neurosurgery 2008;62:564—76.
[3] Penfield W, Boldrey E. Somatic motor and sensory representation in the cerebral cortex of man as studied by electrical stimulation. Brain 1937;60:389—443.
[4] Krings T, et al. Functional magnetic resonance imaging and transcranial magnetic stimulation: complementary approaches in the evaluation of cortical motor function. Neurology 1997;48:1406—16.
[5] Kombos T, Suess O, Funk T, Kern BC, Brock M. Intraoperative mapping of the motor cortex during surgery in and around the motor cortex. Acta Neurochir (Wien) 2000;142:263—8.
[6] Rutten GJ, Ramsey NF. The role of functional magnetic resonance imaging in brain surgery. Neurosurg Focus 2010;28:E4.
[7] Picht T, et al. Preoperative functional mapping for rolandic brain tumor surgery: comparison of navigated transcranial magnetic stimulation to direct cortical stimulation. Neurosurgery 2011.
[8] Forster MT, et al. Navigated transcranial magnetic stimulation and functional magnetic resonance imaging—advanced adjuncts in preoperative planning for central region tumors. Neurosurgery 2011.
[9] Ilmoniemi RJ, Ruohonen J, Karhu J. Transcranial magnetic stimulation—a new tool for functional imaging of the brain. Crit Rev Biomed Eng 1999;27:241—84.
[10] Ruohonen J, Ilmoniemi RJ. Modeling of the stimulating field generation in TMS. Electroencephalogr Clin Neurophysiol 1999;(Suppl. 51):30—40.
[11] Nimsky C, Ganslandt O, Fahlbusch R. Implementation of fiber tract navigation. Neurosurgery 2006;58. ONS-292—303 [discussion ONS-4].
[12] Cedzich C, Taniguchi M, Schafer S, Schramm J. Somatosensory evoked potential phase reversal and direct motor cortex stimulation during surgery in and around the central region. Neurosurgery 1996;38:962—70.
[13] Taniguchi M, Cedzich C, Schramm J. Modification of cortical stimulation for motor evoked potentials under general anesthesia: technical description. Neurosurgery 1993;32:219—26.
[14] Bland JM, Altman DG. Measuring agreement in method comparison studies. Stat Methods Med Res 1999;8:135—60.
[15] Krings T, et al. Functional MRI for presurgical planning: problems, artefacts, and solution strategies. J Neurol Neurosurg Psychiatry 2001;70:749—60.
[16] Hou BL, et al. Effect of brain tumor neovasculature defined by rCBV on BOLD fMRI activation volume in the primary motor cortex. Neuroimage 2006;32:489—97.
[17] Lehericy S, et al. Correspondence between functional magnetic resonance imaging somatotopy and individual brain anatomy of the central region: comparison with intraoperative stimulation in patients with brain tumors. J Neurosurg 2000;92:589—98.
[18] Yetkin FZ, et al. Functional MR activation correlated with intraoperative cortical mapping. AJNR Am J Neuroradiol 1997;18:1311—5.
[19] Ruohonen J, Karhu J. Navigated transcranial magnetic stimulation. Neurophysiol Clin 2010;40:7—17.
[20] Brasil-Neto JP, et al. Optimal focal transcranial magnetic activation of the human motor cortex: effects of coil orientation, shape of the induced current pulse, and stimulus intensity. J Clin Neurophysiol 1992;9:132—6.
[21] Krings T, et al. Stereotactic transcranial magnetic stimulation: correlation with direct electrical cortical stimulation. Neurosurgery 1997;41:1319—25.
[22] Levy WJ, Amassian VE, Schmid UD, Jungreis C. Mapping of motor cortex gyral sites non-invasively by transcranial magnetic stimulation in normal subjects and patients. Electroencephalogr Clin Neurophysiol 1991;(Suppl 43):51—75.
[23] Suess O, et al. Evaluation of a DC pulsed magnetic tracking system in neurosurgical navigation: technique, accuracies, and influencing factors. Biomed Tech (Berl) 2007;52:223—33.
[24] Hastreiter P, et al. Strategies for brain shift evaluation. Med Image Anal 2004;8:447—64.
[25] Duffau H. New concepts in surgery of WHO grade II gliomas: functional brain mapping, connectionism and plasticity—a review. J Neurooncol 2006;79:77—115.
[26] Martino J, Taillandier L, Moritz-Gasser S, Gatignol P, Duffau H. Re-operation is a safe and effective therapeutic strategy in recurrent WHO grade II gliomas within eloquent areas. Acta Neurochir (Wien) 2009;151:427—36.
[27] Robles SG, Gatignol P, Lehericy S, Duffau H. Long-term brain plasticity allowing a multistage surgical approach to World Health Organization grade II gliomas in eloquent areas. J Neurosurg 2008;109:615—24.
[28] Willems PW, Taphoorn MJ, Burger H, Berkelbach van der Sprenkel JW, Tulleken CA. Effectiveness of neuronavigation in resecting solitary intracerebral contrast-enhancing tumors: a randomized controlled trial. J Neurosurg 2006;104:360—8.

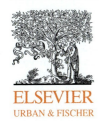
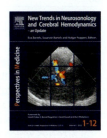

Bartels E, Bartels S, Poppert H (Editors):
New Trends in Neurosonology and Cerebral Hemodynamics — an Update.
Perspectives in Medicine (2012) 1, 65—72

journal homepage: www.elsevier.com/locate/permed

Endovascular sono-lysis using EKOS system in acute stroke patients with a main cerebral artery occlusion — A pilot study

Martin Kuliha[a], Martin Roubec[a], Táňa Fadrná[a], Daniel Šaňák[b], Roman Herzig[b], Tomáš Jonszta[c], Daniel Czerný[c], Jan Krajča[c], Václav Procházka[c], David Školoudík[a,b,*]

[a] Department of Neurology, University Hospital and Ostrava University Medical School, Ostrava, Czech Republic
[b] Department of Neurology, Faculty of Medicine and Dentistry, Palacký University and University Hospital Olomouc, Olomouc, Czech Republic
[c] Department of Radiology, University Hospital, Ostrava, Czech Republic

KEYWORDS
Stroke;
Sono-lysis;
Sonothrombolysis;
Arterial occlusion;
Recanalization;
Therapy

Summary

Aim: Sono-lysis is a new therapeutic procedure for arterial recanalization. The aim of the study was to confirm the safety and efficacy of intravascular sono-lysis using EKOS system with 3F microcatheter EkoSonic and 2.05—2.35 MHz ultrasound frequencies.

Methods: Nine patients admitted to the stroke unit with acute middle cerebral artery (MCA) or basilar artery (BA) occlusion were enrolled to the study. Treatment using EKOS system started within 8 h after stroke onset. Neurological deficit on admission (using NIHSS), after 24 h and after 7 days, MCA/BA recanalization at the end of intervention, occurrence of symptomatic intracerebral hemorrhage (SICH), and 3-month clinical outcome (using Modified Rankin score — mRS) were evaluated.

Results: Nine patients were included in the pilot study (6 males, 3 females; age 51—80, mean 65 ± 10.4 years) with NIHSS 10—33 (median 19.0) points on admission. Five patients suffered from MCA occlusion, 4 patients from BA occlusion. Complete/partial recanalization at the end of EKOS treatment was achieved in 3 (33%)/4 (44%) patients, resp. Median NIHSS values at the end of EKOS treatment/24 h/7 days after stroke onset were 17.0/12.0/6.0 points, resp. No SICH was detected on control computed tomography. Four (44%) patients were independent at 3 months (mRS 0—3); median mRS was 4.

Conclusions: According to the results of the presented pilot study, EKOS system seems to be a new treatment option for acute stroke patients.
© 2012 Elsevier GmbH. All rights reserved.

---

* Corresponding author at: Department of Neurology, University Hospital Ostrava, 17. listopadu 1790, CZ-708 52 Ostrava, Czech Republic. Tel.: +420 597375613; fax: +420 597375604.
E-mail address: skoloudik@hotmail.com (D. Školoudík).

2211-968X/$ — see front matter © 2012 Elsevier GmbH. All rights reserved.
doi:10.1016/j.permed.2012.02.055

Introduction

Stroke is one of the most frequent causes of mortality, morbidity and disability of population in developed countries [1,2]. Ischemic stroke (IS) is the most common type of stroke which constitutes about 80% of all strokes.

The most often cause of IS is an acute occlusion of cerebral arteries which can be demonstrated in more than 70% of patients in the first 3—6 h after onset of symptoms [3]. Very high mortality during the first month, which ranges between 10% and 17% and even up to 75% in patients with expansive ischemia, documents the importance of IS [4]. Finally, only about 30% of IS patients are independent after 3 months [2].

The independent prognostic factors of IS are not only comorbidities and complications but especially location of cerebral artery occlusion and time to recanalization. Early recanalization [within 6 h after onset of symptoms] is associated with a significantly higher chance of self-sufficiency after 90 days with a significant reduction of mortality [5]. In the last decade, the number of methods using to acceleration of artery recanalization strongly increased. In addition to pharmacological methods, especially intravenous (IVT) and intra-arterial thrombolysis (IAT) [6—8], mechanical (neuro-interventional) methods (i.e. percutaneous transluminal angioplasty with stenting, Merci Retriever®, Penumbra®, Solitaire® stent, sono-lysis, EKOS®, EPAR®, LATIS®, Amplaplatz Goose-Neck Snare®, Attractor-18® or Neuronet® were tested and introduced into clinical practice similarly as in the treatment of heart ischemic syndromes [9—13].

Data from the meta-analysis of 53 clinical trials (including 2066 patients) suggests that early recanalization is present only in 24.1% patients without specific treatment (spontaneous recanalization), 46.2% patients treated with IVT, 63.2% patients treated with IAT, 67.5% of patients treated with combined IVT—IAT and in up to 83.6% patients treated with mechanical methods [5]. Nevertheless, the use of these methods only in specialized centers represents the main limitation.

Sono-lysis is one of the methods used for the acceleration of recanalization of the occluded intracranial artery.

Mechanisms of the effects of sono-lysis

Although the complex effect of ultrasound on the acceleration of thrombus lysis is not yet fully understood, it is assumed that the ultrasonic waves accelerate enzymatic fibrinolysis by primarily non-thermal mechanisms — increasing the transport of fibrinolytic agents into the thrombus by mechanical disruption of its structure [14], direct activation of fibrinolytic enzymes, either mechanical breaking of the complex molecules, in which fibrinolytic enzymes are inactivated by binding to their inhibitors, or irritation of the endothelium with increased production of fibrinolytic enzymes [15,16], transient peripheral (capillary) vasodilatation caused probably by increased production of nitrite oxide in the endothelium [17,18]. Radiation force and acoustic cavitation are the next possible and discussed mechanical effects of ultrasound [19].

In vitro and in vivo studies

Different frequencies (20 kHz to 3.4 MHz) and intensities of ultrasound with different effects have been used in various in vitro studies [20,21]. Low frequency (about 20 kHz) and high intensity ultrasound lead to a rapid and efficient lysis of thrombi into microscopic fragments primarily by direct mechanical effect although the signs of activation of fibrinolytic lysis were also observed. These studies even demonstrated the ability of ultrasound to disrupt both fibrous and calcified atherosclerotic plaques [15,22—26]. Unfortunately thermal impairment and perforation of vascular walls were observed as side effects.

Unlike low-frequency ultrasonic waves, the high frequency ultrasound (0.5—3.4 MHz) with ultrasound intensities higher than $1 W/cm^2$ led primarily to the increase of fibrinolytic-induced fibrinolysis [27—32]. Sono-lysis in these studies accelerated lysis of thrombus in the presence of a fibrinolytic. Without the presence of fibrinolytics, neither lysis nor mechanical thrombus fragmentation were observed.

Similar results were found also in in vivo studies with animal models [25,26,33,34]. Sono-lysis using ultrasound with low frequencies and high intensities in dog models of femoral and coronary artery resulted to recanalization of thrombosis without the use of fibrinolytic agents. However, histological signs of damage to the vascular wall were found in some models. Sono-lysis effect was demonstrated in studies in combination with a systemic administration of thrombolytics (recombinant tissue plasminogen activator — rt-PA, urokinase, streptokinase) [35,36]. Ishibashi et al. [37] studied the effect of high-frequency ultrasound with a frequency of 490 kHz and low-intensity ($0.13 W/cm^2$) in a rabbit femoral thrombosis model to test the combined application of ultrasound-lysis with monteplase. Percentage of recanalization in combination therapy has increased from 16.7 to 66.7%.

Clinical studies in patients with acute IS

CLOTBUST trial (Combined Lysis of Thrombus in Brain ischemia using transcranial Ultrasound and Systemic TPA) was the first randomized study testing the therapeutic effect of ultrasound (sono-lysis) in patients with acute IS [38]. In this study, all patients with acute MCA occlusion were treated with IVT. Patients were randomized to the sono-lysis group with additional therapeutic transcranial Doppler insonation with 2 MHz probe for 2 h, and control group. In sono-lysis group, there was a threefold higher chance for a complete recanalization of the occluded arteries than in the control (rt-PA only) group without the increase of the risk of symptomatic intracerebral hemorrhage (SICH).

Similar results were published by Eggers et al. [39], who used sono-lysis (transcranial duplex probe with a frequency of 1.8—4 MHz) in IVT treated patients. A higher rate of complete recanalization and better early outcome and clinical status after 3 months (mRS 0—1: 21% vs. 0%) were achieved in the treatment group than in control group. However, a higher incidence of SICH (15.7% vs. 5.6%) in patients receiving sono-lysis was observed. In a multicenter case—control Thrombotripsy study, the sono-lysis in patients with acute MCA occlusion was performed using transcranial

2 MHz duplex probe [40]. Length of insonation was maximum of 45 min. Percentage of arterial recanalization was significantly higher in the sono-lysis group compared to the control group (69% vs. 8% at 6 h after onset of symptoms), as well as a good clinical outcome after 90 days (mRS 0—2: 61.5% vs. 32.7%). Sono-lysis effect was more evident in the group of patients contraindicated to IVT than in IVT treated patients. Percentage of SICH was similar in the treated and control groups (3.8%).

The effect of sono-lysis in IS patients contraindicated to IVT was also described by other authors [41,42]. Eggers et al. [41] published a set of patients with acute IS and MCA occlusion treated with sono-lysis using 2 MHz duplex transcranial probe. They detected higher number of at least partial arterial recanalization and National Institutes of Health Stroke Scale (NIHSS) improvement of more than 4 points in the treated group.

In the next study, patients with acute MCA occlusion were randomized into three treatment groups — 20 patients were treated with IVT within 3 h since stroke onset, 10 patients received IAT and 10 patients were treated by 60-min sono-lysis using 2 MHz transcranial duplex probe in the 6-h time window. The study demonstrated superior efficacy and safety of sono-lysis when compared to the IVT [43]. During the first 24 h, a clinical improvement was observed in only 45% of patients treated with IVT, but in up to 70% of patients treated with sono-lysis or IAT. The incidence of SICH was 5% in the IVT group, 0% in the sono-lysis group and 20% in the IAT group.

In later sono-lysis studies, the additive effect of echocontrast agents has been tested. The first study with Levovist® (galactose based air microbubbles, Schering, Germany) and Sonovue® (sulphurhexafluoride microbubbles, Bracco, Italy) demonstrated an increase in the percentage of arterial recanalization and better clinical improvement in acute IS patients treated with sono-lysis in combination with echocontrast agent [44]. This study demonstrated also the safety of echocontrast agent use. SICH occurred in 3.3% in the Levovist® group and in 2.1% in the Sonovue® group.

Better improvement of neurological symptoms as well as the improvement of the flow signal in the occluded arteries were showed in the study of Perren et al., using sono-lysis with 2 MHz transcranial duplex probe in combination with Sonovue® in patients with acute MCA occlusion treated with IVT [45].

The pilot randomized clinical trial with the new generation echocontrast agent (perfluten-lipid microspheres) demonstrated additive effect of echocontrast agent in patients treated with IVT and sono-lysis [46]. Percentage of complete recanalization within 2 h after therapy start was 50% in the group treated with a combination of IVT, sono-lysis and echocontrast agent in comparison with 18% in the control group selected from the CLOTBUST study. Asymptomatic intracerebral hemorrhage was found in 25% of patients in the treatment group and in 33% in the control group. A higher percentage of asymptomatic hemorrhagic transformation was also associated with a higher percentage of recanalization and better clinical status outcome in this study. No SICH was detected. Similar results with higher recanalization rate, higher percentage of good clinical outcome and also higher number of asymptomatic hemorrhagic transformation were found by Dinia et al., who used the combination of IVT, sono-lysis and administration of echocontrast agent [47]. This result supported the hypothesis that the finding of asymptomatic hemorrhagic transformation of ischemic lesion is a marker of early reperfusion and it is associated with a higher chance of good clinical outcome.

These promising results were tested in the TUCSON (Transcranial Ultrasound in Clinical Sonothrombolysis) study. Sono-lysis using 2 MHz transcranial Doppler probe in combination with an echocontrast agent MRX-801 (perfluten-lipid microspheres, ImaRx Therapeutics, Inc., USA) as adjunctive therapy to IVT was used [48]. Although the study showed that administration of a dose of 1.4 ml of MRX-801® in 90-min continuous infusion during the IVT combined with sono-lysis is safe, the study was discontinued due to the higher SICH risk in higher dose of echocontrast agent.

Explanation of the effect of sono-lysis in the humans required several studies. The authors demonstrated a direct effect of sono-lysis on the fibrinolytic system in both healthy volunteers and IS patients using transcranial 2 MHz duplex probe [15,16,49]. In healthy volunteers, 1-h sono-lysis of MCA or radial artery led to the decrease of fibrinolysis inhibitors (PAI-1 antigen, plasminogen activity and alpha-2 antiplasmin) levels [16,49]. Similar results were obtained in patients with acute IS. Also t-PA antigen was increased in sono-lysis group in comparison with a control group. These findings were more evident in patients treated with IVT in combination with sono-lysis than in sono-lysis group only. There were no significant differences in the number of SICH between the groups. This study demonstrated that activation of the fibrinolytic system is one of the therapeutic effects of ultrasound.

On the contrary to the studies with diagnostic frequencies, studies with lower frequency (300 kHz) ultrasound led to the increased risk of intracranial bleeding and blood—brain barrier breakdown.

TRUMBI (TRanscranial low-frequency Ultrasound Mediated thrombolysis in Brain Ischemia) study used low-frequency ultrasound (300 kHz, the intensity of 700 mW/cm^2) for 90 min for sono-lysis in patients with acute cerebral artery occlusion treated with IVT. The study was early terminated due to the extreme increase in the risk of SICH and of subarachnoid hemorrhage [50]. One of the hypotheses explains the increased risk of bleeding in the study by the abnormal permeability of the blood—brain barrier in humans caused by low frequency ultrasound. Multiple reflecting and focusing of ultrasonic waves within the skull, which can significantly increase the intensity of ultrasound applied in some areas of the brain, represent another option. The increased risk could also contributed to the excessive activation of the endogenous fibrinolytic system in combination with IVT.

Reinhard et al. [51] demonstrated that 60-min sono-lysis using an ultrasound frequency of 300 kHz leads to the increased permeability of the blood—brain barrier. The study was also prematurely terminated after the inclusion of 4 patients.

Clinical studies with endovascular sono-lysis

EKOS system® is the first system that allows the application of endovascular ultrasound-lysis, using a catheter

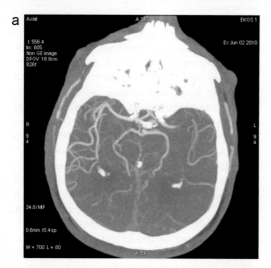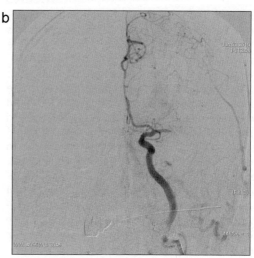

Figure 1 Occlusion of middle cerebral artery detected by computed tomography angiography (a) and digital subtraction angiography (b).

for intra-arterial administration of drugs (e.g. thrombolytics) terminated with the emitter of ultrasonic waves. It emits ultrasound waves with the frequency between 1.7 and 2.35 MHz and with the emitted intensity of 400 mW/cm^2 into the thrombus. The first clinical studies with endovascular sono-lysis were used for the coronary arteries. In the ACUTE (Analysis of Coronary Ultrasound Thrombolysis Endpoints in Acute Myocardial Infarction) study, the low-frequency (45 kHz) ultrasound with a high intensity (18 W/cm^2) was used in acute coronary artery occlusion [52]. Complete recanalization was achieved in 87% patients. No side effects were observed during the therapy and 80% of patients showed clinical improvement.

Other studies showed the effect of endovascular ultrasound-lysis by EKOS system in patients with deep venous thrombosis of lower extremities and in patients with pulmonary embolism [53—56].

Mahon et al. [57] published the first experience with endovascular sono-lysis using the EKOS system in patients with acute IS. They used a combination of IAT using rt-PA with endovascular ultrasound applied continuously for 60 min in 10 patients with MCA occlusion and in 4 patients with BA occlusion. Partial or complete recanalization was detected in 57% patients and there were no adverse effects observed during the therapy.

The authors also performed a prospective mono-centric study aimed to confirm a safety and efficacy of intravascular sono-lysis using EKOS system® with 3F microcatheter EkoSonic and 2.05—2.35 MHz ultrasound frequencies for the recanalization of brain arteries in acute stroke patients within an 8-h time window.

Material and methods

The pilot, prospective, observational, single center study of consecutive patients presenting with acute stroke symptoms and radiologically confirmed MCA or BA occlusion was performed. The entire study was conducted in accordance with the Helsinki Declaration of 1975 (as revised in 1983, 2004 and 2008). It was approved by the Local Ethics Committee of University Hospital Ostrava. All subjects signed informed consent. In case of technical problems with regard to signing, their signature was also verified by an independent witness.

Patients with (1) acute IS, (2) NIHSS score of 10—24 points on admission, (3) MCA or BA occlusion detected by computed tomography (CT) angiography and digital subtraction angiography (DSA) (Fig. 1a and b), (4) admitted and treated within 8 h since stroke onset, and with (5) signed informed consent were consecutively enrolled to the study during 12 months.

Exclusion criteria were (1) previous disability, (2) intracranial bleeding or tumor on brain CT, (3) infarction on brain CT in more than 2/3 of the MCA territory, and (4) partial or complete recanalization of brain artery after IVT treatment detected using transcranial duplex sonography.

A physical examination, blood samples, electrocardiogram, chest X-ray, and standard neurologic evaluation by a certified neurologist using the NIHSS were performed on admission followed by brain CT and CT angiography (CTA) of cervical and intracranial arteries. Patients underwent standard treatment [58,59]. Patients who fulfilled SITS-MOST criteria [60] for IVT were treated using rt-PA intravenously (0.9 mg/kg) within 4.5 h since stroke onset. Secondary preventive therapy was administered according to the European Stroke Organisation guidelines [59].

Endovascular sono-lysis using EKOS system

The interventional procedure started with arterial puncture via femoral approach. At the beginning of the procedure, heparin was administered intraarterially (50 IU/kg). Then, the 6F sheath insertion was performed with standard Seldinger technique. All patients underwent 4-vessel diagnostic angiography with 4 or 5F pre-shaped catheters inserted over the 0.035 in. diameter hydrophilic wires. The 6F guiding catheter was introduced subsequently into the target brain supplying vessel over the same hydrophilic wire and microcatheter with a support of a 0.014 in./300 microwire was advanced behind the occluded intracranial vessel segment. Occlusion of MCA or BA was classified according to the Thrombolysis in Cerebral Ischemie (TICI)

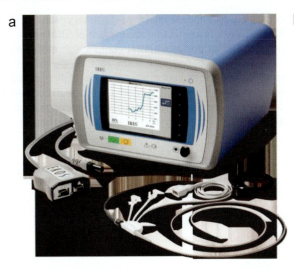 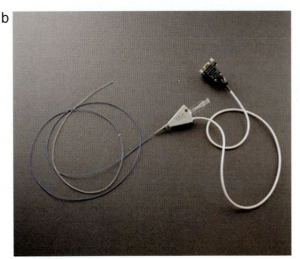

Figure 2 EKOS system.

criteria. The intraluminal position of the microcatheter was always checked. All catheters were continuously flushed with heparinized saline. The microcatheter was then replaced with the EKOS endovascular catheter terminated with the emitter of ultrasonic waves and connected to the central unit. The EndoWave System manufactured by EKOS Corporation (Bothell, WA, USA) was used (Fig. 2a and b). It consists of a 5.2F, 106 cm long infusion catheter, an ultrasound core wire, and a control unit with catheter interface cables. The ultrasound wire delivers pulsed high frequency (1.7—2.1 MHz) and low-intensity (400 mW/cm^2) ultrasound waves. Special care was taken for the location of a tip of the catheter into the occluded segment of the artery (Fig. 3). Both the insonation and the local administration of tPA directly into the thrombus were simultaneously started. In this study, a dose of 15 mg/h of tPA was delivered by an infusion pump with a maximal calculated total dosage not exceeding 20 mg of tPA.

Patients with partial recanalization after EKOS treatment were further treated by angioplasty and stent implantation.

Radiological and clinical evaluation

The recanalization status at the end of DSA was evaluated by blinded independent radiologist using the TICI criteria. TICI IIc and III were evaluated as complete recanalization (Fig. 4), TICI IIa and IIb were evaluated as partial recanalization.

Neurological and physical examinations were done before therapy start and 24 h, 30 and 90 days after the start of treatment. Certified neurologist performed evaluation of neurological symptoms using NIHSS in all visits. Modified Rankin score was used for the evaluation of disability at days

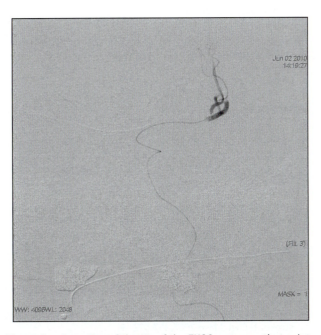 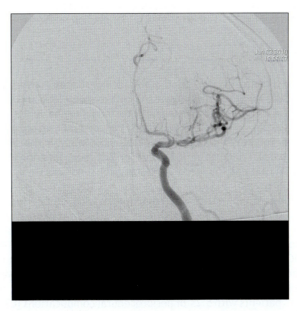

Figure 3 Insertion of the tip of the EKOS system catheter into the occluded segment of the artery.

Figure 4 Complete recanalization at the end of sono-lysis using EKOS system.

30 and 90. Good clinical outcome was defined as a mRS 0—3, poor clinical outcome as a mRS 4—6.

All adverse events were recorded. All changes in physical examinations, worsening of neurological symptoms (>4 points in NIHSS) and all disorders prolonging or requiring hospitalization were recorded as adverse events.

Intracranial bleeds detected in the control brain CT examination 24 h after therapy onset were recorded. Intracranial bleeding with worsening of neurological symptoms > 4 points in the NIHSS were evaluated as SICH (ECASS 3 criteria). Other intracranial bleeds were evaluated as asymptomatic intracranial hemorrhage (AICH).

In the control brain CT scan, detected brain edema associated with worsening of neurological symptoms > 4 points in the NIHSS was evaluated as "symptomatic".

Statistical analysis

Data with a normal distribution was reported as mean ± standard deviation. All parameters not fitting to a normal distribution were presented as median and range. Statistical analyses were performed using SPSS 14.0 software (SPSS Inc., Chicago, IL, USA).

Results

Nine patients (6 males, 3 females) were included in the pilot study. The age range was 51—80, mean 65.0 ± 10.4 years. NIHSS on admission was 10—33 with median of 19.0 points. Five patients suffered from MCA occlusion, 4 patients form BA occlusion. Mean time onset-to-treatment was 282 ± 184 min.

Complete recanalization at the end of EKOS treatment was achieved in 3 (33%) and partial in 4 (44%) patients, resp. Mean time between diagnostic angiography and artery recanalization was 108.1 ± 39.9 min. No SICH or symptomatic brain edema were detected on control CT.

Median NIHSS at the end of EKOS treatment was 17.0 points. After 24 h, the median NIHSS was 12.0 and 7 days after stroke onset 6.0 points, resp. Four (44%) patients were independent at 3 months (mRS 0—3); median mRS was 4.

Discussion

The results of the pilot study demonstrated safety of endovascular sono-lysis using the EKOS system. SICH and also malignant infarction were not detected in any patient.

Partial or complete recanalization of brain artery was achieved in 77% patients in the presented study. In the similar study, Mahon et al. [57] achieved any recanalization only in 57% patients treated by endovascular sono-lysis using the EKOS system.

Presented results are comparable with other studies using mechanical methods for brain artery recanalization. In the MultiMerci study the partial or complete recanalization was achieved in 55% patients with 9.8% occurrence of SICH [61]. Higher recanalization rate was demonstrated in the study with Penumbra system. Partial recanalization was achieved in 54% patients and complete recanalization in 33% patients with 5.7% of periprocedural complications [62]. However, the highest recanalization rates were achieved using the Solitaire stents. In the recent studies, partial or complete recanalization of brain artery was achieved in 88—90% patients with the occurrence of SICH of 2—17% and less than 8% of periprocedural complications [63—66].

Although the recanalization rate in published studies using new devices was quite high and still increasing, the number of independent patients did not exceed 60%. 44% patients in the presented study were independent 90 days after stroke onset. In the previously mentioned studies, 31—59% patients were independent at day 90 with mRS 0—3 [61—66].

Several limitations of the presented study should be mentioned. This was a single center observational pilot study. The main goal was to assess the safety of endovascular sono-lysis. Evaluation of artery recanalization is still very subjective even though the vascular status was evaluated by blinded radiologist in the presented study.

In the future, the randomized multicenter study has to be performed to confirm a potential effect of endovascular sono-lysis on the acceleration of artery recanalization.

Conclusion

Sono-lysis is a promising method of treatment of acute IS. This is a relatively safe treatment with a high efficacy in the acceleration of cerebral arteries recanalization. A good availability and a low price are the advantages of transcranial sono-lysis, but its use is limited by the quality of the temporal bone window and the availability of an experienced sonographer. Also endovascular sono-lysis seems to be safe and effective. It is not dependent on the bone window quality, but it is limited by the availability of interventional radiologist. Further double-blind randomized studies are needed to confirm the safety and efficacy of sono-lysis, and especially to determine the optimal frequency, intensity and character of the ultrasonic waves.

Acknowledgements

The study was supported by grant of the Internal Grant Agency of the Ministry of Health of the Czech Republic number NT/11386-5/2010.

References

[1] Feigin VL, Lawes CM, Bennett DA, Anderson CS. Stroke epidemiology: a review of population-based studies of incidence, prevalence, and case-fatality in the late 20th century. Lancet Neurol 2003;2:43—53.

[2] Rosamond W, Flegal K, Furie K, Go A, Greenlund K, Haase N, et al. Heart disease and stroke statistics—2008 update: a report from the American Heart Association Statistics Committee and Stroke Statistics Subcommittee. Circulation 2008;117:e25—146.

[3] Fieschi C, Argentino C, Lenzi GL, Sacchetti ML, Toni D, Bazzao L. Clinical and instrumental evaluation of patients with ischemic stroke within the first six hours. J Neurol Sci 1989;91:311—21.

[4] van der Worp HB, van Gijn J. Clinical practice. Acute ischemic stroke. N Engl J Med 2007;357:572—9.

[5] Rha JH, Saver JL. The impact of recanalization on ischemic stroke outcome: a meta-analysis. Stroke 2007;38:967—73.

[6] Blakeley JO, Llinas RH. Thrombolytic therapy for acute ischemic stroke. J Neurol Sci 2007;261:55—62.

[7] Brott T, Bogousslavsky J. Treatment of acute ischemic stroke. N Engl J Med 2000;343:710—22.

[8] The National Institute of Neurological Disorders and Stroke rt-PA Stroke Study Group. Tissue plasminogen activator for acute ischemic stroke. N Engl J Med 1995;333:1581—7.

[9] Smith WS, Sung G, Starkman S, Saver JL, Kidwell CS, Gobin YP, et al. Safety and efficacy of mechanical embolectomy in acute ischemic stroke: results of the MERCI trial. Stroke 2005;36:1432—8.

[10] Chopko BW, Kerber C, Wong W, Georgy B. Transcatheter snare removal of acute middle cerebral artery thromboembolism: technical case report. Neurosurgery 2000;46:1529—31.

[11] Kerber CW, Barr JD, Berger RM, Chopko BW. Snare retrieval of intracranial thrombus in patients with acute stroke. J Vasc Interv Radiol 2002;13:1269—74.

[12] Fourie P, Duncan IC. Microsnare-assisted mechanical removal of intraprocedural distal middle cerebral arterial thromboembolism. AJNR Am J Neuroradiol 2003;24:630—2.

[13] Schumacher HC, Meyers PM, Yavagal DR, Harel NY, Elkind MS, Mohr JP, et al. Endovascular mechanical thrombectomy of an occluded superior division branch of the left MCA for acute cardioembolic stroke. Cardiovasc Intervent Radiol 2003;26:305—8.

[14] Francis CW, Blinc A, Lee S, Cox C. Ultrasound accelerates transport of recombinant tissue plasminogen activator into clots. Ultrasound Med Biol 1995;21:419—24.

[15] Skoloudík D, Fadrná T, Roubec M, Bar M, Zapletal O, Blatný J, et al. Changes in hemocoagulation in acute stroke patients after one-hour sono-thrombolysis using a diagnostic probe. Ultrasound Med Biol 2010;36:1052—9.

[16] Skoloudík D, Fadrná T, Bar M, Zapletalová O, Zapletal O, Blatný J, et al. Changes in haemocoagulation in healthy volunteers after a 1-hour thrombotripsy using a diagnostic 2—4 MHz transcranial probe. J Thromb Thrombolysis 2008;26:119—24.

[17] Suchkova VN, Baggs RB, Francis CW. Effect of 40-kHz ultrasound on acute thrombotic ischemia in a rabbit femoral artery thrombosis model: enhancement of thrombolysis and improvement in capillary muscle perfusion. Circulation 2000;101:2296—301.

[18] Bardoň P, Skoloudík D, Langová K, Herzig R, Kaňovský P. Changes in blood flow velocity in the radial artery during 1-hour ultrasound monitoring with a 2-MHz transcranial probe—a pilot study. J Clin Ultrasound 2010;38(November—December (9)):493—6.

[19] Harvey EN. Biological aspects of ultrasonic waves, a general survey. Biol Bull 1930;59:306—25.

[20] Siddiqi F, Blinc A, Braaten J, Francis CW. Ultrasound increases flow through fibrin gels. Thromb Haemost 1995;73:495—8.

[21] Braaten JV, Goss RA, Francis CW. Ultrasound reversibly disaggregates fibrin fibers. Thromb Haemost 1997;78:1063—8.

[22] Siegel RJ, Fishbein MC, Forrester J, Moore K, DeCastro E, Daykhovsky L, et al. Ultrasonic plaque ablation. A new method for recanalization of partially or totally occluded arteries. Circulation 1988;78:1443—8.

[23] Rosenschein U, Bernstein JJ, DiSegni E, Kaplinsky E, Bernheim J, Rozenzsajn LA. Experimental ultrasonic angioplasty: disruption of atherosclerotic plaques and thrombi in vitro and arterial recanalization in vivo. J Am Coll Cardiol 1990;15:711—7.

[24] Hong AS, Chae JS, Dubin SB, Lee S, Fishbein MC, Siegel RJ. Ultrasonic clot disruption: an in vitro study. Am Heart J 1990;120:418—22.

[25] Ariani M, Fishbein MC, Chae JS, Sadeghi H, Michael AD, Dubin SB, et al. Dissolution of peripheral arterial thrombi by ultrasound. Circulation 1991;84:1680—8.

[26] Steffen W, Fishbein MC, Luo H, Lee DY, Nita H, Cumberland DC, et al. High intensity, low frequency catheter-delivered ultrasound dissolution of occlusive coronary artery thrombi: an in vitro and in vivo study. J Am Coll Cardiol 1994;24:1571—9.

[27] Francis CW, Onundarson PT, Carstensen EL, Blinc A, Meltzer RS, Schwarz K, et al. Enhancement of fibrinolysis in vitro by ultrasound. J Clin Invest 1992;90:2063—8.

[28] Lauer CG, Burge R, Tang DB, Bass BG, Gomez ER, Alving BM. Effect of ultrasound on tissue-type plasminogen activator-induced thrombolysis. Circulation 1992;86:1257—64.

[29] Luo H, Nishioka T, Fishbein MC, Cercek B, Forrester JS, Kim CJ, et al. Transcutaneous ultrasound augments lysis of arterial thrombi in vivo. Circulation 1996;94:775—8.

[30] Harpaz D, Chen X, Francis CW, Meltzer RS. Ultrasound accelerates urokinase-induced thrombolysis and reperfusion. Am Heart J 1994;127:1211—9.

[31] Harpaz D, Chen X, Francis CW, Marder VJ, Meltzer RS. Ultrasound enhancement of thrombolysis and reperfusion in vitro. J Am Coll Cardiol 1993;21:1507—11.

[32] Olsson SB, Johansson B, Nilsson AM, Olsson C, Roijer A. Enhancement of thrombolysis by ultrasound. Ultrasound Med Biol 1994;20:375—82.

[33] Trübestein G, Engel C, Etzel F, Sobbe A, Cremer H, Stumpff U. Thrombolysis by ultrasound. Clin Sci Mol Med 1976;3(Suppl.):697—8.

[34] Rosenschein U, Frimerman A, Laniado S, Miller HI. Study of the mechanism of ultrasound angioplasty from human thrombi and bovine aorta. Am J Cardiol 1994;74:1263—6.

[35] Tachibana S. Application of ultrasonic vibration for boosting fibrinolytic effect of urokinase in rats. Blood Vessel 1985;16:46—9.

[36] Riggs PN, Francis CW, Bartos SR, Penney DP. Ultrasound enhancement of rabbit femoral artery thrombolysis. Cardiovasc Surg 1997;5:201—7.

[37] Ishibashi T, Akiyama M, Onoue H, Abe T, Furuhata H. Can transcranial ultrasonication increase recanalization flow with tissue plasminogen activator. Stroke 2002;33:1399—404.

[38] Alexandrov AV, Molina CA, Grotta JC, Garami Z, Ford SR, Alvarez-Sabin J, et al. Ultrasound-enhanced systemic thrombolysis for acute ischemic stroke. N Engl J Med 2004;351:2170—8.

[39] Eggers J, Koch B, Meyer K, König I, Seidel G. Effect of ultrasound on thrombolysis of middle cerebral artery occlusion. Ann Neurol 2003;53:797—800.

[40] Skoloudik D, Bar M, Skoda O, Vaclavik D, Hradilek P, Allendoerfer J, et al. Safety and efficacy of the sonographic acceleration of the middle cerebral artery recanalization: results of the pilot thrombotripsy study. Ultrasound Med Biol 2008;34:1775—82.

[41] Eggers J, Seidel G, Koch B, König IR. Sonothrombolysis in acute ischemic stroke for patients ineligible for rt-PA. Neurology 2005;64:1052—4.

[42] Cintas P, Le Traon AP, Larrue V. High rate of recanalization of middle cerebral artery occlusion during 2-MHz transcranial color-coded Doppler continuous monitoring without thrombolytic drug. Stroke 2002;33:626—8.

[43] Sanak D, Herzig R, Skoloudik D, Horák D, Zapletalova J, Köcher M, et al. The safety and efficacy of continuous transcranial duplex Doppler monitoring of middle cerebral artery occlusion in acute stroke patients: comparison of TCDD and thrombolysis in MCA recanalization. J Neuroimaging 2010;20:58—63.

[44] Rubiera M, Ribo M, Delgado-Mederos R, Santamarina E, Maisterra O, Delgado P, et al. Do bubble characteristics affect recanalization in stroke patients treated with microbubble-enhanced sonothrombolysis. Ultrasound Med Biol 2008;34:1573—7.

[45] Perren F, Loulidi J, Poglia D, Landis T, Sztajzel R. Microbubble potentiated transcranial duplex ultrasound enhances IV thrombolysis in acute stroke. J Thromb Thrombolysis 2008;25:219—23.

[46] Alexandrov AV, Mikulik R, Ribo M, Sharma VK, Lao AY, Tsivgoulis G, et al. A pilot randomized clinical safety study of sonothrombolysis augmentation with ultrasound-activated

perfluten-lipid microspheres for acute ischemic stroke. Stroke 2008;39:1464—9.
[47] Dinia L, Rubiera M, Ribo M, Maisterra O, Ortega G, del Sette M, et al. Reperfusion after stroke sonothrombolysis with microbubbles may predict intracranial bleeding. Neurology 2009;73:775—80.
[48] Molina CA, Barreto AD, Tsivgoulis G, Sierzenski P, Malkoff MD, Rubiera M, et al. Transcranial ultrasound in clinical sonothrombolysis [TUCSON] trial. Ann Neurol 2009;66:28—38.
[49] Školoudík D, Fadrná T, Bar M, Zapletalová O, Zapletal O, Blatný J, et al. Changes in fibrinolytic system after continual Doppler monitoring in healthy volunteers. Cesk Slov Neurol N 2009;5:446—52.
[50] Daffertshofer M, Gass A, Ringleb P, Sitzer M, Sliwka U, Els T, et al. Transcranial low-frequency ultrasound-mediated thrombolysis in brain ischemia: increased risk of hemorrhage with combined ultrasound and tissue plasminogen activator: results of a phase II clinical trial. Stroke 2005;36:1441—6.
[51] Reinhard M, Hetzel A, Krüger S, Kretzer S, Talazko J, Ziyeh S, et al. Blood—brain barrier disruption by low-frequency ultrasound. Stroke 2006;37:1546—8.
[52] Rosenschein U, Roth A, Rassin T, Basan S, Laniado S, Miller HI. Analysis of coronary ultrasound thrombolysis endpoints in acute myocardial infarction [ACUTE trial]. Results of the feasibility phase. Circulation 1997;95:1411—6.
[53] Ganguli S, Kalva S, Oklu R, Walker TG, Datta N, Grabowski EF, et al. Efficacy of lower-extremity venous thrombolysis in the setting of congenital absence or atresia of the inferior vena cava. Cardiovasc Intervent Radiol 2011;(August).
[54] Grommes J, Strijkers R, Greiner A, Mahnken AH, Wittens CH. Safety and feasibility of ultrasound-accelerated catheter-directed thrombolysis in deep vein thrombosis. Eur J Vasc Endovasc Surg 2011;41(4):526—32.
[55] Shah KJ, Scileppi RM, Franz RW. Treatment of pulmonary embolism using ultrasound-accelerated thrombolysis directly into pulmonary arteries. Vasc Endovascular Surg 2011;45(6):541—8.
[56] Lin PH, Annambhotla S, Bechara CF, Athamneh H, Weakley SM, Kobayashi K, et al. Comparison of percutaneous ultrasound-accelerated thrombolysis versus catheter-directed thrombolysis in patients with acute massive pulmonary embolism. Vascular 2009;17(Suppl. 3):S137—47.
[57] Mahon BR, Nesbit GM, Barnwell SL, Clark W, Marotta TR, Weill A, et al. North American clinical experience with the EKOS MicroLysUS infusion catheter for the treatment of embolic stroke. AJNR Am J Neuroradiol 2003;24:534—8.
[58] The European Stroke Initiative Executive Committee and the EUSI Writing Committee. European Stroke Initiative recommendations for stroke management — update 2003. Cerebrovasc Dis 2003;16:311—37.
[59] The European Stroke Organisation (ESO) Executive Committee and the ESO Writing Committee. Guidelines for management of ischaemic stroke and transient ischaemic attack 2008. Cerebrovasc Dis 2008;25:457—507.
[60] Toni D, Lorenzano S, Puca E, Prencipe M. The SITS-MOST registry. Neurol Sci 2006;27(Suppl. 3):260—2.
[61] Smith WS, Sung G, Saver J, Budzik R, Duckwiler G, Liebeskind DS, et al. Mechanical thrombectomy for acute ischemic stroke: final results of the Multi MERCI trial. Stroke 2008;39:1205—12.
[62] Tarr R, Hsu D, Kulcsar Z, Bonvin C, Rufenacht D, Alfke K, et al. The POST trial: initial post-market experience of the Penumbra system: revascularization of large vessel occlusion in acute ischemic stroke in the United States and Europe. J Neurointerv Surg 2010;2:341—4.
[63] Machi P, Costalat V, Lobotesis K, Lima Maldonado I, Vendrell JF, Riquelme C, et al. Solitaire FR thrombectomy system: immediate results in 56 consecutive acute ischemic stroke patients. J Neurointerv Surg 2011;(April) [Epub ahead of print].
[64] Stampfl S, Hartmann M, Ringleb PA, Haehnel S, Bendszus M, Rohde S. Stent placement for flow restoration in acute ischemic stroke: a single-center experience with the Solitaire stent system. AJNR Am J Neuroradiol 2011;32:1245—8.
[65] Castaño C, Dorado L, Guerrero C, Millán M, Gomis M, Perez de la Ossa N, et al. Mechanical thrombectomy with the Solitaire AB device in large artery occlusions of the anterior circulation: a pilot study. Stroke 2010;41:1836—40.
[66] Roth C, Papanagiotou P, Behnke S, Walter S, Haass A, Becker C, et al. Stent-assisted mechanical recanalization for treatment of acute intracerebral artery occlusions. Stroke 2010;41:2559—67.

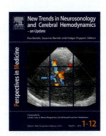

Bartels E, Bartels S, Poppert H (Editors):
New Trends in Neurosonology and Cerebral Hemodynamics — an Update.
Perspectives in Medicine (2012) 1, 73—76

journal homepage: www.elsevier.com/locate/permed

Act on Stroke — Optimization of clinical processes and workflow for stroke diagnosis and treatment

Bernd M. Hofmann [a,*], Udo Zikeli [a], E. Bernd Ringelstein [b]

[a] Siemens AG, Healthcare Sector, Erlangen, Germany
[b] Department of Neurology, University of Münster, Münster, Germany

KEYWORDS
Stroke;
Process optimization;
Outcome;
Quality of care

Summary In the Helsingborg Declaration the continuum of care consisting of pre-, intra- and posthospital organization of stroke services combined with evaluation of outcome measures and dedicated quality assessments was considered as key for best outcome. Despite the evidence of such measures there are still striking disparities in organized stroke care all over Europe. Aim of this paper is to describe current concepts used for process optimization in stroke care and to evaluate if methodologies used in industry provide additional benefit in order to address this issue.

We describe the transfer of a commonly accepted industrial maturity model to stroke care addressing structural, process and outcome quality. Moreover, this tool can be used to compare different stroke services and provides valuable information for their optimization by transferring best practices from ''best in class'' services as well as for prioritization of improvement measures.
© 2012 Elsevier GmbH. All rights reserved.

Introduction

The burden of stroke is high due to its high incidence, mortality and morbidity [1—4]. In order to reduce this burden, the Helsingborg Declaration has postulated the present and future European goals of stroke care. As a major component of the chain of care, stroke unit treatment was considered essential, and was therefore nominated the ''backbone'' of integrated stroke services. This is clear scientific evidence that outcomes in stroke patients managed in dedicated stroke units are better than those managed in general medical wards [5]. Within one year, stroke unit care leads to significantly reduced death or poor outcome [6]. As a logical consequence, basic requirements were defined for successful stroke unit care, which are multi-professional team approach, acute treatment combined with early mobilization and rehabilitation, as well as an exclusive admission of patients with stroke syndromes to that ward [6]. Moreover, the continuum of stroke care was considered as the key for best outcome consisting of prehospital, intrahospital and posthospital organization of stroke services, also considering secondary prevention, as well as step down rehabilitation after stroke, including measures for evaluation of stroke outcome and dedicated quality assessment [5]. However, there are still striking disparities in organized stroke unit care all over Europe [7—10], and no generally accepted definition of a stroke unit in terms of state-of-the-art requirements of facilities, personal and processes does exist. In order to solve this problem, there are constraints in the

* Corresponding author at: Siemens AG Healthcare Sector, H CX CRM-VA HCC NEURO, Allee am Roethelheimpark 3a, 91058 Erlangen, Germany. Tel.: +49 9131843374.
E-mail address: bernd.m.hofmann@siemens.com (B.M. Hofmann).

European Stroke Organization to define a terminology and shared requirements on a European stroke unit (Ringelstein, personal communication). Hospitals should be encouraged to compete for the best solution, and the most engaged ones should serve as guides and frontiers for stroke unit development. In addition, a recent consensus paper [11] requested to improve and develop the systems of international cooperation in stroke research, and to implement key elements into clinical pathways which are identified to be beneficial in stroke treatment. Moreover, it was postulated to identify and implement standardized clinical and surrogate assessments and to accelerate the capacity to address unmet needs. This could be done by scanning other areas of science in order to enhance the likelihood of generating new ideas and concepts.

In industries the optimization of infrastructure and processes and the determination of so-called key performance indicators in order to proof the efficacy of improvement measures is standard since many years. By extending the above stroke-related requests, the aim of this paper is to evaluate whether concepts can be transferred from industry to healthcare in order to support optimization processes in stroke unit care.

Methodology

In a first step, current concepts used worldwide for the optimization of stroke treatment were analyzed regarding their efficacy. Possible reasons for suboptimal results from these measures were extracted. In a second step, generally available methodologies for process optimization used in industry were analyzed with respect to their transfer into healthcare systems. In particular, we analyzed which requirements have to be met by those methodologies in order to be transferred successfully, how the relevant clinical and scientific content could be identified and implemented as basis for optimization. We also elaborated how clinical and scientific evidence of the content and improvement potentials could be ensured.

Results

Clinical guidelines were found to be the most important sources for optimizing stroke care and have to be obeyed in all circumstances. This is due to their scientific and clinical evidence. Some hospitals, however, do not support to implement them into clinical routine in an effective matter jeopardizing their impact. Programs monitoring guideline adherence are addressing this issue but do not provide enough support for systematic implementation.

Several national certification programs are based on guidelines, but rather assess the structural quality of a stroke service than the process and the improvement of treatment quality and clinical outcome; although it has been shown in a recent publication that certification efforts can lead to better clinical outcome [12]. A new certification program proposed by the European Stroke Organization will overcome some of the above mentioned shortages and will monitor outcome parameters. Guidance for hospitals willing to improve their processes, however, will still be required for a sufficient implementation of clinical guidelines into routine processes.

The effect of programs measuring quality or performance indicators is still under debate [13] and they often focus too much on the formal fulfillment of requirements like prescription and dispensation of anticoagulants, or statins as well as the early rehabilitation assessment, but are not helpful in defining how to increase the performance level [14]. The underlying processes to ensure the fulfillment of given requirements and regulations have to be defined and implemented by the hospital staff.

Quality management systems like ISO, EFQM and TQM evaluate structures and processes but do not assess the related outcome. They were first used in industry and transferred to healthcare systems thereafter. The necessity that an individual organization has to define its own quality goals, as well as the processes to achieve them, could be considered as a weakness. Moreover, those programs are addressing entire hospitals rather than specific diseases or functional units.

Pure industrial process optimization programs are addressing processes without considering best practices from other organizations. After defining their own quality goals, the processes to achieve them have to be developed by the organization itself.

Finally, process consulting is helpful in order to solve individual problems, and best practice transfer is the basis of this type of optimization. Most consulting projects are very long lasting, however, and put a high burden of the organization regarding human resources.

According to our experience, all above-mentioned programs are addressing relevant parts of clinical process optimization in stroke care. None of them provides a holistic solution, however. Reviewing the literature, Donabedian [15] has defined three different qualities in medical care describing the basis for optimization in stroke care. The *structural quality* is covered by guideline adherence. In this context it is important that the guidelines are defined by the medical societies and based on clinical and scientific evidence. However, the guidelines have to be implemented into clinical processes resulting in a positive impact on *process quality*. By combining both efforts, the quality of care is expected to increase but this effect has to be monitored in order the proof *outcome quality*.

In order to address these three qualities, a methodology for process optimization in stroke care has to include all the relevant clinical guidelines and to reflect the organizational structure which is defined by specific guidelines. Moreover, such a methodology has to have the capability to support optimization of clinical processes addressed by management consulting tools. Additionally, transfer of best practices will be helpful in achieving this goal. Our focus should be on support processes as well, which contributes in improving the process quality, e.g. providing optimized imaging infrastructure. An essential part is also to measure quality parameters thus addressing structural, procedural and outcome performance indicators.

Keeping all these requirements in mind, so called ''process maturity models'' seem to best meet our needs. They are generally accepted in software industry or aeronautics. The calculation of a provider's maturity level which is an integral part allows even benchmarking between hospitals and can be used to define best practices and to facilitate their transfer. Thereafter, Process improvements can be derived from those best practices best practices. Combining this methodology with intelligent approaches for simulation, prioritization between different improvement measures becomes possible.

Because industrial maturity models are based on a virtual best practice combination composed of real-world practice elements from various organizations, the question arises how this principle can be applied to healthcare systems. In our clinical maturity model named "Act on Stroke", we implemented all relevant clinical guidelines, as well as latest results in stroke research based on clinical and scientific evidence. We performed best practice visits in institutions well known for their excellent stroke service and included experience from more than 400 consulting projects in healthcare. In the end, our data resulted in a clinical maturity model addressing optimized stroke care.

Best practice visits and pilot projects in hospitals with experienced department heads in stroke care were performed and provided further promising results which again were introduced into the methodology. Indeed, heads of the departments certified that all relevant strengths and weaknesses of their services have been identified by using this clinical maturity model. Proposals for process improvements have also been helpful to them. Meanwhile, the first regular projects have been carried out successfully, and the results are currently in preparation for publication.

Discussion

For more than 40 years, maturity models have been helpful in software industry in order to improve processes and, as a consequence, leading to better outcomes. This principle has been used for the optimization of clinical processes, as well. Healthcare is dealing with human beings, however, has and the applicability of industrial processes had to be discussed carefully.

The content for the definition of the virtual best practice is of clinical and scientific relevance, and it has to be specified who defines it. From our point of view this should be done as a joint venture by experienced stroke physicians in cooperation with specialists experienced in process optimization. Care has to be taken that the patient's needs and the adherence to clinical guidelines are the most important and that the maturity level is respecting this. A not yet fully solved problem is how to deal with improvement measures to processes or requirements not yet based on clinical evidence. It has been shown [16,17] that improvement of key measures lead to better outcome even if they are as such not based on large randomized trials. The fact that some requirements are based on clinical evidence while others are not, has to be met by the particular methodology of "Act on Stroke" and a solution for this issue has been implemented.

In contrast to the linear nature of industrial processes, processes in healthcare are more complex and can be influenced by hard to control parameters. For this reason, it is not always possible to directly assess the impact of a single optimization measure, because a given factor influencing a certain process does not do so in different hospitals. As a consequence, the efficacy of our model has to be proven first in pilot projects, in particular with respect to clinical outcomes.

The authors have developed a clinical maturity model providing answers to the above mentioned questions. They carried out several pilot projects for proof of principle and with the intention of individual process optimization. A detailed description of the methodology and the encouraging results of the first projects are currently under evaluation and will be published in a separate paper.

Conclusion

Industry can provide useful tools for supporting the optimization of quality of care and outcome in stroke treatment. This can be achieved by a standardized and unbiased assessment of hospital infrastructure, improved processes of stroke care and comparison of outcome performance from "best in class" services.

References

[1] Feigin VL, Lawes CM, Bennett DA, Barker-Collo SL, Parag V. Worldwide stroke incidence and early case fatality reported in 56 population-based studies: a systematic review. Lancet Neurology 2009;8(4):355—69.

[2] Lloyd-Jones D, Adams R, Carnethon M, De Simone G, Ferguson TB, Flegal K, et al. Heart disease and stroke statistics—2009 update: a report from the American Heart Association Statistics Committee and Stroke Statistics Subcommittee. Circulation 2009;119(3):480—6.

[3] Lopez AD, Mathers CD, Ezzati M, Jamison DT, Murray CJ. Global and regional burden of disease and risk factors 2001 systematic analysis of population health data. Lancet 2006;367(9524):1747—57.

[4] Truelsen T, Piechowski-Jozwiak B, Bonita R, Mathers C, Bogousslavsky J, Boysen G. Stroke incidence and prevalence in Europe: a review of available data. European Journal of Neurology 2006;13(6):581—98.

[5] Kjellstrom T, Norrving B, Shatchkute A. Helsingborg Declaration 2006 on European stroke strategies. Cerebrovascular Diseases (Basel, Switzerland) 2007;23(2—3):231—41.

[6] Seenan P, Long M, Langhorne P. Stroke units in their natural habitat: systematic review of observational studies. Stroke; A Journal of Cerebral Circulation 2007;38(6):1886—92.

[7] Grieve R, Hutton J, Bhalla A, Rastenyte D, Ryglewicz D, Sarti C, et al. A comparison of the costs and survival of hospital-admitted stroke patients across Europe. Stroke; A Journal of Cerebral Circulation 2001;32(7):1684—91.

[8] Leys D, Cordonnier C, Debette S, Hacke W, Ringelstein EB, Giroud M, et al. Facilities available in French hospitals treating acute stroke patients: comparison with 24 other European countries. Journal of Neurology 2009;256(6):867—73.

[9] Leys D, Ringelstein EB, Kaste M, Hacke W. Facilities available in European hospitals treating stroke patients. Stroke; A Journal of Cerebral Circulation 2007;38(11):2985—91.

[10] Ringelstein EB, Meckes-Ferber S, Hacke W, Kaste M, Brainin M, Leys D. European stroke facilities survey: the German and Austrian perspective. Cerebrovascular Diseases (Basel, Switzerland) 2009;27(2):138—45.

[11] Hachinski V, Donnan GA, Gorelick PB, Hacke W, Cramer SC, Kaste M, et al. Stroke: working toward a prioritized world agenda. Cerebrovascular Diseases (Basel, Switzerland) 2010;30(2):127—47.

[12] Lichtman JH, Jones SB, Wang Y, Watanabe E, Leifheit-Limson E, Goldstein LB. Outcomes after ischemic stroke for hospitals with

and without Joint Commission-certified primary stroke centers. Neurology 2011;76(23):1976–82.
[13] Fonarow GC, Gregory T, Driskill M, Stewart MD, Beam C, Butler J, et al. Hospital certification for optimizing cardiovascular disease and stroke quality of care and outcomes. Circulation 2010;122(23):2459–69.
[14] Fonarow GC, Reeves MJ, Smith EE, Saver JL, Zhao X, Olson DW, et al. Characteristics, performance measures, and in-hospital outcomes of the first one million stroke and transient ischemic attack admissions in get with the guidelines-stroke. Circulation: Cardiovascular Quality and Outcomes 2010;3(3):291–302.
[15] Donabedian A. Evaluating the quality of medical care. Milbank Memorial Fund Quarterly 1966;44(3 Suppl):166–206.
[16] Bradley EH, Herrin J, Wang Y, Barton BA, Webster TR, Mattera JA, et al. Strategies for reducing the door-to-balloon time in acute myocardial infarction. The New England Journal of Medicine 2006;355(22):2308–20.
[17] Lindsberg PJ, Happola O, Kallela M, Valanne L, Kuisma M, Kaste M. Door to thrombolysis: ER reorganization and reduced delays to acute stroke treatment. Neurology 2006;67(2):334–6.

Telestroke — How does that work?

Sandra Boy

Department of Neurology, University of Regensburg, Bezirksklinikum Regensburg, Universitätsstrasse 84, 93053 Regensburg, Germany

KEYWORDS
Stroke;
Telemedicine;
TEMPiS network

Summary The significance of cerebrovascular disorders is steadily increasing due to the demographic changes in western industrial societies. Therefore the implementation of telemedical networks seems tempting to improve deliverance of specialised stroke care in non-urban areas. Networks like TEMPiS, located in the rural area of south-eastern Bavaria, have shown to deliver high experienced stroke therapy to underserved areas.

Mandatory for a high quality of supply is the appropriate technical equipment. Moreover, beside the teleconsultations, a continuous training should be performed. Mobile solutions allow more flexibility for the teleconsultants.
© 2012 Elsevier GmbH. All rights reserved.

Introduction

Cerebrovascular disorders, specifically ischemic stroke, remain the third most common cause of death and leading cause of disability [1]. Its significance is steadily increasing due to the demographic changes in western industrial societies. The introduction of IV thrombolysis with recombinant tissue plasminogen activator (rtPA) more than a decade ago was a milestone in stroke therapy; however, still only a minority of patients all over Europe and the world benefit from this treatment, especially due to the narrow time window [2—5]. Moreover, thrombolysis as well as stroke-unit treatment, which also has been proven to be beneficial in stroke treatment [6], needs expertise and experience. Especially rural areas are lacking of this expertise. Therefore the implementation of telemedical networks seems tempting to improve deliverance of specialised stroke care in non-urban areas. Several studies have shown, that remote neurological examination via videoconferencing is reliable and feasible [7—11]. Also the accuracy of teleradiologic assessment of computerized tomography (CT) scans in acute stroke by neurologists with access to Digital Imaging and Communications in Medicine (DICOM) format data has been shown [12].

In essence, the implementation of telemedical networks more patients should be able to reach a hospital providing specialised stroke care more quickly and the quality of stroke care in these hospitals should be improved due to the close cooperation between stroke centres and network hospitals.

The TEMPiS-Network

In Germany, Bavaria is a typical example for a rural area with only a few specialised stroke units. However, in congested urban areas the density of stroke units appears adequate, the south-eastern part of Bavaria, a very non-urban area, lacks adequate stroke unit care.

Therefore the Telemedic Pilot Project for Integrative Stroke Care (TEMPiS) Network was founded with the aim to provide modern stroke management and advanced stroke expertise in these rural areas. It was supported by the Bavarian health insurance companies, the Bavarian State Ministry for Employment and Social Order, Family and Women, and the German Stroke Foundation.

E-mail address: sandra.boy@medbo.de

It consists of a cooperation of two academic hospitals (Department of Neurology, University of Regensburg, Bezirksklinikum Regensburg and Klinikum Harlaching, Städtisches Klinikum München GmbH) specialised in acute stroke care with 12 (meanwhile 15) community hospitals serving for acute stroke care in the local population.

Before implementation of the network in 2003, none of these community hospitals provided specialised stroke care. Each community hospital implemented a stroke ward, consisting of up to eight beds, about half of them equipped with monitors. Community hospitals in the network formed stroke teams consisting of doctors, nurses, physiotherapists, occupational therapists, and speech therapists. All members of the stroke team underwent continuous medical training beginning with a 4-day course based on international stroke treatment guidelines. This was followed by onsite visits of specialised stroke nurses and stroke neurologists for individual training. Additionally, the stroke teams had centrally conducted courses in transcranial Doppler sonography, swallowing disorders and dysphagia treatment.

A 24 h teleconsultation service is currently provided by the two stroke centres. The telemedical system consists of a digital network including a 2-way video conference and CT/MRI-image transfer using a high-speed-data transmission (transferring the pictures of the CT-scan within seconds). Stroke experts are contacted while the patient is still in the emergency department. The expert, using the 2-way video conference, can talk to the patient directly and examine the patient with the help of the local physician. Within minutes the expert can now decide whether or not a thrombolysis therapy is indicated. This service has a job chart with colleagues who are in the process of advanced specialist training in neurology and have got at least 1 year of experience in acute stroke unit management. They work in 24 h shifts located in the stroke centres [13–15].

Effectiveness of TEMPiS

To investigate the effectiveness of telemedical stroke networking, five community hospitals without pre-existing specialised stroke care were compared to network hospitals in a non-randomised, open intervention study. The five community hospitals were matched individually to the network hospitals. Between 2003 and 2005 stroke patients who were admitted consecutively to one of the participating hospitals, were included in the study. Patients in network and control hospitals were assessed in the same manner and were followed up for vital status, living situation, and disability at 3 months. Poor outcome was defined by death, institutional care, or disability (Barthel index <60 or modified Rankin scale >3).

After 3 months there was a substantial difference of about 10% on patient's risk of death, institutionalisation, or severe disability between those treated in the network hospitals compared with those receiving usual care. Thrombolytic therapy was provided in about 5% of patients of the network compared with 0.4% of those in control hospitals. This means that use of rtPA in network hospitals was increased 10-fold. Safety data showed that administration of rtPA within the TEMPiS network is safe. The rate of symptomatic haemorrhage of 9% and in-hospital mortality of 10% is in line with other safety data outside clinical trials [14–16].

But effectiveness was not only shown in comparison with community hospitals but as well with stroke centres. Between 2003 and 2004, 170 patients received rtPA in the network hospitals and 132 patients in the two stroke centres. Baseline data of these patients were comparable. Mortality rates as well as good functional outcome after 6 months did not differ in patients treated in network community hospitals or in stroke centres [17].

Mobile solutions

Teleconsultation may not be limited to workstations in the hospital requiring the continuous presence of a stroke neurologist in the hospital since TEMPiS provides an immediate answer to stroke calls made from network hospitals and start of the video conference within 3 min. Since mobile network computers are increasingly available, we investigated the quality of mobile versus stationary telemedical stroke consultation.

Between June and August 2007 a total of 223 teleconsultations with video-examination were conducted. Significant differences were assessed for teleconsultants' ratings of video and audio quality with better results for the hospital-based system and worse audio quality for the ratings from doctors in the local hospitals for the mobile teleconsultations. However, the overall quality of the teleconsultations taking the patient perspective was not different and the clinical relevance of teleconsultations was rated high for both forms of teleconsultations.

Therefore mobile teleconsultation using the available European mobile network technology provides good feasibility and stability.

Whether a mobile or a hospital based solution is preferred may also depend on individual structures of networks and the frequency of teleconsultations. As during nighttimes the number of teleconsultations is lower [18], here the mobile solution may be favoured in order to reduce hospital nights of teleconsultants and costs of staffing [19].

Technical requirements

Telemedic stroke care should provide more than just expert phone care or teleradiology but combine real-time video conference and electronic transmission of cerebral imaging data.

Phone based stroke and rtPA care only have been shown to lead to a poorer outcome and higher mortality compared to patients treated in specialised stroke wards [20].

For high quality and stable videoconferences connections with a stable bandwidth of at least 300 kb/s and cameras with remote control, rotation and zoom functions should be used. For adequate assessment of CT or MRI scans digital data (DICOM), which provide better quality and allows post processing of the images, should be obtained. In community hospitals and even more important in stroke centres large monitors with a high resolution are needed [21]. After every single teleconsultation a written report should be sent to the remote hospital and be preserved just like the standards for in-patient documents.

TEMPiS today

To date more than 6000 patients suffering from stroke have been treated in the 15 hospitals of the TEMPiS-network every year. Meanwhile the TEMPiS has emerged from a scientific stroke research project to regular patient care, and the health insurances cover the costs by reimbursing the remote hospitals, which in turn finance the costs of the consulting stroke centres. Since 2003, more than 25,000 teleconsultations have been performed and more than 2200 patients received thrombolysis. In Germany today the percentage of acute stroke patients receiving rtPA is about 10 percent (www.dsg-info.de), whereas in the TEMPiS network it is 13.8%.

In addition, the TEMPiS-network not only provides telemedical advice. The ongoing stroke education, provided to the network hospitals due to on-site visits with ward rounds, standardised clinical procedures, actualised every year and updates, performed twice a year in order to update knowledge concerning new therapeutic options.

The network also provides training courses for young clinicians in network hospitals regarding acute stroke therapy. Hereby face-to-face contact is facilitated, which lowers the barriers to requests for a teleconsultation and transports stroke knowledge in both directions. Quality assurance is given by follow-up presentations in critical patients.

But not only rtPA treatment in acute stroke is improved in rural areas. As there are new options in acute stroke therapy like neuroradiological interventions as thrombectomy and treatment of complications like hemicraniectomy in malignant infarctions, therapies just available in specialised stroke centres, patients in rural areas can profit from telemedic networks as well. Due to the videoconference and assessment of CT and MRI images patients requiring more than standard stroke care can be identified and transferred to stroke centres with the opportunity to provide these therapeutic options.

Summary

In summary, only a minority of stroke patients all over Europe receive thrombolytic and specialised stroke unit therapy. Due to telemedic approaches like the TEMPiS-network, patients, especially in rural areas can now receive highly specialized stroke treatment. Therefore a high quality of the technical equipment is needed and beside the teleconsultations a continuous training should be performed to achieve high quality.

References

[1] Heart disease and stroke statistics – 2006 update. Dallas: American Heart Association; 2006.
[2] Clark WM, Wissman S, Albers GW, Jhamandas JH, Madden KP, Hamilton S. Recombinant tissue-type plasminogen activator (alteplase) for ischemic stroke 3 to 5 hours after symptom onset. The Atlantis study: a randomized controlled trial. Alteplase thrombolysis for acute noninterventional therapy in ischemic stroke. JAMA 1999;282:2019–26.
[3] Albers GW, Olivot JM. Intravenous alteplase for ischaemic stroke. Lancet 2007;369:249–50.
[4] Hacke W, Kaste M, Bluhmki E, Brozman M, Davalos A, Guidetti D, et al. Thrombolysis with alteplase 3 to 4.5 hours after acute ischemic stroke. N Engl J Med 2008;359:1317–29.
[5] Alberts MJ, Brass LM, Perry A, Webb D, Dawson DV. Evaluation times for patients with in-hospital strokes. Stroke 1993;24:1817–22.
[6] Organised inpatient (stroke unit) care for stroke. Cochrane Database Syst Rev; 2007 [CD000197].
[7] Meyer BC, Raman R, Chacon MR, Jensen M, Werner JD. Reliability of site-independent telemedicine when assessed by telemedicine-naive stroke practitioners. J Stroke Cerebrovasc Dis 2008;17:181–6.
[8] Shafqat S, Kvedar JC, Guanci MM, Chang Y, Schwamm LH. Role for telemedicine in acute stroke. Feasibility and reliability of remote administration of the NIH stroke scale. Stroke 1999;30:2141–5.
[9] Meyer BC, Lyden PD, Al-Khoury L, Cheng Y, Raman R, Fellman R, et al. Prospective reliability of the stroke doc wireless/site independent telemedicine system. Neurology 2005;64:1058–60.
[10] Wang S, Lee SB, Pardue C, Ramsingh D, Waller J, Gross H, et al. Remote evaluation of acute ischemic stroke: reliability of national institutes of health stroke scale via telestroke. Stroke 2003;34:e188–91.
[11] Handschu R, Littmann R, Reulbach U, Gaul C, Heckmann JG, Neundorfer B, et al. Telemedicine in emergency evaluation of acute stroke: interrater agreement in remote video examination with a novel multimedia system. Stroke 2003;34:2842–6.
[12] Johnston KC, Worrall BB. Teleradiology assessment of computerized tomographs online reliability study (tractors) for acute stroke evaluation. Telemed J E Health 2003;9:227–33.
[13] Audebert HJ, Wimmer ML, Schenkel J, Ulm K, Kolominsky-Rabas PL, Bogdahn U, et al. Telemedicine stroke department network. Introduction of a telemedicine pilot project for integrated stroke management in south Bavaria and analysis of its efficiency. Nervenarzt 2004;75:161–5.
[14] Audebert HJ, Kukla C, Clarmann von Claranau S, Kuhn J, Vatankhah B, Schenkel J, et al. Telemedicine for safe and extended use of thrombolysis in stroke: the telemedic pilot project for integrative stroke care (TEMPiS) in Bavaria. Stroke 2005;36:287–91.
[15] Audebert HJ, Schenkel J, Heuschmann PU, Bogdahn U, Haberl RL. Effects of the implementation of a telemedical stroke network: the telemedic pilot project for integrative stroke care (TEMPiS) in Bavaria, Germany. Lancet Neurol 2006;5:742–8.
[16] Audebert HJ, Kukla C, Vatankhah B, Gotzler B, Schenkel J, Hofer S, et al. Comparison of tissue plasminogen activator administration management between telestroke network hospitals and academic stroke centers: the telemedical pilot project for integrative stroke care in Bavaria/Germany. Stroke 2006;37:1822–7.
[17] Schwab S, Vatankhah B, Kukla C, Hauchwitz M, Bogdahn U, Furst A, et al. Long-term outcome after thrombolysis in telemedical stroke care. Neurology 2007;69:898–903.
[18] Vatankhah B, Schenkel J, Furst A, Haberl RL, Audebert HJ. Telemedically provided stroke expertise beyond normal working hours. The telemedical project for integrative stroke care. Cerebrovasc Dis 2008;25:332–7.
[19] Audebert HJ, Boy S, Jankovits R, Pilz P, Klucken J, Fehm NP, et al. Is mobile teleconsulting equivalent to hospital-based telestroke services? Stroke 2008;39:3427–30.
[20] Frey JL, Jahnke HK, Goslar PW, Partovi S, Flaster MS. TPA by telephone: extending the benefits of a comprehensive stroke center. Neurology 2005;64:154–6.
[21] Telestroke AH. Effective networking. Lancet Neurol 2006;5:279–82.

Ultrasound fusion imaging

Jeffrey Stoll

Siemens Ultrasound, Mountain View, CA, USA

KEYWORDS
Fusion;
CT;
MRI;
Biopsy;
Workflow

Summary Confident interpretation of image data is critical for the success of complex cases. By enabling the simultaneous live navigation of reference series, such as CT, MRI and PET, side-by-side with live ultrasound, fusion imaging enables the physician to directly correlate anatomy between modalities. This display facilitates interpretation of ultrasound and communication of findings.
© 2012 Elsevier GmbH. All rights reserved.

Ultrasound fusion is an emerging technique in the field of abdominal imaging with translation possibilities to neuroradiology. This technique involves the co-registered display of live ultrasound with a reference series from another modality, such as CT, MRI or PET [1,2]. As the ultrasound exam is performed the fusion system continuously generates reformatted planes from the reference series matching the oblique imaging planes of the ultrasound transducer. The reformatted planes are displayed either as an overlay or side-by-side with the live ultrasound (Figs. 1 and 2). This display enhances interpretation of ultrasound by enabling a direct comparison with the reference images from the same view angle.

The combined use of different modalities for definitive diagnosis is common. Ultrasound, for instance, is useful to assess indeterminate lesions identified in CT or MRI. A confident diagnosis can be made if a clear correlation can be made between ultrasound and the preceding series. However, if a physician is not confident that ultrasound has found the correct lesion, the case may be further referred to another modality with increased time, cost and potentially mixed results. Fusion imaging enables greater confidence in establishing a clear correlation between modalities by visualizing the same anatomy from the same view angle. Ultrasound is also useful for guiding biopsies for definitive diagnosis. Once again, clear correlation with CT or MRI is required to confidently target a specific lesion. Fusion imaging also has potential as a training tool, similarly allowing trainees to better understand ultrasound in the context of CT or MRI.

Fusion imaging makes use of a tracking system to localize ultrasound transducers and other devices relative to the patient. Optical and electromagnetic systems are available, the latter being most commonly used. Various software tools are also used to bring the reference series into alignment with the tracking system for fusion display [3–6]. Research into these tools has been ongoing for approximately 20 years. Clinical implementation of fusion imaging has suffered, however, due to the time required to achieve adequate alignment using traditional methods. Recent advancements in automatic image analysis may potentially reduce this time greatly.

Tracking sensors are also incorporated into some interventional devices such as introducers and ablation needles, enabling the display of needle location as an overlay on live ultrasound images (Fig. 2). This display can be useful for overcoming difficulties in visualizing needles during ultrasound-guided procedures [7]. Such devices may allow procedures to be completed more quickly and with fewer placement attempts, particularly for more complex cases (Fig. 3).

E-mail addresses: jeffrey.stoll@siemens.com, jeff.stoll@gmail.com

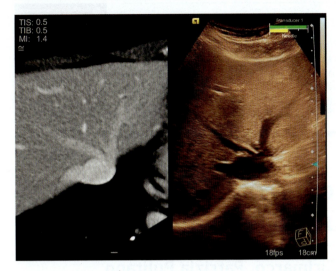

Figure 1 Ultrasound (right) fused with a contrast CT of the liver (left). The ultrasound image is taken from an oblique plane showing the hepatic vasculature. The same vasculature is visualized in the same anatomical plane from the CT.

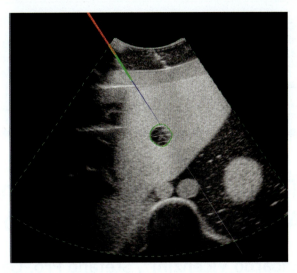

Figure 3 Needle spatial tracking data overlaid graphically on live ultrasound images. The colors indicate parts of the needle behind and in front of the ultrasound image. The display enables the physician to orient the needle with respect to the image.

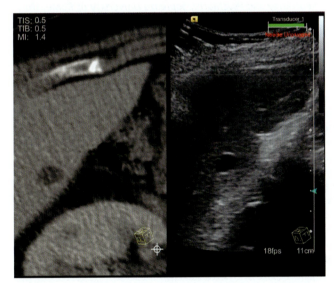

Figure 2 Ultrasound fusion images showing a liver cyst. Fusion imaging enables correlation of lesions between ultrasound and other modalities.

Ultrasound fusion imaging can potentially apply to a wide range of specialty disciplines. In neurology, fusion imaging may facilitate the interpretation of vascular imaging, such as for multi-modality characterization of atherosclerosis.

References

[1] Trobaugh JW, Richard WD, Smith KR, Bucholz RD. Frameless stereotactic ultrasonography: method and applications. Computerized Medical Imaging and Graphics 1994;18:235—46.
[2] Helck A, D'Anastasi M, Notohamiprodjo M, Thieme S, Sommer W, Reiser M, et al. Multimodality imaging using ultrasound image fusion in renal lesions. Clinical Hemorheology and Microcirculation 2012;50(1):79—89.
[3] Arbel T, Morandi X, Comeau RM, Collins DL. Automatic non-linear MRI-ultrasound registration for the correction of intra-operative brain deformations. Computer Aided Surgery 2004;9(4):123—36.
[4] Penney GP, Blackalla JM, Hamadyb MS, Sabharwalb T, Adamb A, Hawkes DJ. Registration of freehand 3D ultrasound and magnetic resonance liver images. Medical Image Analysis 2004;8(1):81—91.
[5] Lange T, Eulenstein S, Hünerbein M, Schlag P. Vessel-based non-rigid registration of MR/CT and 3D ultrasound for navigation in liver surgery. Computer Aided Surgery 2003;8(5):228—40.
[6] Wein W, Brunke S, Khamene A, Callstrom MR, Navab N. Automatic CT-ultrasound registration for diagnostic imaging and image-guided intervention. Medical Image Analysis 2008;12(5):577—85.
[7] Stippel DL, Böhm S, Beckurts TK, Brochhagen HG, Hölscher AH. Experimental evaluation of accuracy of radiofrequency ablation using conventional ultrasound or a third-dimension navigation tool. Archives of Surgery 2002;387(7):303—8.

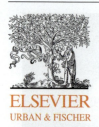
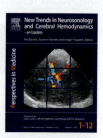

Threedimensional imaging of carotid arteries: Advantages and pitfalls of ultrasound investigations

Edoardo Vicenzini*, Stefano Pro, Gaia Sirimarco, Patrizia Pulitano, Oriano Mecarelli, Gian Luigi Lenzi, Vittorio Di Piero

Stroke Unit — Neurosonology, Neurophysiology Unit, Department of Neurology and Psychiatry, Sapienza University of Rome, Italy

KEYWORDS
3D ultrasound;
Carotid arteries imaging;
Extracranial carotid arteries tortuosity and kinking;
Carotid stenosis

Summary
Objectives: To describe normal and pathological findings with three-dimensional (3D) ultrasound of the carotid bifurcation.
Methods: Patients admitted to our ultrasound laboratory for vascular screening were submitted to standard carotid duplex and to 3D ultrasound reconstruction of the carotid bifurcation. Volume 3D scans were performed manually, on the axial plane, and the software presented the volume rendering from the inward blood flow signal detected with the Power Color Mode.
Results: Forty normal subjects, 7 patients with caliber alterations (4 carotid bulb ectasia and 3 internal carotid lumen narrowing), 45 patients with course variations (tortuosities and kinkings) and 35 patients with internal carotid artery stenosis of various degrees have been investigated.
Conclusions: 3D ultrasound is a feasible technique. It can improve carotid axis general imaging through a global image presentation "at a glance", visualizing caliber variations and vessels course. Imaging of stenosis from inward flow can be provided, but complete stenosis characterization requires the assessment of plaque morphology and vessel wall.
© 2012 Elsevier GmbH. All rights reserved.

Introduction

Several specialists use three-dimensional (3D) ultrasound (US) as adjuvant imaging technique in their clinical practice, from cardiologists to gynecologists [1–5]. The virtual 3D image presentation may be useful also for surgeons, to better study anatomical boundaries of the structures to be submitted to surgical procedures [6,7]. For carotid arteries, it has been applied to study carotid plaque morphology, surface and volume during atherosclerosis progression [8–13].

Recently we have published the possibility of 3D US bifurcation imaging in other conditions than carotid stenosis [14], easily visualizing bifurcation anatomy changes of the caliber and vessels course modifications.

Materials and methods

Patients admitted to our US laboratory for vascular screening were submitted to standard carotid duplex and to 3D US reconstruction of the carotid bifurcation. Forty normal subjects, 7 patients with caliber alterations (4 carotid bulb ectasia and 3 internal carotid lumen narrowing), 45 patients with course variations (tortuosities and kinkings) and 35 patients with ICA stenosis of various degrees have been investigated.

* Corresponding author at: Department of Neurology and Psychiatry, Sapienza University of Rome, Viale dell'Università 30, 00185 Rome, Italy. Tel.: +39 06 49914705; fax: +39 06 49914194.
E-mail address: edoardo.vicenzini@uniroma1.it (E. Vicenzini).

2211-968X/$ — see front matter © 2012 Elsevier GmbH. All rights reserved.
http://dx.doi.org/10.1016/j.permed.2012.03.005

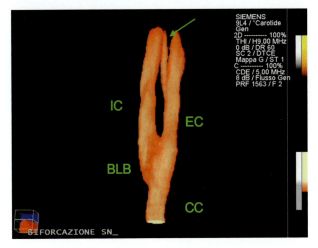

Figure 1 US 3D reconstruction of normal bifurcation. IC: internal carotid artery; EC: external carotid artery; BLB: carotid bulb; CC: common carotid artery. Green arrow indicates the superior thyroidal artery.

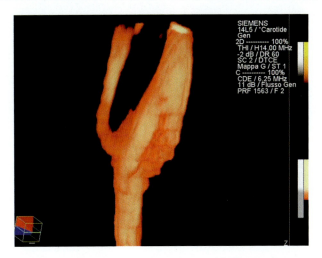

Figure 2 US 3D reconstruction of carotid bulb ectasia.

3D US data acquisition

The Siemens S2000 US system with high frequency linear probes (9, 14 and 18 MHz) and proprietary 3D/4D reconstruction software (v 1.6) have been used.

3D volume scans were recorded manually. After fixing the proximal tract of the common carotid artery (CC) in the center of the display in the transversal plane, a test axial scanning was performed, from proximal CC to distal internal carotid artery (ICA) — at approximately 1 cm per second speed — to adjust the visualization. The 3D ultrasound software was then switched on to record the volume scan: the Power box was set to the orthogonal 90° angle position; Pulse Repetition Frequency (PRF), color gain and color persistence were adjusted during a second test axial scan, in order to reduce artifacts due to the inward flow color signal overlapping the vessel wall and to minimize color ''flashing'' due to the blood pulsatility. The features of the software ''axial reconstruction'' and ''medium resolution'' — that is set for a length of 10 cm to be scanned in 12 s — were selected. Data acquisition was then started and stopped manually; a bar control displayed on the screen the feedback for maintaining a constant straight direction and scan velocity. At the end of the scan, the 3D ultrasound ''volume rendering'' reconstruction of the acquired volume set was started on the system. After the global 3D image presentation, B-Mode imaging was excluded and Color Magnification (Color Priority) adjusted to optimize the final visualization of the vessels.

Results

Visualization of the normal bifurcation

Threedimensional US reconstruction in normal subjects allows a good visualization of the carotid bifurcation. In Fig. 1 (Clip 1), an example is reported: all the extracranial carotid arteries are easily identifiable (CC: common carotid artery; IC: internal carotid artery; EC: external carotid artery; green arrow: superior thyroidal artery), with the possibility of rotating the image through different planes.

Caliber variations

Carotid bulb ectasia

The vessel dilatation, characterized by a fusiform enlargement (usually 1—1.5 cm of antero-posterior diameter), usually involving the distal tract of the common carotid artery and extending through the bulb to the internal carotid artery origin, can be easily recognized. Moreover, the 3D reconstruction, rotating in the different planes, allows a better global identification of the anatomy (Fig. 2). However, the reconstruction images have always to be considered with caution for final diagnostic decisions, as flow disturbances can cause several artifacts in the post-processing image reconstruction: final 3D pictures cannot be considered alone and without the previous or concomitant mandatory analysis of the bidimensional images.

Course variations — tortuosities and kinkings

Extracranial vessels course abnormalities are frequent and generally asymptomatic in the general population [15]. According to their angle in respect to the vessel, they can be classified in ''tortuosities'' and ''kinkings'', when changes in the vessel course are greater than 90°. Even though these alterations are asymptomatic and without clinical relevance in the normal subject, tortuosities and kinkings have to be identified prior to surgical procedures, since they may hinder — for example — the intravascular positioning of a stent, while the anatomical approach and clamping of the internal carotid artery may be easier during endarterectomy [16]. Bidimensional standard US imaging with Duplex, Color and Power Doppler easily reveal the changes of the blood flow direction according to the vessel direction change. While in the bidimensional images it is usually necessary to repeatedly correct the color box insonation angle or to adjust the probe orientation to obtaining optimal complete vessel recognition, the 3D reconstruction can be of help to gain the whole visualization ''at a glance'' [to view the figure, please visit the online supplementary file].

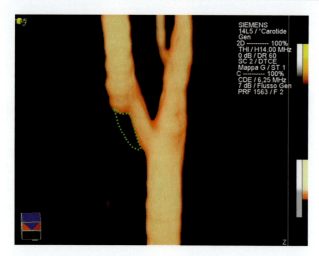

Figure 3 US 3D reconstruction of moderate internal carotid stenosis. Green dotted lines show plaque contour, designed according to bidimensional imaging.

Internal carotid artery stenosis

3D imaging of carotid stenosis have been performed with different techniques: (1) by the 3D reconstruction of the internal carotid artery plaque structure from either the US B-Mode and/or from the vessel wall parenchymal (CT/MRI) imaging; (2) by the 3D reconstruction of the inner residual lumen, visualized with the Power Doppler or with other imaging techniques. These two methods may have their own disadvantages, fundamentally represented by the possibility of under interpretation of the stenosis in case 2, because the vessel considered as normal reference is — actually — only supposed-to-be-so, not being the vessel wall directly visualized. In Fig. 3 (Clip 3), the 3D reconstruction of a cases of internal carotid artery stenosis is presented. Note as the visualization of the "missing part" of the vessel lumen in 3D US, reconstructed on the basis of the residual flow. Increased blood flow velocities may induce an underestimation of the stenosis in the 3D ultrasound reconstruction, because the image is computed on the base of the flow signal — increased in this case — from the inward flow. Identification of the degree of carotid stenosis has represented a cornerstone for the comprehension of stroke pathophysiology in stroke history [17,18]. Nonetheless, it has to be kept in mind that the evaluation of the degree of stenosis must always include the study of the vessel wall and cannot be excluded, also for its importance in analyzing plaque morphology, to identify the "unstable plaque" [19].

Diagnostic pitfalls

In this study, only the 3D reconstruction of the residual lumen detected with Power mode was applied. This method, even though images presented may seem impressive, have to be considered with caution, similarly to all the techniques that reconstruct imaging only from the inward flow. This is particularly true in cases of internal carotid stenosis, because if the plaque is not considered, degree quantification is based on the comparison of what we only suppose to be normal, and hence it may be underestimated.

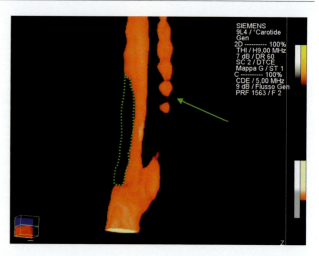

Figure 4 US 3D reconstruction of moderate internal carotid stenosis (green dotted lines). Green arrow shows the typical artifact in 3D US reconstruction in case of low diastolic flow due to high-resistive pattern in the external carotid artery. The absence of signal may be erroneously misinterpreted as a vessel occlusion.

Moreover, in these cases of the 3D US reconstruction, the blood flow pulsating at each cardiac cycle or the acoustic shadow of calcific plaques may create further artifacts: even if the persistence color setting is set to maximal values, blood flow slowing or stopping during diastole — especially in cases of very high resistive patterns as in the external carotid artery — induce the reduction or absence of signal, an artifact difficult to be eliminated even performing the scan as slow as possible (Fig. 4).

Conclusions

Threedimensional ultrasound is a feasible technique when performed by experienced examiners. It can help in the general carotid axis imaging, better presenting the vessels course and the caliber variations "at a glance". Three-dimensional US reconstructions from the inward flow can also provide imaging of stenosis, but its quantification must always take into account the assessment of plaque morphology and vessels wall, by the exact knowledge of the bidimensional images and of hemodynamic patterns.

Appendix A. Supplementary data

Supplementary data associated with this article can be found, in the online version, at doi:10.1016/j.permed.2012.03.005.

References

[1] De Castro S, Yao J, Pandian NG. Three-dimensional echocardiography: clinical relevance and application. Am J Cardiol 1998;18:96G—102G.
[2] Badano LP, Dall'Armellina E, Monaghan MJ, Pepi M, Baldassi M, Cinello M, et al. Real-time three-dimensional echocardiography: technological gadget or clinical tool? J Cardiovasc Med (Hagerstown) 2007;8:144—62.

[3] Shen O, Yagel S. The added value of 3D/4D ultrasound imaging in fetal cardiology: has the promise been fulfilled? Ultrasound Obstet Gynecol 2010;35:260—2.
[4] Dückelmann AM, Kalache KD. Three-dimensional ultrasound in evaluating the fetus. Prenat Diagn 2010;30:631—8.
[5] Grigore M, Mare A, Grigore M, Mare A. Applications of 3-D ultrasound in female infertility. Applications of 3-D ultrasound in female infertility. Rev Med Chir Soc Med Nat Iasi 2009;113:1113—9.
[6] Kalmantis K, Dimitrakakis C, Koumpis C, Tsigginou A, Papantoniou N, Mesogitis S, et al. The contribution of three-dimensional power Doppler imaging in the preoperative assessment of breast tumors: a preliminary report. Obstet Gynecol Int 2009:530579.
[7] Pfister K, Rennert J, Greiner B, Jung W, Stehr A, Gössmann H, et al. Pre-surgical evaluation of ICA-stenosis using 3D power Doppler, 3D color coded Doppler sonography, 3D B-flow and contrast enhanced B-flow in correlation to CTA/MRA: first clinical results. Clin Hemorheol Microcirc 2009;41:103—16.
[8] Rosenfield K, Boffetti P, Kaufman J, Weinstein R, Razvi S, Isner JM. Three-dimensional reconstruction of human carotid arteries from images obtained during noninvasive B-mode ultrasound examination. Am J Cardiol 1992;70:379—84.
[9] Delcker A, Diener HC. Quantification of atherosclerotic plaques in carotid arteries by three-dimensional ultrasound. Br J Radiol 1994;67:672—8.
[10] Landry A, Ainsworth C, Blake C, Spence JD, Fenster A. Manual planimetric measurement of carotid plaque volume using three-dimensional ultrasound imaging. Med Phys 2007;34:1496—505.
[11] Egger M, Spence JD, Fenster A, Parraga G. Validation of 3D ultrasound vessel wall volume: an imaging phenotype of carotid atherosclerosis. Ultrasound Med Biol 2007;33:905—14.
[12] Chiu B, Beletsky V, Spence JD, Parraga G, Fenster A. Analysis of carotid lumen surface morphology using three-dimensional ultrasound imaging. Phys Med Biol 2009;54:1149—67.
[13] Schminke U, Motsch L, Hilker L, Kessler C. Three-dimensional ultrasound observation of carotid artery plaque ulceration. Stroke 2000;31:1651—5.
[14] Vicenzini E, Galloni L, Ricciardi MC, Pro S, Sirimarco G, Pulitano P, et al. Advantages and pitfalls of three-dimensional ultrasound imaging of carotid bifurcation. Eur Neurol 2011;65:309—16.
[15] Stanciulescu R, Ispas A, Filipoiu F, Bordei P, Galaman L, La Marca G, et al. Anatomical variations of the carotid arteries: kinking, coiling, and tortuosity. Anatomical and functional considerations. IJAE 2010;115:161—8.
[16] Faggioli G, Ferri M, Gargiulo M, Freyrie A, Fratesi F, Manzoli L, et al. Measurement and impact of proximal and distal tortuosity in carotid stenting procedures. J Vasc Surg 2007;46:1119—24.
[17] North American Symptomatic Carotid Endarterectomy Trialists' Collaborative Group. The final results of the NASCET trial. N Engl J Med 1998;339:1415—25.
[18] European Carotid Surgery Trialists' Collaborative Group. Randomised trial of endarterectomy for recently symptomatic carotid stenosis: final results of the MRC European Carotid Surgery Trial (ECST). Lancet 1998;351:1379—87.
[19] Hennerici MG. The unstable plaque. Cerebrovasc Dis 2004;17(Suppl. 3):17—22.

Four-dimensional ultrasound imaging in neuro-ophthalmology

Ekaterina Titianova [a,b,*], Sylvia Cherninkova [c], Sonja Karakaneva [a], Boyko Stamenov [d]

[a] *Clinic of Functional Diagnostics of Nervous System, Military Medical Academy, 3 Georgi Sofiiski str., 1606 Sofia, Bulgaria*
[b] *Medical Faculty, Sofia University, 1 Koziak str., 1407, Sofia, Bulgaria*
[c] *Clinic of Neurology, University Hospital "Alexandrovska", 1 Georgi Sofiiski str., 1431 Sofia, Bulgaria*
[d] *Department of Neurology, Pleven Medical University, 8 G. Kochev str., 5800 Pleven, Bulgaria*

KEYWORDS
4D ultrasound imaging;
Optic disc swelling;
Optic nerve edema;
Retinal detachment;
Macular degeneration

Summary

Purpose: To demonstrate diagnostic abilities of space—time (4D) ultrasound imaging in patients with eye pathology and some neuro-ophthalmic syndromes.
Methods: Fifteen healthy controls and 15 patients with eye pathology (papilledema, retinal detachment, macular degeneration and intraocular metastasis) were studied by multimodal (color duplex, B-flow and 3D/4D imaging) sonography.
Results: Normal optic disc resulted in a smooth and sharp contour without swelling. Papilledema was presented as a hyperechoic prominence into the vitreous. On its side the optic sheath diameter was increased in association with the degree of optic disc swelling. The retinal detachment was imaged as a hyperechoic undulating membrane, the neovascular macular degeneration — as a hyperechoic membrane behind the retina, and the intraocular metastasis — as irregular unifocal formation into the vitreous.
Conclusions: The 4D neuro-ophthalmo-sonology helps for the quick and non-invasive volume imaging of the type, size, location and severity of optic disc and optic nerve edema and its differentiation from other types of eye lesions.
© 2012 Elsevier GmbH. All rights reserved.

Introduction

The conventional ultrasound methods are widely used in ophthalmology for evaluating the eye structures (lens, vitreous, chambers, retina, optic discs and optic nerves) and eye circulation (ophthalmic arteries and veins) mainly in the presence of cataract or other processes, hindering the ophthalmoscopy [1—3]. Recently the volume 3D/4D eye ultrasound imaging in adults has been introduced [4] which provides additional information for the structural and functional eye changes in normal and pathological conditions.

The aim of the study was to demonstrate the diagnostic abilities of 4D ultrasound imaging in patients with eye pathology and neuro-ophthalmic syndromes.

* Corresponding author at: Clinic of Functional Diagnostics of Nervous System, Military Medical Academy, 3 Georgi Sofiiski str., 1606 Sofia, Bulgaria. Tel.: +359 2 9225454.
E-mail addresses: titianova@yahoo.com (E. Titianova), s_cherninkova@abv.bg (S. Cherninkova), s_karakaneva@abv.bg (S. Karakaneva), bb_stamenov@abv.bg (B. Stamenov).

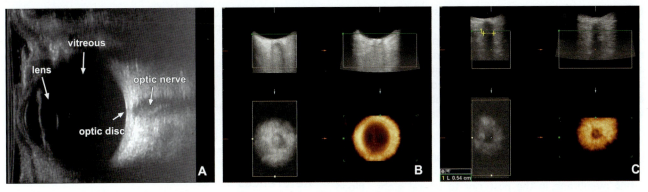

Figure 1   Normal B-mode sonogram of the eye (A), 4D optic disc (B) and optic nerve (C) images.

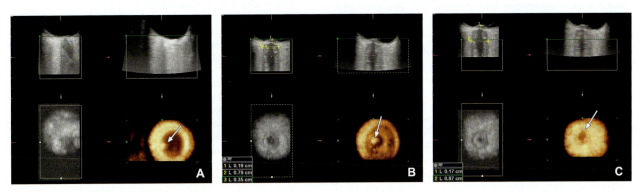

Figure 2   Space—time imaging of mild (A) and severe (B) optic disc swelling, associated with optic nerve edema (C).

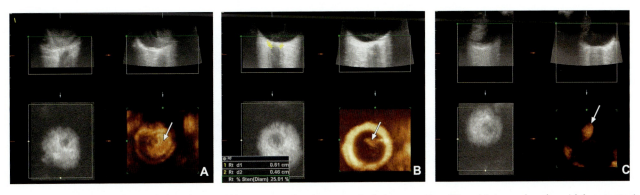

Figure 3   4D imaging of retinal detachment (A), wet macular (neovascular) degeneration (B) and intraocular choroidal metastasis (C).

Materials and methods

Fifteen healthy controls (10 women and 5 men, mean age 47 ± 10 years, age range 21—69 years) and 15 patients (9 women and 6 men, mean age 45 ± 17 years, age range 21—84 years) with visual problems were studied: 10 patients with papilledema, 3 patients with retinal detachment, 1 man with macular degeneration and 1 man with right intraocular choroidal metastasis. Multimodal sonography (color duplex, B-flow and 3D/4D imaging) was used for the evaluation of eye morphology and circulation (Logic 7, GE). The optic nerve sheath was measured 3 mm distal to the optic disc [5].

Results

The normal eye had a typical circular hypoechoic B-mode image with well seen structures inside: a thin hypoechoic cornea (parallel to the eyelid), anechoic anterior and posterior chambers (filled with liquid), anechoic lens, hyperechoic iris and ciliary body (linear structures extending from the peripheral globe towards lens) and relatively echolucent vitreous. The normal retina was not able to be differentiated from the choroidal layers. The optic nerve caused a hypoechoic shadow away from the globe. The same structures had also a typical 4D ultrasound image — the optic disc had a sharp contour without swelling into the vitreous and the optic nerves were with relatively symmetrical sheath diameters on both sides (Fig. 1).

In the presence of optic nerve head pathology we found relatively specific 4D images. Papilledema was presented as a contoured hyperechoic prominence into the vitreous. Its degree correlated with the severity of edema, measured by ophthalmoscopy. On the same side the optic sheath diameter was increased in association with the degree of optic disc swelling (Fig. 2).

The space—time imaging contributed for the quick distinguish of neuro-ophthalmic syndromes from other ophthalmic lesions. Retinal detachment was seen as a hyperechoic undulating membrane in the posterior to lateral globe. Blood vessels had grown up from the choroid behind the retina in the case of wet macular (neovascular) degeneration producing hyperechoic membrane into the vitreous. The choroidal metastasis was imaged as a heterogenic irregular unifocal formation within the lateral part of the affected vitreous with a feeding vessel connecting the formation with the choroidea (Fig. 3).

Discussion

Our study shows that space—time ultrasound imaging gives additional information for the type, location and severity of the eye structures and allows their real time volume assessment in normal and disease conditions. All available 4D ultrasound data in the literature are for studying fetal behavior and prenatal eye movements during pregnancy [6], therefore we could not compare our findings with other volume ultrasound ophthalmic studies in adults.

Conclusions

The 4D neuro-ophthalmo-sonology helps for the quick volume imaging of the type, size, location and severity of optic disc and optic nerve edema and its differentiation from other ophthalmic lesions. It may be helpful in avoiding the need from lumbar puncture, CT or MRI.

References

[1] Restori M, McLeod D, Wright JE. Diagnostic ultrasound in ophthalmology. J R Soc Med 1980;73:273—8.
[2] Fledelius HC. Ultrasound in ophthalmology. Ultrasound Med Biol 1997;23:365—75.
[3] Stone MB. Ultrasound diagnosis of papilledema and increased intracranial pressure in pseudotumor cerebri. Am J Emerg Med 2009;27:376.
[4] Titianova E, Cherninkova S, Karakaneva S. Four-dimensional (4D) ultrasound imaging of optic nerves and optic discs. Neurosonol Cerebral Hemodyn 2009;5:13—6.
[5] Sutherland A, Morris DS, Owen CG, Bron AJ, Roach RC. Optic nerve sheath diameter, intracranial pressure and acute mountain sickness on Mount Everest: a longitudinal cohort study. Brit J Sport Med 2008;42:183—8.
[6] Kurjak A, Predojević M, Stanojević M, Talić A, Honemeyer U, Kadić AS. The use of 4D imaging in the behavioral assessment of high-risk fetuses. Imag Med 2011;3:557—69.

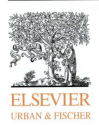
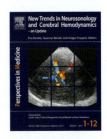

Bartels E, Bartels S, Poppert H (Editors):
New Trends in Neurosonology and Cerebral Hemodynamics — an Update.
Perspectives in Medicine (2012) 1, 89—93

journal homepage: www.elsevier.com/locate/permed

Clinical application of laser Doppler flowmetry in neurology

Zlatka Stoyneva*

15 Acad. Ivan Geshov Str., St. Ivan Rilsky University Hospital, 1404 Sofia, Bulgaria

KEYWORDS
Laser Doppler flowmetry;
Clinical application;
Neurology

Summary Laser Doppler flowmetry is a contemporary method for microcirculatory investigation used in different medical fields including neurology.
Aim: To present principles and clinical application of laser-Doppler method in neurology and related pathologies.
Methods: The diagnostic value was studied by evaluating systematic literature and personal experience. It is based on Doppler principle and uses a laser-generated monochromatic light beam, a fiber-optic probe and sensitive photodetectors. The tissue perfusion of a sample volume is calculated by multiplying the number of moving blood cells and their velocity and is presented in perfusion units.
Results: A high diagnostic value was established in studying microcirculation and its autoregulation using a battery of functional tests for evaluation of vasomotor response mediated by sympathetic neural, axon-reflex, receptor or endothelial mechanisms. It has clinical significance in assessment of Raynaud's phenomenon, distal autonomic neuropathy of the small C fibers due to diabetes mellitus, peripheral arterial occlusive disease, systemic autoimmune diseases, chronic venous insufficiency, peripheral neuropathies, for medical expertise of occupational diseases as hand-arm vibration syndrome, toxic neuropathies, etc. By iontophoretic transducer different drugs or substances might be applied locally to test an effect, physiological or pathophysiological mechanisms. Unlike the contemporary ultrasound investigations it studies the blinded sphere for neurosonology — microcirculation and its autoregulation.
Conclusions: Laser Doppler flowmetry is a valuable and reliable method for diagnostics of microcirculation and perfusion, for assessment of autoregulation and effect of treatment, for experimental studies and research. In combination with ultrasound sonography it gives a thorough information for both macro- and microcirculation.
© 2012 Elsevier GmbH. All rights reserved.

---

* Corresponding author. Tel.: +359 2 9525934.
E-mail address: zlatka_stoyneva@yahoo.com

2211-968X/$ — see front matter © 2012 Elsevier GmbH. All rights reserved.
http://dx.doi.org/10.1016/j.permed.2012.03.009

Introduction

Laser Doppler flowmetry (LDF) is a contemporary noninvasive method for microvascular investigation used in different medical fields including neurology.

The Doppler shift of the laser beam is the carrier of the information about microcirculatory blood flow.

Many studies have proved reliable correlations between LDF and clearance of 133Xe [1], fluorescence flowmetry [2], venous occlusion plethysmography and heat thermal clearance [3] as methods for microcirculatory investigations. Unlike plethysmography and isotope clearance techniques LDF monitors and records sudden microcirculatory changes and reflex responses to sympathetic vasomotor stimuli [4] giving a reproducible parameter of sympathetic vasomotor control [5].

The aim of the study was to present the principles and clinical application of laser-Doppler method in neurology and related pathologies.

Methods

The diagnostic value of LDF was studied by evaluating the systematic literature and our personal experience submitting some data for illustration.

Results

The working of LDF is based on Doppler principle using a laser-generated monochromatic light beam, a transducer with optic fibers and sensitive photodetectors. The light beam is reflected and scattered by the moving blood cells undergoing a change of the wave length (Doppler shift), dependent on the number and velocities of the cells in the investigated sample volume but not on the direction of their movement [6]. The scattered laser beam is perceived by detectors with the help of optic fibers. The signals are analyzed giving values to the number of the cells and their velocities and perfusion is their product.

The depth of penetration of laser beam depends on the tissue characteristics and its vascularisation, on the length of the light wave, the distance between the optic fibers. So the penetration of light source with wave length 633 nm is less than that with 780 nm. By investigation of the skin the depth is from 0.5 to 1.5 mm, and the sample volume is about 1 mm^3. Only the movement in microvessels but not in the bigger blood vessels contributes to the perfusion value because the vessel wall is enough to exclude the greatest part of the laser beam.

Calibration of different apparatuses makes their values equal.

LDF of the skin is easiest to access noninvasively and thus global skin blood flow including both nutritious (capillaries) and thermoregulatory (arterioles, venules and their shunts) microvessels is investigated. The information about thermoregulatory blood flow prevails because the blood flow from the richly sympathetically innervated arterio-venular anastomoses and subpapillary plexus contribute predominantly to the laser-doppler signal, especially of the volar site of the hand and plantar site of the feet. About 90—98% of the finger pulp flow passes through arteriovenular anastomoses [7].

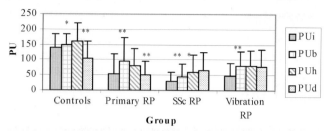

Figure 1 Finger pulp perfusion during venoarteriolar test in Raynaud's phenomenon patients [16]. PU — perfusion units at a finger pulp; PUi — initial perfusion; PUb — basal perfusion at 32 °C; PUh — perfusion at heart level; PUd — perfusion in the dependent hand; Controls — group of healthy controls, Primary RP — primary RP group; SSc RP — secondary RP group due to sclerodermy; Vibration RP — secondary vibration-induced RP group; *$p < 0.05$; **$p < 0.0001$ in relation to previous perfusion value according to Wilcoxon matched pairs signed rank test.

Registration of initial skin perfusion in controlled standard laboratory conditions is measured at first with the natural superficial skin temperature of the patient and then the perfusion is recommended to be measured at 32—33° Celsius superficial skin temperature in order to make skin perfusion at a definite site between different persons comparable.

The accuracy and sensitivity of LDF is improved by applying standardized functional tests [8]. Monitoring of microvascular responses to autonomic vasomotor stimuli is a recognized method for functional diagnosis and assessment of peripheral dysautonomy and function of small unmyelinated autonomic fibers [9].

Thus in orthostatic test constriction of skin precapillary and arteriolar sphincters and microvessels due to the increased sympathetic mediation induces a decrease of skin blood flow. Posture changes of the limbs below heart level activate sympathetic venoarteriolar axon-reflex mechanisms and cause increased skin microvascular resistance like in orthostatism with decrease of skin perfusion. Testing of veno-arteriolar reflex at the finger pulp by LDF is an indicator of unmyelinated autonomic C fiber function [8] and pure postganglionic sympathetic nervous activity [10]. It is more sensitive method for assessment of autonomic dysfunction than the sympathetic skin response [11].

Vasoconstrictor response is changed in the limbs of patients with peripheral arterial occlusive disease [12], diabetic [13] or venous hypertensive microangiopathy [14]. In diabetics type 2 and patients with chronic venous insufficiency a primary defect of venoarteriolar axon-reflex is speculated [7]. Dysregulation of feedback mechanisms between venules, identifying the transmural pressure and arterioles, controlling precapillary resistance is found in secondary Raynaud's phenomenon, too [15,16] (Fig. 1).

Inspiratory tests of Valsalva, deep breathing, deep inspiration with abdominal arrest induce sympathetic vasoconstriction activity with significant decrease of skin perfusion. Peripheral microvascular resistance is significantly decreased in diabetes mellitus.

By cold test a somatic afferent part consisted of pain and temperature nerve fibers in the skin and a sympathetic efferent vasoconstrictor part of the reflex arch is evaluated. The effectiveness of the response after cold stress test with temperature below 15° Celsius might be an index of a sympathetic vasoconstrictor activity [17,18].

Tests of isometric muscular constriction and emotional stress also induce sympathetic skin vasoconstriction [19,20].

By heating test an axon-reflex mediated thermoregulatory microvascular vasodilation is studied as a result of activation of heat-induced nociceptors even at a lack of conscious perception of heat-induced pain [21]. The release of vasoactive peptides from primary nociceptor afferents cause an initial local heat-induced vasodilation at temperatures above 40° Celsius followed by a sustained plateau phase induced by nitric oxide. Thermoregulatory vasomotor responses are abnormal in Raynaud's phenomena (Fig. 2) and diabetic foot (Fig. 3).

Reactive hyperemia test is mediated by local endothelial dependent vasodilator factors with significant decrease of skin vascular resistance and sudden increase of skin perfusion in healthy persons (Fig. 4). Microcirculatory vasodilator reactivity in response to ischemia reflects functional integrity of terminal vessels and assesses microvascular endothelial dependent dilator capacity in physiological and pathological conditions.

Vascular responses to drugs or chemical substances as physiological or pathophysiological mechanisms in different diseases can be studied experimentally by using an iontophoresis system for delivering minute volumes of a substance non-invasively in a controlled fashion together with LDF.

Along with other spheres of application LDF is a valuable method in neurology to diagnose small fiber neuropathy

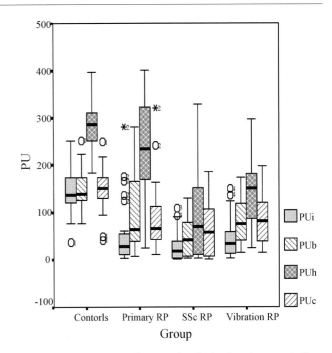

Figure 2   Perfusion at finger pulps during heating test in Raynaud's phenomenon patients [22]. PU — perfusion units at a finger pulp; PUi — initial perfusion; PUb — basal perfusion at 32 °C; PUh — perfusion at 44 °C; PUc — perfusion back to 32 °C; Controls — group of healthy controls; Primary RP — primary RP group; SSc RP — secondary RP group due to sclerodermy; Vibration RP — secondary vibration-induced RP group.

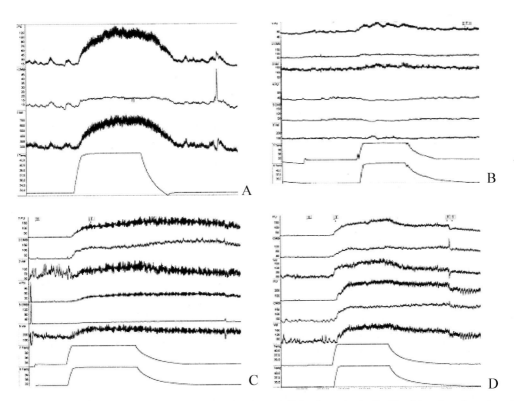

Figure 3   Heating test applied to tiptoes in a healthy person (A) and diabetic patients (B—D) with reduced or absent responses to heating and/or cooling [23].

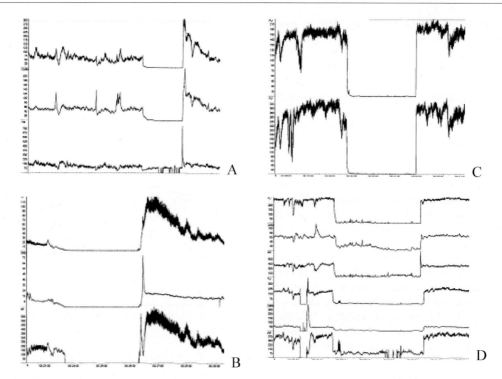

Figure 4 Reactive hyperemia test applied to tiptoes in healthy persons (A, B) and diabetic patients (C, D)[23].

and distal acral vasomotor dysautonomia as an idiopathic or secondary manifestation of polyneuropathies, radiculopathies, mononeuropathies, reflex sympathetic dystrophy, neurovascular syndromes caused by diabetes mellitus, thyroid dysfunction, rheumatic diseases, amyloidosis, lepra, AIDS, venous limb insufficiency, neuropathic pain or occupationally induced by overstrain, vibration, microtrauma, toxic exposure, etc.

The method is valuable to follow up the effect of applied therapy. It is reliable and with very good reproducibility.

A laser Doppler blood perfusion imager is created scanning tissue with a low-power laser beam and colour-coded images of the blood perfusion in the microvasculature.

Conclusions

Unlike the contemporary ultrasound investigations laser Doppler flowmetry studies the blinded sphere for neurosonology, i.e. microcirculation and its autoregulation. Laser Doppler flowmetry is a valuable, easy to use, non-expensive microcirculatory method of investigation which in combination with ultrasound sonography gives thorough information for both macro- and microcirculation.

- Laser-generated monochromatic light beam is directed towards the surface of the investigated tissue by a probe with optic fibers. The tissue perfusion of the investigated sample volume monitored by the flowmeter is calculated automatically by multiplying the number of the moving blood cells and their velocity and is presented in perfusion units (PU).
- Laser beam penetrates tissues, so monitoring of perfusion is noninvasive. for assessment of the integrity of constrictor microcirculatory mechanisms. Afterwards with increased skin flux, decreased venoarteriolar response and increased skin filtration inducing edema
- Using functional reflex vasomotor tests contribute for differentiation of primary from secondary Raynaud's phenomenon. diabetic distal sympathetic neuropathy and microangiopathy; small fiber neuropathy; polyneuropathies or radiculopathies with autonomic dysfunction., distal sympathetic neuropathy, neurovascular syndromes, toxic neuropathies and microvascular reflex vasomotor reactivity and evaluation of microcirculatory vasomotor response mediated by sympathetic neural, axon-reflex, receptor or endothelial mechanisms;
- It is reliable to follow up the effect of applied therapy.
- Measurements are less dynamic than with the probe-based single-point laser Doppler monitor but the microcirculation can be studied over a larger area.
- Laser Doppler flowmetry not only measures and monitors microvascular blood flow but also evaluates microcirculation and its autoregulation.

References

[1] Tur E, Tur M, Maibach HI, Guy RH. Basal perfusion of the cutaneous microcirculation: measurements as a function of anatomic position. Journal of Investigative Dermatology 1983;81:442—6.
[2] Proano E, Svensson L, Perbeck L. Correlation between the uptake of sodium fluorescein in the tissue and xenon-133 clearance and laser Doppler fluxmetry in measuring changes in skin circulation. International Journal of Microcirculation: Clinical and Experimental 1997;17:22—8.
[3] Saumet JL, Dittmar A, Leftheriotis G. Non-invasive measurement of skin blood flow: comparison between plethysmography, laser-doppler flowmeter and heat thermal clearance

method. International Journal of Microcirculation: Clinical and Experimental 1986;5:73—83.
[4] Oberg PA. Laser-Doppler flowmetry. Biomedical Engineering 1990;18:125—63.
[5] Hilz MJ, Hecht MJ, Berghoff M, Singer W, Neundoerfer B. Abnormal vasoreaction to arousal stimuli-an early sign of diabetic sympathetic neuropathy demonstrated by laser Doppler flowmetry. Journal of Clinical Neurophysiology 2000;17:419—25.
[6] Oberg PA. Blood flow measurements. Linkoping University: CRC Press; 1999.
[7] Nuzzaci G, Evangelisti A, Righi D, Giannico G, Nuzzaci I. Is there any relationship between cold-induced vasodilatation and vasomotion? Microvascular Research 1999;57:1—7.
[8] Wahlberg E, Olofsson P, Swedenborg J, Fagrell B. Level of arterial obstruction in patients with peripheral arterial occlusive disease (PAOD) determined by laser Doppler fluxmetry. European Journal of Vascular Surgery 1993;7:684—9.
[9] Abbot NC, Beck JS, Mostofi S, Weiss F. Sympathetic vasomotor dysfunction in leprosy patients: comparison with electrophysiological measurement and qualitative sensation testing. Neuroscience Letters 1996;206:57—60.
[10] Birklein F, Riedl B, Neundorfer B, Handwerker HO. Sympathetic vasoconstrictor reflex pattern in patients with complex regional pain syndrome. Pain 1998;75:93—100.
[11] Wilder-Smith A, Wilder-Smith E. Electrophysiological evaluation of peripheral autonomic function in leprosy patients, leprosy contacts and controls. International Journal of Leprosy and Other Mycobacterial Diseases 1996;64:433—40.
[12] Creutzig A, Caspary L, Alexander K. Disturbances of skin microcirculation in patients with chronic arterial occlusive disease and venous incompetence. VASA 1988;17:77—83.
[13] Rayman G, Hassan A, Tooke JE. Blood flow in the skin of the foot related to posture in diabetes mellitus. British Medical Journal 1986;292:87—90.
[14] Belcaro G, Laurora G, Cesarone MR, De Sanctis MT, Incandela L. Microcirculation in high perfusion microangiopathy. Journal of Cardiovascular Surgery 1995;36:393—8.
[15] Edwards CM, Marshall JM, Pugh M. Cardiovascular responses evoked by mild cool stimuli in primary Raynaud's disease: the role of endothelin. Clinical Science (London) 1999;96:577—88.
[16] Stoyneva Z. Laser Doppler-recorded venoarteriolar reflex in Raynaud's phenomenon. Autonomic Neuroscience 2004;116:62—8.
[17] Kurvers HA, Tangelder GJ, De-Mey JG, Slaaf DW, Beuk RJ, van-den-Wildenberg FA, et al. Skin blood flow abnormalities in a rat model of neuropathic pain: result of decreased sympathetic vasoconstrictor outflow? Journal of the Autonomic Nervous System 1997;63:19—29.
[18] Hodges GJ, Traeger 3rd JA, Tang T, Kosiba WA, Zhao K, Johnson JM. Role of sensory nerves in the cutaneous vasoconstrictor response to local cooling in humans. American Journal of Physiology Heart and Circulatory Physiology 2007;293:H784—9.
[19] Tuck RR, McLeod JG. Vasomotor function and dysfunction. In: Asbury AK, McHaun GM, McDonald WI, editors. Diseases of the Nervous System. Clinical Neurobiology, I—II, 2nd ed. London, Toronto, Montreal, Sydney, Tokyo, Philadelphia: WB Saunders Co.; 1992. p. 468—88.
[20] Stanton AW, Levick JR, Mortimer PS. Assessment of noninvasive tests of cutaneous vascular control in the forearm using a laser Doppler meter and a Finapres blood pressure monitor. Clinical Autonomic Research 1995;5:37—47.
[21] Tew GA, Klonizakis M, Moss J, Ruddock AD, Saxton JM, Hodges GJ. Role of sensory nerves in the rapid cutaneous vasodilator response to local heating in young and older endurance-trained and untrained men. Experimental Physiology 2011;96:163—70.
[22] Stoyneva Z. Raynaud's Phenomenon. Sofia: AEM AMS Infopress; 2006. p. 252 (in Bulgarian).
[23] Stoyneva Z. Diabetic Peripheral Neuropathy. Sofia: AEM AMS Infopress; 2004. p. 260 (in Bulgarian).

3. Stroke Prevention, Diagnostics and Therapy

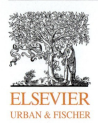

Bartels E, Bartels S, Poppert H (Editors):
New Trends in Neurosonology and Cerebral Hemodynamics — an Update.
Perspectives in Medicine (2012) 1, 94—99

journal homepage: www.elsevier.com/locate/permed

The role of extracranial ultrasound in the prevention of stroke based on the new guidelines

Brigitta Léránt, László Csiba*

University of Debrecen, Medical and Health Science Centre, Department of Neurology, 22 Móricz Zsigmond Str. Debrecen 4032 Hungary

KEYWORDS
Ultrasound;
Carotid stenosis;
Stroke;
Prevention;
Guideline

Abstract Extracranial ultrasonography is recommended to use as a baseline non-invasive method in the initial evaluation of either asymptomatic or symptomatic patients to define the possible stenosis on carotid artery.

The latest 2011 guidelines specify the sequence of examinations with certain classification of recommendations and level of evidence.

Carotid duplex ultrasonography plays an important role both in primary and secondary prevention of stroke and the results found determine the use of further investigations and management of patients with extracranial carotid and vertebral artery disease. In case of diagnostic uncertainty other brain imaging methods, like computed tomography angiography, magnetic resonance angiography and catheter-based angiography can be chosen to assess vascular lesions.

Carotid duplex ultrasound serves not only diagnostic purposes but can also be useful in the follow up processes. It is widely used for control examinations after revascularization procedures of the carotid or vertebrobasilar arteries.

By the establishment of indications of revascularization procedures degree of carotid stenosis is a major factor which therefore requires accuracy of the assessment. Carotid duplex ultrasound has some difficulties in this question. This diagnostic uncertainty is tried to be solved by improving the criteria system of stenosis grading in internal carotid artery.

The aim of this article is to give an overview about the importance and role of extracranial duplex ultrasonography in stroke prevention based on the latest guidelines.
© 2012 Published by Elsevier GmbH.

Abbreviations: CABG, coronary artery bypass graft; CAS, carotid artery stenting; CEA, carotid endarterectomy; CTA, computed tomography angiography; DSA, digital subtraction angiography; HT, hypertension; ICA, internal carotid artery; MRA, magnetic resonance angiography; NASCET, North American Symptomatic Carotid Endarterectomy Trial; US, ultrasound; PAD, peripheral artery disease; TIA, transient ischemic attack.

* Corresponding author. Tel.: +36 52 255 255; fax: +36 52 453 590.
E-mail addresses: lerant.brigi@gmail.com (B. Léránt), csiba@dote.hu (L. Csiba).

1. Introduction

Stroke is currently the third leading cause of death and the biggest single cause of major disability worldwide. Each year more than 700,000 people experience a new or recurrent stroke and on average someone dies every 4 min of a stroke [1]. Despite the diagnostic and treatment development in medicine the recovery rate from stroke is poor.

The well-documented and modifiable risk factors including e.g. hypertension, smoking, diabetes, obesity or dyslipidemia lead to both structural and hemodynamic alterations of the extra- and intracranial vessels. The most common structural consequence is the progression of atherosclerotic processes. The presence of an atherosclerotic lesion in the carotid bulb or in the extracranial internal carotid artery (ICA) is associated with elevated stroke risk [2]. Several mechanisms are attributable to the increased risk of cerebrovascular events including decrease in the blood flow resulting from critical stenosis or occlusion, or the stenotic lesion can also be the source of thromboembolic events.

Regarding the severity of the disease and the very short time for successful intervention after the attack early recognition and prevention are the only chance for patients to survive and to retain their quality of life. Prevention, monitoring of cardiovascular risk factors is therefore an important public health concern [3].

The latest 2011 guidelines specify the role of extracranial duplex ultrasound (US) in the diagnostic processes during the initial evaluation of the patients.

The aim of this article is to summarize the indications of duplex US and the recommended sequence of examinations both in primary and secondary stroke prevention based on 2011 ASA/ACCF/AHA/AANN/AANS/ACR/ASNR/CNS/SAIP/SCAI/SIR/SNIS/SVM/SVS Guideline on the Management of Patients With Extracranial Carotid and Vertebral Artery Disease [4].

2. Primary vascular prevention

2.1. Classification of recommendations and level of evidence

Table 1 shows the classification of recommendations and level of evidence used in the latest guidelines.

2.2. The role of carotid ultrasound in primary prevention

The presence of hemodynamically significant atherosclerotic lesion on carotid artery is often identified in the background of ischemic stroke. Regarding the long process of the development of atherosclerosis, recognition of subclinical forms is of great importance in the primary prevention of cerebrovascular events.

The latest guideline [4] recommends the use of carotid duplex US in asymptomatic patients with the following limitations and conditions.

The routine screening of asymptomatic patients with carotid duplex US is not recommended if no clinical signs or risk factors for atherosclerosis can be detected (Class III, Level of Evidence: C).

The examination is also not beneficial in case of patients with neurological and psychiatric conditions which are unrelated to focal ischemic lesions, such as brain tumours, motor neuron diseases, infection and inflammation of the brain, epilepsy (Class III, Level of Evidence: C).

Standard physical examination contains auscultation of the cervical arteries. If during the examination of an asymptomatic patient presence of carotid bruit is revealed, it is reasonable to perform the measurement to detect the hemodynamically significant carotid stenosis (Class IIa, Level of Evidence: C).

In asymptomatic patients with 2 or more risk factors including hypertension (HT), smoking, hyperlipidemia, family history of manifested atherosclerosis before the age of 60 years and ischemic stroke in a first-degree relative, duplex US may be considered (Class IIb, Level of Evidence: C).

The same recommendation can be applied in case of asymptomatic patients with symptomatic peripheral artery disease (PAD), coronary artery disease or atherosclerotic aortic aneurysm (Class IIb, Level of Evidence: C).

Fig. 1 summarizes the diagnostic approach of asymptomatic patients.

Beside the diagnostic aim of carotid duplex US, this method is proven to be useful in the follow up as well. In case of a stenosis greater than 50% it is reasonable to repeat the examination annually to assess the progression or regression of the vascular alteration and the effect of therapeutic interventions. Less frequent control measurements are acceptable after stability establishment or in case of a change of patient's candidacy for further intervention (Class IIa, Level of Evidence: C).

The establishment of the degree of carotid stenosis by duplex US and angiography (magnetic resonance angiography — MRA, computed tomography angiography — CTA, digital subtraction angiography — DSA) is an important part of the indication of carotid reconstruction surgery in asymptomatic patients. Prophylactic carotid revascularization may be considered in highly selected asymptomatic patients if the degree of stenosis reaches at least 60% by angiography and 70% by duplex US (Class IIb, Level of Evidence: B) [5,6].

Elective coronary artery bypass graft (CABG) surgery makes previous carotid duplex US reasonable in patients with the following conditions: older than 65 years, history of cigarette smoking, PAD, left main coronary stenosis, history of stroke, TIA or carotid bruit (Class IIa, Level of Evidence: C).

3. Secondary vascular prevention

3.1. Carotid duplex US in secondary stroke prevention

Among survivors of ischemic stroke or TIA after the immediate management further investigations should be performed to assess the cause and pathophysiology of the event. The possible origin of ischemic stroke includes intra- or extracranial-artery atherosclerotic infarction, cardiac embolism, small-vessel disease, hypercoagulable state, dissection, sickle cell disease or it can be an infarct of undetermined cause.

As initial evaluation all patients with the symptoms of TIA or ischemic stroke should have non-invasive brain imaging (Class I, Level of Evidence: C).

As a first step duplex US is recommended to detect carotid stenosis for patients with acute, focal neurological symptoms, which reflect the insufficient supply of certain brain territories from the left or right ICA (Class I, Level of Evidence: C).

Table 1 Classification of recommendations and level of evidence.

May be considered	Class I	Class IIa	Class IIb	Class III no benefit or Class III harm		
	Benefit >> risk Procedure/Treatment should be performed/administered	Benefit >> risk Additional studies with focused objectives needed	Benefit ≥ risk Additional studies with broad objectives needed; additional registry data would be helpful		Procedure/test Not helpful	Treatment No proven benefit
				COR III: No benefit		
		It is reasonable to perform procedure/administer treatment	Procedure/treatment may be considered	CORIII: Harm	Excess cost w/o benefit or harmful	Harmful to patients
Level A						
Multiple populations evaluated	•Recommendation that procedure or treatment is useful/effective	•Recommendation in favour of treatment or procedure being useful/effective	•Recommendation's usefulness/efficacy less well established	•Recommendation that procedure or treatment is not useful/effective and may be harmful		
Data derived from multiple randomized clinical trials or meta-analyses	•Sufficient evidence from multiple randomized trials or meta-analyses	•Some conflicting evidence from multiple randomized trials or meta-analyses	•Greater conflicting evidence from multiple randomizes trials or meta-analyses	•Sufficient evidence from multiple randomized trials or meta-analyses		
Level B						
Limited populations evaluated	•Recommendation that procedure or treatment is useful/effective	•Recommendation in favour of treatment or procedure being useful/effective	•Recommendation's usefulness/efficacy less well established	•Recommendation that procedure or treatment is not useful/effective and may be harmful		
Data derived from a single randomized trial or nonrandomized studies	•Evidence from single randomized trial or nonrandomized studies	•Some conflicting evidence from single randomized trial or nonrandomized studies	•Greater conflicting evidence from single randomized trial or nonrandomized studies	•Evidence from single randomized trial or nonrandomized studies		
Level C						
Very limited populations evaluated	•Recommendation that procedure or treatment is useful/effective	•Recommendation in favour of treatment or procedure being useful/effective	•Recommendation's usefulness/efficacy less well established	•Recommendation that procedure or treatment is not useful/effective and may be harmful		
Only consensus opinion of experts, case studies, or standard of care	•Only expert opinion, case studies, or standard of care	•Only diverging expert opinion, case studies, or standard of care	•Only diverging expert opinion, case studies, or standard of care	•Only expert opinion, case studies, or standard of care		

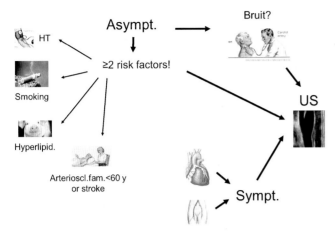

Fig. 1 Diagnostic recommendations of asymptomatic patients.

If duplex US cannot be obtained or does not result in clear and diagnostic results, MRA or CTA is indicated as further imaging tools in the detection of carotid stenosis (Class I, Level of Evidence: C).

Correlation of findings detected by different non-invasive methods is very important in the aspect of quality assurance in every laboratory.

When extra- or intracranial vascular alterations are found with such severity which cannot explain the neurological symptoms, further investigation should be performed to reveal the possible cardiac origin by means of echocardiography (Class I, Level of Evidence: C). Echocardiography serves as the gold standard in the examination of these patients. Detection of the source of cardiac embolism is of great importance regarding that this mechanism accounts for 15—30% of ischemic stroke or TIA [7,8].

Fig. 2 shows the diagnostic steps recommended in patients with symptoms of ischemic stroke or TIA.

3.2. Investigations if carotid reconstruction is planned

When the result of carotid duplex US raises the need for carotid reconstruction, further angiographic examinations (MRA, CTA, catheter-based contrast angiography) can be beneficial to assess the severity of the stenosis and to detect additional intrathoracic and intracranial vascular lesions not seen by duplex US (Class IIa, Level of Evidence: C).

The angiographic method chosen is influenced by other conditions of the patient (Fig. 3).

In patients with extensive arteriosclerosis and renal insufficiency MRA without contrast material is reasonable to be performed (Class IIa, Level of Evidence: C).

DSA may also be considered in case of renal dysfunction because of the advantage of limiting the amount of potentially nephrotoxic contrast material (Class IIb, Level of Evidence: C).

When MRA is contraindicated, e.g. in patients with claustrophobia or implanted pacemaker, CTA can be effective for patient's evaluation (Class IIa, Level of Evidence: C).

When duplex US, CTA, or MRA suggests complete carotid occlusion, catheter-based contrast angiography might be reasonable to decide whether carotid lumen is suitable for revascularization procedure (Class IIb, Level of Evidence: C).

3.3. Non-invasive control after CEA/CAS

Carotid endarterectomy (CEA) is the gold standard for the treatment of carotid atherosclerosis. It is recommended if the degree of stenosis is more than 70% measured by non-invasive methods (Class I, Level of Evidence A) [9], or more than 50% with catheter angiography (Class I, Level of Evidence: B) [10] in symptomatic patients (TIA or ischemic stroke within the past 6 months) at average or low surgical risk with an anticipated perioperative stroke or mortality rate less than 6%.

Carotid artery stenting (CAS) is an alternative method of CEA, which might be considered for patients with severe (>70%) stenosis, especially if the stenosis is difficult to access surgically (Class IIb, Level of Evidence: B) [11].

Non-invasive control of the extracranial arteries can be useful 1 month, 6 months and annually after revascularization (CEA/CAS) to ascertain the patency and to exclude the development of ipsi- or contralateral lesions (Class IIa, Level of Evidence: C).

3.4. Non-invasive imaging in vertebrobasilar insufficiency

Vertebral artery atherosclerosis is responsible for approximately 20% of posterior circulation stroke, which can be an underestimation because of the difficult visualization of vertebral arteries by ultrasonography [12].

The symptoms of vertebral artery disease include dizziness, vertigo, diplopia, tinnitus, blurred vision, perioral numbness, ataxia, bilateral sensory deficits and syncope.

After clinical history and examination of the patient non-invasive imaging is needed in the initial evaluation process.

In patients with symptoms suggesting posterior circulation deficits MRA or CTA should be preferred over ultrasonography to detect vertebral artery disease (Class I, Level of Evidence: C).

If the location and degree of stenosis cannot be defined with certainty by these non-invasive methods and the

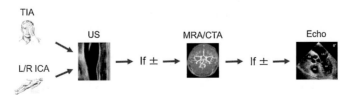

Fig. 2 Sequence of investigations in patients with symptoms of ischemic stroke or TIA (± nondiagnostic results).

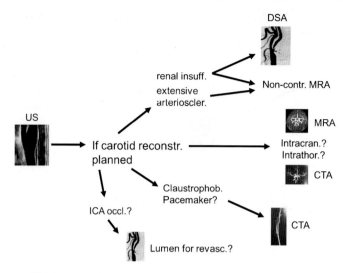

Fig. 3 Examinations if carotid reconstruction is planned.

patient with vertebrobasilar insufficiency symptoms may be a candidate to undergo revascularization procedure, catheter-based contrast angiography is reasonable to assess the pathoanatomy of the artery (Class IIa, Level of Evidence: C).

After vertebral artery revascularization non-invasive control of extracranial vertebral arteries is probably indicated 1 month, 6 months and then annually after the procedure (Class IIa, Level of Evidence: C).

4. Difficulties in stenosis grading

The patients' selection for surgical or endovascular intervention is based on the degree of carotid stenosis, therefore an accurate assessment is required by means of non-invasive imaging and in some cases by catheter-based angiography.

Several methods can be used during catheter-based angiography for stenosis measurement, but the most frequently used one is the NASCET (North American Symptomatic Carotid Endarterectomy Trial) [13], which define the degree of stenosis by measuring the minimal residual lumen at the level of the stenosis, then comparing it with the diameter of the more distal ICA, where the arterial walls become parallel.

The diameter of the artery cannot be assessed directly by carotid duplex ultrasound. This method uses blood flow velocity to indicate the severity of stenosis. Duplex ultrasound may be insensitive to distinguish high-grade stenosis from complete occlusion [14].

The severity of stenosis measured by ultrasound can be categorized into 2 groups: 50—69% stenosis when flow velocity exceeds the normal value due to plaque formation, and 70—99% stenosis in case of more severe atherosclerotic alterations. In case of 50—69% stenosis the peak systolic velocity is in range of 125—230 cm/s and a plaque can be seen in the ultrasound picture. The ratio of peak systolic velocities of internal to common carotid artery is between 2 and 4, while the end-diastolic velocity of ICA reaches 40—100 cm/s.

In case of >70% stenosis the peak systolic velocity exceeds 230 cm/s in ICA, the ratio of this value of internal to common carotid artery is above 4 and end-diastolic velocity accelerates above 100 cm/s in ICA [15].

The velocities of 70% and less severe stenosis overlap, which results in difficulties in the degree grading and which therefore indicates the use of other vascular imaging methods as well.

Several factors can reduce the accuracy of ultrasound measurements, like obesity, vascular tortuosity, high carotid bifurcation or in situ carotid stents and it is also influenced by operator expertise.

Because of the some diagnostic uncertainty new efforts tend to be invested to improve the accuracy of these measurements. The multi-parametric German ''DEGUM ultrasound criteria'', which contained Doppler and imaging criteria combination, have been revised and transferred to NASCET measurement. The criteria are categorized into main and additional groups, in combination if which the accuracy of carotid stenosis grading by ultrasonography can be improved [16].

5. Discussion

In 2011 a new guideline was published by ASA/ACCF/AHA/AANN/AANS/ACR/ASNR/CNS/SAIP/SCAI/SIR/SNIS/SVM/SVS [4] which specifies the principles of the management of patients with symptomatic or asymptomatic carotid and vertebral artery disease.

The importance of non-invasive imaging methods in the diagnostic routine is evident. Extracranial duplex ultrasound combining 2-dimensional real-time imaging with Doppler measurements is widely used as one of the initial diagnostic tools in patients' evaluation regarding its cost-effectiveness, repeatability and safety.

The 2011 guideline defines the place of carotid duplex US in the sequence of initial examinations both in asymptomatic patients and in patients with symptoms of stroke, TIA or vertebrobasilar insufficiency.

With different classification of recommendations and level of evidence extracranial duplex US is still present and play an important role both in diagnosis and thus in primary and secondary prevention of cerebrovascular events and in the follow up of patients. The results gained from duplex US determine the use of other imaging methods (MRA, CTA, catheter-based angiography) which ensure a more accurate mapping of patients' vascular lesions and are an important part of patients' selection for revascularization.

The diagnostic uncertainty in case of carotid duplex US caused by difficulties in stenosis grading can be improved by using main and additional criteria system proposed by the Revision of DEGUM ultrasound criteria [16].

References

[1] Lloyd-Jones D, Adams RJ, Brown TM, Carnethon M, Dai S, De Simone G, et al. Heart disease and stroke statistics — 2010 update: a report from the American Heart Association. Circulation 2010;121:e46—215.

[2] Spagnoli LG, Mauriello A, Sangiorgi G, Fratoni S, Bonanno E, Schwartz RS, et al. Extracranial thrombotically active carotid plaque as a risk factor for ischemic stroke. Journal of the American Medical Association 2004;292: 1845—52.

[3] Goldstein LB, Bushnell CD, Adams RJ, Appel LJ, Braun LT, Chaturvedi S, et al. Guidelines for the primary prevention of stroke: a guideline for healthcare professionals from the American Heart Association/American Stroke Association. Stroke 2011;42:517—84.

[4] Brott TG, Halperin JL, Abbara S, Bacharach JM, Barr JD, Bush RL, et al. ASA/ACCF/AHA/AANN/AANS/ACR/ASNR/CNS/SAIP/SCAI/SIR/SNIS/SVM/SVS guideline on the management of patients with extracranial carotid and vertebral artery disease. A report of the American College of Cardiology Foundation/American Heart Association Task Force on Practice Guidelines, and the American Stroke Association, American Association of Neuroscience Nurses, American Association of Neurological Surgeons, American College of Radiology, American Society of Neuroradiology, Congress of Neurological Surgeons, Society of Atherosclerosis Imaging and Prevention, Society for Cardiovascular Angiography and Interventions, Society of Interventional Radiology, Society of NeuroInterventional Surgery, Society for Vascular Medicine, and Society for Vascular Surgery. Circulation 2011;124:e54—130, 2011.

[5] Halliday A, Mansfield A, Marro J, Peto C, Peto R, Potter J, et al. Prevention of disabling and fatal strokes by successful carotid endarterectomy in patients without recent neurological symptoms: randomised controlled trial. Lancet 2004;363:1491—502.

[6] Executive Committee for the Asymptomatic Carotid Atherosclerosis Study. Endarterectomy for asymptomatic carotid artery stenosis. JAMA 1995;273:1421—8.

[7] Pepi M, Evangelista A, Nihoyannopoulos P, Flachskampf FA, Athanassopoulos G, Colonna P, et al. Recommendations for echocardiography use in the diagnosis and management of cardiac sources of embolism: European Association of Echocardiography (EAE) (a registered branch of the ESC). European Journal of Echocardiography 2010;11:461—76.

[8] Doufekias E, Segal AZ, Kizer JR. Cardiogenic and aortogenic brain embolism. Journal of the American College of Cardiology 2008;51:1049—59.

[9] Barnett HJ, Taylor DW, Eliasziw M, Fox AJ, Ferguson GG, Haynes RB, et al. Benefit of carotid endarterectomy in patients with symptomatic moderate or severe stenosis. North American Symptomatic Carotid Endarterectomy Trial Collaborators. New England Journal of Medicine 1998;339:1415—25.

[10] Randomised trial of endarterectomy for recently symptomatic carotid stenosis: final results of the MRC European Carotid Surgery Trial (ECST). Lancet 1998; 351:1379—87.

[11] Yadav JS, Wholey MH, Kuntz RE, Fayad P, Katzen BT, Mishkel GJ, et al. Protected carotid-artery stenting versus endarterectomy in high-risk patients. New England Journal of Medicine 2004;351:1493—501.

[12] Borhani Haghighi A, Edgell RC, Cruz-Flores S, Zaidat OO. Vertebral artery origin stenosis and its treatment. Journal of Stroke and Cerebrovascular Diseases 2011;20:369—76.

[13] North American Symptomatic Carotid Endarterectomy Trial Collaborators. Beneficial effect of carotid endarterectomy in symptomatic patients with high-grade carotid stenosis. New England Journal of Medicine 1991;325:445—53.

[14] Thanvi B, Robinson T. Complete occlusion of extracranial internal carotid artery: clinical features, pathophysiology, diagnosis and management. Postgraduate Medical Journal 2007;83:95—9.

[15] Braun RM, Bertino RE, Milbrandt J, Bray M, Society of Radiologists in Ultrasound Consensus Criteria to a Single Institution Clinical Practice. Ultrasound imaging of carotid artery stenosis: application of the Society of Radiologists in Ultrasound Consensus Criteria to a Single Institution Clinical Practice. Ultrasound Quarterly 2008;24:161—6.

[16] Arning C, Widder B, von Reutern GM, Stiegler H, Görtler M. Revision of DEGUM ultrasound criteria for grading internal carotid artery stenoses and transfer to NASCET measurement. Ultraschall in der Medizin 2010;31:251—7.

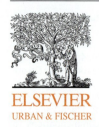
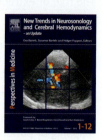

Bartels E, Bartels S, Poppert H (Editors):
New Trends in Neurosonology and Cerebral Hemodynamics — an Update.
Perspectives in Medicine (2012) 1, 100—103

journal homepage: www.elsevier.com/locate/permed

Optimized prevention of stroke: What is the role of ultrasound?

Dirk Sander[a,b,*]

[a] Department of Neurology, Benedictus Krankenhaus Tutzing, Germany
[b] Department of Neurology, Klinikum rechts der Isar, Technische Universität München, Germany

KEYWORDS
Stroke prevention;
Ultrasound;
Carotid stenosis;
Ankle—brachial index

Summary Major cardio- and cerebrovascular events often occur in individuals without known preexisting cardiovascular disease. The prevention of such events, including the accurate identification of those at risk, remains a serious public health challenge. Scoring equations to predict those at increased risk have been developed using cardiovascular risk factors, but they tend to overestimate the risk in low-risk populations and underestimate it in high-risk populations. This overview discusses the possible role of ultrasound for an optimized prevention of stroke and focusses on (1) the importance of embolic signals in asymptomatic carotid stenosis, (2) the detection of unstable carotid plaques using duplex ultrasonography, and (3) the role of the ankle—brachial index for the stroke risk prediction in the acute stage and for secondary prevention.
© 2012 Elsevier GmbH. All rights reserved.

Introduction

Despite the improvements in acute stroke therapy as well as effective secondary prevention measures, stroke remains the most important disease for permanent disability and is the second frequent cause of death worldwide [1]. The risk factors for stroke are well known and were subdivided into non-modifiable (e.g. age, sex, genetic predisposition) and modifiable catergories (e.g. hypertension, smoking, diabetes). The INTERSTROKE study [2] shows that 5 risk factors (history of hypertension or blood pressure >160/90 mm Hg, smoking, waste-to-hip ratio, physical inactivity and diet-risk score) explain 83.4% of the stroke risk in the population.

However, major cardio- and cerebrovascular events often occur in individuals without known preexisting cardiovascular disease. The prevention of such events, including the accurate identification of those at risk, remains a serious public health challenge [3]. Scoring equations to predict those at increased risk have been developed using cardiovascular risk factors, but they tend to overestimate the risk in low-risk populations and underestimate it in high-risk populations [4]. An important prerequisite for the use of surrogate parameters for risk prediction particularly in the primary care setting is that these parameters add substantial incremental value in risk prediction beyond the traditional Framingham-type risk scores or give a better estimate to select high-risk patients for invasive procedures, e.g. carotid endarterectomy (CEA). This overview discusses the possible role of ultrasound for an optimized prevention of stroke and focusses on (1) the detection of unstable carotid plaques using duplex ultrasonography, (2) the importance of embolic signals in asymptomatic carotid stenosis (ACS), and (3) the

* Corresponding author at: Department of Neurology, Benedictus Krankenhaus Tutzing & Feldafing, Dr.-Appelhans-Weg 6, 82340 Feldafing, Germany. Tel.: +49 8157 28140; fax: +49 8157 28141.
E-mail address: D.Sander@mac.com

2211-968X/$ — see front matter © 2012 Elsevier GmbH. All rights reserved.
doi:10.1016/j.permed.2012.02.029

role of the ankle—brachial index for the stroke risk prediction in the acute stage and for secondary prevention.

Detection of embolic signals in asymptomatic carotid stenosis

Due to the improvements of medical management in patients with high-grade ACS, there is uncertainty as how to best manage these patients. New studies demonstrate, that a well-treated patient with ACS has an annual risk of ipsilateral stroke of only 0.3% [5]. Therefore, 80 patients with an ACS must be treated by a CEA to prevent one disabling stroke. Consequently, the cost-effectiveness of CEA in patients with ACS has been questioned [6]. Nevertheless, ACS accounts for a large burden of stroke, and the majority of ipsilateral strokes are unheralded [7]. Identification of the group of ACS patients at higher risk would improve both risk-benefit and cost-benefit ratios for CEA. Several methods to identify such a high-risk group have been suggested, including ultrasonic detection of asymptomatic embolization. If clinical embolism is a good predictor of the subsequent stroke risk, asymptomatic cerebral emboli might also predict clinical stroke risk [8]. Transcranial Doppler ultrasound (TCD) is a non-invasive technique that can be used to detect circulating emboli. Several studies evaluated the association between detection of embolic signals and new ischemic events in patients with ACS [9—11] and reported different results. Recently a large prospective and multi-center study (ACES, Asymptomatic Carotid emboli Study) evaluated the relationship between asymptomatic emboli and stroke risk in 467 patients with an ACS of at least 70% [8]. The detection of emboli was associated with an increased risk for ipsilateral TIA and stroke (HR 2.54, 95% CI 1.2—5.36) and in particular for ipsilateral stroke (HR 5.57, 95% CI 1.61—19.32) during 2 years of follow-up even after adjusting for antiplatelet therapy, degree of stenosis, and other risk factors. The absolute annual risk of ipsilateral stroke or TIA between baseline and 2 years was 7.13% in patients with embolic signals and 3.04% in those without, and for ipsilateral stroke was 3.62% in patients with embolic signals and 0.70% in those without. The authors performed a meta-analysis with all studies available including 1144 patients. The hazard ratio for the risk of ipsilateral stroke for those with embolic signals compared with those without was 6.63 (95% CI 2.85—15.44) with no heterogeneity between studies ($p = 0.33$).

If TCD is to be used as a clinical tool for risk stratification, improved methods of automated detection of embolic signals are needed [8]. TCD recording itself is simple, non-invasive, and widely used in clinical practice worldwide. However, review of data for the presence of embolic signals is time consuming and relies on trained observers. Automated systems have been developed that have high sensitivity and specificity for detecting the higher intensity embolic signals seen in patients with symptomatic stenosis [12]. However, these systems were less sensitive to the lower intensity embolic signals found in ACS [13]. Therefore new systems are needed that enable an automatic detection of emboli even at lower signal intensity levels with an improved sensitivity and specificity.

Conclusion

- Detection of asymptomatic embolization on TCD can be used to identify patients with ACS who are at a higher risk of stroke and TIA.
- Assessment of the presence of embolic signals on TCD might be useful in the selection of patients with ACS who may benefit from CEA.
- Better systems are needed that enable an automatic detection of emboli even at lower signal intensity levels with an improved sensitivity and specificity.

Unstable plaque

A number of prospective studies have examined associations between ultrasonic plaque characteristics and stroke risk in ACS. Associations have been detected with a number of features including texture heterogeneity, echolucency, and surface irregularities [14]. A limited number of studies have used a simple measure of echolucency and these have shown conflicting results. More recently, data from ACES demonstrated that plaque morphology assessed using a simple visual rating scale predicts ipsilateral stroke in ACS [14]. 435 subjects with ACS $\geq$ 70% were included and followed-up for 2 years. A 4-point visual rating scale was applied to the plaques and they were classified as echolucent (37.7%) or echogenic. Plaque echolucency at baseline was associated with an increased risk of ipsilateral stroke alone (HR 6.43, 95% CI 1.36—30.44). A combination of plaque echolucency and ES positivity at baseline was associated with an increased risk of ipsilateral stroke alone (HR 10.61, 95% CI 2.98—37.82). The combination of ES detection and plaque morphology allows a greater prediction than either measure alone and identifies a high-risk group with an annual stroke risk of 8%, and a low-risk group with a risk of <1% per year. These data show that the combination of 2 measures of plaque instability may identify a high-risk group of patients with ACS that may benefit from a CEA.

Conclusion

- Plaque morphology assessed using a simple and clinically applicable, visual rating scale predicts ipsilateral stroke risk in ACS.
- The combination of asymptomatic emboli detection and plaque morphology allows a greater prediction than either measure alone and identifies a high-risk group with an annual stroke risk of 8%.

Ankle-brachial index (ABI)

Peripheral arterial disease (PAD) is increasingly recognized as a clinically important marker of atherosclerotic disease due to its association with cardiovascular disease incidence and mortality. Determination of the ABI, which is the ratio of systolic pressure at the ankle to that in the arm, is quick, easy to measure and a noninvasive method used to establish the presence of PAD. The equipment is inexpensive — a handheld Doppler sonograph costs less than 400 EUR. The procedure is simple, taking less than 10—15 min, and can

Table 1 Meta-analysis for the association between an pathological ABI (<0.9) and new vascular events according to [21].

Outcome	Age- and sex-adjusted risk		
	No. of studies	Relative risk (95% CI)	Test for heterogenicity
Overall mortality	14	4.0 (3.7—4.3)	$P = 0.002$
Vascular events	11	2.8 (2.6—3.1)	$P < 0.001$
Stroke/TIA	8	2.3 (2.0—2.7)	$P = 0.025$
CHD	8	2.4 (2.1—2.7)	$P < 0.001$

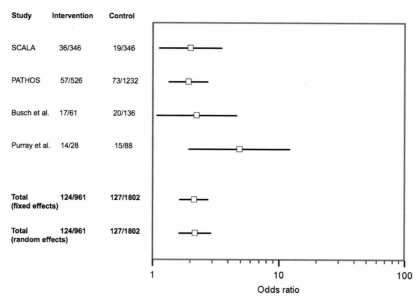

Figure 1 Meta-analysis of four trials showing the predictive value of low ABI (<0.9) for new cardiovascular events (stroke, MI or death) in patients with acute stroke.

be performed by a suitably trained nurse or health care professional.

A reduced ABI has been shown to identify patients at risk for cardiovascular events (Table 1). Patients with stroke or transient ischemic attack often had PAD. However, it is still unclear whether PAD is also a good predictor for future cerebrovascular disease. A recent meta-analysis demonstrated a pooled multivariate adjusted relative risk of 1.35 (95% confidence interval, CI 1.10—1.65) for stroke in patients with an ABI < 0.9 [15].

Meves et al. [16] analyzed the association between PAD, either symptomatic or asymptomatic (defined as an ABI < 0.9), and the future stroke risk in 6880 patients from the German Epidemiological Trial on Ankle—Brachial Index (getABI), a large and prospective cohort study of a typical primary care sample of unselected elderly patients. During the 5-year follow-up period, 183 patients had a stroke. In patients with PAD ($n = 1429$) compared to those without PAD ($n = 5392$), the incidence of all stroke types, with the exception of hemorrhagic stroke, was about doubled (for fatal stroke tripled). The corresponding adjusted hazard ratios were 1.6 (95% CI 1.1—2.2) for total stroke, 1.7 (95% CI 1.2—2.5) for ischemic stroke, 0.7 (95% CI 0.2—2.2) for hemorrhagic stroke, 2.5 (95% CI 1.2—5.2) for fatal stroke and 1.4 (95% CI 0.9—2.1) for nonfatal stroke. Lower ABI categories were associated with higher stroke rates. Besides high age, previous stroke and diabetes mellitus, PAD was a significant independent predictor for ischemic stroke. The stroke risk was similar in patients with symptomatic ($n = 593$) as compared to asymptomatic ($n = 836$) PAD.

Interestingly, recent studies that analyzed the prognostic impact of low ABI values (<0.9) on stroke recurrence and cardiovascular events in acute stroke patients revealed comparable results (Fig. 1). Purroy et al. [17] observed an increased stroke recurrence rate (32.1 vs. 13.6%, $p < 0.001$) and more vascular events (50 vs. 70%, $p < 0.001$) in patients with low ABI values. Similar results were seen in the SCALA trial [18] that examined 852 patients from 85 neurological stroke units throughout Germany as well as the PATHOS study [19] from Italy with 755 acute stroke patients. Busch et al. [20] described an increased risk for stroke, myocardial infarction or death in acute stroke patients with a low ABI < 0.9 (relative risk 2.2; 95% CI 1.1—4.5).

Conclusion

- An ABI < 0.9 is an independent predictor of stroke recurrence in acute stroke.
- The detection of PAD defined as an ABI < 0.9 identifies high-risk patients for further vascular events; the vascular

risk including stroke is clearly increased even in subjects with asymptomatic PAD.
- Elderly patients in the primary care setting should be screened for (asymptomatic) PAD to enable consequent treatment of modifiable cardiovascular risk factors to reduce the risk of ischemic stroke and other vascular events; however, whether this screening is cost-effective remains to be established.

References

[1] Goldstein LB, Bushnell CD, Adams RJ, Appel LJ, Braun LT, Chaturvedi S, et al. Guidelines for the primary prevention of stroke: a guideline for healthcare professionals from the American Heart Association/American Stroke Association. Stroke 2011;42:517—84.

[2] O'Donnell MJ, Xavier D, Liu L, Zhang H, Chin SL, Rao-Melacini P, et al. Risk factors for ischaemic and intracerebral haemorrhagic stroke in 22 countries (the INTERSTROKE study): a case—control study. The Lancet 2010;376:112—23.

[3] Greenland P, Smith SCJ, Grundy SM. Improving coronary heart disease risk assessment in asymptomatic people: role of traditional risk factors and noninvasive cardiovascular tests. Circulation 2001;104:1863—7.

[4] Brindle P, Beswick A, Fahey T, Ebrahim S. Accuracy and impact of risk assessment in the primary prevention of cardiovascular disease: a systematic review. Heart 2006;92:1752—9.

[5] Marquardt L, Geraghty OC, Mehta Z, Rothwell PM. Low risk of ipsilateral stroke in patients with asymptomatic carotid stenosis on best medical treatment: a prospective, population-based study. Stroke 2010;41:e11—7.

[6] Abbott AL. Medical (nonsurgical) intervention alone is now best for prevention of stroke associated with asymptomatic severe carotid stenosis: results of a systematic review and analysis. Stroke 2009;40:e573—83.

[7] Inzitari D, Eliasziw M, Gates P, Sharpe BL, Chan RK, Meldrum HE, et al. The causes and risk of stroke in patients with asymptomatic internal-carotid-artery stenosis. North American Symptomatic Carotid Endarterectomy Trial Collaborators. N Engl J Med 2000;342:1693—700.

[8] Markus HS, King A, Shipley M, Topakian R, Cullinane M, Reihill S, et al. Asymptomatic embolisation for prediction of stroke in the Asymptomatic Carotid Emboli Study (ACES): a prospective observational study. Lancet Neurol 2010;9:663—71.

[9] King A, Markus HS. Doppler embolic signals in cerebrovascular disease and prediction of stroke risk: a systematic review and meta-analysis. Stroke 2009;40:3711—7.

[10] Spence JD, Tamayo A, Lownie SP, Ng WP, Ferguson GG. Absence of microemboli on transcranial Doppler identifies low-risk patients with asymptomatic carotid stenosis. Stroke 2005;36:2373—8.

[11] Abbott AL, Chambers BR, Stork JL, Levi CR, Bladin CF, Donnan GA. Embolic signals and prediction of ipsilateral stroke or transient ischemic attack in asymptomatic carotid stenosis: a multicenter prospective cohort study. Stroke 2005;36:1128—33.

[12] Cullinane M, Reid G, Dittrich R, Kaposzta Z, Ackerstaff R, Babikian V, et al. Evaluation of new online automated embolic signal detection algorithm, including comparison with panel of international experts. Stroke 2000;31:1335—41.

[13] Cullinane M, Kaposzta Z, Reihill S, Markus HS. Online automated detection of cerebral embolic signals from a variety of embolic sources. Ultrasound Med Biol 2002;28:1271—7.

[14] Topakian R, King A, Kwon SU, Schaafsma A, Shipley M, Markus HS, et al. Ultrasonic plaque echolucency and emboli signals predict stroke in asymptomatic carotid stenosis. Neurology 2011;77:751—8.

[15] Heald CL, Fowkes FG, Murray GD, Price JF. Risk of mortality and cardiovascular disease associated with the ankle—brachial index: systematic review. Atherosclerosis 2006;189: 61—9.

[16] Meves SH, Diehm C, Berger K, Pittrow D, Trampisch HJ, Burghaus I, et al. Peripheral arterial disease as an independent predictor for excess stroke morbidity and mortality in primary-care patients: 5-year results of the getABI study. Cerebrovasc Dis 2010;29:546—54.

[17] Purroy F, Coll B, Oro M, Seto E, Pinol-Ripoll G, Plana A, et al. Predictive value of ankle brachial index in patients with acute ischaemic stroke. Eur J Neurol 2010;17:602—6.

[18] Weimar C, Goertler M, Rother J, Ringelstein EB, Darius H, Nabavi DG, et al. Predictive value of the Essen Stroke Risk Score and Ankle Brachial Index in acute ischaemic stroke patients from 85 German stroke units. J Neurol Neurosurg Psychiatry 2008;79:1339—43.

[19] Agnelli G, Cimminiello C, Meneghetti G, Urbinati S. Low ankle—brachial index predicts an adverse 1-year outcome after acute coronary and cerebrovascular events. J Thromb Haemost 2006;4:2599—606.

[20] Busch MA, Lutz K, Rohl JE, Neuner B, Masuhr F. Low ankle—brachial index predicts cardiovascular risk after acute ischemic stroke or transient ischemic attack. Stroke 2009;40:3700—5.

[21] Banerjee A, Fowkes FG, Rothwell PM. Associations between peripheral artery disease and ischemic stroke: implications for primary and secondary prevention. Stroke 2010;41:2102—7.

Measuring the degree of internal carotid artery stenosis

Gerhard-Michael von Reutern*

Ambulantes Kardiologisches Zentrum, Neurologische Praxis, Kuechlerstrasse 2, 61231 Bad Nauheim, Germany

KEYWORDS
Carotid stenosis;
Degree of stenosis;
Doppler ultrasound;
Duplex sonography;
Peak systolic velocity

Summary The use of ultrasonic methods to evaluate carotid disease differs from country to country. Most popular is the criterion of flow velocity in the stenosis, a criterion influenced by multiple other factors than narrowing of the artery. On the other side angiography does not reliably measure area reduction, responsible for the hemodynamic effect of a stenosis. Therefore correlations of velocity and the degree of stenosis as measured by angiography were never satisfying. In a recent international consensus a multiparametric approach has been proposed aiming to reduce possible errors. This article illustrates some of the possible errors measuring flow velocity with Doppler ultrasound and discusses the background for using multiple criteria. Ultrasound can be used for clinical decision making. This is possible in a clear cut high degree stenosis and in low degree disease. The advantage of Doppler ultrasound is to describe best the hemodynamic consequences of vessel narrowing. This may yield important additional information in combination with other imaging modalities.
© 2012 Elsevier GmbH. All rights reserved.

Introduction

In 1986, the first German guideline for measuring the degree of carotid stenosis with sonography based on an intersociety consensus was published [15]. At that time, continuous wave (CW) Doppler sonographic was the prevailing methodology. As part of duplex sonography B-Mode imaging was added as rather poor method for correcting the orientation of the Doppler beam and placement of the sample volume. CW Doppler criteria for estimating the degree of narrowing were mainly based on hemodynamic parameters. Later duplex criteria were established in accordance with the established CW Doppler sonographic criteria. The stenotic signal was categorised using descriptive terms and broad Doppler shift categories.

In North America, documentation through imaging is of special importance because of the division of duties between technician (examining) and physician (reading). Soon duplex sonography replaced C-Mode Doppler imaging and the simple "Doppler ophthalmic test" as one of the hemodynamic parameters became unpopular. Aiming to improve quantification of a stenosis the intrastenotic peak systolic velocity PSV (instead of Doppler frequencies) were recorded after correction for the angle of insonation. Several correlations between PSV and the degree of stenosis measured by X-ray angiography were published [10] and a consensus for threshold values based on a meta-analysis was published [4]. However all correlations between PSV and angiography showed a considerable scatter. Therefore the NASCET group [2] and recently the AHA did not recommend carotid surgery in symptomatic patients based on duplex sonography alone [8].

Abbreviations: ECST, the European Carotid Surgery Trial; NASCET, the North American Symptomatic Carotid Endarterectomy Trial.
* Tel.: +49 1715856099.
E-mail address: g.v.reutern@gmx.de

Table 1 Set of main and secondary criteria. For further details see Ref. [10].

Main criteria
  (1) B-Mode and color imaging
  (2) Mean or threshold values of peak systolic velocities in the stenosis
  (3) Poststenotic velocity
  (4) Appearance of collateral flow (ophthalmic artery, circle of Willis)
Secondary criteria
  (5) Prestenotic reduced flow in the CCA
  (6) Poststenotic flow disturbances, severity and length
  (7) End diastolic flow velocity in the stenosis
  (8) Carotid ratio (ICA/CCA velocities)

In Germany, as in other European countries the local diameter narrowing (ESCT method) was popular whereas in the US the distal diameter of the internal carotid artery (ICA) was taken as denominator (distal diameter narrowing, NASCET method). The ESCT method results in higher degrees of stenosis especially in the range of up to 70% stenosis [11]. This opened the possibility of misuse by measuring following the ESCT method and recommending carotid surgery following the NASCET criterion of 70%. In consequence new intersociety guidelines were published in Germany [1] very similar to the first ones [15], but using the NASCET method as the morphologic correlate. In addition the role of color coded imaging for detecting low degree disease and total occlusion was added, as well as PSV values. Recently a similar consensus was reached by the Neurosonology Research Group (NSRG) of the WFN [10]. Both of these guidelines emphasize the difference between main or primary and additional criteria. They are listed in Table 1. This article shall outline the background of grading a stenosis and especially focus on the weighting of these ultrasonic criteria as main and secondary.

Two different methods to grade a stenosis

A stenosis can be graded following its morphologic or hemodynamic effect. The morphologic aspect is measured in mm or as percent diameter reduction. Additional features can be described as precise location or shape of the plaque, regular or irregular. The hemodynamic effect can be measured as local flow velocity at the level of a plaque or stenosis [13], pressure drop or reduced flow volume. Doppler ultrasound in its clinical application cannot measure the two last parameters directly, but make estimations by measuring prestenotic side to side differences, the appearance of collateral flow, the poststenotic pulsatility and velocity of flow and flow disturbances [6]. Both the morphologic parameters and the hemodynamic parameters can be translated to each other, i.e. ''a hemodynamic relevant stenosis corresponds to a $\geq$70% stenosis (NASCET)'', or ''in a 80% stenosis collateral flow via the circle of Willis is highly probable''. In general the final diagnosis will be expressed in % diameter reduction, as it is the tradition with angiography. In mild degrees of stenosis duplex sonography describes both the morphology and local hemodynamic as well. With increasing severity a precise morphologic description is more difficult due to calcium shadowing and reverberation. Hemodynamic parameters are however more useful. Angiography will have fewer problems to show the stenotic canal in a high degree stenosis, but the hemodynamic evaluation is less reliable or needs special techniques such as contralateral injection. In addition the more hemodynamically oriented ultrasonography and the more morphologically orientated angiography have both technical limitations, as it will be described in detail below. Therefore a perfect correlation between these different approaches is not possible. It has to be kept in mind, that the prognosis and therefore the rational for decisions are only indirectly linked with diameter reduction or pressure drop but with plaque instability, thrombus formation and embolisation. The final diagnosis in % stenosis is only a surrogate parameter for the risk of an imminent ischemic event whichever technique is used.

Limitations of angiography

X-ray angiography was the method chosen for the carotid surgery trials run in the second half of the 80s and published in the early 90s. They provided conclusive evidence for the benefit of surgery [9]. The problem of angiographic measurements is that the diameter is measured, but the hemodynamic effect of a stenosis is due to the degree of area reduction. This is one important reason for a good deal of the discrepancies between ultrasonic and angiographic measurements. The area of stenosis is seldom concentric, often semicircular or oval shaped. Especially a high degree stenosis may have a very irregular opening making it completely illusive to estimate area reduction by measuring the diameter. This irregular aspect can often only be realised by the surgeon during endarterectomy.

Limitations of ultrasonography

Spectral analysis

The most popular parameter is the peak systolic velocity (PSV) in the stenosis. The envelope of the Doppler spectrum is chosen instead of the instant mean Doppler shift and converted to velocity. The envelope of the spectrum is more reproducible than the instant mean especially in systole. The highest frequencies in systole are recorded from those streamlines with the highest velocities and with the smallest angle of incidence (Doppler angle). That means that at the outlet of a stenosis with diverging streamlines the best Doppler angle may not be parallel to the vessel axis (Fig. 1). Helical flow organisation and disturbances due to tortuosity are further factors making a correct angle estimation difficult or impossible even using color flow as a guide. The possible error converting Doppler shift to velocity increases with increasing Doppler angle due to the cosine function (Doppler equation). Therefore the variability of velocity estimations is higher compared to simple frequency recordings. Beside disturbed flow technical factors have to be considered. Intrinsic spectral broadening is due to beam spreading [7]. For recording Doppler signals with a linear probe a series of transducer elements are pulsed to generate and direct the wave-front. As a consequence the recorded

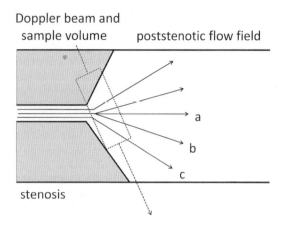

Figure 1 Possible error calculating velocity in disturbed flow. Schematic poststenotic flow field with diverging flow lines. The sample volume (dotted lines) is set immediately at the outlet of a stenosis. Each flow line represents the same velocity. The highest Doppler frequency (envelope of the spectral waveform) will be recorded from the flow line (c) due to the small angle of incidence. Overestimation of peak velocity (PSV) results if it is calculated using the angle of insonation (a) or (b). In practice the sample volume often covers the canal and the outlet of a stenosis.

spectrum is composed of signals originating from different angles of insonation creating spectral broadening [12]. All this may lead to considerable overestimation of velocities in the stenosis. This ''error'' is highly variable depending on the individual circumstances (flow and insonation). On the other hand underestimation of PSV can result from insufficient gain or a low wall filter. In this case the sample volume contains few fast moving blood cells (jet) and many slow ones (eddies) the signal amplitude of the fast ones may be too small in relation to the slow ones being displayed [6].

Hemodynamic influences

Velocity in a stenosis (PSV) depends not only on area restriction but also on the resulting pressure drop. This pressure drop is smaller in case of good collateral supply to the irrigated territory [14]. This results in a reduced flow volume and flow velocity in the severely stenosed artery. On the contrary very high velocities can be recorded from the same degree of stenosis when there is no collateral supply available. A contralateral occlusion leads also to increased velocities in a stenosis [5] but only in case of functioning cross flow. The highest velocities will be seen in 80—90% stenoses. In near occlusion, velocities are lower and variable [1,14,15]. Therefore the PSV alone cannot differentiate between a moderately stenosed artery and a nearly occluded one.

Grading carotid stenosis by means of Doppler duplex sonography needs a multiparametric approach

PSV for grading a stenosis has only a limited value. Therefore additional criteria are mandatory. The method is combining these criteria in grading carotid stenosis in well defined categories: the first question to ask is whether a stenosis has any hemodynamic effect. This happens in a stenosis of ≥ 70 NASCET [14]. The most important sign is reversal of flow in the ophthalmic artery and in the ipsilateral anterior cerebral artery signifying collateral flow (criterion 4, Table 1). This does not differentiate a stenosis from occlusion of the ICA, but in case of stenosis this indicates undoubtedly a severe and hemodynamically relevant one. PSV is high (criterion 2) except in near occlusion or in the rare condition of additional severe intracranial stenosis. Among the severe, $\geq 70\%$ stenoses criterion 3 (poststenotic flow velocity, beyond flow disturbances) allows a further differentiation because with increasing narrowing flow volume and velocity are decreasing [14]. This is not found in a stenosis below 70% [14]. The guidelines [1,10] differentiate within the group of high degree stenoses ($\geq 80\%$) those with a poststenotic velocity drop to $\leq 30 \, cm/s$ as very high (90%). A side to side comparison of the waveform and velocities of the distal ICA is helpful to make clear not only the reduction of PSV but also a reduced poststenotic pulsatility on the side of the stenosis. In case there is no sign of hemodynamic compromise, a stenosis may be moderate (50—60%) or of lower degree. With a moderate stenosis there is still a considerable local increase of velocities, whereas this is not the case in low degree stenosis. This last category is best demonstrated by B-Mode ultrasound with the unique advantage to demonstrate wall thickening with high spatial resolution. The width of the stenotic canal can often be measured in higher degrees of stenosis as well with B-mode imaging. The diameter can then be related to the distal one for measuring the degree of stenosis following the NASCET method, but this is only possible with excellent conditions for insonation. Color Doppler is helpful in delineating plaques of low echogenicity or proving absence of flow in the occluded ICA. But it does not allow precise diameter measurements due to its low frame rate and a huge influence of the gain. Grading of stenoses above 50% is the basis of clinical decisions. Combining morphologic and several hemodynamic features allows a reliable description of at least four classes of stenosis. Such a multiparametric approach avoids severe misclassification as is done with a simplified PSV criterion or its derivates alone (end diastolic velocities in the stenosis, ratio of velocities ICA/CCA). Secondary criteria may be helpful in supporting the diagnosis as the extend of flow disturbances being most pronounced in a 70—80% stenosis and diminishing together with a reduced flow volume in very a high degree stenosis

Is it justified to use ultrasonography as the only method to decide about interventions on the internal carotid artery?

In a high degree stenosis the hemodynamic effect is shown by the appearance of collateral flow, which is driven by the poststenotic pressure drop. Another effect is a poststenotic decrease of velocity and pulsatility of flow. All these effects can be measured reliably by extra- and intracranial Doppler duplex sonography. The question is whether the trial result that surgery is highly beneficial in case of a symptomatic $\geq 70\%$ NASCET stenosis as measured by angiography can be translated into: beneficial in case of a ''hemodynamically relevant stenosis'' because 70% stenosis is the threshold from which a pressure drop and decreased poststenotic flow can be observed. This seems reasonable but is so far not accepted as level one evidence. [8]. A meta-analysis of studies correlating PSV and percent of stenosis as measured by angiography showing a considerable disagreement was the background of not accepting ultrasonography. The old concept of a multiparametric diagnosis was not considered. However it has been used and taught over decades. New technical elements have been continuously introduced. But there is a lack of well designed and large studies for this concept, including all these new techniques. In older publications e.g. the definition for measuring the degree of stenosis (NASCET or ECST) is missing. This is one of the reasons why, they do not add very much to the evidence. Even with such new studies some disagreement between methods will persist as explained above. Clinically most useful would be to repeat randomized carotid surgery trials with ultrasonography as criterion for decision in symptomatic patients. However it is ethically not justified to randomize for this question again. With an asymptomatic carotid stenosis the decision about invasive measures is more delicate and controversial as the risks of angiography is small but real. Nevertheless recent recommendations of the AHA accepted duplex sonography for indicating invasive treatment of asymptomatic patients [3]. This makes evident the dependence of consensus recommendations on the time and design of selected studies.

How to proceed in practice?

Training, quality control and certification are prerequisites before using Doppler duplex sonography for decision making. Documentation has to be comprehensive and conclusive. These prerequisites are the same as for other methods. Vascular ultrasonography is non-invasive but not "quick and easy".

In case of definitely low or high degree disease as shown by using several main criteria, decisions may be based directly on the sonographic diagnosis. Then angiography is not justified (risk and expenses) just for additional documentation. In case of a symptomatic patient with a diagnosis in between both of these situations the decision may be based on additional imaging with angiography (intraarterial, CTA, MRA) in case of unfavourable insonation conditions or contradictory findings.

The presently available guidelines shall provide a common terminology and promote the diagnosis based on a set of weighted criteria.

Acknowledgement

The author thanks Alfred Persson M.D. (Wellesley Massachusetts) for kindly reviewing the text.

References

[1] Arning C, Widder B, von Reutern GM, Stiegler H, Gortler M. Revision of DEGUM ultrasound criteria for grading internal carotid artery stenoses and transfer to NASCET measurement. Ultraschall Med 2010;31:251—7.
[2] Eliasziw M, Rankin RN, Fox AJ, Haynes RB, Barnett HJM, North American Symptomatic Carotid Endarterectomy Trial (NASCET) Group. Accuracy and prognostic consequences of ultrasonography in identifying severe carotid artery stenosis. Stroke 1995;26:1747—52.
[3] Goldstein LB, Bushnell CD, Adams RJ, Appel LJ, Braun LT, Chaturvedi S, et al. Guidelines for the primary prevention of stroke: a guideline for healthcare professionals from the American Heart Association/American Stroke Association. Stroke 2011;42:517—84.
[4] Grant EG, Benson CB, Moneta GL, Alexandrov AV, Baker JD, Bluth EI, et al. Carotid artery stenosis: gray-scale and Doppler US diagnosis—Society of Radiologists in Ultrasound Consensus Conference. Radiology 2003;229:340—6.
[5] Henderson RD, Steinman DA, Eliasziw M, Barnett HJ. Effect of contralateral carotid artery stenosis on carotid ultrasound velocity measurements. Stroke 2000;31:2636—40.
[6] Kaps M, von Reutern GM, Stolz E, von Büdingen HJ. Ultraschall in der Neurologie, 2 Auflage. Stuttgart, New York: Thieme; 2005.
[7] Kremkau FW. Diagnostic ultrasound, principles and instruments. 5th ed. Philadelphia: W.B. Saunders Company; 1998.
[8] Latchaw RE, Alberts MJ, Lev MH, Connors JJ, Harbaugh RE, Higashida RT, et al. Recommendations for imaging of acute ischemic stroke: a scientific statement from the American Heart Association. Stroke 2009;40:3646—78.
[9] North American Symptomatic Carotid Endarterectomy Trial (NASCET) Collaborators. Beneficial effect of carotid endarterectomy in symptomatic patients with high-grade carotid stenosis. N Engl J Med 1991;325:445—53.
[10] von Reutern GM, Goertler MW, Bornstein NM, Del Sette M, Evans DH, Hetzel A, et al. Recommendations for grading carotid stenosis by means of ultrasonic methods. Stroke 2012;43:916—21.
[11] Rothwell PM, Gibson RJ, Slattery J, Sellar RJ, Warlow CP. Equivalence of measurements of carotid stenosis. A comparison of three methods on 1001 angiograms. European Carotid Surgery Trialists' Collaborative Group. Stroke 1994;25:2435—9.
[12] Thrush JA, Evans DH. Intrinsic spectral broadening: a potential cause of misdiagnosis of carotid artery disease. J Vascular Invest 1995;1:187—92.
[13] Spencer MP, Reid JM. Quantification of carotid stenosis with continuous-wave (C-W) Doppler ultrasound. Stroke 1979;10:326—30.
[14] Spencer MP. Hemodynamics of arterial stenosis. In: Spencer MP, editor. Ultrasonic diagnosis of cerebrovascular disease. Dordrechts: Martinus Nijhoff Publishers; 1987.
[15] Widder B, von Reutern GM, Neuerburg-Heusler D. Morphologic and Doppler sonographic criteria for determining the degree of stenosis of the internal carotid artery. Ultraschall Med 1986;7:70—5.

Early ultrasound imaging of carotid arteries in the acute ischemic cerebrovascular patients

Maria Fabrizia Giannoni [a,*], Edoardo Vicenzini [c], Enrico Sbarigia [b], Vittorio Di Piero [c], Gian Luigi Lenzi [c], Francesco Speziale [b]

[a] Dept "Paride Stefanini", Vascular Ultrasound Investigations Unit, Sapienza University of Rome, Italy
[b] Dept "Paride Stefanini" Vascular Surgery, Italy
[c] Dept Neurological Sciences, Sapienza, University of Rome, Italy

KEYWORDS
Acute cerebral ischemia;
Unstable carotid plaques;
Ultrasonography;
Contrast enhanced ultrasound;
Carotid surgery;
Timing of carotid surgery

Summary

Background and purpose: The early identification of ischemic stroke pathophysiology may lead to different diagnostic and therapeutical strategies. In 1/3 of patients, stroke is related to carotid disease, when a vulnerable plaque evolves with surface rupture and local apposition of highly embolic/thrombotic material. This being a rapidly evolving dynamic process, the value of its early identification may be underestimated. With the diffusion of high-resolution ultrasound equipments, the possibility of identifying these features of plaque vulnerability has become easily available. These plaque characteristics have to be always considered in the patient management, in order to avoid further worsening of neurological conditions or to prevent recurrent events, and to choose the appropriate strategies.

Methods: Early ultrasonography was performed with high frequency probes (9, 15, 18 MHz) in patients admitted to emergency area for acute ischemic symptomatology from carotid stenosis.

Results: In 8 patients admitted to the emergency area few hours after the onset of neurological symptoms, we detected peculiar plaque characteristics closely related to the neurological events and at high risk of further embolic events with local thrombosis, surface plaque rupture and carotid floating thrombi. All these cases were successfully submitted to emergency carotid endarterectomy repair.

Conclusions: Timing of carotid endarterectomy has always been debated in stroke patients' clinical management, depending on several factors. All imaging techniques contribute to the identification of plaque morphology features, but early admission of stroke patients to the emergency areas and early US have a crucial leading role in detecting plaque rupture and dynamic changes in real-time. Peculiar characteristics of high unstable plaques allow the identification of those lesions at particularly high risk of further embolic events according to their fragile characteristics that may benefit from early surgery.
© 2012 Elsevier GmbH. All rights reserved.

* Corresponding author at: Dept "Paride Stefanini", Vascular Ultrasound Investigation Unit, Vascular Surgery, Policlinico Umberto I, Viale del Policlinico 155 00161 Rome, Italy. Tel.: +39 6 49970660; fax: +39 49970652.
E-mail address: mariafabrizia.giannoni@uniroma1.it (M.F. Giannoni).

Introduction

Vulnerable atherosclerotic plaque rupture with surface apposition of thrombotic material is the predominant pathological substrate of acute cerebrovascular events, accounting for 30% of all strokes [1]. In acute ischemic stroke patients, in addition to standard imaging techniques aimed at the decision whether to perform thrombolysis, early ultrasound investigation is fundamental to detect potential embolic carotid source in order to avoid further embolization by means of carotid surgery.

The aim of this report is to evaluate the possibility of early detection of these carotid plaque features with ultrasound and to discuss the implications of this diagnosis in order to plan the most appropriate strategy in acute cerebrovascular ischemic patients.

Material and methods

All patients referred to the emergency area for the onset of acute ischemic neurological symptoms were subjected to Duplex Ultrasonography (DUS) (Siemens Sequoia 512 and Siemens S2000 apparatus), according to the conventional methodology and standard AHA and European Guidelines with high-resolution probes (9, 15, 18 MHz), Tissue Harmonics and Spatial Compound. DUS was performed immediately after brain imaging. No patients with ipsilateral (middle cerebral artery) occlusion or an ischemic area > 1/3 of the Middle Cerebral Artery area underwent carotid endarterectomy.

Results

We report 8 patients (M: 6, F: 2, mean age 64.7 yrs, range 53—78 yrs), referred to the emergency area for the onset of acute neurological symptoms occurred no more than 6 h before, in whom we detected with US immediately performed after brain CT scan, plaque features of high risk of further embolic events, as mobile thrombus over plaque ruptures.

Symptoms included: hemiparesis ($n = 5$), amaurosis fugax ($n = 3$), language impairment ($n = 3$). Three patients had a combination of the symptoms.

Mean NIHSS on admission was 4 (min: 0, max: 8). Cerebral Magnetic Resonance Imaging with diffusion-weighted sequences documented the presence of ischemic areas in 7 patients in the corresponding omolateral carotid territory.

All patients presented hemodynamic internal carotid stenosis consistent with the clinical symptoms. Heterogeneous, mostly hypoechoic, complicated plaques were detected in all cases. Moreover, high-resolution B-Mode imaging performed with high frequency probes and spatial compound to better visualize plaque surface and texture, demonstrated an extensive rupture of the surface with structure fissurations (Fig. 1), intraoperatively confirmed. Ultrasound B-Mode imaging also allowed the detection of an abnormal motion of the soft parts of the plaques, in particular nearby the sites of plaque rupture. In two cases, real-time B-Mode imaging demonstrated an endothelial floating flap represented by the ruptured cap of the plaque, mobile in the lumen, and thus confirming the high potential embolic risk of these lesions (Fig. 2). Mobile clots were also visualized from the surface at the site of plaque rupture in two cases (Fig. 3). Contrast ultrasound imaging detected a high density of microvessels in the plaque tissue consisting with relevant neoangiogenesis, as already described elsewhere [2,3] in acute symptomatic plaques.

Furthermore, contrast ultrasound allowed a better visualization of the plaque extension and surface, better demonstrating the rupture extended deeply from the surface to the core of the plaque. In one case, a small ulceration with a mobile clot was also identified.

All patients were immediately and successfully submitted to CEA: mean NIHSS at discharge was 2 (min: 0, max: 4).

Discussion

Stroke remains a leading cause of disability and death worldwide [4]. About one-third of ischemic strokes arise from

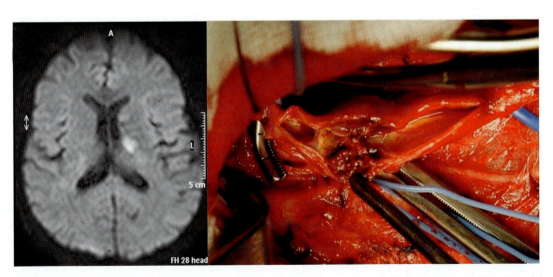

Figure 1 Left side MRI: cerebral ischemic lesion. Right side: intraoperative macroscopic findings ultrasound imaging of the ruptured plaque with the mobile flap (Clip 1).

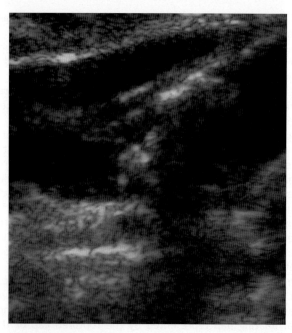

Figure 2 Ultrasonography: hypoechoic, mobile thrombus in the distal anterior part of the plaque (right side of the image) (Clip 2).

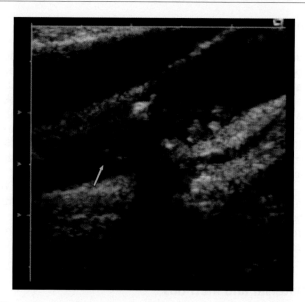

Figure 3 Ultrasonography: hypoechoic, mobile thrombus in the proximal part of the plaque (left side of the image) (Clip 3).

carotid atherosclerotic plaques, embolization representing the main pathophysiological explanation. For this reason, the identification of vulnerable lesions represents the fundamental step to select patients at risk of cerebrovascular ischemic events from carotid disease where the surgical procedure is indicated. This is a particularly relevant hot topic in literature since optimal management of asymptomatic carotid stenosis still remains controversial [5], while the beneficial effect of CEA is recognized worldwide in symptomatic patients for hemodynamic stenosis. However, the timing of surgery in acute cerebrovascular events is still controversial. At present, early CEA is indeed the most appropriate strategy to prevent further carotid cerebrovascular events.

Moreover, in particular, the aim of this short report is to focus on the utility of evaluating acute symptomatic lesions in the early phase, due to the possible detection of peculiar morphological aspects: plaque rupture is an unstable, very common event, detected in our experience in all cases admitted to the emergency area few hours from onset of symptomatology.

The behavior of acute symptomatic plaques in the early phase is often underestimated, while an early and accurate evaluation may be helpful to plan the most appropriate strategy to prevent further cerebrovascular events. Further efforts have to be performed to make a greater awareness in patients so that they arrive in specialized areas as soon as possible: this is a crucial node. The onset of neurological symptomatology must be considered as an emergency condition.

Advances of arterial imaging, through conventional radiological imaging (CT and MR Angiography) [6,7] as well as with ultrasonography [8], converge to achieve more detailed information regarding the identification of these plaques. Summarizing, peculiar plaque characteristics such as severe degree of stenosis, low GSM and surface ulceration are important predictors of plaque vulnerability and there are clear evidences that acute symptomatic plaques are always complicated, with low echogenicity and with relevant surface alterations. However, acute symptomatic plaques in the very early phase have peculiar characteristics that are possible to detect with careful US investigations. Their incidence is often underestimated while an accurate evaluation may be helpful to plan the most appropriate strategy to prevent further cerebrovascular events. Acute symptomatic lesions have specific morphological aspects, and plaque rupture is a true adverse extremely unstable and common event in our experience in early phase. Data collected from recent studies indirectly confirm this condition: in the very acute stroke phase or in patients with transient ischemic attacks, the risk of recurrency is significantly higher and CEA significantly reduces the absolute risk of ipsilateral ischemic stroke [9,10]. As recently indicated by Wardlow et al. [11], ''increasing delays to endarterectomy prevented fewer strokes''. In our experience, early ultrasonography performed with high resolution B-Mode imaging in real-time, quickly revealed in all these symptomatic plaques harmful characteristics, different from surface irregularities and chronic ulcerations, or low echogenicity or low GSM.

Early admission to emergency-specific areas represents the early care in hospitalized centers and the 24 h availability of diagnostic facilities and operating rooms and vascular teams is a fundamental step to get a significant improvement of acute stroke patients prognosis. In conclusion, ultrasound vascular imaging is a key component of the evaluation of early ischemic carotid diseases. Acute symptomatic plaques are a well-defined entity that require early and accurate real-time evaluation, mandatory to thoroughly assess their unstable behavior, rare, but highly risk condition. US imaging, with high-resolution probes, harmonic imaging and spatial compound, has the unique capability to assess these particular features in real-time, where immediate surgery may reduce further stroke risk.

Conclusions

Timing of carotid endarterectomy has always been debated in stroke patients' clinical management, depending on several factors, i.e. blood-brain-barrier breaking, neurological severity, entity of cerebral damage. All imaging techniques contribute to the identification of plaque morphology unstable features, but early US has a crucial leading role in detecting plaque rupture and dynamic changes in real-time, allowing the identification of those lesions at particularly high risk of further embolic events for their fragile characteristics and that may benefit from CEA performed early.

Acute symptomatic plaques require early and accurate real-time evaluation, mandatory to thoroughly assess their unstable behavior and successfully treat them.

Appendix A. Supplementary data

Supplementary data associated with this article can be found, in the online version, at doi:10.1016/j.permed.2012.02.045.

References

[1] Peeters W, Hellings WE, de Kleijn DP, de Vries JP, Moll FL, Vink A, et al. Carotid atherosclerotic plaques stabilize after stroke: insights into the natural process of atherosclerotic plaque stabilization. Arterioscler Thromb Vasc Biol 2009;29:128–33.

[2] Vicenzini E, Giannoni MF, Puccinelli F, Ricciardi MC, Altieri M, Di Piero V, et al. Detection of carotid adventitial vasa vasorum and plaque vascularization with ultrasound cadence contrast pulse sequencing technique and echocontrast agent. Stroke 2007;38:2841–3.

[3] Giannoni MF, Vicenzini E, Citone M, Ricciardi MC, Irace L, Laurito A, et al. Contrast carotid ultrasound for the detection of unstable plaques with neoangiogenesis: a pilot study. Eur J Vasc Endovasc Surg 2009;37:722–7.

[4] Rigby H, Gubitz G, Phillips S. A systematic review of caregiver burden following stroke. Int J Stroke 2009;4:285–9.

[5] Markus HS, King A, Shipley M, Topakian R, Cullinane M, Reihill S, et al. Asymptomatic embolisation for prediction of stroke in the Asymptomatic Carotid Emboli Study (ACES): a prospective observational study. Lancet Neurol 2010;9:663–71.

[6] Sadat U, Weerakkody RA, Bowden DJ, Young VE, Graves MJ, Li ZY, et al. Utility of high resolution MR imaging to assess carotid plaque morphology: a comparison of acute symptomatic, recently symptomatic and asymptomatic patients with carotid artery disease. Atherosclerosis 2009;207:434–9.

[7] Wintermark M, Arora S, Tong E, Vittinghoff E, Lau BC, Chien JD, et al. Carotid plaque computed tomography imaging in stroke and non-stroke patients. Ann Neurol 2008;64:149–57.

[8] Vicenzini E, Giannoni MF, Ricciardi MC, Toscano M, Sirimarco G, Di Piero V, et al. Non-invasive imaging of carotid arteries in stroke: the emerging value of real-time, high resolution ultrasound in carotid occlusion due to cardiac embolism. J Ultrasound Med 2010;29:1635–41.

[9] Coull AJ, Lovett JK, Rothwell PM, on behalf of the Oxford Vascular Study. Population based study of early risk of stroke after transient ischaemic attack or minor stroke: implications for public education and organisation of services. BMJ 2004;328:326.

[10] Eliasziw M, Kennedy J, Hill MD, Buchan AM, Barnett HJ, North American Symptomatic Carotid Endarterectomy Trial Group. Early risk of stroke after a transient ischemic attack in patients with internal carotid artery disease. Can Med Assoc J 2004;170(March):1105–9.

[11] Wardlaw JM, Stevenson MD, Chappell F, Rothwell PM, Gillard J, Young G, et al. Carotid artery imaging for secondary stroke prevention: both imaging modality and rapid access to imaging are important. Stroke 2009;40:3511–7.

How to treat an asymptomatic carotid stenosis? The view of the neurologist

Dirk Sander [a,b,*], Michael Valet [a,b]

[a] Department of Neurology, Benedictus Krankenhaus Tutzing, Technische Universität München, Germany
[b] Department of Neurology, Klinikum rechts der Isar, Technische Universität München, Germany

KEYWORDS
Stroke prevention;
Asymptomatic carotid stenosis;
Medical treatment;
Carotid endarterectomy;
Carotid stenting

Summary The optimal treatment strategy for patients with asymptomatic carotid artery stenosis (ACS) is still a matter of debate. Based on a simplistic view, all stenosed vessels should be cleaned, and the earlier the better. Due to the improvements of medical management in patients with high-grade ACS, there is uncertainty as how to best manage these patients. Consequently, the cost-effectiveness of CEA in patients with ACS has been questioned. Therefore, the question arises how best medical treatment changes the risk of stroke in patients with ACS. This overview discussed the therapeutic options for ACS from a neurological point of view.
© 2012 Elsevier GmbH. All rights reserved.

Introduction

Asymptomatic significant (>50%) carotid stenosis (ACS) is a frequent finding in the aging population. The prevalence of moderate stenosis (50–70%) increases from 3.6% for those <70 years to 9.3% in those 70 years and above. The prevalence of severe (70–99%) stenosis is 1.7% [1].

The optimal treatment strategy for patients with ACS is still a matter of debate. Based on a simplistic view, all stenosed vessels should be cleaned, the earlier the better. This is the rationale behind an approach to treat even asymptomatic patients. The therapeutic effectiveness of a carotid endarterectomy (CEA) in high-grade ACS has been demonstrated in large trials, but the number needed to treat (NNT) is high. On the other hand, CEA is not free of complications, the frequency of which depends on

* Corresponding author at: Department of Neurology, Benedictus Krankenhaus Tutzing & Feldafing, Dr. Appelhans-Weg 682340 Feldafing, Germany. Tel.: +49 8157 28140; fax: +49 8157 28141.
E-mail address: D.Sander@mac.com (D. Sander).

center and surgeon. Unlike symptomatic carotid stenosis, ACS carries a low risk for ipsilateral stroke [2]. The data from CEA trials are more than 20 years old and medical treatment of risk factors (e.g. statins, ACE inhibitors) has changed considerably. In the current best medical treatment (BMT) approach the risk of stroke is therefore even smaller and the number needed to treat by CEA increases. Consequently, the cost-effectiveness of CEA in patients with ACS has been questioned [3]. Recently carotid artery stenting (CAS) became a new ''bloodless'' option. Unfortunately, the comparison between CEA and CAS resulted in conflicting conclusions.

This overview discussed the therapeutic options for ACS from a neurological point of view.

CEA vs. CAS vs. BMT

Whether CEA and CAS are comparable treatment options in ACS or whether a revascularization is better than BMT is currently investigated in the ongoing SPACE-II trial [4], including patients with >70% carotid stenosis that were randomized into 3 arms (CEA, CAS, BMT) as well as in the ACST-2 trial

2211-968X/$ — see front matter © 2012 Elsevier GmbH. All rights reserved.
doi:10.1016/j.permed.2012.02.025

that plans to recruit 5000 patients and follow them up for at least 5 years [5].

CEA vs. CAS

The CREST ("carotid revascularization endarterectomy vs. stenting trial") and SAPPHIRE ("stenting and angioplasty with protection in patients at high risk for endarterectomy") are 2 randomized trials comparing CEA and CAS.

The North-American CREST trial showed a comparable 30-day complication rate for CEA (3.7%) and PTA (3.1%) in the subgroup of patients with ACS [6]. The 4-year risk (any peri-procedural stroke or death, ipsilateral post-procedural stroke) was increased in CAS (4.5%) as compared to CEA (2.7%). However, this difference was not statistically significant (RR 1.86; 95% CI 0.95—3.66, p=0.07) but CREST was not powered for subgroup analysis.

In the SAPPHIRE study, the 30-day risk of MI, stroke, or death was 5.4% for CAS, and 10.2% for CEA (not significantly different). Of note, these complication rates are higher for asymptomatic individuals compared with symptomatic participants within the same trial, and probably exceed the threshold of 3% [7]. For this reason, a persistent criticism of this trial remains that the enrolled patients should not have undergone revascularization at all, given the trial's perioperative complication rates [8].

Current practice of CAS and CEA in the US for asymptomatic stenosis was recently examined, and in-hospital complication rates were presented [9]. CAS was associated with increased odds of stroke or death (OR 1.28, 95% CI 1.03—1.58).

CAS vs. BMT

Neither SAPPHIRE nor CREST address the question now posed by improvements in BMT, namely whether patients with ACS should undergo any revascularization procedure.

CEA vs. BMT

Two trials, ACAS ("asymptomatic carotid atherosclerosis study") and ACST ("asymptomatic carotid surgery trial"), randomized asymptomatic patients with angiographically confirmed stenosis >60% (ACAS) or stenosis >50% on ultrasonography studies (ACST) to CEA vs. a BMT group (or BMT/deferred CEA in the case of ACST). Despite slight differences in entry criteria and analysis, overall outcomes were fairly similar, with a slightly less than 5% decrease in stroke/death over 5 years. The larger number of patients enrolled into ACST and its longer follow-up period provide a more specific understanding of the modest gains of CEA vs. BMT, as follows: (1) of the 4.1% absolute reduction in stroke/death over 5 years, only half of this benefit came from preventing disabling strokes/death (a net gain < 0.5% per year); (2) after 5 years, no further benefit accrues, with a net gain of only 4.6% at 10 years (CEA vs. BMT lines parallel each other after 5 years); (3) no benefit exists for patients older than 75 years; (4) women derive less benefit (reaching statistical significance only at 10 years); and (5) patients on a regimen of lipid-lowering agents have less benefit [8].

Given the underwhelming gains achieved by CEA in asymptomatic patients relative to symptomatic patients, benefit was critically dependent on an extremely low perioperative complication rate, with 3% set as the threshold margin for perioperative stroke/death.

However, significant improvements in BMT have occurred over time, especially in the use of lipid-lowering drugs such as statins, which were used in only 10% of patients in the ACST at trial initiation and in 80% at 10-year follow-up. The SMART ("second manifestation of arterial disease") trial showed that in patients with an ACS >50% the annual stroke risk was only 0.8% even in patients with an increased vascular risk [10]. Marquard et al. [11] demonstrated in a population-based trial from Oxford that a well-treated patient with ACS >50% has an annual risk of ipsilateral stroke of only 0.34%. Recent data from the asymptomatic arm of the CREST trial revealed a 30-day peri-procedural risk of 3.1% for TEA and an ipsilateral 4-year stroke risk (excluding the peri-procedural period) of 1.3% [12]. Similar results were obtained from an analysis of registry data from the US which showed, that a benefit of CEA (if any) may be seen only after several years [13]. A recent meta-analysis [3] including 11 studies with 3724 patients with ACS done between 1983 and 2003 revealed that rates of ipsilateral and any-territory stroke and TIA, with medical intervention alone, have fallen significantly since the mid-1980s and show a gradual reduction in the average annual risk from approximately 2.5% in the mid-1980s to approximately 1% by 2008, with recent estimates overlapping those of operated patients in randomized trials. Additionally, current medical intervention alone was estimated at least 3—8 times more cost-effective [14].

ACS is associated with an increased overall vascular risk

The ACS patient has an increased overall vascular risk: In the SMART study the MI risk was 3.6% per year and thus 4 times higher than the stroke risk [10]. The PRECORIS study [15] assessed the prevalence of ≥50% asymptomatic coronary artery disease (CAD) in 274 patients with ischemic stroke or TIA using cardiac CTA. The prevalence of ≥50% asymptomatic CAD was 18% Asymptomatic CAD was independently associated with traditional risk factors assessed individually and through the Framingham Risk Score (OR 2.6; 95% CI 1.0—7.6 for a 10-year risk of coronary heart disease of 10—19%; and OR 7.3; 95% CI 2.8 to 19.1 for a 10-year risk of coronary heart disease ≥20%), the presence of at least one ≥50% cervicocephalic artery stenosis (OR, 4.0 95% CI 1.4—11.2) and other factor including alcohol consumption and ankle brachial index. In every category of Framingham risk, prevalence of CAD was strongly related to the degree of cervicocephalic stenosis (Fig. 1). Therefore, detection of an ACS should lead to a cardiac workup and to an optimal treatment of vascular risk factors [2].

Risk stratification

Asymptomatic embolization

Several methods to identify such a high-risk group have been suggested, including ultrasonic detection of asymptomatic

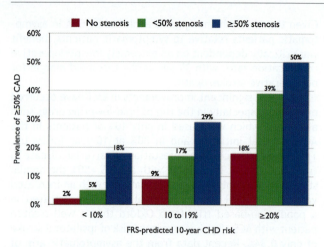

Figure 1 Prevalence of asymptomatic CAD according to severity of cervicocephalic stenosis and Framingham risk score (FRS)-predicted 10-year CHD risk group. According to [15].

embolization. If clinical embolism is a good predictor of the subsequent stroke risk, asymptomatic cerebral emboli might also predict clinical stroke risk [16]. Transcranial Doppler ultrasound (TCD) is a non-invasive technique that can be used to detect circulating emboli. Several studies evaluated the association between detection of embolic signals and new ischemic events in patients with ACS [17—19] and reported different results. Recently a large prospective and multi-center study (ACES, asymptomatic Carotid emboli Study) evaluated the relationship between asymptomatic emboli and stroke risk in 467 patients with an ACS of at least 70% [16]. The detection of emboli was associated with an increased risk for ipsilateral TIA and stroke (HR 2.54, 95% CI 1.2—5.36) and in particular for ipsilateral stroke (HR 5.57, 95% CI 1.61—19.32) during 2 years of follow-up even after adjusting for antiplatelet therapy, degree of stenosis, and other risk factors. The absolute annual risk of ipsilateral stroke or TIA between baseline and 2 years was 7.13% in patients with embolic signals and 3.04% in those without, and for ipsilateral stroke was 3.62% in patients with embolic signals and 0.70% in those without. The authors performed a meta-analysis with all studies available including 1144 patients. The hazard ratio for the risk of ipsilateral stroke for those with embolic signals compared with those without was 6.63 (95% CI 2.85—15.44) with no heterogeneity between studies ($p = 0.33$).

Detection of echolucent plaque using ultrasound

More recently, data from ACES demonstrated that plaque morphology assessed using a simple visual rating scale predicts ipsilateral stroke in ACS [20]. 435 subjects with ACS ≥70% were included and followed-up for 2 years. A 4-point visual rating scale was applied to the plaques and they were classified as echolucent (37.7%) or echogenic. Plaque echolucency at baseline was associated with an increased risk of ipsilateral stroke alone (HR 6.43, 95% CI 1.36—30.44). A combination of plaque echolucency and ES positivity at baseline was associated with an increased risk of ipsilateral stroke alone (HR 10.61, 95% CI 2.98—37.82). The combination of ES detection and plaque morphology allows a greater prediction than either measure alone and identifies a high-risk group with an annual stroke risk of 8%, and a low-risk group with a risk of <1% per year. These data show that the combination of 2 measures of plaque instability may identify a high-risk group of patients with ACS that may benefit from a CEA.

Magnetic resonance imaging (MRI) of plaque

MRI is a non-invasive method of plaque measurement that does not involve ionizing radiation. Examination of plaque under different contrast weighting (black blood: T1, T2, proton density-weightings, and magnetization prepared rapid gradient echocardiography or bright blood: time of flight) allows characterization of individual plaque components, including lipid-rich necrotic core, fibrous cap status, hemorrhage, and calcification [21]. A few small prospective studies have been done to investigate characteristics of carotid artery plaque on MRI that are associated with disease progression and future cardiovascular events. One study [22] examined patients with symptomatic and asymptomatic carotid disease to determine whether fibrous cap thinning or rupture as identified on MRI were associated with a history of recent transient ischemic attack or stroke. When compared with patients with a thick fibrous cap, patients with a ruptured cap were 23 times more likely to have had a recent transient ischemic attack or stroke. An increased risk of ipsilateral cerebrovascular events has also been reported over a mean follow-up period of 38.2 months in asymptomatic patients who had 50—79% carotid stenosis and the presence of a thin or ruptured fibrous cap, intraplaque hemorrhage, or a larger lipid-rich necrotic core [23]. At this time there are no published prospective population data to evaluate the role of MRI findings in risk assessment of asymptomatic adults. A number of large-scale studies are ongoing [21].

Conclusion

- Patients with ACS have a high overall vascular risk. A cardiac workup and an optimal treatment of vascular risk factors should be done.
- CEA is an evidenced-based therapeutic option. However, most data come from the 90s of the last century. Actually, the available data for CAS are not sufficient to judge the role of CAS as compared to TEA and BMT.
- BMT has led to a significant reduction of stroke risk (<1% per year) in patients with ACS, Therefore, the indication or a CEA should be done with restraint and based on life expectancy, sex, and comorbidity.
- Detection of echolucent plaques using duplex ultrasonography, embolic signals using TCD or unstable plaques using MRI criteria identifies high-risk patients for stroke and could be helpful for the decision whether a CEA should be done. Otherwise, aggressive medical therapy of risk factors is recommended.

References

[1] de Weerd M, Greving JP, Hedblad B, Lorenz MW, Mathiesen EB, O'Leary DH, et al. Prevalence of asymptomatic carotid artery

stenosis in the general population: an individual participant data meta-analysis. Stroke 2010;41:1294–7.

[2] Goldstein LB, Bushnell CD, Adams RJ, Appel LJ, Braun LT, Chaturvedi S, et al. Guidelines for the primary prevention of stroke: a guideline for healthcare professionals from the American Heart Association/American Stroke Association. Stroke 2011;42:517–84.

[3] Abbott AL. Medical (non-surgical) intervention alone is now best for prevention of stroke associated with asymptomatic severe carotid stenosis: results of a systematic review and analysis. Stroke 2009;40:e573–83.

[4] Reiff T, Stingele R, Eckstein HH, Fraedrich G, Jansen O, Mudra H, et al. Stent-protected angioplasty in asymptomatic carotid artery stenosis vs. endarterectomy: SPACE2—a three-arm randomized-controlled clinical trial. Int J Stroke 2009;4:294–9.

[5] Hirt L, Halliday A. Controversies in neurology: asymptomatic carotid stenosis—intervention or just stick to medical therapy. The argument for carotid endarterectomy. J Neural Transm 2011;118:631–6.

[6] Silver FL, Mackey A, Clark WM, Brooks W, Timaran CH, Chiu D, et al. Safety of stenting and endarterectomy by symptomatic status in the carotid revascularization endarterectomy vs. stenting trial (CREST). Stroke 2011;42:675–80.

[7] Brott TG, Halperin JL, Abbara S, Bacharach JM, Barr JD, Bush RL, et al. 2011 ASA/ACCF/AHA/AANN/AANS/ACR/ASNR/CNS/SAIP/SCAI/SIR/SNIS/SVM/SVS guideline on the management of patients with extracranial carotid and vertebral artery disease: executive summary. A report of the American College of Cardiology Foundation/American Heart Association Task Force on Practice Guidelines, and the American Stroke Association, American Association of Neuroscience Nurses, American Association of Neurological Surgeons, American College of Radiology, American Society of Neuroradiology, Congress of Neurological Surgeons, Society of Atherosclerosis Imaging and Prevention, Society for Cardiovascular Angiography and Interventions, Society of Interventional Radiology, Society of NeuroInterventional Surgery, Society for Vascular Medicine, and Society for Vascular Surgery. Circulation 2011;124:489–532.

[8] Young KC, Jain A, Jain M, Replogle RE, Benesch CG, Jahromi BS. Evidence-based treatment of carotid artery stenosis. Neurosurg Focus 2011;30:E2.

[9] Young KC, Jahromi BS. Does current practice in the United States of carotid artery stent placement benefit asymptomatic octogenarians? AJNR Am J Neuroradiol 2011;32:170–3.

[10] Goessens BMB, Visseren FLJ, Kappelle LJ, Algra A, van der Graaf Y. Asymptomatic carotid artery stenosis and the risk of new vascular events in patients with manifest arterial disease: the SMART study. Stroke 2007;38:1470–5.

[11] Marquardt L, Geraghty OC, Mehta Z, Rothwell PM. Low risk of ipsilateral stroke in patients with asymptomatic carotid stenosis on best medical treatment: a prospective, population-based study. Stroke 2010;41:e11–7.

[12] Brott TG, Hobson RW, Howard G, Roubin GS, Clark WM, Brooks W, et al. Stenting vs. endarterectomy for treatment of carotid-artery stenosis. New Engl J Med 2010;363:11–23.

[13] Woo K, Garg J, Hye RJ, Dilley RB. Contemporary results of carotid endarterectomy for asymptomatic carotid stenosis. Stroke 2010;41:975–9.

[14] Streifler JY. Asymptomatic carotid stenosis: intervention or just stick to medical therapy—the case for medical therapy. J Neural Transm 2011;118:637–40.

[15] Calvet D, Touze E, Varenne O, Sablayrolles JL, Weber S, Mas JL. Prevalence of asymptomatic coronary artery disease in ischemic stroke patients: the PRECORIS study. Circulation 2010;121:1623–9.

[16] Markus HS, King A, Shipley M, Topakian R, Cullinane M, Reihill S, et al. Asymptomatic embolization for prediction of stroke in the asymptomatic carotid emboli study (ACES): a prospective observational study. Lancet Neurol 2010;9:663–71.

[17] King A, Markus HS. Doppler embolic signals in cerebrovascular disease and prediction of stroke risk: a systematic review and meta-analysis. Stroke 2009;40:3711–7.

[18] Spence JD, Tamayo A, Lownie SP, Ng WP, Ferguson GG. Absence of microemboli on transcranial Doppler identifies low-risk patients with asymptomatic carotid stenosis. Stroke 2005;36:2373–8.

[19] Abbott AL, Chambers BR, Stork JL, Levi CR, Bladin CF, Donnan GA. Embolic signals and prediction of ipsilateral stroke or transient ischemic attack in asymptomatic carotid stenosis: a multicenter prospective cohort study. Stroke 2005;36:1128–33.

[20] Topakian R, King A, Kwon SU, Schaafsma A, Shipley M, Markus HS, et al. Ultrasonic plaque echolucency and emboli signals predict stroke in asymptomatic carotid stenosis. Neurology 2011;77:751–8.

[21] Greenland P, Alpert JS, Beller GA, Benjamin EJ, Budoff MJ, Fayad ZA, et al. 2010 ACCF/AHA guideline for assessment of cardiovascular risk in asymptomatic adults: executive summary. JAC 2010;56:2182–99.

[22] Yuan C, Zhang SX, Polissar NL, Echelard D, Ortiz G, Davis JW, et al. Identification of fibrous cap rupture with magnetic resonance imaging is highly associated with recent transient ischemic attack or stroke. Circulation 2002;105:181–5.

[23] Takaya N, Yuan C, Chu B, Saam T, Underhill H, Cai J, et al. Association between carotid plaque characteristics and subsequent ischemic cerebrovascular events: a prospective assessment with MRI—initial results. Stroke 2006;37:818–23.

Medical management of asymptomatic carotid stenosis

Marek Jauss*

Department of Neurology, Oekumenisches Hainich Klinikum, Muehlhausen, Thüringen, Germany

KEYWORDS
Asymptomatic;
Carotid stenosis;
Medical treatment;
Primary prevention

Summary Operative treatment of asymptomatic carotid stenosis is well established since results of Asymptomatic Carotid Atherosclerosis Study (ACAS) trial and Asymptomatic Carotid Surgery Trial (ACST) were published. However, advances in medical treatment and recent trials that revealed success of "best medical treatment" over interventional treatment for stenosis of brain supplying arteries have raised the question, if "best medical treatment" should be considered as first option in case of asymptomatic carotid stenosis.
© 2012 Elsevier GmbH. All rights reserved.

Operative treatment of asymptomatic carotid stenosis

Arterioarterial embolism is one of the most common stroke etiologies. Although screening for carotid artery disease in patients with lack of symptoms of cerebrovascular disease on a routine base is not recommended, these patients are identified in many ways, particularly by a general physician, who examines the origin of a carotid bruit or by an angiologist screening for additional manifestations of arteriosclerosis in patients with peripheral arterial occlusive disease. When asymptomatic carotid stenosis is diagnosed, operative treatment of carotid stenosis is well established since results of the Asymptomatic Carotid Atherosclerosis Study (ACAS) trial [1] and the Asymptomatic Carotid Surgery Trial (ACST) [2] were published.

Drawbacks of operative treatment of asymptomatic carotid stenosis

However, due to low absolute risk reduction of 1.2% the efficacy of surgical intervention has been questioned by means of calculations leading to a disclosure of costs of up to 580.000 AUS$ for one stroke prevented with prophylactic TEA in case of asymptomatic stenosis [3]. Costs may be even higher, taking into account, that the periprocedural complication rate of less than 3% in the multicenters trials was not confirmed in postapproval registries [4,5]. A recent meta analysis went even further and calculated the difference in estimated fatal and disabling stroke-free survival in case of endarterectomy in patients with asymptomatic severe carotid stenosis as less than 4 days over the course of 5 years [6].

Benefits of best medical treatment in asymptomatic carotid stenosis

Rate for ipsilateral stroke in untreated carotid stenosis has been declined from 3.3% [7] in 1985 to 0.6% [8] in 2007. A recent meta analysis concluded, that this observation was not due to reduced incidence of risk factors but rather due

* Correspondence address: Department of Neurology, Oekumenisches Hainich Klinikum, Justus-Liebig-University of Giessen, Pfafferode 102, D-99974 Mühlhausen, Germany.
E-mail address: marek.jauss@neuro.med.uni-giessen.de

to improved medical treatment (particularly hypertensive drugs and statines) [9].

At least for high-risk asymptomatic patients with poor 5-year survival (e.g., those with previous vascular surgery, claudication, cardiac disease, an abnormal electrocardiogram, diabetes mellitus, or older age) medical treatment was recommended since many years [10]. Recent guidelines state that selection of asymptomatic patients for carotid revascularization should be guided by an assessment of comorbid conditions, life expectancy, and other individual factors and should include a thorough discussion of the risks and benefits of the procedure with an understanding of patient preferences brott [11].

Further evidence for efficacy of best medical treatment was gained by evaluation of the SAMMPRIS trial [12]. In this trial (although focused on intracranial instead of extracranial stenosis) a strict medical management according to a previous published regimen [13,14] was able to mask any probable effect of additional interventional treatment of stenosis of intracranial arteries.

Table 1 Aggressive medical treatment (according to the SAMMPRIS trial) [12].

Aspirin, at a dose of 325 mg/day
Management of
  Elevated systolic blood pressure
    Aim: systolic blood pressure of less than 140 mm Hg
  (<130 mm Hg in patients with diabetes)
  Elevated low-density lipoprotein [LDL] cholesterol levels
    Aim: LDL cholesterol level of less than 70 mg/dl
  (1.81 mmol/l)
  Diabetes
  Elevated non-high-density lipoprotein [non-HDL]
  cholesterol levels
Reduce/quit
  Smoking
  Excess weight
  Insufficient exercise (with the help of a lifestyle modification program)

Specification of best medical treatment in asymptomatic carotid stenosis

Best medical treatment may be specified [15] as weight and girth loss by means of dietary counseling, lipid-lowering therapy (aimed at low-density lipoprotein level <2.6 mmol/l and a triglyceride <1.7 mmol/l and high-density lipoprotein level >1.0 mmol/l), smoking cessation (if applicable), blood pressure below 140/90 mm Hg (in case of diabetes or kidney disease, below 130/80 mm Hg) by means of antihypertensive agents and screening for diabetes and treatment (if applicable) with a target glycated hemoglobin level of less than 7% and a moderate-intensity aerobic physical exercise program ($\geq$30 min most days of the week) however, treadmill testing should be performed in case of suspected coronary heart disease, that is present with high incidence in patients with carotid artery disease [16].

"Pleiotropic" effects of best medical treatment in asymptomatic carotid stenosis

Best medical treatment in patients is able to reduce also incidence of stroke due to other causes beside stenosis of carotid artery as proven by the aggressive medical treatment at the SPARCL study [17] that had reduced the chance of a fatal stroke from 1.7% (placebo) to 1% (80 mg atorvastatin) at 5 years independent from type of stroke. Remarkably there was an additional reduction of absolute risk for cardiovascular events including myocardial infarction from 29% (placebo) to 22.4% (80 mg atorvastatin) at 5 years. Therefore when interventional or operative treatment of asymptomatic stenosis of carotid artery is preferred over best medical treatment, more patients will die from ischemic heart disease, which is only preventable with medical therapy and not from either procedure in this particular risk group (Table 1).

A note of caution

However, an elevated risk for stroke compared to the general population remains in patients with asymptomatic carotid stenosis. Therefore education of this particular risk group about the symptoms of transient ischemic attack and stroke is necessary. In contrast to limited effect of large mass media public awareness campaigns about stroke symptoms [18], the effect may be even improved by direct contact with the physician and knowledge of the particular finding of an asymptomatic carotid stenosis and the positive effect of best medical treatment.

References

[1] Executive Committee for the Asymptomatic Carotid Atherosclerosis Study. Endarterectomy for asymptomatic carotid artery stenosis. JAMA 1995;273:1421—8.
[2] Halliday A, Mansfield A, Marro J, Peto C, Peto R, Potter J, et al. Prevention of disabling and fatal strokes by successful carotid endarterectomy in patients without recent neurological symptoms: randomised controlled trial. Lancet 2004;363:1491—502.
[3] Hankey GJ. Stroke: how large a public health problem, and how can the neurologist help? Arch Neurol 1999;56:748—54.
[4] Wolff T, Guirguis-Blake J, Miller T, Gillespie M, Harris R. Screening for carotid artery stenosis: an update of the evidence for the U.S. preventive services task force. Ann Intern Med 2007;147:860—70.
[5] Feasby TE, Kennedy J, Quan H, Girard L, Ghali WA. Real-world replication of randomized controlled trial results for carotid endarterectomy. Arch Neurol 2007;64:1496—500.
[6] Arazi HC, Capparelli FJ, Linetzky B, Rebolledo FP, Augustovski F, Wainsztein NA. Carotid endarterectomy in asymptomatic carotid stenosis: a decision analysis. Clin Neurol Neurosurg 2008;110:472—9.
[7] Johnson JM, Kennelly MM, Decesare D, Morgan S, Sparrow A. Natural history of asymptomatic carotid plaque. Arch Surg 1985;120:1010—2.
[8] Goessens BM, Visseren FL, Kappelle LJ, Algra A, van der Graaf Y. Asymptomatic carotid artery stenosis and the risk of new vascular events in patients with manifest arterial disease: the SMART study. Stroke 2007;38:1470—5.

[9] Abbott AL. Medical (nonsurgical) intervention alone is now best for prevention of stroke associated with asymptomatic severe carotid stenosis: results of a systematic review and analysis. Stroke 2009;40:e573–83.

[10] Cohen SN, Hobson RW, Weiss DG, Chimowitz M. Death associated with asymptomatic carotid artery stenosis: long-term clinical evaluation. VA cooperative study 167 group. J Vasc Surg 1993;18:1002–9.

[11] Brott TG, Halperin JL, Abbara S, Bacharach JM, Barr JD, Bush RL, et al. ASA/ACCF/AHA/AANN/AANS/ACR/ASNR/CNS/SAIP/SCAI/SIR/SNIS/SVM/SVS guideline on the management of patients with extracranial carotid and vertebral artery disease: executive summary. J Neurointerv Surg 2011;2011(3):100–30.

[12] Chimowitz MI, Lynn MJ, Derdeyn CP, Turan TN, Fiorella D, Lane BF, et al. Stenting versus aggressive medical therapy for intracranial arterial stenosis. N Engl J Med 2011;365:993–1003.

[13] Chaturvedi S, Turan TN, Lynn MJ, Kasner SE, Romano J, Cotsonis G, et al. Risk factor status and vascular events in patients with symptomatic intracranial stenosis. Neurology 2007;69:2063–8.

[14] Gordon NF, Salmon RD, Franklin BA, Sperling LS, Hall L, Leighton RF, et al. Effectiveness of therapeutic lifestyle changes in patients with hypertension, hyperlipidemia, and/or hyperglycemia. Am J Cardiol 2004;94:1558–61.

[15] Sila CA, Higashida RT, Clagett GP. Clinical decisions. Management of carotid stenosis. N Engl J Med 2008;358:1617–21.

[16] Adams RJ, Chimowitz MI, Alpert JS, Awad IA, Cerqueria MD, Fayad P, et al. Coronary risk evaluation in patients with transient ischemic attack and ischemic stroke: a scientific statement for healthcare professionals from the Stroke Council and the Council on Clinical Cardiology of the American Heart Association/American Stroke Association. Circulation 2003;108:1278–90.

[17] Amarenco P, Bogousslavsky J, Callahan III A, Goldstein LB, Hennerici M, Rudolph AE, et al. High-dose atorvastatin after stroke or transient ischemic attack. N Engl J Med 2006;355:549–59.

[18] Lecouturier J, Rodgers H, Murtagh MJ, White M, Ford GA, Thomson RG. Systematic review of mass media interventions designed to improve public recognition of stroke symptoms, emergency response and early treatment. BMC Public Health 2010;10:784.

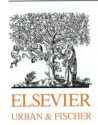
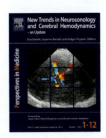

When to perform transcranial Doppler to predict cerebral hyperperfusion after carotid endarterectomy?

Claire W. Pennekamp[a], Selma C. Tromp[b,*], Rob G. Ackerstaff[b], Michiel L. Bots[c], Rogier V. Immink[d], Wilco Spiering[e], Jean-Paul P. de Vries[f], Jaap Kappelle[g], Frans L. Moll[a], Wolfgang F. Buhre[d], Gert J. de Borst[a]

[a] Department of Vascular Surgery, University Medical Center Utrecht, Utrecht, The Netherlands
[b] Department of Clinical Neurophysiology, St. Antonius Hospital, Nieuwegein, The Netherlands
[c] Department of Primary Care, University Medical Center Utrecht, Utrecht, The Netherlands
[d] Department of Anesthesiology, University Medical Center Utrecht, Utrecht, The Netherlands
[e] Department of Vascular Medicine, University Medical Center Utrecht, Utrecht, The Netherlands
[f] Department of Vascular Surgery, St. Antonius Hospital, Nieuwegein, The Netherlands
[g] Department of Neurology and Julius Center for Health Sciences, University Medical Center Utrecht, Utrecht, The Netherlands

KEYWORDS
Cerebral hyperperfusion syndrome;
Transcranial Doppler;
Carotid endarterectomy

Summary Cerebral hyperperfusion syndrome (CHS) after carotid endarterectomy (CEA) is a potential life-threatening disease. Identification of patients at risk for CHS commonly takes place with use of intra-operative transcranial Doppler (TCD), but is associated with both false positive and false negative results. We aimed to determine the diagnostic value for predicting CHS, by adding a TCD measurement in the early post-operative phase after CEA.

We retrospectively included 72 patients who underwent CEA between January 2004 and August 2010 and in whom both intra- and post-operative TCD of the ipsilateral middle cerebral artery monitoring were performed. Twelve patients (17%) had an intra-operative mean blood flow velocity (V_{mean}) increase >100% and 13 patients (18%) a post-operative V_{mean} increase of >100%. In 5 patients (7%) CHS was diagnosed; 2 of those had an intra-operative V_{mean} increase of >100% and all 5 a post-operative V_{mean} increase >100%. This results in a positive predictive value of 17% for the intra-operative and 38% for the post-operative measurement.

In conclusion, a post-operative increase of the mean velocity in the ipsilateral middle cerebral artery of >100% as measured by TCD is superior to an intra-operative velocity increase, for the identification of patients at risk for the development of CHS after CEA.
© 2012 Elsevier GmbH. All rights reserved.

* Corresponding author at: Department of Clinical Neurophysiology, St Antonius Hospital, P.O. Box 2500, 3430 EM Nieuwegein, The Netherlands. Tel.: +31 30 6092452; fax: +31 30 6092327.
E-mail address: s.tromp1@antoniusziekenhuis.nl (S.C. Tromp).

Introduction

Cerebral hyperperfusion syndrome (CHS) after carotid endarterectomy (CEA) is a potential life-threatening disease. It is defined by a combination of symptoms, including headache, vomiting, neurological deficit or seizures, and at least a doubling of pre-operative cerebral blood flow. CHS can occur during the first few days up to four weeks after CEA in 1—3% of patients [1]. If not recognized and treated adequately in time (i.e., strict blood pressure control), hemorrhagic stroke may occur, which subsequently leads to death in up to 40% of patients [2].

The generally accepted definition of post-operative cerebral hyperperfusion in the context of CEA is defined as an increase in cerebral blood flow (CBF) of >100% over baseline [3]. This occurs in approximately 10% of CEA patients [4] and has been associated with a tenfold higher risk for post-operative intra-cerebral hemorrhage in patients operated under general anesthesia [3,5]. Changes in CBF are correlated with changes in the mean blood velocity (V_{mean}) in the ipsilateral middle cerebral artery (MCA) as measured with TCD [6,7]. Currently, during CEA under general anesthesia, an increase in V_{mean} of >100% three minutes after declamping the ICA, compared to the pre-clamping V_{mean} is the most commonly used predictor of CHS [2,8—10]. However, intra-operative TCD monitoring is associated with both false negative and false positive results [2,11]. Therefore, a more precise method is needed to predict which patients are at risk for CHS [12].

This study aimed to assess the predictive values of TCD monitoring regarding the development of CHS, by introducing an additional TCD measurement in the first two post-operative hours.

Methods

Patients who underwent CEA between January 2004 and August 2010 in the St. Antonius Hospital, Nieuwegein, The Netherlands, were retrospectively included. All patients who underwent CEA for a high degree ICA stenosis and in whom both intra- and post-operative TCD monitoring were performed were included.

Surgery was performed under general anesthesia and all patients received the same anesthetic regimen. An intra-luminal shunt was used selectively in case of EEG asymmetry or a decrease of >60% of V_{mean} measured by TCD [13].

For the TCD registration, a pulsed Doppler transducer (Pioneer TC4040, EME, Überlingen, Germany), gated at a focal depth of 45—60 mm, was placed over the temporal bone to insonate the main stem of the MCA ipsilateral to the treated carotid artery. The TCD transducer was fixed with a head frame and V_{mean} was recorded continuously.

V_{mean} values at the following time points were used for further analysis. For the pre-operative V_{mean} (V1), a TCD measurement was performed 1—3 days prior to operation. During operation, the pre-clamping V_{mean} (V2) was registered 30 s prior to carotid cross-clamping. The post-declamping V_{mean} (V3) was determined three minutes after declamping. An additional post-operative V_{mean} (V4) was measured within the first 2 h after surgery on the recovery ward. The intra-operative increase of V_{mean} was defined

Table 1 Patient characteristics.

Patient characteristics	N = 72; mean ± SD
Age (years)	68.4 (± 10.1)
Gender (male)	53 (74%)
Site (right)	36 (50%)
Symptomatic	62 (86%)
Shunt use	22 (31%)
Post-operative hypertension	19 (26%)
Cerebral hyperperfusion syndrome	5 (7%)

and calculated as $(V3 - V2)/V2 \times 100\%$. For calculating the post-operative increase of V_{mean} the following formula was used $(V4 - V1)/V1 \times 100\%$. The positive (PPV) and negative predictive values (NPV) of both intra-operative and post-operative increase of V_{mean} were calculated.

All patients with post-operative hypertension, i.e. blood pressure (BP) >160 mmHg systolic (absolute), >20% above the pre-operative BP, or BP risen above the individual restriction in patients with an intra-operative V_{mean} increase >100%, underwent strict individualized BP control during the early post-operative period with intravenous labetalol (first choice) or clonidine (second choice).

CHS was diagnosed if the patient developed headache, confusion, seizures, intracranial hemorrhage or focal neurological deficits in the presence of post-operative cerebral hyperperfusion (defined as >100% increase of the pre-operative V_{mean}) after a symptom-free interval.

Results

Of the 560 patients undergoing CEA during the time of the study, 72 (13%) received both intra- and post-operative TCD monitoring and were included for the present analysis. See Table 1 for patient characteristics. The majority of patients were symptomatic (86%). About a third of the patients required the use of an intra-luminal shunt because of either EEG asymmetry or a decrease of >60% of V_{mean} measured by TCD.

Twelve patients (17%) had an intra-operative V_{mean} increase >100%. Post-operatively, V_{mean} increase >100% was found in the 13 patients (18%).

During all TCD measurements no significant increase in BP was found after declamping compared to the pre-clamping systolic BP or when the post-operative measurement was compared to the pre-operative systolic BP.

Of all 72 patients, 19 patients (26%) developed post-operative hypertension and 5 patients (7%) suffered from CHS. All patients with CHS had hypertension during the post-operative phase. The overall 30-day rate of death/stroke was 1%.

TCD measurements and clinical outcome

Of 12 patients with an intra-operative increase of V_{mean} > 100%, 2 patients developed CHS. On the other hand, in 60 patients who had an intra-operative increase less than 100%, 3 patients suffered from CHS. This results in a PPV of 17% (2/12) and NPV of 95% (57/60) in the prediction of CHS (Table 2).

Table 2 Cross tables for predictive values of intra- or post-operative TCD measurements for the occurrence of CHS.

	CHS+	CHS−	PPV (%)	NPV (%)
Intra-operative increase				
>100%	2 (3%)	10 (14%)	17	95
<100%	3 (4%)	57 (79%)		
Post-operative increase				
>100%	5 (7%)	8 (11%)	38	100
<100%	0 (0%)	59 (82%)		

CHS+: number of patients who developed CHS (%); CHS−: number of patients who did not develop CHS (%); PPV: positive predictive value (%); NPV: negative predictive value (%).

With respect to the post-operative TCD measurements 5 of the 13 patients with at least a doubling of post-operative V_{mean} developed CHS. In the subgroup of 59 patients with a post-operative increase of less than 100% CHS did not occur. This results in a PPV of 38% (5/13) and a NPV of 100% (59/59) for the development of CHS.

Discussion

In the present retrospective study, as previously published, an increase in V_{mean} measured with post-operative TCD is superior in predicting the development of CHS to the commonly used increase in V_{mean} measured three minutes after declamping versus pre-clamping value [12]. The PPV of the post-operative measurement in the prediction of CHS is more than two times higher than the PPV of the intra-operative measurement (38% and 17% respectively). Moreover, absence of doubling of the V_{mean} at the post-operative measurement completely excluded the development of CHS (NPV 95% vs. 100% for the intra-operative and post-operative measurements, respectively). Therefore, with post-operative measurement fewer patients will be treated unnecessarily by strict intravenous antihypertensive medication. These observations need confirmation in larger patients cohorts, with special focus on the optimal threshold of post-operative CHS prediction.

In our study, only 5 of all patients developed CHS. The low incidence of CHS hampers the interpretation of our results. However, the incidence in our group of patients (7%) is relatively high compared to other series. This might be explained by the fact that in our referral hospital a selected group of patients with relatively severe hemodynamic compromise are treated, which is also reflected in the relatively high number of patients in whom a shunt was used (31%). In addition, data were collected retrospectively, and were more likely to be complete (i.e., including post-operative measurements) in patients with an intra-operative V_{mean} increase of >100%, or in patients who developed post-operative hypertension. However, prospectively collected data in another large vascular training hospital show similar results and thus confirm our findings [12]. A multicenter prospective study to optimize the post-operative TCD-measurements will start in 2012.

Conclusion

Besides the commonly used intra-operative TCD monitoring, additional TCD measurement in the early post-operative phase is useful to predict CHS in patients that underwent CEA under general anesthesia. By measuring V_{mean} in the post-operative instead of only in the intra-operative phase, both the positive and negative predictive value of TCD for development of CHS after CEA can be improved. Therefore, we recommend a baseline measurement before the administration of anesthetics and a post-operative measurement within two hours after surgery.

References

[1] van Mook WN, Rennenberg RJ, Schurink GW, van Oostenbrugge RJ, Mess WH, Hofman PA, et al. Cerebral hyperperfusion syndrome. Lancet Neurol 2005;4(December (12)):877—88.

[2] Dalman JE, Beenakkers IC, Moll FL, Leusink JA, Ackerstaff RG. Transcranial Doppler monitoring during carotid endarterectomy helps to identify patients at risk of postoperative hyperperfusion. Eur J Vasc Endovasc Surg 1999;18(September (3)):222—7.

[3] Sundt Jr TM, Sharbrough FW, Piepgras DG, Kearns TP, Messick Jr JM, O'Fallon WM. Correlation of cerebral blood flow and electroencephalographic changes during carotid endarterectomy: with results of surgery and hemodynamics of cerebral ischemia. Mayo Clin Proc 1981;56(September (9)):533—43.

[4] Ogasawara K, Yukawa H, Kobayashi M, Mikami C, Konno H, Terasaki K, et al. Prediction and monitoring of cerebral hyperperfusion after carotid endarterectomy by using single-photon emission computerized tomography scanning. J Neurosurg 2003;99(September (3)):504—10.

[5] Piepgras DG, Morgan MK, Sundt Jr TM, Yanagihara T, Mussman LM. Intracerebral hemorrhage after carotid endarterectomy. J Neurosurg 1988;68(April (4)):532—6.

[6] Aaslid R, Markwalder TM, Nornes H. Noninvasive transcranial Doppler ultrasound recording of flow velocity in basal cerebral arteries. J Neurosurg 1982;57(December (6)):769—74.

[7] Poulin MJ, Robbins PA. Indexes of flow and cross-sectional area of the middle cerebral artery using doppler ultrasound during hypoxia and hypercapnia in humans. Stroke 1996;27(December (12)):2244—50.

[8] Jansen C, Sprengers AM, Moll FL, Vermeulen FE, Hamerlijnck RP, van Gijn J, et al. Prediction of intracerebral haemorrhage after carotid endarterectomy by clinical criteria and intra-operative transcranial Doppler monitoring. Eur J Vasc Surg 1994;8(May (3)):303—8.

[9] Powers AD, Smith RR. Hyperperfusion syndrome after carotid endarterectomy: a transcranial Doppler evaluation. Neurosurgery 1990;26(January (1)):56—9.

[10] Jorgensen LG, Schroeder TV. Defective cerebrovascular autoregulation after carotid endarterectomy. Eur J Vasc Surg 1993;7(July (4)):370—9.

[11] Ogasawara K, Inoue T, Kobayashi M, Endo H, Yoshida K, Fukuda T, et al. Cerebral hyperperfusion following carotid endarterectomy: diagnostic utility of intraoperative transcranial Doppler ultrasonography compared with single-photon emission computed tomography study. AJNR Am J Neuroradiol 2005;26(February (2)):252—7.

[12] Pennekamp CWA, Tromp SC, Ackerstaff RGA, Bots ML, Immink RV, Spiering W, et al. Prediction of cerebral hyperperfusion after carotid endarterectomy with Transcranial Doppler. Eur J Vasc Endovasc Surg 2012 (January (18)), [Epub ahead of print].

[13] Jansen C, Moll FL, Vermeulen FE, van Haelst JM, Ackerstaff RG. Continuous transcranial Doppler ultrasonography and electroencephalography during carotid endarterectomy: a multimodal monitoring system to detect intraoperative ischemia. Ann Vasc Surg 1993;7(January (1)): 95—101.

Predictors of carotid artery in-stent restenosis

Katrin Wasser[a], Sonja Gröschel[a], Janin Wohlfahrt[a], Klaus Gröschel[b],*

[a] Department of Neurology, University of Göttingen, Robert-Koch-Str. 40, 37075 Göttingen, Germany
[b] Department of Neurology, University of Mainz, Langenbeckstr. 1, 55131 Mainz, Germany

KEYWORDS
Carotid artery stenosis;
Stent;
Angioplasty;
Restenosis;
Stroke;
Carotid ultrasound

Summary

Background: Carotid angioplasty and stenting (CAS) is increasingly being used as a treatment alternative to endarterectomy (CEA), especially in patients aged <70 years with significant carotid artery stenosis. However, an in-stent restenosis (ISR) might endangering the long-term efficacy of CAS. The aim of this article was to review the current literature regarding incidence and clinical significance as well as predictors of in-stent restenosis.
Methods: We conducted a systematic review of the literature to identify all studies on the abovementioned factors.
Results: 3 randomized-controlled trials comparing CAS and CEA and 13 single centre studies fulfilled our inclusion criteria. The occurrence of ISR after CAS ranged from 2.7 to 33% and was detected within the first year in most of the studies. The clinical impact as well as the therapeutic consequence of ISR remains unclear, but many baseline characteristics (age, prior CEA or radiation), procedural (insufficient stent deployment, stent dimensions, inflammatory marker) and follow-up factors (reduced HDL, diabetes mellitus) could be found to identify patients at special risk for ISR. A wide heterogeneity related to the definition and their corresponding ultrasound criteria for ISR was observed.
Conclusions: A close follow-up is suggested especially in those patients with predictors of an ISR. The wide range of ISR ultrasound definitions urges the need for an implementation of generally valid criteria in ISR diagnosis. Against the background of the unknown clinical significance of ISR and a lacking established treatment modality these findings should be taken into account when offering CAS as a treatment alternative to CEA.
© 2012 Published by Elsevier GmbH.

Introduction

Atherosclerotic stenosis of the internal carotid artery is known as a major risk factor for disabling stroke or death leading to enormous socioeconomic problems. The standard therapy for a symptomatic stenosis of the internal carotid artery has been a carotid endarterectomy (CEA) in combination with best medical treatment of concomitant cerebrovascular risk factors. In recent years, carotid angioplasty and stenting (CAS) has widely been used as a treatment of first choice in many patients, despite the fact that the randomized controlled trials and subsequent meta-analyses could not prove a general superiority of CAS over CEA [1–6]. However, the results of the aforementioned trials have been interpreted very controversely resulting in conflicting recommendations in various current guidelines.

* Corresponding author. Tel.: +49 6131 173105; fax: +49 6131 17473105.
E-mail address: klaus.groeschel@unimedizin-mainz.de (K. Gröschel).

In the American guidelines, for instance, the authors concluded that CAS could be used as an equivalent treatment modality to CEA in medium risk patients with a symptomatic carotid stenosis [7], whereas elsewhere, CEA still is advocated as the first treatment of choice [8]. Despite this ongoing current debate, there is accumulating evidence that a subgroup of patients aged <70 years may profit from a CAS intervention [3–5,9]. Because the clinical long-term outcome is of crucial importance especially in younger patients, the occurrence of an in-stent restenosis (ISR) could be one factor endangering the long-term efficacy and safety of CAS. Unfortunately, data concerning the rate and clinical impact of ISR during long-term follow-up are still sparse and show conflicting results [3,10,11] which may in part be attributable to different definitions of an ISR during ultrasound follow-up investigations [12,13].

This article briefly summarizes the currently available long-term data of randomized controlled trials comparing CAS and CEA and of several single centre studies regarding the incidence and clinical impact of ISR as well as clinical predictors for ISR.

Methods

A MEDLINE search was conducted by two independent reviewers (K.W. and J.W.) using the following keyword searches: "carotid artery", "stent", and "restenosis". As a key feature before retrieving a full text article after investigating a potentially beneficial abstract, the studies had to fulfil the following criteria: (1) studies had to be published between January 2000 and October 2011 in a journal which is indexed within the MEDLINE database, (2) the follow-up of the patients had to be performed for at least six months, (3) the occurrence of carotid in-stent restenosis had to be mentioned within the text, (4) articles had to be written in English and (5) at least 100 stented carotid arteries had to be investigated. If there was more than one publication about the same patient cohort, the most recent one or rather the publication with the longest follow-up time was used.

After retrieving the full-text article of abstracts which met the above mentioned criteria, the following data, if available, were extracted in a predefined data sheet: (1) number of arteries that were treated by CAS, (2) follow-up time, (3) baseline characteristics of patients (age, proportion of male patients), (4) amount and definition of ISR, (5) clinical complications of ISR, divided into stroke and death and (6) clinical factors which had been identified to predict the occurrence of an ISR during follow-up. After all relevant data had been extracted by the two reviewers, disagreements were resolved by consensus with the help of a third independent investigator (K.G.)

Results

We could identify 3 randomized, controlled studies (CAVATAS [14,15], SPACE [1,16] and EVA-3S [2,17]) and 13 [18–30] smaller single centre studies that fulfilled our inclusion criteria and reported incidence, clinical significance and predictors of recurrent in-stent stenosis after stent-protected angioplasty of significant internal carotid artery stenosis.

Detailed description of randomized trials of CAS versus CEA

Carotid and Vertebral Artery Transluminal Angioplasty Study (CAVATAS) [14,15] was the first completed, prospective multicentre trial (24 centres in Europe, Australia and Canada) comparing endovascular versus surgical treatment of patients with symptomatic (96.4%) and asymptomatic carotid artery stenosis. CEA was performed in 253 patients, whereas 251 patients received endovascular treatment (mainly angioplasty alone). This study excluded high-risk patients, and stents were used selectively, when available, and in only 26% of cases ($n = 55$). During a median carotid ultrasound follow-up time of 4 years patients undergoing endovascular treatment were found to suffer significantly more often from severe restenosis ($\geq 70\%$) or occlusion than patients after CEA [15]. When comparing balloon angioplasty alone to angioplasty and stenting, those patients who were treated with a stent ($n = 50$) had a significantly lower risk of developing restenosis of $\geq 70\%$ (adjusted hazard ratio 0.43, 0.19–0.97; $p = 0.04$). Regarding the clinical complications in patients with a restenosis, the incidence of ipsilateral stroke or transient ischemic attack was significantly higher in patients with a restenosis $\geq 70\%$ (cumulative 5-year incidence 22.7% vs. 10.9%, $p = 0.04$) compared to those with no ISR. Current or past smoking turned out to be independently associated with a higher incidence of restenosis [15].

The *Stent-Supported Percutaneous Angioplasty of the Carotid Artery vs. Endarterectomy Trial* (SPACE) assessed non-inferiority of CAS to CEA and randomized 1183 patients (CAS $n = 605$; CEA $n = 595$) with a symptomatic carotid artery stenosis as assessed with duplex ultrasound ($\geq 50\%$ according to NASCET criteria, or $\geq 70\%$ according to ECST criteria) at 35 centres in Austria, Germany and Switzerland [1]. The type of stent and use of a protection system were chosen at the discretion of the interventionalist. Restenosis during follow-up were observed more frequently in those patients treated with CAS (4.6% vs. 10.7%, $p < 0.001$) compared to CEA [16]. The majority of the recurrent stenosis occurred within the first 6 months after the initial treatment (CAS $n = 28$ (51.9%), CEA $n = 12$ (52.2%)). Furthermore, additional new ISR were observed even after 24 months of follow-up after carotid stenting whereas no new recurrent restenosis was found after CEA beyond 2 years of follow-up. Because a predefined definition of ISR was not used during the study period and the definition of an ISR depends on the local criteria of each center, a slight overestimation of ISR might be possible [16].

Endarterectomy versus angioplasty in patients with symptomatic severe carotid stenosis (EVA-3S) trial [2] was carried out to demonstrate non-inferiority of CAS compared with CEA and enrolled 527 patients with $\geq 60\%$ symptomatic carotid stenosis at 30 centres in France. In 507 patients (CAS $n = 242$, CEA $n = 265$) serial long-term carotid ultrasound follow-up was performed during a mean follow-up time of 2.1 years [17]. Although the development of a moderate stenosis (≥ 50–69%) within 3 years was found to differ significantly between the groups with a higher proportion after CAS compared to CEA (12.5% vs. 5.0%, $p = 0.02$), the incidence of a high-grade restenosis $\geq 70\%$ showed no significant difference between the two groups (3.3% vs. 2.8%). A clinical impact of an ISR on ipsilateral stroke or death during follow-up could not be observed. Advanced age was a clinical risk factor, which could be identified to be predictive for developing carotid restenosis [17].

To date, to the best of our knowledge, no data about rates of restenosis have yet been published by the other commonly known large randomized controlled studies comparing CEA and CAS especially the International Carotid Stenting Study (ICSS) [31], the Carotid Revascularization Endarterectomy vs. Stenting Trial (CREST) [4], and the Stenting and Angioplasty with Protection in Patients at High Risk for Endarterectomy study (SAPPHIRE) [11,32].

Within the analysed non-randomised trials, there was a wide range concerning the amount of treated patients. The smallest study included 100 patients [33]; the largest number of CAS patients was enrolled in the study of Setacci et al. ($n = 814$) [25]. In the vast majority, patients aged 60 years or over with roughly two-thirds male sex were included in the reviewed studies. The relevant data which were extracted are delineated in Table 1. The diagnostic tool used to detect an ISR was serial duplex ultrasound in all studies ($n = 13$). A confirmatory diagnostic procedure such as CTA or conventional angiography had been carried out after ultrasound in ten studies [19,21–27,29,30]. Notably, there was a wide variation concerning the ultrasound criteria applied for the detection of an ISR between the studies. As one of the main key features for the detection of a restenosis, a cut-off peak systolic velocity is mentioned [19,22,24,26,28–30] sometimes in addition to other criteria such as end-diastolic velocity or the ICA/CCA index [18,20,21,23,25,27].

Although the minority of the studies reported concise details about the exact time point of ISR occurrence, most ISR were found to occur within the first year (median: 8 months, IQR: 7–9) after CAS [16,18,20,21,26,29,30]. There was a broad range concerning the clinical complications for patients with ISR between 0% [21,22,24,26,29] and 25% [30] for stroke and from 0% [19,21–23,25,26,29] to 11.1% [18] for death, respectively.

Common baseline characteristics like advanced age [19], female gender [19], prior revascularization treatment, [23,25,27,34,35] the treatment of a radiogenic stenosis [23] or prior neck cancer [21] could be found to be predictive for ISR development. Furthermore, some cardiovascular risk factors such as smoking [17], lowered HDL cholesterol, [26] diabetes mellitus [22] or elevated HbA1c [18,36] could be identified as predictors for ISR, too. In addition to traditional cardiovascular risk factors, periprocedural elevated inflammatory markers were found to play a major role in ISR development [20,30]. Finally, several procedure-related factors such as stent dimensions [30], implantation of multiple stents [19,28], or an insufficient dilatation effect of CAS [19,20,28] could be identified to promote ISR.

Discussion

Recurrent stenosis after CEA was first described by Stoney and String in 1976 [37] and turned out to be associated with a higher rate of periprocedural complications during a secondary operation [9]. Soon after CAS had received broader acceptance as a potential alternative treatment option for patients with severe carotid artery stenosis, first reports about ISR were published in the late 1990s [38–40]. Since then, the awareness for detecting an ISR has increased further and was more frequently considered in published case series. Within one of the most recent meta-analyses, a 180% increase in the risk of intermediate to long-term carotid restenosis was observed after CAS as compared to CEA. [41] Since CAS is currently widely used as a treatment alternative to CEA, it is necessary to contribute to the ongoing controversial discussion regarding the incidence, clinical significance and appropriate therapeutic management of ISR in order to ameliorate long-term efficacy.

With regard to the etiology of ISR, there may be some similar mechanisms to recurrent stenosis after coronary artery stenting. First of all, an endothelial injury which is caused e.g. by balloon inflation and stent placement, seems to play a major role for the developing of ISR, both after CAS or coronary artery stenting. This damage could initiate a cascade of inflammational processes, which finally leads to a neointimal proliferation and a concentric vessel lumen reduction. Like Schillinger et al. [20] we were recently able to support the notion of an inflammatory cascade as a main cause for ISR by showing that elevated periprocedural inflammation markers are significantly correlated with the development of an ISR [30]. The initial injury of the endothelial layer caused by balloon inflation, guide-wire manipulation or stent placement might explain why additional procedural factors could be identified within our literature review to influence the occurrence of ISR: the use of multiple stents during CAS [19,28] or even wider and longer stent dimensions by their own [30] could be identified to be associated with a higher incidence of ISR. Potential endothelial injuries by either an amplified sheer force of the stent, a more pronounced abrasion or higher inflation pressure during the procedure are some of the discussed issues accountable for restenosis.

Despite the heterogeneity of the analysed studies, one of the most common findings was the time during which an ISR could be detected as it seems to develop most frequently within the first year after a CAS intervention [16,18,20,21,26,29,30]. This fact suggests the assumption that rather an intimal hyperplasia than an atherosclerotic burden is the main driven pathologic factor for an early restenosis.

Although different diagnostic tools and criteria were chosen to determine the presence of an ISR, the incidence is surprisingly constant throughout most of the publications under review. The rate of moderate ($\geq$50%) and high-grade ISR ($\geq$70%) varies between 6.7–13.9% and 2.7–6.3%, respectively (see Table 1). Notably, this rate is higher as compared to those with a preceding CEA treatment within some of the randomised trials [16,42], which has led to a keen discussion on the long-term durability of a CAS procedure [10]. Against the background that there is no established treatment standard for patients with an ISR, this should be considered before a CAS intervention is recommended as the preferred treatment modality. The surgical treatment of an ISR remains an exception since it is technically demanding and might be associated with periprocedural complications [43]. In most of the cases, a redo-PTA or CAS is currently performed after ISR, which seems to be associated with an acceptable rate of periprocedural complications [29,30,35].

As a method of first choice to diagnose ISR, preferably a non-invasive technique should be chosen to avoid a potential

Table 1 Main characteristics of all studies included.

First author (year)	Number of treated arteries, male patients	Mean follow-up time [mo], range	Mean age (years) ± SD	Definition of ISR, DUS criteria (cm/s)	Proportion of ISR (%) during follow-up	Time to detection of ISR [months]	Complications of ISR-patients (%) during follow-up	Independent predictors of ISR
Willfort-Ehringer (2002)	303, 70%	12[b], 6–24[a]	70 ± 9	≥70% ICA/CCA >4	3.0	<12	Stroke 22.2 Death 11.1	Elevated HbA1c at baseline
Khan (2003)	209, 71%	<12, n.g.	72% >75	≥50% PSV ≥140	6.7	n.g.	Stroke 0.4 Death 0.0	Age >75 y Female gender Multiple stent deployment Suboptimal CAS result
Schillinger (2003)	108, 68%	6, n.g.	ISR 62, r60-76 N-ISR 70, r65-76	≥50% PSV ≥150 +ICA/CCA >2.5	13.9	≤6	Stroke 13.3 Death 6.7	Prior CAS Suboptimal CAS result Elevated CRP after CAS
Skelly (2006)	109, 55%	5[b], 0–30	70 ± 9	≥60% PSV ≥170 ≥80% ≥60% + EDV ≥145	≥60% 11.0 ≥80% 4.6	≥60% 7 ≥80% 7, r 1–9	ISR ≥60% Stroke 0 Death 0	Prior neck cancer
Lal (2007)	255, n.g.	19.3, n.g.	ISR 71.8	≥40% PSV ≥140	33.3	n.g.	Stroke 0.0 Death 0.0	Diabetes mellitus Worsening of suggested ISR pattern
Younis (2007)	399, 67%	24, 6–99	70 ± 3.5	≥80% EDV-ICA/CCA >5.4	3.8	24.5 r 5–90	Stroke 20.0 Death 0.0	Prior CEA Radiogenic stenosis
AbuRhama (2008)	144, 51%	20, 1–78	70, r 40–88	≥50% PSV ≥224 cm/s ≥80% PSV ≥325 cm/s	≥50% 7.6 ≥80% 5.6	n.g.	ISR ≥50% Stroke 0.0 Death n.g.	n.g.
Setacci (2008)	814, 64%	45, 0–73	73 ± 8	≥50% PSV ≥175 ≥70% PSV ≥300, EDV ≥140	≥50% 9.0 ≥70% 2.7	n.g.	ISR ≥70% Stroke 9.0 Death 0.0	Prior CEA
Topakian (2008)	102, 66%	12, n.g.	66 ± 9	≥50% PSV ≥180 cm/s	9.8	≤12	Stroke 0.0 Death 0.0	Postprocedural low HDL cholesterol
Zhou (2008)	282, n.g.	32, 6–48	69, r 55–87	≥70% PSV ≥125, EDV <140	6.3	n.g.	Stroke 11.1 Death n.g.	Prior CEA
Cosottini (2010)	200, 74%	26[b], 0–99	72 ± 8	≥50% PSV ≥220 cm/s	11.5	n.g.	Stroke 13.0 Death 8.7	Suboptimal CAS result Multiple stent deployment
Takigawa (2010)	113, 86%	28.6, 12–67	70 ± 7	≥50% PSV ≥150 cm/s	11.3	9 ± 3	Stroke 0 Death 0	Cilostazol
Wasser (2011)	210, 72%	33.4[b], 15–54[a]	68[b] ± 10	≥70% PSV ≥300 cm/s	5.7	9[b], 3–17[a]	Stroke 25.0 Death 8.3	Leukocyte count after CAS Stent length Stent width

DUS, duplex ultrasound; PSV, peak systolic velocity; EDV, end diastolic velocity; ICA/CCA, index of PSV of ICA and CCA; NISR, group of patients without ISR r, range; n.g., not given.
[a] Interquartile range.
[b] Median.

harm for the patient during the essential long-term follow-up. In this context, serial duplex ultrasound investigations seem to best fulfil the requirements for long-term follow-up and have been used in all studies retrieved for the current review. As a secondary validation method, high-grade ISR could be confirmed by CT angiography in some selected cases. Since duplex ultrasound has turned out to lead to a reliable ISR diagnosis whereas conventional angiography is known to be an invasive procedure possibly linked with potentially dangerous complications such as stroke or bleedings, a conventional angiography should only be considered in those patients with a symptomatic or high-grade ISR, who are likely to be treated afterwards or within the same angiographic session.

A fact which could reduce the value of duplex ultrasound as a first choice method for serial follow-up investigations is the generally lacking agreement of exact ultrasound criteria to grade an ISR. Considering the peak systolic velocity (PSV) as the most commonly used duplex criterion, a considerable distribution of cut-off values could be observed. For example, the cut-off PSV for the diagnosis of an ISR of $\geq 50\%$ varied from ≥ 140 cm/s in one study [19], over a PSV ≥ 175 cm/s in the publication of Setacci et al. [25] and a PSV ≥ 220 cm/s in the study by Cosottini et al. [28] up to a PSV ≥ 224 cm/s by AbuRahma et al. [24]. Despite the fact that ultrasound criteria have to be adapted to each local high quality ultrasound laboratory, the wide range of values between the studies urges the need for an implementation of generally valid ultrasound criteria in ISR diagnosis [12,13].

There is currently a very controversial discussion on the clinical impact of ISR. Amongst others, the results from the SPACE study have encouraged those claiming that restenosis might be a relatively benign pathology [16,44]. On the other hand, especially long-term follow-up data raise concern that patients with ISR could be suffering from a higher complication rate in comparison to patients without ISR [30]. Since CAS is often recommended the treatment of choice in younger patients (<70a) [3–5,9] it is of greatest interest to evaluate the complication rates of ISR in the long run. By now, the results regarding the incidence and clinical complications of ISR of the randomized controlled trials comparing CAS and CEA [4,6,11] are eagerly awaited.

The unresolved clinical impact of ISR further highlights the importance to identify independent risk factors which are predictive for an ISR. These would be helpful to detect those patients in which a tight follow up is necessary. Advanced age [17,19] has been found to be predictive for an ISR, which would further contribute to the recommendation of choosing a CEA as a first treatment of choice especially in elderly patients [3,5]. CAS is frequently recommended in patients with a restenosis after CEA because a redo-CEA sometimes appears to be technically difficult and might bear a higher periprocedural risk than the initial operation [7] or in patients with a radiogenic stenosis [45]. When considering the optimal treatment option for those patient subgroups, one should take into account though that a CAS procedure because of a CEA-restenosis or radiation-induced stenosis is also associated with a higher rate of ISR [20,23,34,35]. An insufficient result after a CAS procedure, e.g. due to insufficient stent adaptation, could be shown to be associated with a higher risk of ISR occurrence [19,20,28]. Therefore, to ameliorate the long-term benefit of a CAS, it is a worthwhile aim to pursue a perfect stent adaptation to the vessel lumen. The fact that an aggressive postdilation bears the risk of distal embolization and microvascular injury, which may itself initiate neointimal hyperplasia complicates the procedure. Furthermore, the characteristics of the stent deployed are of special interest regarding the incidence of ISR. Usually, the selection of the stent length and width are based on angiographic findings in order to appropriately cover the stenosis. However, narrower and longer stents were correlated with a higher ISR risk [28,30]. It is conceivable that a stent with a larger diameter results in a reduced flow-velocity, less turbulences and thus in less frequent ISR. A longer stent, which is used to cover longer lesions, probably represents the presence of a high plaque burden and has repeatedly been identified as an independent predictor for periprocedural complications [46,47]. Although it is clear that mainly anatomical conditions lead to the selection of a specific stent, it is recommendable to choose the shortest but widest stent as possible in order to minimize the risk of ISR development and to closely follow-up those patients in whom a longer, narrower stent has been used.

After a successful CAS, a stringent monitoring of cardiovascular risk factors seems to be essential. Not only with regard to primary and secondary stroke prevention, but also especially in the context of ISR development, several publications show a correlation between the presence of cardiovascular risk factors, such as tobacco use [17,42], diabetes mellitus [18,22], e.g. represented by an elevated HbA1c [36], low HDL cholesterol [26], and the occurrence of an ISR.

Conclusions

ISR after CAS is frequently observed within the first year of follow-up and might be associated with a higher risk for clinical complications. Against the light that a CAS intervention is frequently recommended as an alternative treatment strategy to CEA especially in patients aged <70 years, a tight and long-lasting follow-up is warranted. Particularly patients who are of advanced age, treated for a radiogenic stenosis or a recurrent stenosis after CEA, or with the presence of cardiovascular risk factors such as tobacco use, diabetes mellitus or a dyslipoproteinemia or certain procedure-related factors (a narrow or long stent, insufficient stent adaptation after CAS or the use of multiple stents) are prone to develop an ISR. A significant heterogeneity especially regarding the exact duplex criteria to identify an ISR has been observed between the reviewed studies thus supporting the need to establish commonly accepted criteria for ISR-grading. With respect to the possible clinical relevance of an ISR and a lacking commonly accepted treatment strategy, all efforts should be made to carefully follow-up especially those patient subgroups at risk for ISR in order to further develop an optimized treatment strategy.

References

[1] Ringleb PA, Allenberg J, Bruckmann H, Eckstein HH, Fraedrich G, Hartmann M, et al. 30 day results from the SPACE trial of stent-protected angioplasty versus carotid endarterectomy

in symptomatic patients: a randomised non-inferiority trial. Lancet 2006;368:1239—47.
[2] Mas JL, Chatellier G, Beyssen B, Branchereau A, Moulin T, Becquemin JP, et al. Endarterectomy versus stenting in patients with symptomatic severe carotid stenosis. N Engl J Med 2006;355:1660—71.
[3] Economopoulos KP, Sergentanis TN, Tsivgoulis G, Mariolis AD, Stefanadis C. Carotid artery stenting versus carotid endarterectomy: a comprehensive meta-analysis of short-term and long-term outcomes. Stroke 2011;42:687—92.
[4] Brott TG, Hobson RW, Howard G, Roubin GS, Clark WM, Brooks W, et al. Stenting versus endarterectomy for treatment of carotid-artery stenosis. N Engl J Med 2010;363:11—23.
[5] Bonati LH, Dobson J, Algra A, Branchereau A, Chatellier G, Fraedrich G, et al. Short-term outcome after stenting versus endarterectomy for symptomatic carotid stenosis: a preplanned meta-analysis of individual patient data. Lancet 2010;376:1062—73.
[6] Ederle J, Dobson J, Featherstone RL, Bonati LH, van der Worp HB, de Borst GJ, et al. Carotid artery stenting compared with endarterectomy in patients with symptomatic carotid stenosis (International Carotid Stenting Study): an interim analysis of a randomised controlled trial. Lancet 2010;375:985—97.
[7] Brott TG, Halperin JL, Abbara S, Bacharach JM, Barr JD, Bush RL, et al. 2011 ASA/ACCF/AHA/AANN/AANS/ACR/ASNR/CNS/SAIP/SCAI/SIR/SNIS/SVM/SVS guideline on the management of patients with extracranial carotid and vertebral artery disease: executive summary. A report of the American College of Cardiology Foundation/American Heart Association Task Force on Practice Guidelines, and the American Stroke Association, American Association of Neuroscience Nurses, American Association of Neurological Surgeons, American College of Radiology, American Society of Neuroradiology, Congress of Neurological Surgeons, Society of Atherosclerosis Imaging and Prevention, Society for Cardiovascular Angiography and Interventions, Society of Interventional Radiology, Society of NeuroInterventional Surgery, Society for Vascular Medicine, and Society for Vascular Surgery. Circulation 2011;124:489—532.
[8] The Carotid Stenting Guidelines Committee: An Intercollegiate Committee of the RACP (ANZAN, CSANZ), RACS (ANZSVS) and RANZCR. Guidelines for patient selection and performance of carotid artery stenting. Intern Med J 2011; 41:344—7.
[9] Kastrup A, Gröschel K. Carotid endarterectomy versus carotid stenting: an updated review of randomized trials and subgroup analyses. Acta Chir Belg 2007;107:119—28.
[10] Rothwell PM. Poor outcomes after endovascular treatment of symptomatic carotid stenosis: time for a moratorium. Lancet Neurol 2009;8:871—3.
[11] Gurm HS, Yadav JS, Fayad P, Katzen BT, Mishkel GJ, Bajwa TK, et al. Long-term results of carotid stenting versus endarterectomy in high-risk patients. N Engl J Med 2008;358:1572—9.
[12] Gröschel K, Riecker A, Schulz JB, Ernemann U, Kastrup A. Systematic review of early recurrent stenosis after carotid angioplasty and stenting. Stroke 2005;36:367—73.
[13] Nederkoorn PJ, Brown MM. Optimal cut-off criteria for duplex ultrasound for the diagnosis of restenosis in stented carotid arteries: review and protocol for a diagnostic study. BMC Neurol 2009;9:36.
[14] Investigators C. Endovascular versus surgical treatment in patients with carotid stenosis in the Carotid and Vertebral Transluminal Angioplasty Study (CAVATAS): a randomised trial. Lancet 2001;357:1729—37.
[15] Bonati LH, Ederle J, McCabe DJ, Dobson J, Featherstone RL, Gaines PA, et al. Long-term risk of carotid restenosis in patients randomly assigned to endovascular treatment or endarterectomy in the Carotid and Vertebral Artery Transluminal Angioplasty Study (CAVATAS): long-term follow-up of a randomised trial. Lancet Neurol 2009;8:908—17.
[16] Eckstein HH, Ringleb P, Allenberg JR, Berger J, Fraedrich G, Hacke W, et al. Results of the Stent-Protected Angioplasty versus Carotid Endarterectomy (SPACE) study to treat symptomatic stenoses at 2 years: a multinational, prospective, randomised trial. Lancet Neurol 2008;7:893—902.
[17] Arquizan C, Trinquart L, Touboul PJ, Long A, Feasson S, Terriat B, et al. Restenosis is more frequent after carotid stenting than after endarterectomy: the EVA-3S study. Stroke 2011;42:1015—20.
[18] Willfort-Ehringer A, Ahmadi R, Gschwandtner ME, Haumer M, Lang W, Minar E. Single-center experience with carotid stent restenosis. J Endovasc Ther 2002;9:299—307.
[19] Khan MA, Liu MW, Chio FL, Roubin GS, Iyer SS, Vitek JJ. Predictors of restenosis after successful carotid artery stenting. Am J Cardiol 2003;92:895—7.
[20] Schillinger M, Exner M, Mlekusch W, Rumpold H, Ahmadi R, Sabeti S, et al. Acute-phase response after stent implantation in the carotid artery: association with 6-month in-stent restenosis. Radiology 2003;227:516—21.
[21] Skelly CL, Gallagher K, Fairman RM, Carpenter JP, Velazquez OC, Parmer SS, et al. Risk factors for restenosis after carotid artery angioplasty and stenting. J Vasc Surg 2006;44:1010—5.
[22] Lal BK, Kaperonis EA, Cuadra S, Kapadia I, Hobson RW. Patterns of in-stent restenosis after carotid artery stenting: classification and implications for long-term outcome. J Vasc Surg 2007;46:833—40.
[23] Younis GA, Gupta K, Mortazavi A, Strickman NE, Krajcer Z, Perin E, et al. Predictors of carotid stent restenosis. Catheter Cardiovasc Interv 2007;69:673—82.
[24] AbuRahma AF, Abu-Halimah S, Bensenhaver J, Dean LS, Keiffer T, Emmett M, et al. Optimal carotid duplex velocity criteria for defining the severity of carotid in-stent restenosis. J Vasc Surg 2008;48:589—94.
[25] Setacci C, Chisci E, Setacci F, Iacoponi F, de Donato G. Grading carotid intrastent restenosis: a 6-year follow-up study. Stroke 2008;39:1189—96.
[26] Topakian R, Sonnberger M, Nussbaumer K, Haring HP, Trenkler J, Aichner FT. Postprocedural high-density lipoprotein cholesterol predicts carotid stent patency at 1 year. EurJ Neurol 2008;15:179—84.
[27] Zhou W, Felkai DD, Evans M, McCoy SA, Lin PH, Kougias P, et al. Ultrasound criteria for severe in-stent restenosis following carotid artery stenting. J Vasc Surg 2008;47:74—80.
[28] Cosottini M, Michelassi MC, Bencivelli W, Lazzarotti G, Picchietti S, Orlandi G, et al. In stent restenosis predictors after carotid artery stenting. Stroke Res Treat 2010, 2010, pii: 864724.:864724.
[29] Takigawa T, Matsumaru Y, Hayakawa M, Nemoto S, Matsumura A. Cilostazol reduces restenosis after carotid artery stenting. J Vasc Surg 2010;51:51—6.
[30] Wasser K, Schnaudigel S, Wohlfahrt J, Psychogios MN, Knauth M, Gröschel K. Inflammation and in-stent restenosis: the role of serum markers and stent characteristics in carotid artery stenting. PLoS One 2011;6:e22683.
[31] International Carotid Stenting Study investigators, Ederle J, Dobson J, Featherstone RL, Bonati LH, van der Worp HB, et al. Carotid artery stenting compared with endarterectomy in patients with symptomatic carotid stenosis (International Carotid Stenting Study): an interim analysis of a randomised controlled trial. Lancet 2010;375:985—97.
[32] Yadav JS, Wholey MH, Kuntz RE, Fayad P, Katzen BT, Mishkel GJ, et al. Protected carotid-artery stenting versus endarterectomy in high-risk patients. N Engl J Med 2004;351: 1493—501.
[33] AbuRahma AF, Bates MC, Eads K, Armistead L, Flaherty SK. Safety and efficacy of carotid angioplasty/stenting in 100

consecutive high surgical risk patients: immediate and long-term follow-up. Vasc Endovascular Surg 2008;42:433—9.
[34] Setacci C, Pula G, Baldi I, de Donato G, Setacci F, Cappelli A, et al. Determinants of in-stent restenosis after carotid angioplasty: a case-control study. J Endovasc Ther 2003;10:1031—8.
[35] Zhou W, Lin PH, Bush RL, Peden EK, Guerrero MA, Kougias P, et al. Management of in-sent restenosis after carotid artery stenting in high-risk patients. J Vasc Surg 2006;43:305—12.
[36] Willfort-Ehringer A, Ahmadi R, Gessl A, Gschwandtner ME, Haumer A, Lang W, et al. Neointimal proliferation within carotid stents is more pronounced in diabetic patients with initial poor glycaemic state. Diabetologia 2004;47:400—6.
[37] Stoney RJ, String ST. Recurrent carotid stenosis. Surgery 1976;80:705—10.
[38] Diethrich EB, Ndiaye M, Reid DB. Stenting in the carotid artery: initial experience in 110 patients. J Endovasc Surg 1996;3:42—62.
[39] Yadav JS, Roubin GS, Iyer S, Vitek J, King P, Jordan WD, et al. Elective stenting of the extracranial carotid arteries. Circulation 1997;95:376—81.
[40] Theron JG, Payelle GG, Coskun O, Huet HF, Guimaraens L. Carotid artery stenosis: treatment with protected balloon angioplasty and stent placement. Radiology 1996;201:627—36.
[41] Bangalore S, Kumar S, Wetterslev J, Bavry AA, Gluud C, Cutlip DE, et al. Carotid artery stenting vs carotid endarterectomy: meta-analysis and diversity-adjusted trial sequential analysis of randomized trials. Arch Neurol 2011;68:172—84.
[42] McCabe DJ, Pereira AC, Clifton A, Bland JM, Brown MM. Restenosis after carotid angioplasty, stenting, or endarterectomy in the Carotid and Vertebral Artery Transluminal Angioplasty Study (CAVATAS). Stroke 2005;36:281—6.
[43] van Haaften AC, Bots ML, Moll FL, de Borst GJ. Therapeutic options for carotid in-stent restenosis: review of the literature. J Vasc Interv Radiol 2010;21:1471—7.
[44] Naylor AR. Stenting versus endarterectomy: the debate continues. Lancet Neurol 2008;7:862—4.
[45] Tallarita T, Oderich GS, Lanzino G, Cloft H, Kallmes D, Bower TC, et al. Outcomes of carotid artery stenting versus historical surgical controls for radiation-induced carotid stenosis. J Vasc Surg 2011;53:629—36, e1-5.
[46] Naggara O, Touze E, Beyssen B, Trinquart L, Chatellier G, Meder JF, et al. Anatomical and technical factors associated with stroke or death during carotid angioplasty and stenting: results from the endarterectomy versus angioplasty in patients with symptomatic severe carotid stenosis (EVA-3S) trial and systematic review. Stroke 2011;42:380—8.
[47] Gröschel K, Ernemann U, Schnaudigel S, Wasser K, Nägele T, Kastrup A. A risk score to predict ischemic lesions after protected carotid artery stenting. J Neurol Sci 2008;273:112—5.

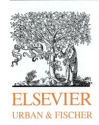
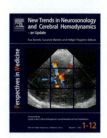

Bartels E, Bartels S, Poppert H (Editors):
New Trends in Neurosonology and Cerebral Hemodynamics — an Update.
Perspectives in Medicine (2012) 1, 129—131

journal homepage: www.elsevier.com/locate/permed

Post-carotid stent ultrasound provides critical data to avoid rare but serious complications

John J. Volpi [a,b,*], Zsolt Garami [b,c], Rasadul Kabir [a], Orlando Diaz-Daza [a,b], Richard Klucznik [a,b]

[a] The Methodist Hospital Neurological Institute, 6560 Fannin, Suite 802, Houston, TX, 77030, USA
[b] The Methodist Hospital Research Institute, 6565 Fannin, Houston, TX, 77030, USA
[c] Methodist DeBakey Heart and Vascular Center, Houston, 6550 Fannin, Suite 1401, TX, 77030, USA

KEYWORDS
Stroke;
Carotid ultrasound;
Carotid stenting

Summary Carotid stenting is a common procedure for revascularization of carotid artery stenosis. In this study, we evaluated the role of carotid ultrasound post carotid stenting. In a retrospective analysis, we identified 45 patients who received post-stent ultrasound. On routine follow-up we measured a range for peak systolic velocity of 33—150 cm/s and end diastolic velocity 11—52 cm/s. We also identified two cases, where immediate post-stent ultrasound provided critical data that required further intervention, and potentially avoided serious complications.
© 2012 Elsevier GmbH. All rights reserved.

Introduction

Carotid stenting is an accepted form of revascularization in the US and many countries based on the recent results of the CREST trial [1]. The choice of follow-up imaging remains variable for post-stent patients and some patients receiving no post-stent imaging. Ultrasound imaging is a cost effective and simple way to evaluate immediate post-stent patients.

Methods

We retrospectively reviewed a database for a 2 year period from 2008 to 2010 for patients who had significant carotid stenosis and underwent carotid stenting, and post-stent carotid ultrasound exam. In stent velocities were measured with a General Electric LOGIQ E9 (Milwaukee, WI) with 9 MHz linear probe that was used to evaluate the post stent carotid artery.

* Corresponding author at: 6560 Fannin, Suite 802, Houston, TX, 77030, USA. Tel.: +1 713 441 3951; fax: +1 713 793 7019.
E-mail address: jjvolpi@tmhs.org (J.J. Volpi).

Results

Forty-five patients (age between 43 and 75 years) were identified, who received post stent ultrasound. We found a mean peak systolic velocity of 83 cm/s and a mean end diastolic velocity of 24 cm/s in this population, with a range peak systolic velocity 33—150 cm/s and end diastolic velocity 11—52 cm/s.

Out of 45, we found 2 cases of immediate complications of stent placement.

Discussion

Case 1: A 77-year-old woman with no focal neurological deficits underwent elective right carotid stenting at an outside institution. Post stent, she complained of neck pain and was lethargic with fluctuating left side weakness. She was transferred to our facility and was found with low flow in the recently stented vessel (Fig. 1). The stent appeared to be patent and fully deployed, but on follow-up angiogram was found to be in the dissected false lumen of

2211-968X/$ — see front matter © 2012 Elsevier GmbH. All rights reserved.
doi:10.1016/j.permed.2012.02.019

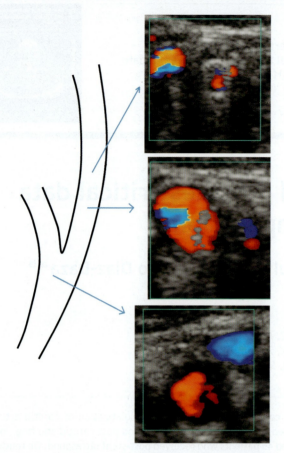

Figure 1 Post Carotid ultrasound. Flow in the right carotid artery did not appear centered in the vessel lumen.

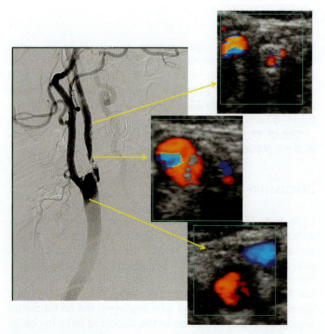

Figure 2 Dissected lumen. The angiogram confirmed that the stent was deployed into a dissected false lumen.

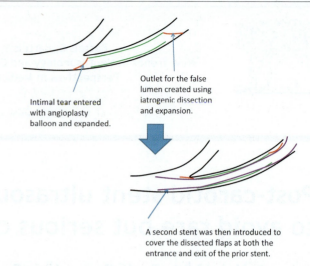

Figure 3 Plan for repair. This treatment approach was used for repair of the stent in the false lumen.

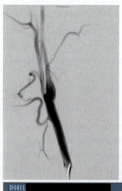

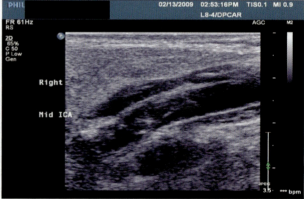

Figure 4 Initial angiogram and post stent ultrasound. The untreated right mid internal carotid artery appeared normal on the routine angiogram, but the post stent ultrasound showed an obvious lumen irregularity.

the carotid (Fig. 2). This was subsequently corrected with no adverse events (Fig. 3).

Case 2: A 40-year-old woman with recent motor vehicle accident and carotid dissection underwent successful stenting of the affected left carotid artery. On her follow-up ultrasound, the stented carotid was normal, but the contralateral (untreated) carotid artery was found to have a new flow-limiting dissection with clot (Fig. 4). This abnormality was not apparent on the initial angiogram during

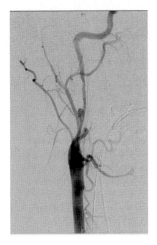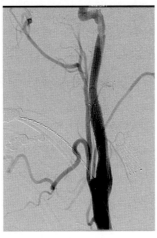

Figure 5 Angiogram and stent. The second angiogram showed an obvious dissection and it was corrected with a second stent.

its injection (Fig. 4). A second angiogram was performed and the dissection was easily identified, and this vessel was also stented subsequently without any adverse events (Fig. 5).

Conclusion

In all patients, post stent ultrasound provides a baseline study for future follow-up. In rare cases, post stent ultrasound can identify potentially serious complications. In our study 2 out of 45 patients (4.4%) were found with a significant abnormality post stenting that could have led to cerebral ischemia. Interestingly, in the CREST study, 4.4% of post stent patients suffered stroke or death. We suggest that post carotid stent ultrasound may yield potentially valuable findings to reduce the risk of imminent stroke.

Reference

[1] Brott TG, Hobson RW, Howard G, Roubin GS, Clark WM, Brooks W, et al. Stenting versus endarterectomy for treatment of carotid-artery stenosis. N Engl J Med 2010;363:11–23.

4. Atherosclerotic Plaque, Intima-Media Thickness

How local hemodynamics at the carotid bifurcation influence the development of carotid plaques

Dieter Liepsch[a,*], Andrea Balasso[b], Hermann Berger[b], Hans-Henning Eckstein[b]

[a] Insitut f. Biotechnik, e.V. Lothstr. 34, 80335, University of Applied Sciences, Munich, Germany
[b] Interdisciplinary Research Laboratory of the Klinikum rechts der Isar der TU München, Germany

KEYWORDS
Carotid artery models;
Flow visualization;
Velocity measurement;
Stents;
Patch plastic

Summary A short introduction is given of how fluid dynamics forces and velocity distribution influence the development of plaque in the carotid bifurcation. The flow parameters are discussed. Flow visualization techniques and also laser-Doppler-anemometer measurements demonstrate the importance of the flow. This will be shown in true-to-scale, physiological accurate models of the carotid arteries. These models have the same compliance as the real blood vessel. Some applications are shown e.g. patches, stents and filters. The most important factors are the flow rate ratio and geometry, unsteady pulsatile flow, wall elasticity and non-Newtonian flow behavior of blood.
© 2012 Elsevier GmbH. All rights reserved.

Introduction

Cell/cell and cell/vessel wall interactions have been the subject of investigation and discussion for more than 40 years. It has been shown that low and high shear regions caused by flow separation regions and oscillatory flow are primarily responsible for chemical reactions which contribute to the formation of arterial plaques.

Most previous shear stress studies have only measured the axial velocity component at a few local points. They calculated the shear stresses with the velocity gradients using a constant viscosity. Accurate three-dimensional or, at least, two-dimensional velocity measurements are necessary to calculate the shear stresses. This is because, at bends and bifurcations, the secondary flow cannot be neglected. Numerical studies very often neglect the real, local viscosity of blood and the compliance of the vessel wall which shows a hysteresis. It is also very important that the non-Newtonian flow behavior of blood be considered, especially in flow separation regions.

We have studied the flow behavior in more than 200 arterial models with a different geometry and different flow rate ratios. The principles of hemodynamics, such as the forces on fluid elements, are important. These forces are

- the volume forces (such as gravity force or centrifugal forces);
- the pressure forces (normal pressure multiplied with the area of the fluid element);
- friction forces (shear stresses multiplied with the surface of the cell fluid element).

Normally, in larger blood vessels, the blood cells are concentrated in the center whereas the plasma flows near the

* Corresponding author at: Fakultät 05, Lothstr. 34, 80335 Germany. Tel.: +49 89 1265 1522; fax: +49 81573160.
E-mail addresses: dliepsch@t-online.de, liepsch@hm.edu (D. Liepsch).

wall. The blood cells are deformed in capillaries where physical/chemical reactions take place. However blood cells are also occasionally transported into these recirculation zones in larger blood vessels, at bends and bifurcations. The cells remain in the recirculation zones over several pulse cycles and are subjected to both high and low shear stresses.

Many papers use the term 'turbulent flow', however a true turbulent flow is found only in the ascending aorta and this is not fully developed because of the entrance length. Everywhere else you will have a nominal, laminar or transitional flow.

The definition for laminar and turbulent flow is:

Laminar flow	The fluid elements move parallel to each other in distinct paths. In all layers the velocity (fluid elements) moves tangentially to the main flow.
Nominal laminar	Small velocity fluctuations are added to laminar flow. This flow is characterized by small velocity disturbances.
Transitional flow	is laminar flow with spatial and temporal velocity disturbances (fluctuations), which decreases relatively quickly distal to the local flow disturbance. It is a flow between laminar and turbulent, where flow disturbances disappear over time.
Turbulent flow	Three-dimensional, spatial and temporal velocity fluctuations are superimposed on the main flow direction. The flow becomes irregular and chaotic.

A fully developed laminar profile creates a parabolic velocity profile (1) and a fully turbulent flow creates a very flat velocity profile (2). The flow behavior can be calculated with a dimensionless parameter called Reynolds number (Re-number). The Re-number can be calculated with the average velocity over the cross section of the vessel, the diameter and the kinematics viscosity. Re = $(u \cdot d / v)$ = (Fig. 1)

For pulsatile flow the Reynolds number should be calculated with a flow rate over one pulse cycle

$$u = V/A \rightarrow Re = \frac{4V \cdot d}{\Pi d^2 v} = \frac{4V}{\Pi d \pi}$$

Normally, you will never find Reynolds numbers higher than 2300 in blood vessels using the above definition. The entrance length is too short and the pulse wave cannot develop into a turbulent flow.

The non-Newtonian flow behavior of blood can be neglected in straight pipes because the profile is only 3—4% different compared to a fully developed paraboloid in a straight pipe (Fig. 1 right, white arrow).

Methods and models

The influence of the bifurcation angle and the stenosis degree were studied.

We used 1:1 true-to scale, elastic silicon rubber models with a compliance similar to that of the arterial wall. This special technique was described in Biorheology 23, 1986.

The surface in the model reproduces the biological vessel surface. The carotid artery models were installed in a physiologically accurate circulatory system.

The fluid was a polyacrylamid mixture and a water solution which shows a flow behavior similar to that of human blood. Only the thixotropic flow behavior could not be simulated (that means the coagulation of blood). The fluid is transparent and has the same refraction index as the model wall. This is important for the laser measurements. The laser light will not be absorbed and the laser beam is not deflected. Measurements were done with 3D-LDA fiber optic system (DANTEC) in a physiological healthy carotid artery

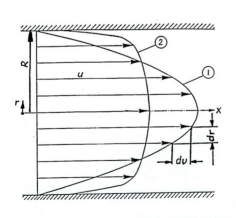
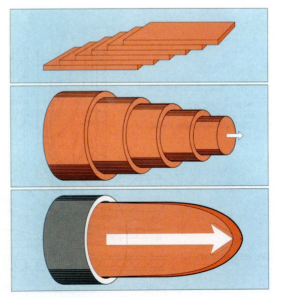

Figure 1 Velocity profile of a laminar and turbulent flow.

model with a bifurcation angel of 37° between the internal and external carotid artery.

In addition to this model, we studied models with a bifurcation angle of 29° and 41° and also with a 90% stenosis in the internal carotid artery, and with a 80% stenosis in the internal and external carotid artery (Fig. S1 — online supplementary file).

The flow rate ratio was mostly 70:30 in the internal to-external carotid artery, but also other flow rate ratios were tested. In earlier studies we used 90°, 60° and 45° bifurcations to study the influence of the different flow parameters separately

- pulsatile, unsteady flow;
- non-Newtonian behavior of blood;
- elasticity of the vessel wall;
- change of blood caused by shear stresses.

We found that the endothelial cell layer was elongated in the flow direction; however in the flow separation area the endothelial cells have a rounded form and are not packed closely together, so small leaks can be found. That means, in this area, material transport from inside into the wall or from outside into the blood can easily occur. At the stagnation point, the endothelial cells are packed closely together and are also around the apex of the inner wall of the flow divider (Fig. 2).

The flow was visualized using dyes for steady flow, and with a photoelasticity apparatus and a birefringent solution to visualize the unsteady pulsatile flow.

Fig. S2 (left) (online supplementary file) demonstrates the influence of the flow rate ratio. The flow separation zone starts at a flow of 30% into the branch and increases with higher flow rate in to the branch. On the right, a short demonstration is shown under pulsatile conditions for a flow rate ratio of 0.3.

It is well known that vessel blockage is caused by the growth of plaque. First, a small atherosclerotic plaque can be found at a bifurcation which creates damage to the intima (ulceration). Fibrin platelet aggregation can be created leading to additional thrombus formation. Finally particles are released from the plaque or parts of the thrombus which can lead to a total blockage of the vessel (thrombus, thrombus emboli). This can be clearly observed with our flow visualization techniques.

Results and applications

Basic flow studies

Fig. 3 shows flow, with a dye, hitting the apex of the carotid bifurcation model. The dye separates into two parts, flowing into the internal and external carotid artery. Because the velocity at the inner side of the internal carotid artery is high, an area with a lower pressure is created on the opposite side; therefore the blue dye spreads out. The flow, however, is still very smooth and therefore, further downstream, the blue dye momentarily spreads over the whole diameter before returning to a smooth laminar flow.

The velocity measurements were done using a laser-Doppler-anemometer. The flow, pressure and velocity curve over one pulse cycle is shown in Fig. S3 (online supplementary file).

Fig. S4 (online supplementary file) shows the axial velocity distribution over one pulse cycle at different phases 2.5 mm distal to the apex. The velocity at the inner wall is very high (up to 1 m/s) and, at the outer wall, very low during the peak systolic phase (60°), as already demonstrated with dyes.

Fig. S5 (online supplementary file) shows the velocity measurements over the cross-section in color, and Fig. S6 (online supplementary file) shows the secondary flow which is very high during peak systolic phase and decreases during the diastolic phase. The velocities in a 90% stenosed model are 4—5 times higher than normal, with velocities

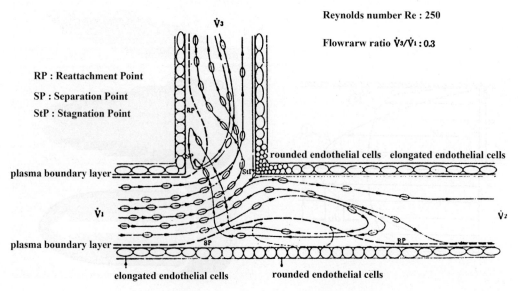

Figure 2 Sketch of the stream paths in a 90° bifurcation such as the left descending coronary artery.

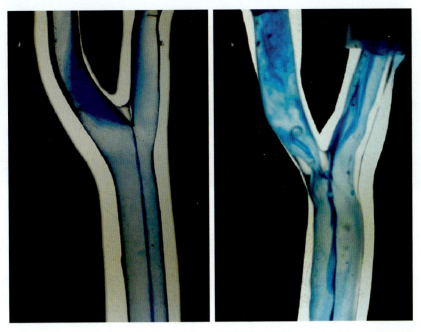

Figure 3 Visualization using a dye in a native and a 90% model with stenoses.

up to 4—5 m/s and with high velocity fluctuations further downstream, just behind the stenosis.

Studies in stents

The fluid dynamic influence of several stents were tested in transparent models. The influence of stents is demonstrated using dyes. Fig. S7 (online supplementary file) shows the angiogram of a stenosed artery (left side and with the inserted stent on the right side. Fig. 4 shows the influence of the stent. The dye spreads slightly into the external carotid artery compared to the healthy model. This is caused by the threads of the stent.

The wire geometry, direction of wires, mesh of wires, the in- and outflow, and the stretching and surface roughness was tested. We tested several stents including covered and uncovered stents. The experiments were carried out with the stents in various positions. Fig. 5 demonstrates the velocity distribution 5 mm distal to the apex in the internal carotid artery model for two different stents compared to a model without a stent.

Other therapeutic procedures in the carotid artery

Surgical procedures in the carotid artery such as endarterectomy for treatment of such conditions as stenosis, aneurysms, thrombosis and cerebral ischemia are risky and may lead to improvement or not. The following study shows the flow and velocity distribution of endarterectomy which is the standard procedure to treat patients with high degree stenosis in the carotid artery (an alternative is to use patch plastics from artificial and biological materials).

Fig. 6 shows a flow, visualized with a dye, at the point marked in the cross-section of the model, in a healthy common carotid artery, a model with a wide patch and a narrow patch. The differences can be clearly seen. The model with the narrow patch shows the same flow behavior as the healthy model; whereas the wide patch creates flow disturbances. Fig. S8 (online supplementary file) shows the pulse cycle. At the beginning of the diastolic phase (90°) a backward flow can be seen in the model with the wide patch. Again, the model with a narrow patch shows flow behavior similar to that in the healthy model. The secondary flow demonstrates this also (Fig. S9 — online supplementary file).

Filters are inserted into the carotid artery before the stent is opened to avoid a particle flow in to the brain. There is controversy in discussions about this procedure because many physicians report that the complication rate is almost the same as without a filter.

Fig. S10 (online supplementary file) demonstrates that particles captured in the filter can escape if the closing of the filter occurs during the diastolic phase. It has been demonstrated that it is crucial that the filter is closed during the systolic phase to prevent this escape.

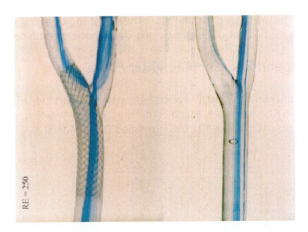

Figure 4 Dye in a healthy model and in a model with a stent.

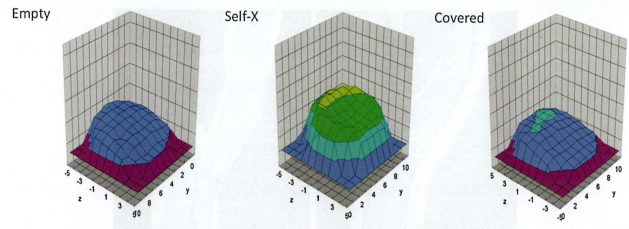

Figure 5 Velocity distribution in the internal carotid artery with two different types of stents.

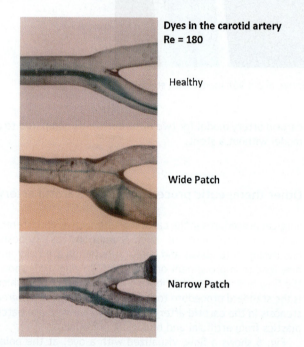

Figure 6 Dye in a healthy model, a model with a wide patch and narrow patch.

Discussion and outlook

From these experiments the following can be clearly seen: All three velocity components have to be measured. The flow rate ratio between the internal and external carotid artery is the most important and significantly influences the flow separation region. The experiments show that particles in flow separation regions sometimes rotate over several pulse cycles before they are washed away. They can, however, suddenly adhere to the wall and remain there. The pulse wave is not strong enough to wash these small deposits away. The procedure of plaque formation starts. More particles are attracted to and adhere to this area and the flow rate ratio is altered because of the higher resistance caused by the deposits. This effect continues and the stenosis enlarges. The geometry only plays a significant role in these regions with larger bifurcation angles, >40°, where a backward flow is created.

In 3D measurements, the calculated shear stresses are up to 20% higher than those found when measuring only the axial velocity component. With an increasing flow rate, the separation region is slightly reduced but the shear stresses increase. 10—16 Pa are the highest shear stresses in a healthy carotid artery and are found just at the apex. Shear stresses higher than 180—250 Pa have been measured in models with 90% stenosis for 100—200 ms.

Downstream of such stenoses, vortices are created where particles can remain over several pulse cycles. They can also adhere to the wall, creating a growing stenosis. Oscillation causes shear stresses between 1—40 Pa in such recirculation zones. Biochemical reactions are released.

It is very important that stents have to be placed precisely. End threads or wires should never reach into the vessel lumen. Filters have to be closed during the systolic phase, so that no particles escape during the diastolic phase, before they can be pulled out. Experimental studies including MRI, ultrasound measurements and new ultrasound imaging which can measure all three velocity components will be increasingly important in the future to aid in training and refinement of diagnostic and therapeutic procedures.

Appendix A. Supplementary data

Supplementary data associated with this article (Figs. S1—S10) can be found, in the online version, at http://dx.doi.org/10.1016/j.permed.2012.04.005.

In vivo wall shear stress patterns in carotid bifurcations assessed by 4D MRI

Andreas Harloff[a,*], Michael Markl[b]

[a] Department of Neurology, University Hospital Freiburg, Breisacher Strasse 64, 79106 Freiburg, Germany
[b] Departments of Radiology and Biomedical Engineering, Northwestern University, 737 N. Michigan Avenue Suite 1600, Chicago, IL 60611, USA

KEYWORDS
Wall shear stress;
Flow-sensitive MRI;
Carotid artery;
Bifurcation;
4D flow MRI

Summary We investigated the distribution of wall shears stress (WSS) within the carotid artery bifurcation of healthy volunteers and patients with internal carotid artery stenosis. WSS was determined by flow-sensitive 4D MRI and correlated with bifurcation angle, vessel tortuosity and the ratio of the diameter of the common (CCA) and internal carotid artery (ICA). Critical WSS occurred at the posterior wall of the physiologically dilated ICA bulb and the incidence of critical WSS values was dependent from individual bifurcation geometry. Moreover, we found that ICA stenosis changed physiological WSS distribution whereas carotid endarterectomy partially restored physiological WSS conditions.
© 2012 Elsevier GmbH. All rights reserved.

Introduction

Wall shear stress (WSS), the friction force of flowing blood that acts on the endothelial wall, can vary considerably throughout the vascular beds and has shown to be altered at the outlet or at the inner curvature of arteries, respectively. In an animal model, Cheng et al. [1] showed that both low and oscillating WSS predispose to the development of atherosclerotic lesions and that oscillatory shear stress causes stable plaques whereas low WSS causes vulnerable lesions. Using computational fluid dynamics Lee et al. [2] demonstrated that individual bifurcation geometry was correlated with the distribution of critical WSS values in healthy volunteers. Data from in vivo studies, however, are sparse. Therefore, we investigated the distribution of WSS along the carotid bifurcations of volunteers and patients using flow-sensitive 4D MRI in vivo [3]. Findings of our previously published study [3] are summarized here in brief.

* Corresponding author. Tel.: +49 761 270 50010.
 E-mail addresses: andreas.harloff@uniklinik-freiburg.de (A. Harloff), mmarkl@northwestern.edu (M. Markl).

Material and methods

64 carotid bifurcations of 32 healthy volunteers and 17 carotid arteries of patients with moderate ICA stenosis or recanalized high-grade ICA stenosis were evaluated. Blood flow velocities were measured using a 3 Tesla MRI system (TIM TRIO, Siemens, Erlangen, Germany) and a combined 12-element head and 6-element neck coil. Temporal and spatial resolution of flow-sensitive 4D MRI that was used for three-dimensional velocity acquisition were 45.6 ms and 1.1 mm × 0.9 mm × 1.4 mm [3]. After postprocessing of raw data and based on a commercially available software (Ensight, CEI, Apex, USA) 7 analysis planes, were positioned along the common (CCA) and internal carotid artery stenosis (ICA) with an inter-slice distance of 4 mm. The use of an in house software (Matlab based Flowtool, The Mathworks, USA) and a lumen segmentation method allowed for individual WSS quantification as described previously [4]. Following the study by Lee et al. [2] individual bifurcation geometry (bifurcation angle, tortuosity and diameter ratio of the CCA and ICA) of healthy volunteers was manually determined by two readers based on time-of-flight MR

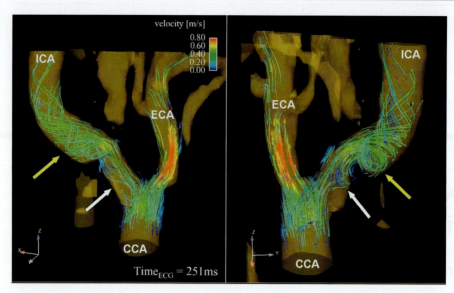

Figure 1 The carotid artery bifurcation of a patient with moderate internal carotid artery (ICA) stenosis is given. Blood flow is visualized using particle traces originating from an emitter plane at the distal common carotid artery (CCA) in early systole (i.e., 251 ms after the R wave of the ECG). Color coding represents absolute velocities in m/s. Accordingly, high velocities are represented by yellow and red and slow velocities by green and blues colors. Left: the stenotic segment of the proximal ICA can be appreciated (white arrow). Moreover, a poststenotic dilatation with the occurrence of a pronounced helical flow pattern in the distal ICA is demonstrated (yellow arrow). The external carotid artery (ECA) is characterized by a flow acceleration at the proximal vessel segment. In addition, a distal branch of the ECA is shown by the vessel contours (gold color, particles are only found at the outlet of the branch). Right: flow visualization of the bifurcation of this patient and at the same time point is presented from a posterior view. The stenotic segment (white arrow) and the pronounced helical pattern of blood flow distal to the ICA stenosis (yellow arrow) are demonstrated.

angiographies. The temporal average over the cardiac cycle of the absolute WSS (N/m^2) and the degree of absolute WSS inversion over the cardiac cycle (oscillatory shear index, OSI in %) were extracted for 12 segments along the vessel circumference. Values of oscillatory and low wall shear stress of all healthy volunteers were pooled and the 10% and 20% highest and lowest values of absolute WSS and OSI of this cohort were defined as critical WSS. The distribution of critical WSS along the bifurcation of healthy volunteers and patients was then displayed and correlated with individual geometrical features [3].

Results and discussion

An example of three-dimensional blood flow visualization in a patient with ICA stenosis and thus significant changes compared to physiological blood flow patterns at the carotid bifurcation is given in Fig. 1. Critical WSS was consistently concentrated in proximal bulb regions of the CCA and ICA and thus at the site where carotid artery plaques typically develop. Multiple regression analysis revealed significant relationships between the vessel walls with critical WSS and the ICA/CCA diameter ratio. The size of regions that were exposed to critically OSI was significantly correlated with all geometrical parameters (bifurcation angle, tortuosity and ICA/CCA diameter ratio). Moderate ICA stenosis altered physiological WSS distribution whereas recanalization of previously high-grade ICA stenosis led to a similar distribution of WSS compared to healthy volunteers [3].

Flow-sensitive 4D MRI demonstrated the distribution of absolute and oscillatory WSS in vivo. Moreover, physiological and pathological blood flow parameter could be identified that were associated with atherosclerotic disease and recanalization procedures. This in vivo MRI technique seems very promising to study the influence of individual bifurcation geometry on local hemodynamics and the development and progression of carotid artery atherosclerosis.

Appendix A. Supplementary data

Supplementary data associated with this article can be found, in the online version, at http://dx.doi.org/10.1016/j.permed.2012.03.019.

References

[1] Cheng C, Tempel D, van Haperen R, van der Baan A, Grosveld F, Daemen MJ, et al. Atherosclerotic lesion size and vulnerability are determined by patterns of fluid shear stress. Circulation 2006;113:2744—53.
[2] Lee SW, Antiga L, Spence JD, Steinman DA. Geometry of the carotid bifurcation predicts its exposure to disturbed flow. Stroke 2008;39:2341—7.
[3] Markl M, Wegent F, Zech T, Bauer S, Strecker C, Schumacher M, et al. In vivo wall shear stress distribution in the carotid artery: effect of bifurcation geometry, internal carotid artery stenosis, and recanalization therapy. Circ Cardiovasc Imaging 2010;3:647—55.
[4] Stalder AF, Russe MF, Frydrychowicz A, Bock J, Hennig J, Markl M. Quantitative 2D and 3D phase contrast MRI: optimized analysis of blood flow and vessel wall parameters. Magn Reson Med 2008;60:1218—31.

Carotid intima-media thickness (cIMT) and plaque from risk assessment and clinical use to genetic discoveries

Susanne Bartels [a,1], Angelica Ruiz Franco [b], Tatjana Rundek [a,*]

[a] Department of Neurology, Miller School of Medicine, University of Miami, Clinical Research Building, Suite #1348, 1120 NW 14th Street, Miami, FL 33136, USA
[b] The Instituto Nacional de Neurología y Neurocirugía Manuel Velasco, Suárez, México City, Mexico

KEYWORDS
Carotid IMT;
Plaque;
Surrogate markers;
Risk factors;
Ultrasound;
Carotid artery

Summary Carotid intima—media thickness (cIMT) and carotid plaque are ultrasound imaging measures of carotid atherosclerosis and strong predictors of future stroke, myocardial infarction and vascular death. The use of ultrasound measures of cIMT and carotid plaque as a screening tool in clinical practice however have been extremely limited by a lack of recognition of its value by medical communities, health care policy makers and a lack of reimbursement by third-party payers engaged in the delivery of vascular imaging services. This review addresses the role of cIMT and plaque in vascular disease risk prediction. Recent data from large population based studies on reclassification of the vascular risk using carotid ultrasound imaging markers is presented. In addition, the common clinical scenarios for the appropriate use of cIMT in clinical setting are summarized according to the recent study conducted by the Society of the Atherosclerosis Imaging and Prevention in collaboration with the International Atherosclerosis Society. This presentation is intended to provide a practical guide for use of cIMT and plaque to clinicians to promote optimal clinical use of cIMT and to researchers to direct cIMT and plaque research towards investigating environmental and genetic factors of a complex disorder — subclinical atherosclerosis — leading to future genetic discoveries and new anti-atherosclerotic therapies.
© 2012 Elsevier GmbH. All rights reserved.

Introduction

Atherosclerosis is a complex inflammatory process underlying the occurrence of heart attacks and most ischemic strokes. Traditional vascular risk factors are important for development of atherosclerosis but interestingly, explain only about 50% of the risk of cardiovascular disease (CVD) and stroke. Current screening strategies are based on these risk factors. However the complexity of stroke and CVD has led to the increasing use of intermediate phenotypes in risk prediction of vascular disease and surrogate outcomes in clinical trials. *Carotid intima—media thickness (cIMT) and carotid plaque* are widely used as intermediate, preclinical phenotypes of vascular disease (Fig. 1). Although individuals with subclinical atherosclerosis have not yet experienced overt vascular disease, they have a greater risk for incident stroke and MI in comparison to individuals without

* Corresponding author. Tel.: +1 305 243 7847; fax: +1 305 243 7081.
E-mail address: trundek@med.miami.edu (T. Rundek).
[1] Current address: Department of Psychiatry and Psychotherapy, Albert-Ludwigs-University Freiburg, Freiburg, Germany.

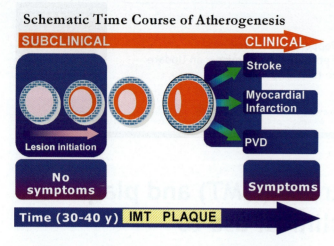

Figure 1 Schematic time course of atherogenesis.

evidence of increased subclinical atherosclerotic disease. Carotid ultrasound imaging measures of carotid plaque and cIMT are proposed as surrogate markers of CVD and stroke as objective indicators of the biological and pathobiological processes of atherosclerosis. They can also serve as surrogate endpoints for clinical vascular outcomes based on epidemiologic, therapeutic, pathophysiologic and other scientific evidence. This review article will provide an overview on the relevant literature regarding the use of cIMT and carotid plaque as surrogate markers in various research investigations and clinical practice.

What is carotid intima—media thickness (cIMT)?

Carotid IMT is a widely accepted imaging surrogate marker of generalized atherosclerosis [1,2]. On ultrasound, cIMT is represented by a double-line pattern on the near and the far wall of the carotid artery (Fig. 2). The two anatomical landmarks which can be measured as the double-line pattern are the lumen—intima and the media—adventitia interfaces [3]. Even without presence of atherosclerosis the intima and the media layer increase with advancing age as a result of adaptive changes to biomechanical parameters, like blood flow and tension on the wall [4]. Since these changes give rise to molecular and cellular pathways, which are also involved in the formation of atherosclerotic plaque, cIMT is related to subclinical atherosclerosis, but should not be used synonymously [5]. According to large studies, such as *The Atherosclerosis Risk in Communities* (ARIC) study, *The Cardiovascular Health Study* (CHS), and *The Rotterdam* study, a correlation between cIMT measurements and risk of cardiovascular events has been established [1,4,6]. Inversely, a connection between the reduction of intima—media progression with lipid-lowering therapies and a reduction of cardiovascular risk shown in clinical trials [7,8] has lead to considering cIMT a surrogate end point for the effect of anti-atherosclerotic therapy [9]. This is an important fact for risk evaluation since cIMT appears at an early stage of atherosclerosis when alterations in treatment can substantially change the course of the disease more effectively. The advantage of measuring the cIMT by high resolution B-mode ultrasonography lies in its rapidly applicable and available, non-invasive and cost-effective nature [3]. Progression of cIMT is therefore an attractive method for use in research as it can be easily assessed to study vascular risk or the therapeutic effects of a specific treatment. Nevertheless, evidence considering cIMT as a surrogate marker for CVD is still a matter of debate [2,10—12].

What is atherosclerosis?

In order to understand the distinctive nature of cIMT and carotid plaque in the risk of stroke and CVD the process of atherosclerosis has to be clearly understood. About 10—20% of ischemic strokes are due to large artery atherosclerosis, mainly located in the extracranial arteries [13]. Atherosclerotic process leads to luminal stenosis, flow restriction and plaque rupture and is therefore a strong predictor of ischemic stroke [14]. Atherosclerosis is a chronic inflammatory process, involving endothelial injury, activation and recruitment of immune-inflammatory cells, smooth muscle cell proliferation, and influx of lipoprotein [15]. Various mediators like chemokines, cytokines, growth factors, proteases, adhesion molecules, hemostasis regulators, and their interactions are involved in the process of plaque growth. Proinflammatory signaling is triggered by oxidized low-density lipoprotein (LDL) or through alterations and remodeling in the extracellular matrix [9,16]. This process leads to different plaque composition with variable vascular risk due to different susceptibility for plaque rupture resulting in artery-to-artery embolization. Depending on the stage of the atherosclerotic changes in the vessel wall there is a variety in plaque morphology. It differs from homogeneous thickening of the wall to hyperechogenic components consisting mainly of fibrous tissue and calcification, and hypoechogenic components representing areas with atheromatous material like lipid deposits, cell debris and necrotic material. Hypoechogenic components are considered more harmful due to their instability [17]. Atherosclerosis predominantly develops at specific sites in the vessel, mainly

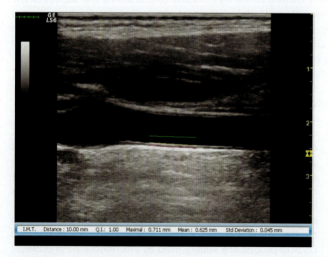

Figure 2 Assessment of carotid IMT.
Measurement of the IMT in the far wall of the common carotid artery (CCA) with an IMT mean of 0.625 ± 0.045 mm. IMT was measured by an automatic edge detection algorithm as represented by the yellow and purple lines (the green line in the lumen of the CCA represents the reference value for the arterial wall echo gradient calculations).

areas with altered blood flow, like bifurcations, branch points and areas of vessel curvature. The mass transport and the shear stress theory are two hypotheses about flow regulated mechanical forces contributing to atherosclerosis. In case of the first theory a low or disturbed blood flow results in an increased uptake of bioactive substances into the vessel wall, whereas in the latter theory mechanical forces of blood flow on the vessel wall, called shear stress, play an important role in protection of endothelial function [16].

Surrogate markers of atherosclerosis

According to the NIH Definition Working Group, surrogate markers act as a substitute for a clinical end point and should be able to predict the desired clinical benefit, respectively the lack of benefit, or harm, based on epidemiologic, therapeutic, pathophysiologic or other scientific evidence [18]. Biological markers are objectively measured and evaluated as an indicator of normal biological or pathogenic processes, or pharmacologic response to a therapeutic intervention. The clinical end point is defined as a variable that reflects how the patient feels, functions, or survives. Alteration of these markers should be displayed in a change of a clinically relevant end point [9]. The interest to use surrogate markers in order to assess the effectiveness of a treatment is increasing rapidly. Traditional biomarkers like blood pressure and serum cholesterol are used widely for risk assessment and in the development of treatment. Despite effective treatments of traditional risk factors, a large number of individuals experience CVD, which shows the need for investigations of other surrogate markers to help in the search for novel therapies [9].

There are numerous risk factors, which are currently used for the screening of atherosclerosis. Besides traditional vascular risk factors like high blood pressure, diabetes, smoking, stress, obesity, and metabolic syndrome, there is a growing list of less traditional and soluble markers such as high LDL or low HDL, CRP, LP (a), homocysteine, LDL particle size, Lp-PLA2, ApoB/ApoA [19]. Additionally, screening for atherosclerosis can be accomplished by imaging methods for arterial structure or function. Among the imaging methods for arterial structure, ultrasound measures of cIMT and plaque are most widely used. Furthermore, aortic and carotid plaque can be assessed by MRI, and the coronary calcium score by electron beam CT (EBCT) [20,21]. Brachial vasoreactivity measured by ultrasound, vascular compliance measured by radial tonometry and microvascular reactivity measured by fingertip tonometry are examples of arterial function tests that have been rapidly developing for the assessment of subclinical atherosclerosis [22,23].

Blood pressure and LDL-cholesterol are FDA-approved surrogate markers of cardiovascular disease while ultrasound measure of cIMT is still awaiting its final approval and validation by the FDA [3,9].

Carotid IMT in epidemiological studies and clinical trials

Carotid IMT has been associated with increased risk of cardiovascular events in large epidemiological studies. In a systematic review and meta-analysis, eight observational population-based studies were examined and showed the significant association of cIMT with risk of CVD [2]. Based on the data from general population, cIMT showed a slightly higher risk for stroke (hazard ratio, HR 1.32; 95% CI, 1.27–1.38) than for myocardial infarction (HR 1.26; 95% CI, 1.21–1.30). However, there are limitations to the interpretation of these results, especially concerning variable methodology, e.g. difference in definitions of carotid segments or the way the measurements were reported. Therefore the importance of following standardized cIMT protocols is emphasized for future studies.

In the clinical trials, a systematic review and meta-analysis of the effect of LDL-lowering by statins on the change of cIMT was examined [24]. Analysis of nine lipid-lowering trials showed a strong correlation between reduction of LDL and cIMT, with each 10% reduction in LDL-cholesterol accounting for a reduction of cIMT by 0.73% per year.

Although the association of cIMT and increased risk of cardiovascular events has been established, there is still a lack of sufficient evidence to show whether lowering of cIMT will translate in the reduction in CVD. Furthermore, subclinical atherosclerosis is to some extend considered a non-causal and nonspecific marker of atherosclerotic complications [2,25]. Diverse approaches for measuring cIMT and a lack of unified criteria for distinguishing early plaque formation from thickening of the cIMT might contribute to the fact of missing evidence on risk prediction. The implementation of standardized methods in the measurement of cIMT is necessary for further investigations since cIMT depicts early atherosclerosis as well as nonatherosclerotic compensatory enlargement, with both phenotypes having a different impact on predicting vascular events [3,25].

Does carotid IMT add to prediction of CVD beyond traditional risk factors?

Current studies on the effect of cardiovascular risk factors in conjunction with measures of atherosclerosis (cIMT and plaque) on risk prediction indicate a small but incremental effect for risk prediction of CVD. In the recent analysis from the community-based ARIC study among 13,145 subjects, approximately 23% individuals were reclassified into a different risk category group after adding information on cIMT and carotid plaque [11]. Adding cIMT to traditional risk factors provided the most improvement in the area under the receiver-operating characteristic curve (AUC), which increased from 0.74 to 0.765. Adding plaque to the cIMT and traditional risk factors had however the best net reclassification index of 10% in the overall population. In the Cardiovascular Health Study, another population-based study among 5888 participants, the elevated CRP was associated with increased risk for CVD only among those individuals who had increased cIMT and plaque detectable on carotid ultrasound. Despite these significant associations with CVD, CRP, cIMT and plaque only modestly improved the prediction of CVD outcomes after accounting for the traditional risk factors [26]. Addition of CRP or subclinical carotid atherosclerosis to conventional risk factors resulted in a modest increase in the ability to predict CVD. In the

NOMAS population, presence of carotid plaque considerably contributed to the better estimation of 10-year Framingham vascular risk [14]. More than a half of individuals in low and moderate FRS categories were reclassified into the higher risk category if carotid plaque was present. Traditional CVD risk prediction schemes need further improvement and cIMT and plaque may help improve CVD risk prediction with a direct implication for the risk stratification and treatment in vascular preventive programs.

Carotid IMT in different carotid artery sites

The localization of atherosclerosis is determined by hemodynamic forces, like shear stress and tensive forces, and additional local predisposing factors [27]. Since these local factors and hemodynamical forces are distributed variably in the carotid vessels there are differences in the distribution and development of cIMT. A population-based study on the association of IMT at various sites and cardiovascular risk factors showed that IMT in the common carotid artery (CCA IMT) is correlated with risk factors for stroke and prevalent stroke. Conversely, intima—media thickness in the bifurcation, together with carotid plaque, were more directly associated with risk factors of ischemic heart disease and prevalent ischemic heart disease [28]. Systolic blood pressure seems to be the most important factor influencing IMT in the common carotid artery, whereas smoking may be more important for IMT in the internal carotid artery (ICA IMT). Both sites of IMT were independently associated with prevalent CVD, with the ICA IMT having a larger area under the ROC (receiver operating characteristic) curve than CCA IMT (0.756 vs. 0.695) [29]. Furthermore, evidence from a population-based study showed variation in the progression of IMT at different arterial sites [30]. Progression rate of ICA IMT was significantly greater compared to IMT in the bifurcation or in the common carotid artery. In addition, ICA IMT correlated better with vascular risk factors than CCA IMT. The results suggest that ICA IMT might be a better measure of CVD than the more frequently investigated CCA IMT.

Carotid atherosclerotic plaque vs. cIMT

Carotid plaque is a distinctive phenotype of atherosclerosis [14]. Carotid IMT, however, is mainly related to hypertension resulting in a hypertrophy of the media layer of the vessel wall [31]. There is evidence of genetic influence on cIMT, whereas carotid plaque is strongly influenced by environmental factors [14,32]. Although cIMT has been associated with increased risk of cardiovascular disease, carotid plaque is a stronger predictor of cardiovascular disease in large population-based studies [33]. Nevertheless, differentiation of early plaque formation from increased cIMT is hard to determine. Although cIMT and plaque share the effect of atherosclerotic risk factors, they have different natural history, patterns of risk factors, and the prediction of vascular events. Since definition of carotid plaque varies, various professional organizations have proposed a standard plaque definition. According to the Mannheim consensus, plaque is defined as a focal structure encroaching into the arterial lumen of at least 0.5 mm or 50% of the surrounding IMT value,

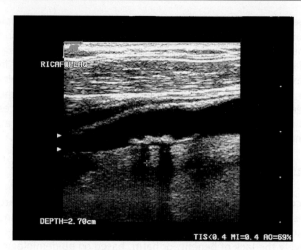

Figure 3 Calcified carotid plaque.

or demonstrates a thickness >1.5 mm as measured from the media—adventitia interface to the intima—lumen interface [3].

Besides presence and plaque size, plaque composition or morphology may be a better predictor or marker of vascular events [34]. Atherosclerosis, including plaque formation, represents a dynamic process involving a complex cascade of inflammatory events from lipid deposition to plaque calcification [35]. There is conflicting evidence about the effect of calcified carotid plaque on cardiovascular events [34,36—38]. Echolucent, fatty plaques are considered more harmful, since they are less stable and therefore more prone to rupture [39]. Individuals with calcified or echodense plaque on the other hand, are less likely to have symptomatic disease [40]. In contrast, a significant association between presence of carotid plaque calcification (Fig. 3.) and increased risk of vascular events was reported in a large population based study [41].

Calcified plaque appeared to be a significant predictor of combined vascular outcomes with a HR of 2.4 [95% CI, 1.0—5.8] when compared to absence of plaque and after adjusting for demographics, mean cIMT, education and risk factors. Another study evaluated the risk of cardiovascular events in the presence of plaque surface irregularities. Irregular plaque surface increased the risk of ischemic stroke by 3-fold. The cumulative 5-year risk for ischemic stroke was over 8% for those with irregular plaque surface compared to those with regular plaque (<3%) [13]. Superficial calcification has been shown to play a role in instability of atherosclerotic plaque [42]. Whether soft, calcified and irregular plaques are different stages of the same process or separate entities is a matter of controversy and longitudinal studies with careful assessments of plaque progression are needed to resolve these issues.

Carotid plaque and risk of CVD in epidemiological studies

Small, non-stenotic carotid plaque is associated with an increased risk of stroke and other vascular events [14]. The predictive power of presence of carotid plaque has been demonstrated in several large observational studies

[13,37,43–45]. In the *Atherosclerosis Risk in Communities* study, a large population based study on 13,123 participants with a mean follow up of 8 years, the presence of carotid plaque was associated with a 2-fold increased risk of ischemic stroke [37]. Carotid plaque was associated with a 1.7-fold increased risk of incident stroke in the *Cardiovascular Health Study* [46] over a mean follow-up time of 3.3 years and with a 1.5-fold increased risk in the *Rotterdam* Study [45] over a mean follow-up time of 5.2 years. In the *Northern Manhattan Study* (NOMAS), presence of plaque was associated with a 2.8-fold [HR 2.76, 95% CI, 2.1–3.63] increased risk of stroke, MI and vascular death during a mean follow up of 6.9 years [14]. Comparison between these studies however is limited due to diverse study populations and different measuring methods of atherosclerotic plaque [14].

Carotid plaque area may be a better measure of atherosclerosis than cIMT or plaque thickness, since evidence suggests that plaque area grows at a double rate in average than it thickens [47]. In the Tromso study, another large population based study, total plaque area was a stronger predictor for the incident ischemic stroke than cIMT [31]. In 3240 men and 3444 women ultrasonographic assessment of plaque area resulted in a HR of 1.23 (95% CI, 1.09–1.38) in men and 1.19 (95% CI, 1.01–1.41) in women for 1 SD increase in square-root-transformed plaque area when adjusted for other cardiovascular risk factors. The multivariable-adjusted HR in the highest quartile of plaque area versus no plaque was 1.73 (95% CI, 1.19–2.52) in men and 1.62 (95% CI, 1.04–2.53) in women. The multivariable-adjusted HR for 1 SD increase in IMT was 1.08 (95% CI, 0.95–1.22) in men and 1.24 (95% CI, 1.05–1.48) in women [31].

Why carotid IMT and plaque are not commonly accepted surrogate endpoints?

A recent large meta-analysis of 18 case–control and cohort studies evaluated the value of cIMT and plaque in the screening for coronary heart disease [10]. It included 2920 individuals with CHD and 41,941 without CHD and showed no benefit of these parameters as a screening tool, since the discrimination between affected and unaffected individuals was insufficient. Similarly, another recent meta-analysis of 41 randomized trials showed that regression or slowed progression of cIMT with cardiovascular drugs did not affect the risk of cardiovascular events [12].

This evidence indicated that cIMT may not completely meet all criteria of a surrogate marker. A marker should be sensitive, available, non-invasive, and easy to evaluate; all of which are characteristics of cIMT and carotid plaque. However, a causal relationship with the clinical outcome would need to be established and these evidences are likely to come from large longitudinal studies in low risk individuals as well as from basic science research. Furthermore, to act as a surrogate marker cIMT should be able to reflect the full therapeutic effect on the clinical outcome which has not been show yet [48]. Some new information will come from an ongoing large multinational meta-regression study investigating individual progression rate of cIMT and risk of vascular outcomes [49].

Who should be screened for carotid IMT and plaque? Current guidelines/appropriate and not appropriate indications

With increasing incidence of CVD and stroke in the population it is important to identify high-risk patients with subclinical manifestation of disease which will benefit from early and aggressive therapy. The Mannheim cIMT consensus states that there is no need to 'treat IMT values' nor to monitor IMT values in individual patients apart from few exceptions [3,50]. The current guideline for the use of carotid IMT in assessment of cardiovascular risk in asymptomatic adults from 2010 gives carotid IMT class IIa rank with a level B for evidence for asymptomatic adults at intermediate risk. They emphasize the importance of following clear recommendations on the use of appropriate scanning and reading imaging ultrasound methodology [51]. Accordingly, the American Society of Echocardiography recommends in their *consensus statement*, the use of carotid IMT assessment should be reserved for individuals with intermediate cardiovascular risk with; e.g. at a 6–20% 10-year risk of cardiovascular disease according to the Framingham Risk Score (FRS). Since some high-risk groups might not be addressed by this approach, there are further clinical circumstances that should be considered: (1) family history of premature CVD in first-degree relative (men <55 years old, women <65 years old); (2) individuals younger than 60 years old with severe abnormalities in a single risk factor (e.g., genetic dyslipidemia) who otherwise would not be candidates for pharmacotherapy; or (3) women younger than 60 years old with at least two CVD risk factors [5].

Appropriate use of measuring carotid IMT in the clinical setting was examined and summarized by the *Society of Atherosclerosis Imaging and Prevention* and the *International Atherosclerosis Society* [52]. To prevent either under- or over-utilization of IMT-measurements, common clinical scenarios, including risk assessment in the absence of known coronary heart disease (CHD), risk assessment in patients with known CHD, and serial carotid IMT imaging for monitoring of CHD risk status, were rated. The conclusion of these professional organizations was that appropriate indications for the use of cIMT is for individuals without CHD with intermediate risk, older, and individuals with metabolic syndrome. The testing of low-risk or very high-risk CHD individuals as well as serial cIMT testing is considered inappropriate use of this method.

Beginning of genetic discoveries

Common vascular risk factors like hypertension, diabetes, hypercholesterolemia, and nicotine play an important role in the development of atherosclerosis. Therefore, the treatment and control of these factors is a major target in prevention of stroke. However, these environmental risk factors contribute only to about half of all cases of atherosclerotic disease [53]. Finding novel risk factors of atherosclerosis is of great importance for prevention of cardiovascular disease [17]. The focus of preventing strategies tends to shift towards the investigation of genetic factors.

Variation in cardiovascular risk in the population is likely to be connected to variability in genes that are involved in the endothelial inflammatory response to oxidized lipids [17]. Identifying factors underlying the variation of subclinical atherosclerosis unexplained by traditional vascular risk factors either deleterious or protective may help targeting preventive strategies. As opposed to traditional thinking, we have found that the traditional vascular risk factors explain only 21% of the variance in the total carotid plaque burden in a multi-ethnic population of NOMAS. The most explanatory risk factors include age, sex, pack-years of smoking, systolic blood pressure, diastolic blood pressure, antihypertensive and lipid-lowering medications, and diabetes mellitus status. An inclusion of less traditional risk factors such as LDL:HDL ratio, homocysteine levels, high school completion, white blood cell count and LDL cholesterol to the traditional model contributed only about additional 2%, explaining 23% of the variance in total carotid plaque burden at best. Therefore variation in subclinical carotid plaque burden is largely unexplained by known vascular risk factors. These results suggest that other unaccounted factors, both environment and genetic, play an important role in the determination of subclinical atherosclerosis. Identification of these genetic and environmental factors underlying unexplained subclinical atherosclerosis is of great importance for successful prevention of stroke and cardiovascular disease, and is in the major focus for future investigations leading to genetic discoveries and new anti-atherosclerotic treatments.

Conclusion

Carotid IMT and carotid plaque are significant predictors of vascular events and 2D ultrasound measurement of cIMT and carotid plaque is an inexpensive way to detect individuals with increased atherosclerotic burden and risk of CVD, evaluate the effects of current and novel therapies and investigate new contributing factors. Many unaccounted factors, both environmental and genetic, may play an important role in the determination of atherosclerosis, underscoring the importance of further cIMT and carotid plaque research investigations for successful prevention and treatment of cardiovascular disease and stroke.

References

[1] Chambless LE, Heiss G, Folsom AR, Rosamond W, Szklo M, Sharrett AR, et al. Association of coronary heart disease incidence with carotid arterial wall thickness and major risk factors: the Atherosclerosis Risk in Communities (ARIC) study, 1987–1993. Am J Epidemiol 1997;146(6):483–94.

[2] Lorenz MW, Markus HS, Bots ML, Rosvall M, Sitzer M. Prediction of clinical cardiovascular events with carotid intima—media thickness: a systematic review and meta-analysis. Circulation 2007:459–67.

[3] Touboul PJ, Hennerici MG, Meairs S, Adams H, Amarenco P, Bornstein N, et al. Mannheim carotid intima—media thickness consensus (2004–2006). An update on behalf of the Advisory Board of the 3rd and 4th Watching the Risk Symposium, 13th and 15th European Stroke Conferences. Cerebrovasc Dis 2007;23(1):75–80.

[4] Bots ML, Hoes AW, Koudstaal PJ, Hofman A, Grobbee DE. Common carotid intima—media thickness and risk of stroke and myocardial infarction: the Rotterdam Study. Circulation 1997;96(5):1432–7.

[5] Stein JH, Korcarz CE, Hurst RT, Lonn E, Kendall CB, Mohler ER, et al. Use of carotid ultrasound to identify subclinical vascular disease and evaluate cardiovascular disease risk: a consensus statement from the American Society of Echocardiography Carotid Intima—Media Thickness Task Force. Endorsed by the Society for Vascular Medicine. J Am Soc Echocardiogr 2008;21(2):93–111 [quiz 89–90].

[6] O'Leary DH, Polak JF, Kronmal RA, Manolio TA, Burke GL, Wolfson Jr SK, et al. Carotid-artery intima and media thickness as a risk factor for myocardial infarction and stroke in older adults. Cardiovascular Health Study Collaborative Research Group. N Engl J Med 1999;340(1):14–22.

[7] Smilde TJ, van Wissen S, Wollersheim H, Trip MD, Kastelein JJ, Stalenhoef AF, et al. Effect of aggressive versus conventional lipid lowering on atherosclerosis progression in familial hypercholesterolaemia (ASAP): a prospective, randomised, double-blind trial. Lancet 2001;357(9256):577–81.

[8] Wiklund O, Hulthe J, Wikstrand J, Schmidt C, Olofsson SO, Bondjers G, et al. Effect of controlled release/extended release metoprolol on carotid intima—media thickness in patients with hypercholesterolemia: a 3-year randomized study. Stroke 2002;33(2):572–7.

[9] Tardif JC, Heinonen T, Orloff D, Libby P. Vascular biomarkers and surrogates in cardiovascular disease. Circulation 2006;113(25):2936–42.

[10] Wald DS, Bestwick JP. Carotid ultrasound screening for coronary heart disease: results based on a meta-analysis of 18 studies and 44,861 subjects. J Med Screen 2009;16(3):147–54.

[11] Nambi V, Chambless L, Folsom AR, He M, Hu Y, Mosley T, et al. Carotid intima—media thickness and presence or absence of plaque improves prediction of coronary heart disease risk: the ARIC (Atherosclerosis Risk In Communities) study. J Am Coll Cardiol 2010;55(15):1600–7.

[12] Costanzo P, Perrone-Filardi P, Vassallo E, Paolillo S, Cesarano P, Brevetti G, et al. Does carotid intima—media thickness regression predict reduction of cardiovascular events? A meta-analysis of 41 randomized trials. J Am Coll Cardiol 2010;56(24):2006–20.

[13] Prabhakaran S, Rundek T, Ramas R, Elkind MS, Paik MC, Boden-Albala B, et al. Carotid plaque surface irregularity predicts ischemic stroke: the northern Manhattan study. Stroke 2006;37(11):2696–701.

[14] Rundek T, Arif H, Boden-Albala B, Elkind MS, Paik MC, Sacco RL, et al. Carotid plaque, a subclinical precursor of vascular events: the Northern Manhattan Study. Neurology 2008;70(14):1200–7.

[15] Naghavi M, Libby P, Falk E, Casscells SW, Litovsky S, Rumberger J, et al. From vulnerable plaque to vulnerable patient: a call for new definitions and risk assessment strategies: Part I. Circulation 2003;108(14):1664–72.

[16] Warboys CM, Amini N, de Luca A, Evans PC. The role of blood flow in determining the sites of atherosclerotic plaques. F1000 Med Rep 2011;3:5.

[17] Gardener H, Beecham A, Cabral D, Yanuck D, Slifer S, Wang L, et al. Carotid plaque and candidate genes related to inflammation and endothelial function in Hispanics from northern Manhattan. Stroke 2011;42(4):889–96.

[18] Biomarkers and surrogate endpoints: preferred definitions and conceptual framework. Clin Pharmacol Ther 2001;69(3):89–95.

[19] Hackam DG, Anand SS. Emerging risk factors for atherosclerotic vascular disease: a critical review of the evidence. JAMA 2003;290(7):932–40.

[20] Saba L, Anzidei M, Sanfilippo R, Montisci R, Lucatelli P, Catalano C, et al. Imaging of the carotid artery. Atherosclerosis 2012;220(2):294–309.
[21] Schmermund A, Baumgart D, Gorge G, Seibel R, Gronemeyer D, Erbel R, et al. Non-invasive visualization of coronary arteries with and without calcification by electron beam computed tomography. Herz 1996;21(2):118–26.
[22] Sitia S, Tomasoni L, Atzeni F, Ambrosio G, Cordiano C, Catapano A, et al. From endothelial dysfunction to atherosclerosis. Autoimmun Rev 2010;9(12):830–4.
[23] Dhindsa M, Sommerlad SM, DeVan AE, Barnes JN, Sugawara J, Ley O, et al. Interrelationships among noninvasive measures of postischemic macro- and microvascular reactivity. J Appl Physiol 2008;105(2):427–32.
[24] Amarenco P, Labreuche J, Lavallee P, Touboul PJ. Statins in stroke prevention and carotid atherosclerosis: systematic review and up-to-date meta-analysis. Stroke 2004;35(12):2902–9.
[25] Touboul PJ, Vicaut E, Labreuche J, Belliard JP, Cohen S, Kownator S, et al. Correlation between the Framingham risk score and intima media thickness: the Paroi Arterielle et Risque Cardiovasculaire (PARC) study. Atherosclerosis 2007;192(2):363–9.
[26] Cao JJ, Arnold AM, Manolio TA, Polak JF, Psaty BM, Hirsch CH, et al. Association of carotid artery intima–media thickness, plaques, and C-reactive protein with future cardiovascular disease and all-cause mortality: the Cardiovascular Health Study. Circulation 2007;116(1):32–8.
[27] Carallo C, Irace C, Pujia A, De Franceschi MS, Crescenzo A, Motti C, et al. Evaluation of common carotid hemodynamic forces. Relations with wall thickening. Hypertension 1999;34(2):217–21.
[28] Ebrahim S, Papacosta O, Whincup P, Wannamethee G, Walker M, Nicolaides AN, et al. Carotid plaque, intima media thickness, cardiovascular risk factors, and prevalent cardiovascular disease in men and women: the British Regional Heart Study. Stroke 1999;30(4):841–50.
[29] Polak JF, Pencina MJ, Meisner A, Pencina KM, Brown LS, Wolf PA, et al. Associations of carotid artery intima–media thickness (IMT) with risk factors and prevalent cardiovascular disease: comparison of mean common carotid artery IMT with maximum internal carotid artery IMT. J Ultrasound Med 2010;29(12):1759–68.
[30] Mackinnon AD, Jerrard-Dunne P, Sitzer M, Buehler A, von Kegler S, Markus HS, et al. Rates and determinants of site-specific progression of carotid artery intima–media thickness: the carotid atherosclerosis progression study. Stroke 2004;35(9):2150–4.
[31] Mathiesen EB, Johnsen SH, Wilsgaard T, Bonaa KH, Lochen ML, Njolstad I, et al. Carotid plaque area and intima–media thickness in prediction of first-ever ischemic stroke: a 10-year follow-up of 6584 men and women: the Tromso Study. Stroke 2011;42(4):972–8.
[32] Juo SH, Lin HF, Rundek T, Sabala EA, Boden-Albala B, Park N, et al. Genetic and environmental contributions to carotid intima–media thickness and obesity phenotypes in the Northern Manhattan Family Study. Stroke 2004;35(10):2243–7.
[33] Spence JD, Eliasziw M, DiCicco M, Hackam DG, Galil R, Lohmann T, et al. Carotid plaque area: a tool for targeting and evaluating vascular preventive therapy. Stroke 2002;33(12):2916–22.
[34] Shaalan WE, Cheng H, Gewertz B, McKinsey JF, Schwartz LB, Katz D, et al. Degree of carotid plaque calcification in relation to symptomatic outcome and plaque inflammation. J Vasc Surg 2004;40(2):262–9.
[35] Fuster V, Moreno PR, Fayad ZA, Corti R, Badimon JJ. Atherothrombosis and high-risk plaque. Part I. Evolving concepts. J Am Coll Cardiol 2005;46(6):937–54.
[36] Burke AP, Taylor A, Farb A, Malcom GT, Virmani R. Coronary calcification: insights from sudden coronary death victims. Z Kardiol 2000;89(Suppl. 2):49–53.
[37] Hunt KJ, Evans GW, Folsom AR, Sharrett AR, Chambless LE, Tegeler CH, et al. Acoustic shadowing on B-mode ultrasound of the carotid artery predicts ischemic stroke: the Atherosclerosis Risk in Communities (ARIC) study. Stroke 2001;32(5):1120–6.
[38] Seeger JM, Barratt E, Lawson GA, Klingman N. The relationship between carotid plaque composition, plaque morphology, and neurologic symptoms. J Surg Res 1995;58(3):330–6.
[39] Wasserman BA, Sharrett AR, Lai S, Gomes AS, Cushman M, Folsom AR, et al. Risk factor associations with the presence of a lipid core in carotid plaque of asymptomatic individuals using high-resolution MRI: the multi-ethnic study of atherosclerosis (MESA). Stroke 2008;39(2):329–35.
[40] Hunt JL, Fairman R, Mitchell ME, Carpenter JP, Golden M, Khalapyan T, et al. Bone formation in carotid plaques: a clinicopathological study. Stroke 2002;33(5):1214–9.
[41] Prabhakaran S, Singh R, Zhou X, Ramas R, Sacco RL, Rundek T, et al. Presence of calcified carotid plaque predicts vascular events: the Northern Manhattan Study. Atherosclerosis 2007;195(1):e197–201.
[42] Xu X, Ju H, Cai J, Cai Y, Wang X, Wang Q, et al. High-resolution MR study of the relationship between superficial calcification and the stability of carotid atherosclerotic plaque. Int J Cardiovasc Imaging 2010;26(Suppl. 1):143–50.
[43] Salonen R, Tervahauta M, Salonen JT, Pekkanen J, Nissinen A, Karvonen MJ, et al. Ultrasonographic manifestations of common carotid atherosclerosis in elderly eastern Finnish men. Prevalence and associations with cardiovascular diseases and risk factors. Arterioscler Thromb 1994;14(10):1631–40.
[44] Kitamura A, Iso H, Imano H, Ohira T, Okada T, Sato S, et al. Carotid intima–media thickness and plaque characteristics as a risk factor for stroke in Japanese elderly men. Stroke 2004;35(12):2788–94.
[45] van der Meer IM, Bots ML, Hofman A, del Sol AI, van der Kuip DA, Witteman JC, et al. Predictive value of noninvasive measures of atherosclerosis for incident myocardial infarction: the Rotterdam Study. Circulation 2004;109(9):1089–94.
[46] Krause KJ. Screening potential elderly preferred markers: exploratory analysis of Cardiovascular Health Study (CHS) data. J Insur Med 2004;36(3):194–9.
[47] Barnett PA, Spence JD, Manuck SB, Jennings JR. Psychological stress and the progression of carotid artery disease. J Hypertens 1997;15(1):49–55.
[48] Boissel JP, Collet JP, Moleur P, Haugh M. Surrogate endpoints: a basis for a rational approach. Eur J Clin Pharmacol 1992;43(3):235–44.
[49] Lorenz MW, Bickel H, Bots ML, Breteler MM, Catapano AL, Desvarieux M, et al. Individual progression of carotid intima media thickness as a surrogate for vascular risk (PROG-IMT): rationale and design of a meta-analysis project. Am Heart J 2010;159(5):730-6.e2.
[50] Touboul PJ, Hennerici MG, Meairs S, Adams H, Amarenco P, Desvarieux M, et al. Mannheim intima–media thickness consensus. Cerebrovasc Dis 2004;18(4):346–9.
[51] Greenland P, Alpert JS, Beller GA, Benjamin EJ, Budoff MJ, Fayad ZA, et al. 2010 ACCF/AHA guideline for assessment of cardiovascular risk in asymptomatic adults: a report of the American College of Cardiology Foundation/American Heart Association Task Force on practice guidelines. J Am Coll Cardiol 2010;56(25):e50–103.
[52] Society of Atherosclerosis Imaging and Prevention Developed in collaboration with the International Atherosclerosis Society. Appropriate use criteria for carotid intima media thickness testing. Atherosclerosis 2011;214(1):43–6.
[53] Lefkowitz RJ, Willerson JT. Prospects for cardiovascular research. JAMA 2001;285(5):581–7.

Arterial wall dynamics

Galina Baltgaile*

Riga Stradina University, Neurological Department, Pilsoņu iela 13, Riga LV-1002, Latvia

KEYWORDS
Arterial wall stiffness;
Distensibility;
Compliance;
Intima—media thickness;
B-mode;
M-mode ultrasound

Summary An early change in arterial wall dynamics introduced as a novel risk factor for cardiovascular events in various populations is discussed in this review.

Distensibility of an artery segment as reflection of the mechanical stress affecting the arterial wall during the cardiac cycle has been intensively studied recent years through the technological development of high-resolution ultrasound systems.

A decrease of arterial distensibility (i.e. increase of arterial wall stiffness) seems to be a common pathological mechanism for many factors associated with cerebrovascular and cardiovascular diseases. It is difficult to define the role of each factor affecting the arterial wall motions dependent mainly on the left ventricle, intra arterial pressure and blood volume, endothelium function, smooth muscle tone and neural control mechanism. The calculations of arterial compliance, elastic modulus, augmentation pressure, stiffness and intima—media thickness may help to identify the role of each mechanism if they are based on high-tech measurements of arterial wall.

The role of nervous regulation of blood vessel's tone in this process is not clear. Our studies show the strong correlation between autonomic imbalance and increase of carotid arterial distensibility in young patients. Various possible relationships between changes in the dynamic artery wall properties and neural regulation are discussed.
© 2012 Elsevier GmbH. All rights reserved.

Methods of analysis of arterial wall motion

It is widely accepted that the early carotid arterial wall disease is a useful predictor of the risk of both ischemic stroke and coronary heart disease in asymptomatic population [1].

The parameters of arterial wall elasticity properties should be employed as a surrogate marker to detect early stage of vascular diseases. Increased artery wall stiffness and decreased arterial distensibility are accepted to be a common pathological mechanism for many factors associated with stroke, arterial hypertension, diabetes mellitus, hyperlipidemia and myocardial infarction [2,3].

* Tel.: +371 29454412; fax: +371 67288769.
E-mail address: baltgaile@gmail.com

Several quantitative or qualitative analysis methods for arterial wall function have been suggested. From them the most popular are the detection of flow-mediated dilatation (FMD) of brachial artery, assessment of peripheral arterial pressure waveforms, measurements of pulse wave velocity (PWV), measurements of arterial distensibility and stiffness with calculation of Young's modulus of elasticity of wall material, wall thickness and blood density.

Flow-mediated vasodilatation (FMD)

In the 1990s, high-frequency ultrasound imaging of the brachial artery to assess endothelium-dependent flow-mediated vasodilation was developed. Although FMD is widely used to provide the information about endothelium function in common it is related to the capacity to respond

Arterial wall dynamics

to different stimuli and confers the ability to self-regulate tone of the brachial artery only [4].

Pulse wave velocity (PWV)

Another assessment of arterial stiffness and compliance can also be performed by measurements of the speed of travel of the pressure pulse wave along the specified distance on the vascular bed. To measure PVW, pulse wave signals are recorded with pressure tonometers positioned over carotid and femoral arteries and are calculated as a ratio of distance and time delay:

$$PWV = \frac{Distance\ (D)}{Time\ delay\ (\Delta T)} m/s$$

Measurement of aortic PWV seems to be the best available non-invasive measurement of aortic stiffness while it is not specific for changes in elastic properties of carotid arteries [5–7,10].

Parameters of arterial wall distensibility and stiffness

Since no precise direct measurement method for the determination of arterial wall elasticity or stiffness has been suggested several indirect methods such as calculation of arterial compliance, Young's modulus of elasticity, stiffness index and arterial distensibility are commonly used.

The different parameters of carotid artery's wall elasticity could be measured by high resolution B-mode and M-mode ultrasound using manual and automatic measurements as well as wall echo-tracking system [8,9]. Development of methods based on ultrasound RF signal, tissue Doppler imaging and other tracking systems helps to increase the accuracy of automatic measurement of vascular wall properties such as IMT, arterial stiffness/distensibility and wall compliance, although even these methods are not free from errors [8,11,12].

The good reproducibility of carotid arteries diameters measured by 2D grayscale imaging, M-mode and A-mode (wall tracking) is proved [13]. However it is also mentioned that very small changes in linear measurements of carotid diameters can have big effects on estimates of arterial mechanical properties such as strain and Young's modulus. Additionally the cross-sectional imaging cannot be used to determine diameter or area of the lumen for a current clinical setting because of inadequate image definition of the lateral walls.

Carotid distensibility measured as changes in arterial diameter or circumferential area in systole and diastole is a reflection of the mechanical stress affecting the arterial wall during the cardiac cycle.

Distensibility can be calculated as $Ds - Dd$

where Ds is end-systolic diameter of artery. Dd is end-diastolic diameter.

$$\text{Distensibility or Wall Strain} = \frac{Ds - Dd}{Dd}$$

$$\text{Cross-sectional distensibility} = \frac{As - Ad}{Ad}$$

where As is the systolic cross-sectional area of artery. Ad is diastolic cross-sectional area.

It is difficult to understand and define the role of each factor influencing the arterial wall dynamics. Vasodilatation and vasoconstriction are dependent upon the left ventricle and intra arterial pressure and blood volume, endothelium function, smooth muscle tone and neural control mechanism.

Could the type of measurement and analysis of arterial wall distensibility help to define the mainly affected part of arterial wall involved in pathological process?

The influence of left ventricle function on a blood pressure could be measured by calculation of total arterial compliance:

$$TAC = \frac{SV}{PP}$$

where SV is left ventricle stroke volume.

Classical compliance is a change in blood volume in response to a given change in expanding pressure:

$$CC = \frac{\Delta V}{\Delta P} - \text{volume change to pressure ratio}$$

Since the distensibility of arterial wall is mainly blood pressure and volume dependent the systolic and diastolic pressure ratio is included in a most of calculations of vessel's elastic properties [14,15].

Wall stress can be defined as the difference in systolic and diastolic blood pressure:

Pulse pressure (PP) = Ps − Pd

The stress/strain relationship can be measured as vessel's diameter (or area) and pressure compliance given by different equations [16,17]. The most frequently used are:

$$\text{Compliance}\ (C)\quad C = \frac{Strain}{PP}$$

Pressure/strain elastic modulus (EM) is calculated as

$$EM = K \times \frac{Ps - Pd}{Strain}$$

where K is conversion factor for mmHg to Nm = 133.3.

Young modulus of elasticity (Y) which reflects the stiffness of an isotropic elastic material and can be defined as a ratio of stress to strain per unit area [18].

$$Y = \frac{\Delta P}{\Delta D} \cdot \frac{Dd}{IMT}$$

where IMT is intima–media thickness.

Stiffness index (β) is calculated as

$$\beta = \ln\frac{Ps}{Pd} \cdot Strain$$

Young elastic modulus (EINC)

$$\text{EINC} = \frac{3(1 = \text{LCSA}/\text{WCSA})}{\text{DIST}}$$

where LSCA — luminal cross-sectional area; WSCA — mean wall cross-sectional area; DIST — cross-sectional distensibility.

There are some beliefs that inclusion of different measurements of wall properties as well as hemodynamic parameters in equation could provide more informative and comprehensive index.

Like EINC-pressure and EINC-stress curves calculated from IMT and from diameter and pressure waveforms could provide more precisely direct information about elastic properties of the wall material that is independent of the vessel's geometry, whereas distensibility gives information on the elastic properties of the artery as a hollow structure [19].

The same could be said about the measure of contribution that the wall reflection makes to systolic arterial pressure. These measurements of reflecting waves coming from periphery to centre are calculated as augmentation pressure (AG) and augmentation index (AI) [20,21].

The disadvantage of above mentioned calculations lies in the comparison of elastic properties of different arteries like the comparison of wall dynamics of carotid artery to changes in blood pressure measured in a brachial artery. Calculations of FMD, PWV, Ai and other stiffness parameters cannot be attributed to carotid artery properties only since brachial, femoral, aortic and internal carotid arterial segments differ in the proportion of elastin—collagen to smooth muscle as well as proportion of endothelium to media layer and neural control.

Thus, the recording of pressure ratio during the cardiac cycle in a brachial artery can provide only indirect information of pressure/strain ratio in carotid artery. Considering this argument, it seems logical to evaluate carotid artery wall dynamics by ultrasound measurements of arterial wall structure and movements in a strictly precised vascular area.

Endothelium, smooth muscle and arterial distensibility

Apart from the blood pressure as the major determinant of vessels stretch the blood flow shear stress could play the important role in arterial distensibility. Endothelial cells are the primary vascular cells exposed to shear stress from the friction of laminar blood flow against the vessels wall. One of possibilities to detect the influence of endothelium and smooth muscle on arterial distensibility or stiffness is the recording of intima—media thickness (IMT) and its relation to vessels diameter (Fig. 1). The most popular are the measurements:

IMT to vessel's radius ratio:

$$\frac{\text{IMT}}{\text{Radius}} = 2 \times \frac{\text{IMT}}{\text{mean internal diameter}},$$

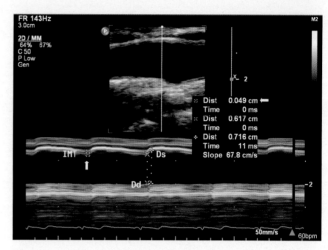

Figure 1 M-mode image of the right bulb of common carotid artery of 24 years old female with normal arterial blood pressure. IMT is 0.049 cm. The artery distension during cardial cycle: Ds − Dd = 0.716 − 0.617 = 0.1 cm, where Ds is marked with + Dd marked with ×.

Mean circumferential wall stress (MCWS) [19]

$$\text{MCWS} = \frac{\text{Mean BP} \times \text{mean internal diameter}}{2 \times \text{IMT}}$$

IMT and MCWS are indicative for changes in both endothelium and smooth muscle wall's layers since even high resolution ultrasound technique can provide the image of intima—media complex [22]. This technique with the phased tracking can obtain the measurements even of minute changes in IMT. From the maximum change in thickness during one heartbeat, the radial strain of each assigned layer in the artery wall (ε_r) is calculated as:

$$\varepsilon_r = \frac{h_{\max} - h_{\min}}{h_{\max}}$$

where $h_{\max}$ and $h_{\min}$ — maximum and minimum thickness of an assigned layer in the wall, respectively [23].

Commonly used the IMT measurement become the marker of early stage of decreased elasticity or increased stiffness of arterial wall. Significant correlations between increased IMT and the presence of arterial hypertension, hyperlipidemia, arterial atherosclerosis, diabetes mellitus and aging had been proven in many studies [24]. IMT and carotid artery stiffness became useful predictors of the risk of cerebrovascular and cardiovascular events [25].

Some results of the correlations between IMT and arterial distensibility indicate that gender- and age-related differences can be manifested even in young, healthy adults and may be identified with techniques that assess carotid distensibility across a range of pressures [26].

Although smooth muscle tone is a key determinant of mechanical properties of arteries its assessment in humans is technically limited and direct contribution of vascular smooth muscle to artery elastic mechanics is controversial [26,27]. Detecting the influence of tone on arterial properties is possible by applying sympathetic/parasympathetic stimulating test to the measurements of wall elastic properties.

Neural stimuli and arterial distensibility

There is the certain association between the changes in carotid arterial distensibility and autonomic imbalance. Some results of investigations suggest that the pathophysiological state of arterial distensibility may modify the autonomic balance. Carotid arterial distensibility is an important determinant of improvement in autonomic nervous regulation after the function of left ventricular wall motion abnormality has been improved [28]. All together both factors — changes in carotid distensibility and changes in left ventricular diastolic filling can influence carotid baroreceptors. Although it is known that baroreceptor sensitivity is reduced with increasing age and in patients with arterial hypertension it is difficult to determine whether this reduction is caused by reduction of arterial distensibility or disturbances in the neural transduction part of baroreflex arc [8]. Some data support the hypothesis that reduction in carotid artery wall elastic properties may lead to low vagal tone. Increased cardiovascular risk associated with low vagal tone may partly be mediated via changes in carotid artery elastic properties [29].

The hypothesis that carotid arteries undergo rapid changes in distensibility on moving from the supine to head-up tilt postures and, subsequently, that this change in carotid distensibility might be associated with concurrent reductions in cardiovagal baroreflex sensitivity had been tested [30]. It might be speculated that the reduction in diameter and maximal distensibility of the carotid region in orthostatic tests alters the interactive effects of the various types of baroreceptor afferents from the carotid sinus that differentially affect blood pressure control. Some findings indicate that sympathetic activation is able to decrease radial arterial compliance in healthy subjects. The reduction in arterial compliance probably resulted from complex interactions between changes in distending blood pressure and changes in radial arterial smooth muscle tone [31].

Values of rates of carotid distention are highly variable in young healthy individuals. There are also findings of carotid sinus distensibility exceeded aortic arch distensibility at the ages<35 whereas this relation was reversed at the ages >35. It could be assumed that this feature may impact on the ability to observe more consistent acute adaptations to postural perturbations [32]. These findings can also be explained by more pronounced effect of nervous regulation on arterial wall motion in young people. Furthermore the fact mentioned in the SMART study that some patients with the low systolic blood pressure had decreased arterial stiffness i.e. increased arterial distensibility coincided with our numerous observations in the practical survey of blood vessels and provoked the question whether it is a consequence of imbalance of autonomic regulation of wall dynamics [2,33].

Material and method

To detect the changes in the carotid artery wall tone we examined 97 young patients (42 men, 55 women from 17 to 35 years of age,) selected from patients who visited our hospital between 2002 and 2005 for clinical examinations. The main complaints were weather dependent and stress related headache, dizziness, excessive sweating, orthostatic light headedness, postural hypotension and fainting in history. All of the clinical routine tests had been done to exclude any disease which could cause above mentioned symptoms. Blood pressure instability during orthostatic test had been detected in the most of cases ($n = 78$) The tendency to low brachial blood pressure (s/d $101/54 \pm 12/9$ mmHg) found in 66 cases and slightly raised brachial blood pressure (s/d $140/75 \pm 9/7$ mmHg) in 12 cases. All patients underwent neck and cerebral blood vessels examination as a part of clinical tests. Results of ultrasound examinations of carotid artery had been compared with the results of the same examination of control group from 25 sex and age matched healthy individuals.

As a part of routine ultrasound examinations blood vessels of neck were examined usual way by 4—7.5 MHz linear probe and cerebral vessels by 3—3.5 MHz sectoral probe using two ultrasound systems — "Applio", Toshiba Medical Systems and "iE-33", Philips. Measurements had been done by one experienced examiner and data from both ultrasound systems had been compared. The small group of 7 patients was observed using both machines.

Ultrasound images of carotid artery were acquired and IMT measurements were done using B-mode regime usual way. Blood flow was examined using Color and Power Doppler mode in a standard regime. To register arterial wall's moving during cardiac cycle the M-mode was applied additionally to B-mode and Color-mode images. With a high M-mode resolution it was possible to define all layers of arterial wall and to measure IMT. All measurements of vessel's IMT and wall movement obtained from B-mode images and M-mode images had been compared and subsequent mean values had been calculated to avoid inevitable errors (Figs. 1 and 2). The area for measurements was carotid bulb dilation. The wall movements were measured as end-systolic (Ds) and end-diastolic (Dd) diameters of carotid artery (Fig. 1).

Results

There was a good comparability of measurements obtained using both ultrasound systems.

IMT of carotid artery of normotensive and hypotensive patients with a signs of autonomic nervous dysfunction did not differ from IMT of healthy controls (mean far wall CCA IMT 0.46 ± 0.07 mm, max -0.53 ± 0.08 mm) while patients with mild hypertension had higher rates of far wall CCA IMT (mean 0.54 ± 0.07 mm, max 0.65 ± 0.09 mm).

The carotid artery distensibility was significantly higher in a patient group as compared with a group of healthy controls: 0.11 ± 0.04 cm and 0.07 ± 0.02 cm respectively. The same change in distensibility in patients with initial mild hypertension was not statistically significant.

The peak systolic blood velocity in carotid artery ($V_{max} \pm sd$ 125 ± 15 cm/s) was increased compared to healthy individuals (V_{max} 87 ± 13 cm/s) Systolic acceleration was accompanied by increase of pulsative index (1.96 ± 0.87) as a result of drop of diastolic velocity (Fig. 2).

Signs of impaired arterial wall tone occurred as vascular bruits and heart tone registered not only in dopplerograms of carotid arteries but also in intracranial arteries were found in 48 of cases. 16 patients had additional mid-diastolic wave as additional wall distention (not exceeded 0.02 ± 0.01 cm) accompanied by high systolic blood flow velocity with a prominent increase of systolic/diastolic velocities ratio. All these patients had significant brachial pressure fall during orthostatic test indicated the lack of autonomic nervous regulation (Fig. 3).

Conclusion and discussion

The strong correlations exist between carotid arterial elastic properties and carotid baroreceptors, cardiovagal baroreflex sensitivity with an impact on arterial blood pressure and stroke volume. We can assume the interdependency between carotid distensibility and autonomic balance. Whereas some studies suggest that reduced elastic properties of carotid arteries cause the reduction of cardiovagal baroreflex sensitivity resulted in changes of hemodynamic, the results of our previous and recent studies show the dependence of carotid arterial distensibility on autonomic neural regulation of wall tone.

The autonomic imbalance in young people was associated with the increase of arterial distensibility, expressed as increase of carotid arterial systolic/diastolic diameter change, sometimes additional arterial mid-diastolic wall motion, accompanied by abnormal distribution of flow velocity during cardiac cycle with the marked systolic flow acceleration and significant increase of systolic/diastolic ratio.

This conclusion coincides with the findings of the decreased arterial stiffness in a young people under the acute sympathetic stimulation of artery. These results may be explained by an unloading of stiffer wall components during active arterial constriction under influence of autonomic stimulation [27]. The further comparable evaluation of patients with different impairment of nervous system could help to determine the role of nervous regulative function on arterial wall dynamics.

Taking into account many basic mechanisms and various factors influencing arterial wall dynamics it is difficult to measure the impact of each of them separately. Arterial wall stiffness or distensibility measurements reflect the dynamics of all structures of the arterial wall as well as dynamics of blood perfusion. Arterial mechanical properties can be calculated in different ways including parameters of various factors affecting wall motion. The development of the high resolution ultrasound tracking techniques makes it possible more accurate measurements of arterial elastic properties which is extremely important for early detection of vascular pathology.

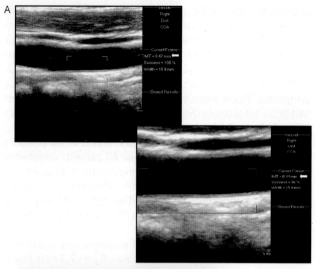
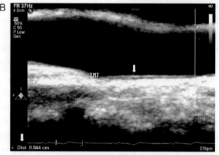

Figure 2 B-mode images of the carotid artery of the same patient. Comparative measurements of IMT: A and B — automatic measurements of mean IMT (0.47 mm, 0.44 mm), C — manual measurement of max IMT (0.44 mm). Compare to IMT measurement by M-mode (0.49 mm) from Fig. 1.

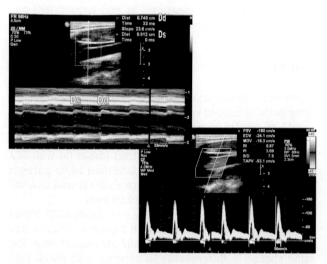

Figure 3 Representative M-mode (A) and color-coded duplex sonographic (B) images of carotid artery (near bulb region) of 18 years old female patient with low blood pressure (90/50 mmHg), and orthostatic intolerance. Increased artery distensibility during cardiac cycle Ds (marked as +) − Dd (marked as ×) = 0.16 cm. Significantly high peak systolic velocity −180 cm/s with diastolic drop: pronounced diastolic notch and significantly increased systolic/diastolic ratio 7.5.

References

[1] Rothwell PM. Carotid artery disease and the risk of ischemic stroke and coronary vascular events. Cerebrovasc Dis 2000;10:21—33.
[2] Dijk JM, Algra A, van der Graaf Y, Grobbee DE, Bots ML, SMART Study Group. Carotid stiffness and the risk of new vascular events in patients with manifest cardiovascular disease. The SMART study. Eur Heart J 2005;26(12):1213—20.

[3] Oliver JJ, Webb DJ. Noninvasive assessment of arterial stiffness and risk of atherosclerotic events. Arterioscler Thromb Vasc Biol 2003;23:554—63.

[4] Corretti C, Anderson TJ, Benjamin EJ, Celermajer D, Charbonneau F, Creager MA, et al. Guidelines for the ultrasound assessment of endothelium-dependent flow-mediated vasodilation of brachial artery. MJ Am Col Cardiol 2002;39(2):257—65.

[5] Boutouyrie R, Laurent S, Benetos A, Gierd XJ, Hoek AP, Safar ME. Opposing effect of aging on distal and proximal large arteries in hypertensives. J Hypertens Suppl 1992;10:S87—91.

[6] Lim MA, Townsend RR. Arterial compliance in the elderly: its effect on blood pressure measurement and cardiovascular outcome. Clin Geriatr Med 2009;25(2):191—205.

[7] Hermeling E, Reesink KD, Hoeks AP, Reneman RS. Potentials and pitfalls of local PWV measurements. Am J Hypertens 2010;23(9):934.

[8] Reneman RS, Meinders JM, Hoeks APG. Non-invasive ultrasound in arterial wall dynamics in humans: what have we learned and what remains to be solved. Eur Heart J 2005;26(10):960—6.

[9] Golemati S, Sassano A, Lever MJ, Bharath AA, Dhanjil S, Nicolaides AN. Carotid artery wall motion estimated from B-mode ultrasound using region tracking and block matching. Ultrasound Med Biol 2003;29(3):387—99.

[10] Soltesz P, Der H, Kerekes G, Szodoray P, Szücs G, Dankó K, et al. A comparative study of arterial stiffness, flow-mediated vasodilatation of the brachial artery, and the thickness of the carotid artery intima—media in patients with systemic autoimmune diseases. Clin Rheumatol 2009;28(6):655—62.

[11] Ramnarine KV, Hartshorne T, Sensier Y, Naylor M, Walker J, Naylor AR, et al. Tissue Doppler imaging of carotid plaque wall motion: a pilot study. Cardiovasc Ultrasound 2003;1:17.

[12] Stadler W, Karl WC, Lees RS. The application of echo-tracking methods to endothelium-dependent vasoreactivity and arterial compliance measurements. Ultrasound Med Biol 1996;22(1):35—42.

[13] Godia EC, Madhok R, Pittman J, Trocio S, Ramas R, Cabral D, et al. Carotid artery distensibility: a reliability study. J Ultrasound Med 2007;26(9):1157—65.

[14] Hickler RB. Aortic and large artery stiffness: current methodology and clinical correlations. Clin Cardiol 1990;13:317—22.

[15] Wada T, Fujishiro K, Fukumoto T, Yamazaki S. Relationship between ultrasound assessment of arterial wall properties and blood pressure. Angiology 1997;48:893—900.

[16] O'Rurke MF, Staessen JA, Viachopoulos C, Duprez D, Plante GE. Clinical applications of arterial stiffness; definitions and reference values. Am J Hypertens 2002;15(5):426—44.

[17] Kuecherer HF, Just A, Kirchheim H. Evaluation of aortic compliance in humans. Am J Physiol Heart Circ Physiol 2000;278(5):H1411—3.

[18] Selzer RH, Mack WJ, Lee PL, Kwong-Fu H, Hodis HN. Improved common carotid elasticity and intima media thickness measurements from computer analysis of sequential ultrasound frames. Atherosclerosis 2001;154(1):185—93.

[19] Bussy C, Boutouyrie P, Lacolley P, Challande P, Laurent S. Intrinsic stiffness of the carotid arterial wall material in essential hypertensives. Hypertension 2000;35(5):1049—54.

[20] Bank AJ, Wilson RF, Kubo SH, Holte JE, Dresing TJ, Wang H. Direct effects of smooth muscle relaxation and contraction on in vivo human brachial artery elastic properties. Circ Res 1995;77(5):1008—16.

[21] Fantin F, Mattocks A, Bulpitt CJ, Banva W, Rajkumar C. Is augmentation index a good measure of vascular stiffness in the elderly? Age Ageing 2007;36(1):43—8.

[22] Hasegawa H, Kanai H, Ichiki M, Tezuka F. Tissue structure of arterial wall revealed with elasticity imaging. J Med Ultrasonics 2007;34(1):73—4.

[23] Yamagishi T, Kato M, Koiwa Y, Hasegswa H, Kanai H. Usefulness of measurement of carotid arterial wall elasticity distribution in detection of early stage atherosclerotic lesions caused by cigarette smoking. J Med Ultrasonics 2006;33:203—10.

[24] Alan S, Ulgen MS, Ozturk O, Alan B, Ozdemir L, Toprak N. Relation between coronary artery disease, risk factors and intima—media thickness of carotid artery, arterial distensibility, and stiffness index. Angiology 2003;54(3):261—7.

[25] Giannattasio C, Mancia G. Arterial distensibility in humans. Modulating mechanisms, alterations in diseases and effects of treatment. J Hypertens 2002;20(10):1889—99.

[26] Myers CW, Ferquahar WB, Forman DE, Williams TD, Dierks DL, Taylor JA. Carotid distensibility characterized via the isometric exercise pressor response. Am J Physiol Heart Circ Physiol 2002;283(6):H2592—8.

[27] Joannides R, Richard V, Moore N, Godin M, Thuille C. Influence of sympathetic tone on mechanical properties of muscular arteries in humans. AJP-Heart 1995;268(February (2)).

[28] Tomiyama H, Nishikawa E, Abe M, Nakagawa K, Fujiwara M, Yamamoto A, et al. Carotid arterial distensibility is an important determinant of improvement in autonomic balance after successful coronary angioplasty. J Hypertens 2000;18(11):1621—8.

[29] Koskinen T, Juonala M, Kähönen M, Jula A, Laitinen T, Keltikangas —Järvinen L, et al. Relations between carotid artery distensibility and heart rate variability. The Cardiovascular Risk in Young Finns Study. Auton Neurosci 2011;161(1—2):75—80.

[30] Steinback CD, O'Leary DD, Bakker J, Cechetto AD, Ladak HM, Shoemaker JK. Carotid distensibility, baroreflex sensitivity, and orthostatic stress. J Appl Phys 2011;99(1):64—70.

[31] Boutouyrie P, Lacolley P, Girerd X, Beck L, Safar M, Laurent S. Sympathetic activation decreases medium-sized arterial compliance in humans. AJP-Heart 1994;267(4):32.

[32] Lénárd Z, Studinger P, Kováts Z, Reneman R, Kollai M. Comparison of aortic arch and carotid sinus distensibility in humans—relation to baroreflex sensitivity. Auton Neurosci 2001;92(1—2):92—9.

[33] Baltgaile G, Timofejeva T. Cerebral vasomotor instability caused by the decrease of vessels wall's tone. Cerebrovasc Dis 2002;S4(13):26.

Morphological, hemodynamic and stiffness changes in arteries of young smokers

Brigitta Lérant[a], Christina Straesser[a], Réka Katalin Kovács[a], László Oláh[a], László Kardos[b], László Csiba[a,*]

[a] University of Debrecen, Medical and Health Science Centre, Department of Neurology, 22 Móricz Zsigmond Str. Debrecen 4032, Hungary
[b] Kenézy Hospital and Outpatient Services, Infection Control Unit, 2-26 Bartók Béla Str. Debrecen 4043, Hungary

KEYWORDS
Smoking;
Intima-media thickness;
Stiffness

Abstract

Aim: The aim of our investigations was to detect the acute and chronic effects of cigarette smoking on arterial wall thickness and stiffness in young, healthy volunteers. We also performed a one-year follow-up to define the possible changes.

Subjects: We recruited 25 non-smoking and 25 smoking university students aged 19—33. Exclusion criteria were any known diseases, abnormally high cholesterol levels and body mass index (BMI) above $30\,kg/m^2$.

Methods: We defined the intima-media thickness on both common carotid arteries by using B-mode ultrasonography and we measured the hemodynamic and stiffness parameters with the help of arteriograph. In case of smokers we also investigated the acute effects after smoking one cigarette. In the follow-up study we measured 15 non-smokers and 13 smokers again.

Results: In the smoking group morphological, stiffness and hemodynamic parameters showed significantly higher values compared to non-smokers. Concerning the acute effects we detected a significant increase in stiffness and hemodynamic parameters after smoking one cigarette. Gender differences were also found in the smoking group. Unadjusted to age, gender and smoking status there was a significant correlation between intima-media thickness and pulse wave velocity. We could not find any progression in smokers after one year, while there was an improvement in intima-media thickness and augmentation index in non-smokers.

Conclusion: Early atherosclerotic processes due to smoking can be detected even at a young age, in healthy university students. One year regular smoking does not result in detectable changes.

© 2012 Elsevier GmbH. All rights reserved.

Abbreviations: Aix, augmentation index; BMI, body mass index; HR, heart rate; IMT, intima-media thickness; PWV, pulse wave velocity; sBP, systolic blood pressure.
* Corresponding author at: University of Debrecen, Medical and Health Science Centre, Department of Neurology, 22 Móricz Zsigmond Str. Debrecen 4032 Hungary. Tel.: +36 52 255 255; fax: +36 52 453 590.
E-mail addresses: lerant.brigi@gmail.com (B. Lérant), tine023@aol.com (C. Straesser), kovacskatireka@yahoo.com (R.K. Kovács), olah@dote.hu (L. Oláh), l.kardos@orvosbiostat.hu (L. Kardos), csiba@dote.hu (L. Csiba).

2211-968X/$ — see front matter © 2012 Elsevier GmbH. All rights reserved.
doi:10.1016/j.permed.2012.02.061

Introduction

Tobacco is one of the most important preventable causes of premature death worldwide. Smoke leads to an increased risk of stroke, heart disease, atherosclerosis and peripheral vascular disease even at the lowest level of exposure. About 5 million tobacco-related deaths occur a year worldwide and it is expected to reach 8 million a year by 2030 [1].

The higher carotid intima-media thickness (IMT) confirms the atherogenic effects of smoking. Several studies attest that there is a dose- and time-dependent relationship between carotid IMT and smoking with the highest value in current smokers, lower in former and the lowest in never smokers [2,3]. The aim of our study was to investigate whether only a few years of smoking results in measurable morphological and stiffness changes on arteries in young healthy students without any other cardiovascular risk factors. Besides the chronic alterations we also measured the acute effects of cigarette smoking on hemodynamic and stiffness parameters.

We intended to define whether any progression could be detected due to smoking after a short period of time by repeating the whole measurement on the same subjects after one year.

Materials and methods

We recruited 25 non-smoking and 25 smoking healthy university students aged 19–33 for our study. Exclusion criteria were any known diseases, abnormally high cholesterol levels and BMI above $30\,kg/m^2$.

Students who have smoked for at least half a year, at least 5 cigarettes per day, belonged to the smoking group. The average duration of smoking was 6.5 years with an amount of 10.2 cigarettes per day. Participants were not allowed to smoke 6 h before the investigations.

After performing laboratory tests we used B-mode ultrasonography to define the intima-media thickness (IMT) on both common carotid arteries and we measured the hemodynamic (heart rate, blood pressure) and stiffness parameters (pulse wave velocity, augmentation index) with an oscillometric method (TensioMed Arteriograph). In case of smokers we repeated the measurement with the arteriograph after smoking one cigarette to detect the acute effects of smoking, too.

We measured the IMT R-syncron, 1 cm before the bifurcation, 6 times on each ultrasound picture, then we calculated an average which was used for the statistical analysis.

Two examiners separately performed the investigations and the subjects were called back after one week to repeat the whole procedure.

In the one-year follow-up we used the same methods and restrictions as in the original study and we measured 15 non-smokers and 13 smokers again. Between-group comparisons were carried out on data averaged over measurement occasions and observers into a single-observation-per-subject structure. The method of comparison was either Student's two-sample t test or Wilcoxon's rank-sum test, subject to normality assumptions being satisfied. Normality was checked using the skewness-kurtosis test. For comparisons of outcomes before and after smoking in smokers

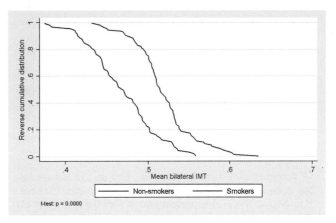

Figure 1 Differences in IMT between non-smokers and smokers. Significant increase can be seen in IMT in the smoking group compared to non-smokers ($p < 0.0001$). (Accepted by Clinical Neuroscience. One part of the results has been accepted by the Hungarian Ideggyógyászati Szemle (Clin Neuroscience). The present form is with the permission of the journal mentioned above. Supported by ETT 407-04/2009.)

Student's paired t test or Wilcoxon's matched-pairs signed-rank test was used, subject to normality assumptions. The relationships between average bilateral IMT and elasticity parameters were modelled using multiple linear regression adjusted for gender and smoking in interaction, and age. For one-year comparisons we used paired t-tests or Wilcoxon matched-pairs signed-ranks tests, subject to normality assumptions being satisfied. Stratification for smoking status was used to eliminate confounding and to reveal effect modification if present.

Results

Significant differences were found in arterial thickness, stiffness and hemodynamic values between smokers and non-smokers.

In our original study mean bilateral carotid IMT was found 0.52 ± 0.034 mm in smokers and 0.46 ± 0.036 mm in non-smokers ($p < 0.0001$). Fig. 1 shows the difference in IMT between the two groups.

The one-year follow-up confirmed this result with values of 0.51 ± 0.033 mm in smokers and 0.44 ± 0.027 mm in non-smokers ($p < 0.01$).

Pulse wave velocity (PWV) also showed significantly higher values in the smoking group compared to non-smokers. As a resting value, after the 6 h prohibition of smoking we measured 7.46 ± 1.1 m/s in smokers and 6.67 ± 0.84 m/s in non-smokers ($p < 0.01$).

After one year we got similar results (8.07 ± 2.1 m/s in smokers, 6.61 ± 0.85 in non-smokers, $p < 0.05$).

Regarding the hemodynamic parameters there was a significant difference in heart rate (HR) due to smoking. The resting value in smokers was found $72 \pm 8.3\,s^{-1}$, while in non-smokers we measured $67 \pm 8.6\,s^{-1}$ ($p < 0.05$). In the one-year follow-up this significance was not confirmed.

As for the acute effects of smoking we detected significant increase in PWV, heart rate and systolic blood pressure

Table 1 The acute effects of smoking one cigarette on stiffness and hemodynamic values[a]. Pulse wave velocity (PWV), heart rate (HR) and systolic blood pressure (sBP) significantly increased due to the inhalation of smoke.

	Before one cigarette	After one cigarette
PWV (m/s)	7.46 ± 1.11	8.05 ± 0.99[*]
HR (s^{-1})	72.5 ± 8.3	83.3 ± 8.2[*]
sBP (Hgmm)	124.9 ± 9.2	132.7 ± 9.7[*]

[*] $p < 0.01$.
[a] Accepted by Clinical Neuroscience. One part of the results has been accepted by the Hungarian Ideggyógyászati Szemle (Clin Neuroscience). The present form is with the permission of the journal mentioned above. Supported by ETT 407-04/2009.

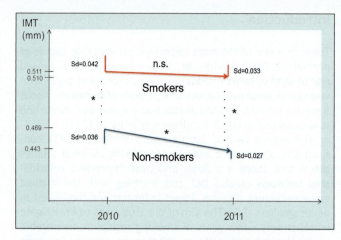

Figure 3 Changes in IMT after one year. No significant differences can be detected in smokers. In non-smokers it decreased significantly ($p = 0.0002$). n.s.: not significant; *$p < 0.05$.

after smoking one cigarette ($p < 0.01$) [Table 1], which was proven by the follow-up too.

Gender differences were also found in stiffness parameters. In our first study and also in the follow-up smoking males showed significantly faster PWV than smoking females ($p < 0.01$), while in case of augmentation index (Aix) we found the opposite ($p < 0.05$). This significance could only be seen in the smoking group.

Investigating the correlation between IMT and pulse wave velocity we found that there is a linear correlation between these two parameters [Fig. 2]. Each 0.1 unit increase in mean bilateral IMT results in a 0.64 m/s faster PWV ($p = 0.0025$). Adjusted to age, gender and smoking status this correlation disappears, which means that there is no cause-consequence relationship between IMT and PWV but if we know the IMT then we can estimate PWV.

Analysing the changes in IMT after one year we found that it remained unchanged in smokers and decreased significantly in non-smokers ($p = 0.0002$) [Fig. 3]. The changes of augmentation index showed similar results.

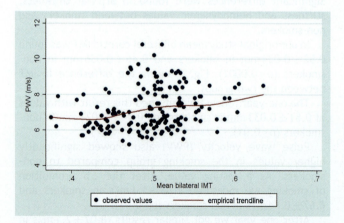

Figure 2 Linear correlation between mean bilateral IMT and PWV unadjusted to age, gender and smoking status. Each 0.1 unit increase in mean bilateral IMT results in a 0.64 m/s faster PWV ($p = 0.0025$). (Accepted by Clinical Neuroscience. One part of the results has been accepted by the Hungarian Ideggyógyászati Szemle (Clin Neuroscience). The present form is with the permission of the journal mentioned above. Supported by ETT 407-04/2009.)

Discussion

Carotid intima-media thickness (IMT), assessed by B-mode ultrasonography, is a sensitive marker for atherosclerosis and can indicate an accelerated disease process in an early stage. Being an independent predictor of stroke and cardiovascular events, IMT is valuable for clarifying CVD risk [4].

According to a 2008 study, subjects with carotid atherosclerosis have a 3-fold higher risk of ischemic stroke independent of other cardiovascular risk factors. Each increase of 1 standard deviation in carotid IMT increases the stroke risk by 43% [5].

The impact of smoking on carotid IMT is verified by several previous studies [6,7], which examined mainly subjects of middle or older age in contrast to our young groups.

Our results approve that only a few years of smoking can cause detectable morphological changes on arterial wall reflected by elevated IMT values in young smokers compared to non-smokers. Besides the wall thickening smoking has chronic effects on stiffness parameters, measured by arteriograph, resulting in faster PWV.

In addition to the long term consequences, several immediate responses are also detectable right after the inhalation of the smoke. Elevated heart rate and systolic blood pressure can be measured, and we also found an increase in PWV, which can be the result of the elevated hemodynamic values or the consequence of smoking directly. Further investigations are needed to clear this question.

According to our follow-up study one year regular smoking does not result in measurable morphological and stiffness changes in young smokers.

Regarding that smoking is a modifiable risk factor for cardio and cerebrovascular events, large forces have to be invested in the cessation of smoking and thus in the prevention of the diseases.

A recent study investigated the impact of smoking cessation on carotid atherosclerosis. According to their results quitting smoking is significantly associated with decreasing risk of the severity of carotid atherosclerosis and plaques [8].

Conclusion

Our results confirm the role of smoking in the progression of atherosclerotic processes and hemodynamic changes which can lead to severe cardio and cerebrovascular consequences and provide evidence for the importance of preventive strategies in young population.

Acknowledgements

The authors would like to thank all of the students participated in the study. We appreciate the help from lab assistance in selecting the candidates.

References

[1] Centers for Disease Control Prevention (CDC). CDC grand rounds: current opportunities in tobacco control. MMWR Morb Mortal Wkly Rep 2010;59:487—92.
[2] Baldassarre D, Castelnuovo S, Frigerio B, Amato M, Werba JP, De Jong A, et al. Effects of timing and extent of smoking, type of cigarettes, and concomitant risk factors on the association between smoking and subclinical atherosclerosis. Stroke 2009;40:1991—8.
[3] Liang LR, Wong ND, Shi P, Zhao LC, Wu LX, Xie GQ, et al. Cross-sectional and longitudinal association of cigarette smoking with carotid atherosclerosis in Chinese adults. Prev Med 2009;49:62—7.
[4] Aguilar-Shea AL, Gallardo-Mayo C, Garrido-Elustondo S, Calvo-Manuel E, Zamorano-Gómez JL. Carotid intima-media thickness as a screening tool in cardiovascular primary prevention. Eur J Clin Invest 2011;41:521—6.
[5] Li C, Engström G, Berglund G, Janzon L, Hedblad B. Incidence of ischemic stroke in relation to asymptomatic carotid artery atherosclerosis in subjects with normal blood pressure. A prospective cohort study. Cerebrovasc Dis 2008;26: 297—303.
[6] Van den Berkmortel FW, Smilde TJ, Wollersheim H, van Langen H, de Boo T, Thien T. Intima-media thickness of peripheral arteries in asymptomatic cigarette smokers. Atherosclerosis 2000;150:397—401.
[7] Fan AZ, Paul-Labrador M, Merz CN, Iribarren C, Dwyer JH. Smoking status and common carotid artery intima-medial thickness among middle-aged men and women based on ultrasound measurement: a cohort study. BMC Cardiovasc Disord 2006; 6:42.
[8] Jiang CQ, Xu L, Lam TH, Lin JM, Cheng KK, Thomas GN. Smoking cessation and carotid atherosclerosis: the Guangzhou Biobank Cohort Study—CVD. J Epidemiol Community Health 2010;64:1004—9.

Breath holding index and arterial stiffness in evaluation of stroke risk in diabetic patients

Iris Zavoreo, Vanja Bašić Kes, Lejla Ćorić, Vida Demarin*

University Department of Neurology, University Hospital Center Sestre Milosrdnice, Zagreb, Croatia

KEYWORDS
Arterial stiffness;
Breath holding index;
Diabetes mellitus

Summary

Background: The aim of the study was to evaluate correlation of breath holding index (BHI) as functional parameter for intracranial subclinical atherosclerotic changes — we have shown in our previous works and arterial stiffness (AS — functional parameter for extracranial subclinical atherosclerotic changes) in diabetic patients with well and poor controlled glucose blood values in correlation with healthy population.

Patients and methods: We included 60 volunteers divided into 3 aged standardized groups — healthy volunteers, patients with well controlled diabetes and patients with poor controlled diabetes. We excluded individuals with moderate and severe carotid stenosis.

Results: There was decreasing trend in BHI values and increasing trend in AS values in diabetic patients, especially with poor regulated blood glucose values ($r = -0.14$ and 1.42; $p < 0.05$).

Conclusion: These results show that decline in BHI as parameter for intracranial microvessel dysfunction is in good correlation with increase of AS as functional parameter of extracranial vascular aging in diabetic patients.

© 2012 Elsevier GmbH. All rights reserved.

Introduction

Stroke is the third most frequent cause of death worldwide and the most frequent cause of permanent disability. There are numerous risk factors for atherosclerosis and stroke, some of them can be modified and some of them not. A large proportion of patients who suffered stroke, either has or is later diagnosed with diabetes (16—24%). Patients with diabetes are at 1.5—3 times the risk of stroke compared with general population and associated mortality and morbidity is greater than in those without this underlying condition. Even patients with metabolic syndrome component have a 1.5-fold increased risk of stroke [1,2]. This is primarily due to increased proatherogenic risk factors — abnormal plasma lipid profiles, hypertension, and hyperglycemia. However, other pathological features associated with diabetes, such as insulin resistance and hyperinsulinemia, also lead to atherosclerotic changes in extracranial and intracranial vessels independently of glycemia or other attendant risk factors. This is particularly expressed in smaller cerebral vessels increasing the incidence of both — overt and silent lacunar infarctions. One of the modifiable risk factors is diabetes mellitus.

Generally, vascular complications of diabetes can be separated into microvascular (diabetic nephropathy, neuropathy and retinopathy) and macrovascular (coronary disease, cerebrovascular disease, peripheral artery disease) complications.

* Corresponding author at: Fellow of Croatian Academy of Sciences and Arts, Head of University Department of Neurology, Sestre Milosrdnice University Hospital, HR-10000, Zagreb, Vinogradska 29, Croatia. Tel.: +385 1 376 82 82; fax: +385 1 376 82 82.
E-mail address: vida.demarin@zg.t-com.hr (V. Demarin).

Atherosclerotic manifestations can be divided in early stages — endothelial dysfunction, increase in arterial stiffness, and increase of intima—media thickness. Later atherosclerotic of blood vessels stages can be recognized as atherosclerotic plaques which provide different grade of vessel lumen stenoses [3].

In addition to atheroma formation, there is a strong evidence of increased platelet adhesion, hypercoagulability, impaired nitric oxide generation and increased free radical formation as well as altered calcium regulation in diabetic patients.

Cerebral autoregulation is the ability to maintain constant cerebral blood flow despite changes in the cerebral perfusion pressure. Breath holding method was introduced in early 90s as reproducible, non-invasive screening method to study cerebral hemodynamic by means of Transcranial Doppler (TCD). It is accurate, specific and sensitive method for evaluation of cerebral vasoreactivity in comparison with other methods (functional magnetic resonance imaging — MR, positron emission tomography — PET, single photon emission computed tomography — SPECT). In our previous works we standardized breath holding index (BHI) values for different age and sex groups [3,4].

Recently pulse pressure amplification and arterial mechanics, most often explored as arterial stiffness (inversely related to arterial strain-measurement of arterial volume load and physiological answer of the body to increased pressure load expressed as pulse pressure) are named as those with greatest sensitivity for vascular event prediction [5—7].

E-tracking is new automatized software for evaluation of the vessel wall functions, it enables monitoring vessel wall biomechanical parameters and early detection of the subclinical extracranial vessel atherosclerotic changes [8,9].

The most efficient stroke management is primary and secondary prevention, optimal prevention would be to recognize atherosclerotic changes in their early subclinical stages. BHI would provide information about intracranial vessel function and arterial stiffness would provide information about extracranial arteries biomechanical characteristics. According to those findings we can recognize atherosclerosis in its subclinical stages and apply principles of primary and secondary prevention [10,11].

Patients and methods

We included 60 volunteers in our study, 20 healthy volunteers and 40 diabetic type 2 patients — 20 with well controlled serum glucose levels and 20 with poor controlled serum glucose levels. All subjects were fully informed about the study and they signed informed consent approved by the Hospital Ethic Committee.

We performed standard laboratory workup, blood pressure measurement, CT scan, Color Doppler and Power Doppler of the main head and neck vessels and Transcranial Doppler, as well as BHI and arterial stiffness (measured by means of e-Tracking software).

All ultrasound measurements were performed in supine position with head elevation of up 45° and side tilt of 30° to the right and to the left.

The TCD examination was performed by TCD DWL Multidop X4 instrument with 2 MHz hand-held pulsed wave Doppler probe. TCD was performed in supine position after 5 min bed rest. Probe was positioned over each transtemporal window, arteries of the Willis circle were insonated by standard protocol and mean blood flow values (MBFV) were recorded. Blood vessels of the vertebrobasilar system were insonated by standard protocol trough the suboccipital window with the same probe, in the sitting position.

Mean velocity of middle cerebral artery (MCA) was continuously monitored during the breath holding test. Baseline was defined as a continuous mean velocity value through 30 s after an initial 5 min resting period — V_{mean}. Subjects were asked to hold their breath for 30 s after normal inspiratory breath to exclude Vasalva maneuver. Subjects who could not hold their breath for 30 s, held their breath as long as they could and that time was taken for the calculations afterwards. MBFV of last 3 s of breath hold period were recorded and taken as V_{max}. This procedure was repeated after 2 min resting period and the mean value of both measurements was taken. For further analysis BHI was calculated as percentage increase in MBFV occurring during breath holding divided by the time (s) for which the subject hold his/her breath [12,13].

Technology of new software application enables calculating of functional indexes of the blood vessel walls during the examination. Aloka is one of the leading companies which developed such software for evaluating patient's vascular status and vascular age at bedside. Evaluation of extracranial blood vessels was performed by Color Doppler Flow Imaging (CDFI) and Power Doppler Imaging (PDI) method by Aloka 5500 Prosound, 7.5 MHz linear probe in a standardized manner (B, D and M mode, and/or combination). In this application we use two waves in order to collect data — pulse wave for Doppler (D mode) information and continuous ultrasonic wave (M mode). These two waves are independent because they are using different angle of insonation (M mode = 90°, D mode <60°). These two waves cross in the middle of the sample volume (angle modification −30° up to +30°), the sample volume is placed in the middle of the arterial lumen (at 1.5 cm in the common carotid artery proximally to the flow divider) and cursors for vessel wall motility monitoring are placed at the border of the tunica media and tunica adventitia at the far and near arterial wall (the first hyperechoic line is representing the border between the vessel lumen and IMT, the second one is representing the border between IMT and adventitia). This software also includes ECG monitoring in order to monitor vessel wall motility during cardiac cycle (systolic and diastolic changes). At the end of the measurement, vessel motility parameters appear in the form of report — arterial stiffness was taken as measure of vessel wall function (blood pressure logarithm/change of vessel wall diameter).

Statistical analysis of different groups of subjects was performed by Student's t test (statistical significance was obtained at $p < 0.05$ value). Variation coefficient was calculated for BHI values as a measure of data dispersion for each group. MBFV and BHI values were compared using Pearson's linear correlation coefficient.

Table 1 Patients data (values are presented as mean values and standard deviations).

	Mean age	Serum glucose levels (mmol/L)	AS	BHI
Controls	55 ± 12	4.63 ± 0.71	6.57 ± 1.14	1.56 ± 0.18
Well controlled diabetic patients	56 ± 11	5.25 ± 0.65	9.21 ± 0.8	1.34 ± 0.09
Poor controlled diabetic patients	58 ± 10	7.84 ± 1.61	12.15 ± 1.16	1.09 ± 0.08

Results

The aim of this study was to evaluate BHI and AS in healthy population in correlation with diabetic patients with good and poor regulated serum glucose levels, groups were aged standardized in order to minimize impact of age as risk factor for vascular aging.

Data did not show any statistically significant differences in BHI and AS values between the left and right side of Willis circle as well as for common carotid artery, and this distinction was excluded from the model. There was no difference in mean BHI and AS values between males and females therefore we presented pooled data — mean BHI and AS values and SD for each group (Table 1). In healthy volunteers all values remain in range between 1.03 and 1.65 — there is decreasing trend in BHI values and increasing trend of AS values depending on glucose control ($p < 0.05$) (Fig. 1).

There was increase in AS in correlation with glucose levels ($r = 1.42$, $p < 0.05$), there was no statistically significant differences between left and right side as well as the sex differences in evaluated model, therefore we presented pooled data. There was statistically significant negative correlation between BHI and serum glucose levels ($r = -0.14$, $p < 0.05$) in all groups, especially in group of diabetic patients with poorly controlled glucose levels.

Discussion

Results of the previous studies have shown that there is no statistically significant differences between BHI in anterior (anterior — ACA and middle cerebral artery — MCA) and posterior circulation (posterior — PCA, vertebral — VA and basilar — BA arteries) in individuals without atherosclerotic plaques on the main head and neck vessels, therefore we measured BHI in MCA. Also, in our previous studies we have standardized BHI measurement method and we have shown that BHI is linear index, therefore there is no difference between short (<27 s) and long (>27 s) measurement times [12—14].

Due to changes that are present as a part of a cardiovascular aging including small vessel pathomorphological changes — amyloid angiopathy, arteriolosclerosis, capillary endothelial and basement membrane changes (increasing of the vessel wall stiffness) we found normal decrease of BHI and increase of AS in healthy population (risk free) according to age and pathological changes of this parameters according to changed glucose metabolism [15]. This data are in correlation with previous studies IRAS (The Insulin Resistance Atherosclerosis Study) has shown that diabetes and glucose intolerance are independent risk factors connected with increase in intima—media thickness (IMT). SANDS trial (The Stop Atherosclerosis in Native Diabetics Study) have shown that reduction in other cerebrovascular risk factors (hypertension, hyperlipoproteinemia) can slower progression of IMT thickening in diabetic patients [16,17].

Previous studies as well as our results suggest that mechanical arterial properties (changes in BHI, AS as functional parameters) are affected first while hemodynamic remains preserved (mean velocities were unchanged due to cerebral autoregulation mechanisms which are preserved in healthy individuals). Our results suggesting that there is a good correlation of BHI as functional parameter which reflect functional state of the intracerebral blood vessels with arterial stiffness as functional parameter for extracranial blood vessels (CCA in our case) in population with diabetes mellitus [10,15—17].

Different pathophysiological mechanisms during the lifetime cause vessel wall aging and subclinical endothelial dysfunction which is the first stage of the atherosclerosis, subtle change of vessel wall before appearance of either vascular remodeling (diameter increase), intima—media thickening or plaque formation. This state is irreversible and it is early marker of atherosclerosis as well as systolic pressure increase and pulse pressure increase. Increased arterial stiffness and decrease in BHI values are normal in advanced age, but in younger individuals this changes are first signs of subclinical atherosclerosis, such individuals should be screened for cerebrovascular risk factors and followed up. In our case we have shown that glucose control is of great importance in diabetic patients in order to prevent vascular aging [3,7,11,15].

We have shown that diabetic patients are at increased risk for cerebrovascular disease, but further studies should be performed in order to evaluate impact of changes in AS and BHI on other clinical manifestations (cognitive decline, every day activities, etc.) in diabetic patients [18,19].

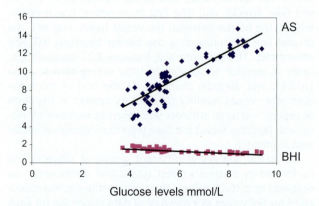

Fig. 1 Correlation between breath holding index and arterial stiffness according to different serum glucose values.

References

[1] Warlow C, Sudlow C, Dennis M, Wardlaw J, Sanderack P. Stroke. Lancet 2003;362:1211—24.

[2] Demarin V, Lovrenčić-Huzjan A, Trkanjec Z, Vuković V, Vargek-Solter V, Šerić V, et al. Recommendations for stroke management 2006 update. Acta Clin Croat 2006;45: 219—85.

[3] Spence JD. New approaches to atherosclerosis based on endothelial function. In: U: Fisher M, Bogousslavsky J, editors. Current review of cerebrovascular disease. Philadelphia: Current Medicine Inc.; 2001. p. 1—14.

[4] Aleksandrov AV. Imaging cerebrovascular disease with ultrasound. Cerebrovasc Dis 2003;16:1—3.

[5] Howard G, Sharrett AR, Heiss G, Evans GW, Chambless LE, Riley WA, et al. Carotid intimal-medial thickness distribution in general populations as evaluated by B-mode ultrasound. ARIC Investigators. Stroke 1993;24:1297—304.

[6] Iglesias del Sol A, Moons KGM, Hollander M, Hofman A, Koustaal PJ, Diederick. Is carotid intima—media thickness useful in cardiovascular disease risk assessment? The Rotterdam study. Stroke 2001;32:1532—8.

[7] Sugioka K, Hozumi T, Sciacca RR, Miyake Y, Titova I, Gaspard G, et al. Impact of aortic stiffness on ischemic stroke in elderly patients. Stroke 2002;33(8):2077—81.

[8] Van Bortel LM, Duprez D, Starmans-Kool MJ, Safar ME, Giannattasio C, Cockcroft J, et al. Clinical applications of arterial stiffness, task force. III. Recommendations for user procedures. AJH 2002;15:445—52.

[9] Niki K, Sugawara M, Chang D, Harada A, Okada T, Sakai R, et al. A new noninasive measurement system for wave intensity: evaluation of carotid arterial wave intensity and reproducibility. Heart Vessels 2000;17:12—21.

[10] Jurasic M-J, Lovrencic-Huzajn A, Roje Bedekovic M, Demarin V. How to monitor vascular aging with ultrasound. J Neurol Sci 2007;257:139—42.

[11] Zavoreo I, Demarin V. Breath Holding Index and arterial stiffness as markers of vascular aging. Curr Aging Sci 2010;3(1):67—70.

[12] Markus HS, Harrison MJG. Estimation of cerebrovascular reactivity using transcranial Doppler, including the use of breath-holding as the vasodilatory stimulus. Stroke 1992;23:668—73.

[13] Zavoreo I, Demarin V. Breath holding indexes in evaluation of cerebral vasoreactivity. Acta Clin Croat 2004;43:15—9.

[14] Gur AY, Bornstein NM. Cerebral vasomotor reactivity of the posterior circulation in patients with carotid occlusive disease. Eur J Neurol 2003;10(1):75—8.

[15] Rajala U, Laakso M, Paivansalo M, PelkonenO, Suramo I, Keinanen-Kiukaanniemi S. Associations of blood pressure with carotid intima—media thickness in elderly Finns with diabetes mellitus or impaired glucose tolerance. J Hum Hypertens 2003;17(10):705—11.

[16] Festa A, D'Agostino Jr R, Tracy RP, Haffner SM. The insulin resistance atherosclerosis study. Circulation 2000;102:42—7.

[17] Evans EL, Ojhita RP, Fischbach LA. Oral hypoglycemic use and the SANDS Trial. JAMA 2008;300(4):389—92.

[18] Demarin V, Bašić Kes V, Morović S, Zavoreo I. Neurosonology: a means of evaluating normal aging versus dementia. Aging Health 2008;4(5):529—34.

[19] Zavoreo I, Kes VB, Morović S, Šerić V, Demarin V. Breath holding index in detection of early cognitive decline. J Neurol Sci 2010;299(December (1—2)):116—9.

Intima-media thickness of the carotid artery in OSAS patients

Silvia Andonova[a,*], Diana Petkova[b], Yana Bocheva[c]

[a] Second Clinic of Neurology, St. Marina University Hospital, Varna, Bulgaria
[b] Clinic of Pneumology and Physiology, St. Marina University Hospital, Varna, Bulgaria
[c] Central Clinical Laboratory, St. Marina University Hospital, Varna, Bulgaria

KEYWORDS
Duplex scanning;
Intima-media thickness;
Obstructive sleep apnea

Summary

Aim: Evaluate the change of intima-media thickness of the carotid artery in patients suffering from obstructive sleep apnea (OSAS).
Materials and methods: The participants of the study were divided into 2 groups: 27 patients suffering from OSAS and a control group of 27 participants (mean age 56.1 ± 1.4 years), having risk factors (RF) for cerebrovascular diseases (CVD) but not OSAS. The morphology of the artery wall — the thickness of the intima media complex (IMT) of the common carotid arteries (CCA), the presence of atherosclerotic plaques, their magnitude, echogenicity and stability were determined with color-coded duplex sonography of the main arteries of the head.
Results: In the OSAS group, CCA-IMT was significantly increased when compared with the non-OSAS patients with RF for CVD, which correlated with the night hypoxemia level. Additionally, the formation of plaques was more pronounced and carotid stenoses were more common in the OSAS patients.
Discussion: These findings are in favor of an independent influence of obstructive sleep apnea on carotid artery atherosclerosis.
© 2012 Elsevier GmbH. All rights reserved.

Introduction

Some present studies show that OSAS is associated with a high risk of cardiovascular and cerebrovascular diseases, because of the high frequency of the risk factors for their appearance [12,13,16]. Epidemiological data say that patients with OSAS often are overweight and have arterial hypertension, they usually smoke and are involved in alcohol abuse [7]. Apneic episodes can induce cardiovascular, hemodynamic and hemorrhagic changes, which are potential promoters for stroke incidence in patients with RF for CVD [4,9]. Experimental studies show that the oxygen desaturation that accompanies the apneic episodes can lead to generative changes of the artery wall [2]. That fact presupposes a connection between OSAS and the progression of the atherosclerotic cerebrovascular disease [10,11], whose early marker is the thickening of the intima media complex of the carotid arteries [6,8].

Some studies show changes of the IMT in patients with OSAS [7]. Some of them find a connection between the level of the night hypoxemia, which is connected to the severity

* Corresponding author at: Department of Neurology, Second Clinic of Neurology with Intensive Care Unit, *St. Marina* University Hospital, 1 *Hristo Smirnenski* St., Varna 9010, Bulgaria.
Tel.: +359 52 978 236.
E-mail address: drsilva@abv.bg (S. Andonova).

of OSAS, and the atherosclerotic changes of the cerebral vessels [14,15].

The aim of this study was to measure the IMT of patients with OSAS, which has been polysomnographically proven. We wanted to compare their results to the IMT of patients with risk factors for CVD, but having no OSAS.

Materials and methods

The patients with OSAS of this study were examined in the center for sleep medicine and noninvasive ventilation, part of the Clinic of Pneumology and Physiology in the St. Marina University Hospital — Varna, using diagnostic polysomnography. Before the examination all the patients were interviewed for having sleep disorder related symptoms — snoring, short stops of breathing, daily sleepiness. Their anthropometric characteristics and co-morbidity were also described.

The diagnostic algorithm consisted of: questioning card for patients with risk for stroke (consensus for primary prevention of ischemic stroke, 2008), detailed somatic and neurologic status, routine laboratory tests — serum glucose — mmol/1, total cholesterol — mmol/1 (enzyme colorimetric determination), triglyceride mmol/l (enzyme determination), HDL — mmol/1 (immune inhibition method), LDL — mmol/1 (Friedewald formula). An electrocardiogram and color-coded duplex sonography of the main arteries of the head were performed for each patient.

The following RF for CVD were considered: non changeable (age and sex) and some changeable — arterial hypertension (AH), diabetes mellitus (DM), dyslipidemia (DL), rhythmic and conductive heart disorders (RCD), overweight. Patients with central or mixed sleep apnea, who have survived myocardial infarction or a stroke, were excluded from the study. For all the patients from the control group the systolic (SAP) and the diastolic (DAP) arterial pressure were taken using the cuff method, while the usual therapy was not stopped. The duration, the severity and the medication of AH were mentioned additionally. The antidiabetic and hypolipidemic drugs taken by the patients were also mentioned.

On the day of the examination, we measured the height (m), using a wall height meter, the body weight (kg) — with calibrated scales — of every patient and we calculated the body mass index (BMI) (kg/m^2) using a standard formula.

Using the WHO criteria [1997], the patients were classified according to their BMI in the following groups: normal weight — BMI 18.5—24.9; overweight — BMI > 25; obese — BMI > 30, extremely obese — BMI > 40 (obesity IV gravity by Bray).

Sleep examination

The sleep analysis included overnight polysomnography, which documented the sleep disturbances and severity of the OSAS according standard criteria [1]. The investigation was performed with MEPAL (MAP, Medizin — Technologie, Martinsried, Germany) monitoring system. According to the known diagnostic standards, the minimal time for examination was 6 h. For the documentation of the sleep, we used standard 16—18 channel polysomnography, including electroencephalogram (C3—A2, C4—A1, O1—A2, O2—A1), electro-oculograms, electromyograms (EMG) of the left/right extremity, electrocardiogram (ECG), heart rate, nasal and oral air flow, thoracic and abdominal movements, registration of snoring, position of the body, pulseoxymetry-monitored oxygen saturation (SaO$_2$) and a polysomnography with video-watching. The sleep phases and arousals were analyzed in conformity with Rechtschaffen and Kales' criteria [14]. All the results were analyzed manually. The breathing was registered by nasal cannulas and combined respiratory inductive plethysmography, which uses composed signal and a thermistor. Apneas and hypopneas were evaluated in accordance with the accepted international criteria [1]. The apnea index (AI) was defined as the number of apneas per hour sleep while hypopnea index (HI) — the number of hypopneas per 1 h sleep. The apnea/hypopnea index (AHI), combined the number of apnea and hypopnea per 1 h sleep. The index of desaturation was defined as episodes of O$_2$ desaturation >3% per hour sleep compared to a stable basic value. The severity of the sleep apnea was graded as: mild, with AHI 5—15 episodes of apnea and hypopnea per hour of sleep; moderate, with AHI 16—30 episodes of apnea and hypopnea per hour of sleep and severe, AHI more than 30 episodes of apnea and hypopnea per hour of sleep.

Neurosonographic examination

The main arteries of the head were examined with color-coded duplex sonography using a 7.5 MHz transducer on Sonix SP (Canada). Real time B-mode imaging was used to measure the thickness of the intima media complex (IMT) of the carotid arteries (mm) with a standard method, using a program for automatic value averaging [2,5,17,18]. The rate of the stenosis was determined with the morphologic method in longitudinal and transversal slice of the examining vessel. They were categorized as: no observable stenosis (1—24%), low grade stenosis (25—49%), moderate stenosis (50—74%), high grade stenosis (75—99%) and thrombosis (100%) [3]. According to their structure the plaques were determined as homogeneous, heterogeneous, mixed and calcified. Their surfaces were evaluated as smooth (regular), rugged (irregular) or having cavities (more than 2 mm concaves and ulcers). Clinically, the plaques were characterized as stable (homogeneous, smooth and fibrous cover) and non-stable (heterogeneous, with inner hemorrhages and cholesterol spots) [1].

Results

Clinical characteristic

The anthropometric, clinical and laboratory examinations of the two groups of patients with OSAS and RF for CVD, and without OSAS are shown in Table 1.

There was no significant difference between the anthropometric parameters and the accompanying cardiovascular and metabolic diseases of the two patient groups. The patients were between 50 and 60 years of age, and all except 1 were overweight males. More than 66% of them suffered from arterial hypertension. In both groups there were more

Table 1 Clinical characteristics.

Parameters	With OSAS (n = 27)	Without OSAS (n = 27)
Age (years)	55.7 ± 1.4 (52–58)	56.1 ± 1.4 (53–59)
Men:women	26/1	26/1
BMI kg m^{-2}	31.9 ± 0.6 (29–34)	29.3 ± 0.5 (28–33)
Arterial hypertension		
% from all patients	69	60
SBP (mm Hg)	136 ± 4 (131–142)	132 ± 4 (127–138)
DBP (mm Hg)	81 ± 3 (78–84)	80 ± 2 (77–83)
treatment (%)	51	44
Cardiac disease (%)	19	23
Smoking (%)	37	60
Years	14.4 ± 3.9 (5.3–22.6)	17.0 ± 3.3 (10.2–26.6)
Diabetes mellitus (%)	20	37
HbA1c %	6.2 ± 0.2 (5.7–6.7)	6.1 ± 0.2 (5.7–6.4)
Treatment (%)	14	26
Hypercholesterolemia (%)	69	52
Total cholesterol (mmol/l)	5.27 ± 1.6	5.16 ± 1.06
LDL (mmol/1)	2.71 ± 0.3	2.60 ± 0.3
HDL (mmol/1)	1.54 ± 0.5	1.56 ± 0.1

SBP, systolic blood pressure; DBP, diastolic blood pressure.

smokers with dyslipidemia, the diabetics were more in the group with no OSAS.

According to the polysomnography analysis, the patients were informed of the disorder findings and the necessity of starting training for ventilation with CPAP (Continuous Positive Airway Pressure)/BiPAP (Bi-Level Positive Airway Pressure)/VPAP (Variable Positive Airway Pressure), so as they could continue with it at home. The mean AHI of the OSAS group was 60.8 ± 36.9 per hour sleep, which corresponds to heavy sleep apnea, the mean oxygen saturation SaO$_2$% was 88.8 ± 6.4, the minimum oxygen saturation — 64.9 ± 14.4 and the index of desaturation — 68.63 ± 32.61.

Neurosonographic examination

The frequency of the atherosclerotic plaques and the mean values of IMT of the common carotid arteries in patients with OSAS were significantly higher compared to the control group (Table 2). There was a correlation between AHI and IMT: the thickening of the IMT in patients with OSAS correlated with the higher AHI ($r = +0.43$, $p < 0.05$) (see Table 3).

Discussion

The study established the same frequency of RF for CVD in both groups, but a greater thickening of IMT of the common carotid artery of the OSAS patients compared to the control group. In the OSAS patients, a significant correlation between the thickening of IMT of the common carotid artery and the severity of the apnea was observed, which corresponded to other authors' conclusions [3,14]. It has been shown that the chronic intermittent hypoxemia is one of the basic factors for atherosclerosis in patients with

Table 2 Sonographic parameters.

Parameters	With OSAS (n = 27)	Without OSAS (n = 27)	p
IMT (mm) left CCA	1.04 ± 0.04 (0.93–1.13)	0.80 ± 0.02 (0.74–0.85)	<0.01
Right CCA	1.03 ± 0.04 (0.92–1.10)	0.79 ± 0.02 (0.74–0.85)	<0.01
Both CCA	1.04 ± 0.04 (0.93–1.12)	0.79 ± 0.02 (0.74–0.85)	<0.01
Plaques Degree of stenosis	Patients n		p
	With OSAS	Without OSAS	
<29%	4	1	<0.05
30–49%	8	5	<0.01
50–74%	3	2	—
75–99%	1	—	—
Total number	59%	30%	<0.05

Table 3 IMT in patients with OSAS in relation to apnea severity.

Apnea severity	Mild AHI episodes/h 5—15	Moderate AHI episodes/h 16—30	Severe AHI episodes/h 30
IMT (mm) left CCA	0.98 ± 0.08 (0.85—1.09)	1.01 ± 0.01 (0.90—1.10)	1.04 ± 0.04 (0.93—1.13)
Right CCA	0.95 ± 0.11 (0.82—1.05)	0.98 ± 0.03 (0.88—1.07)	1.03 ± 0.04 (0.92—1.10)*
Both CCA	0.97 ± 0.10 (0.83—1.07)	1.00 ± 0.02 (0.89—1.08)	1.04 ± 0.04 (0.93—1.12)*

* $p < 0 = 05$ — significant differences between groups.

OSAS [11,15]. In those patients high serum levels of catecholamines, high oxidative stress [7,14], high levels of serum inflammatory markers such as C-reactive protein and cytokines [11], high platelet aggregation and plasma fibrinogen [7] were established. Compared to the controls, patients with OSAS had higher frequency of atherosclerotic plaques and high grade stenosis. This fact should be examined in a bigger group of patients in a future study.

As a conclusion, in OSAS patients a significant thickening of IMT of the common carotid artery was observed, which correlated to the level of the night hypoxemia. That supports the thesis of the role of obstructive sleep apnea as an independent risk factor for CVD.

References

[1] American academy of sleep medicine, sleep related breathing disorders in adults, recommendations for syndrome definition techniques in clinical research. The report of an American academy of sleep medicine task force. Sleep 1999;22: 667—89.

[2] Adaikkappan M, Sampath R, Felix AJW, Sethupathy S. Evaluation of carotid atherosclerosis by B'Mode ultrasonographic study in hypertensive patients compared with normotensive patients. Journal of Radiology and Imaging 2002;12:365—8.

[3] Aminbakhsh A, Mancini GB. Carotid intima-media thickness measurements: what defines an abnormality? A systematic review. Clinical and Investigative Medicine 1999;22:149—57.

[4] Bassetti C, Aldrich MS, Chervin RD, Quint D. Sleep apnea in patients with transient ischemic attack and stroke: a prospective study of 59 patients. Neurology 1996;47:1167—73.

[5] Bots ML, Mulder PG, Van Es GA. Reproducibility of carotid vessel wall thickness measurements: the Rotterdam Study. Journal of Clinical Epidemiology 1994;47:921—30.

[6] Baldassare D, Werba JP, Tremoli E. Common carotid intima-media thickness measurement. A method to improve accuracy and precision. Stroke 1994;25:1588—92.

[7] Dzau VJ. Atherosclerosis and hypertension: mechanisms and interrelationships. Journal of Cardiovascular Pharmacology 1990;15:559—72.

[8] Gainer JL. Hypoxia and atherosclerosis: re-evaluation of an old hypothesis. Atherosclerosis 1987;68:263—6.

[9] Hadjiev D, Lehner H, Jancheva St, Stamenova P, Velcheva I, Manchev I, et al.Stroke. 2001.

[10] Heistad DD. Armstrong. Sick vessel syndrome: recovery of atherosclerotic and hypertensive vessel. Hypertension 1995;26:509—21.

[11] Kiely JL, McNicholas WT. Cardiovascular risk factors in patients with obstructive sleep apnoea syndrome. European Respiratory Journal 2000;16:128—33.

[12] Mohsenin V. Sleep-related breathing disorders and risk of stroke. Stroke 2001;32:1271—8.

[13] Palomaki H. Snoring and the risk of ischemic brain infarction. Stroke 1999;22:1021—5.

[14] Rechtschaffen A, Kales A. A manual of standardized terminology, technique and scoring system for sleep stages of human subjects. Washington, DC: National Institutes of Health; 1968. p. 204.

[15] Titianova E, Stamenova P, Girov K, Petrov I, Velcheva I, Grozdinski L, et al.National consensus of ultrasonographic diagnostic and treatment of extracranial carotid pathology. 2011.

[16] Titianova E, Velcheva I, Karakaneva S, Dimitrov D, Hristova K, Damianov D, et al. Carotid pathology and risk factors for cerebrovasculare disease: clinic, neurosonographic and echocardiographic studies. Neurosonography and Cerebral Haemodynamics 2007;3:77—84.

[17] Titianova E.Ultrasonographic diagnostic in neurology. 2006.

[18] Veller MG. Measurement of the ultrasonic intima-media complex thickness in normal subjects. Journal of Vascular Surgery 1993;17:719—25.

The association of carotid intima-media thickness (cIMT) and stroke: A cross sectional study

Salim Harris

Neurovascular and Neurosonology Division, Neurology Department, Medical Faculty, University of Indonesia, Indonesia

KEYWORDS
cIMT;
Stroke;
Duplex

Summary

Objective: To examine the carotid vessels in stroke and non stroke patients using carotid duplex ultrasonography.

Methods: The author used a cross-sectional approach among 259 patients who were divided into 2 groups: stroke and non-stroke patients. Noninvasive measurements of the intima and media of the common carotid artery were performed with high-resolution ultrasonography to all the patients in both groups.

Results: 259 patients, with age ranging from 31 to 75 years old, were divided into the Stroke group (n = 131) and Non-Stroke group (n = 128). The author found abnormal IMT in both groups, with an occurrence of 130 patients in the Stroke group, and 46 in the Non-Stroke group (P < 0.001).

Conclusion: Increased intima and media thickness of the common carotid artery, measured noninvasively by ultrasonography, are associated with cerebrovascular disease manifested as stroke.

© 2012 Elsevier GmbH. All rights reserved.

Introduction

Stroke is a cerebrovascular disease that results as an impact of chronic diseases that induce pathological changes on the cerebral vessels. Ischemic stroke is the most common type of stroke with a prevalence rate of 85%. Ischemic stroke pathophysiology can be acute such as occlusion by emboli or chronic secondary to atherosclerosis. The early stage of atherosclerosis is vessel injury induced by multiple conditions that directly or indirectly injure the vessels. Hypertension is the most common cause of vessel injury.

Hypertension or high blood pressure is a major risk factor in stroke. It has a stepping gradient in inducing vessel damage that lead to the vessels becoming stiff. In the process of hypertension-induced atherosclerosis, blood vessels become smaller in size, rigid and lose compliance. Elevated blood pressure increases blood flow through the vessels. This induces shear stress elevation that leads to an increase in endothelial-derived relaxing factor (EDRF) production from endothelial cells. This includes nitric oxide, prostaglandin E and prostacyclin. These vasomotor activators induce the superoxide production and reduce the vessels permeability. The endothelial cells in the process of injury will release increased amounts of pro-inflammatory cytokines that will activate the leukocyte. This further induces the elevation of vaso-active substances such as prostacycline and nitric oxide which eventually induce complete endothelial injury.

The increase in intravascular pressure induces stress on the vessel wall in hypertension. This alters the vessel wall thickness through a process called vascular remodeling. Vascular remodeling as a response to high blood pressure leads to the reduction of the diameter of the blood vessel through

E-mail address: dr_salimharris@yahoo.co.id

hypertrophy (hypertrophic outer remodeling or hypertrophic inner remodeling) or through a eutrophic inner remodeling process.

Change in the common-carotid-artery intima—media thickness is believed to be an indicator of generalized atherosclerosis. It has also been adopted as an intermediate end point for determining cardiovascular morbidity and also as a surrogate end point to evaluate the success of lipid lowering drug interventions [4,5]. High-resolution carotid ultrasonography has been used to obtain measurements of the thickness of the tunica intima and media of the carotid arteries. Studies in the western countries have shown not only cross-sectional correlations but also prospective correlations between common-carotid-artery intima—media thickness and the prevalence of cardiovascular and cerebrovascular disease [1—3]. There are still few studies showing an association between increased carotid-artery intima—media thickness and stroke in Asia, especially in Indonesia. In this study, we investigated the hypothesis that carotid-artery intima—media thickness is directly correlated with the incidence of stroke.

Methodology

Subjects and study design

The study subjects were patients in the Cipto Mangunkusumo National Hospital, Jakarta, Indonesia with age ranging from 31 to 75 years old. The patients were categorized into 2 groups, stroke and non stroke groups. There were 131 patients in the stroke group and 128 patients in the non-stroke group. The carotid arteries of all patients were evaluated using high-resolution B-mode ultrasonography using a cross-sectional methodology. One longitudinal image of the common carotid artery was acquired. Measurements were made by readers blinded to all clinical information. The maximal rather than the mean intima—media thickness was used as the key variable in determining the correlation between intima—media thickness and stroke. The maximal intima—media thickness of the common carotid artery is defined as the mean of the maximal intima—media thickness of the near and far wall on both the left and right sides. The intima—media thickness was called abnormal if the thickness was more than 1 mm.

Statistical analysis

Statistical analysis was performed using the software package SPSS for Windows 18.0. Association of the variables was tested using Chi-square statistics. χ^2 statistics and independent t-test were used when appropriate to determine significance of difference among background variables compared.

Results

The base-line characteristics of the 259 patients are given in Table 1.

Other risk factors such as smoking and hypertension were analyzed to rule out the bias in determining the

Table 1 Characteristics of the patients.

Characteristics	Stroke group ($n=131$)	Non-stroke group ($n=128$)
Mean age, y (SD)	58.17 (9.88)	55.15 (11.31)
Male sex (%)	98 (37.84%)	83 (32.04%)
Female sex (%)	33 (12.74%)	45 (17.37%)
Hypertension (%)	88 (33.97%)	72 (27.80%)
Type-2 Diabetes (%)	43 (16.60%)	42 (16.21%)
Dyslipidemia (%)	44 (16.98%)	40 (15.44%)
Smoking (%)	44 (16.98%)	34 (13.12%)

A total of 259 patients (78 women and 181 men) were included in our study. The study population was divided into two groups: stroke patients ($n=131$) and non-stroke patients ($n=128$). The total mean age was 56.65 (10.70) years. Mean age was 58.17 (9.88) years old in the stroke group and 55.15 (11.31) years old in the non-stroke group. There was no statistical difference among the characteristics of the population across both groups, according to sex, hypertension, type 2 diabetes melitus, dyslipidemia and smoking history.

Table 2 The association between IMT and other risk factors with stroke.

Risk factor	Stroke	Non-stroke	P
Hypertension	88	72	0.07
Type-2 Diabetes	43	42	0.99
Dyslipidemia	44	40	0.68
Smoking	44	34	0.22
IMT	97	75	0.008

correlation between IMT and stroke. Using chi-square test for statistical analysis, we found there were no statistical difference between both group according to hypertension and smoking. We can therefore conclude that the correlation of IMT and stroke were statistically significant ($P=0.008$) (Table 2).

Discussion

Many journals have previously reported on the positive correlation between cardiovascular risk factors and carotid artery intima—media thickness, and the positive correlation between carotid-artery intima—media thickness and the incidence of myocardial infarction and stroke amongst Caucasian people [6,7]. This study shows the strong association of the intima—media thickness and stroke ($P=0.008$) in the Indonesian population. This direct correlation exists because intima—media thickness is a marker of generalized atherosclerosis. This pathologic vascular phenomenon plays an important role in the pathogenesis of cerebro and cardiovascular events such as stroke, and explains the association between IMT and stroke [9,10].

Five other studies have previously explored the possible correlation between carotid-artery intima—media thickness and the incidence of cardiovascular events. Three of these studies reported results using measurements of the common carotid artery. Salonen and Salonen, in a study of 1257 middle-aged Finnish men, observed an association between common carotid-artery intima—media thickness and cardiac events. This observation was based on a one-year follow-up and a total of 24 events. The Rotterdam Elderly Study was a single-center, prospective study of disease and disability in the elderly involving 7983 subjects 55 years of age or older. They performed a case-control study in a subgroup of their population that showed an association between common-carotid-artery intima—media thickness and the risk of myocardial infarction and stroke [6—8].

The differences between their study and this study may be explained by the race of population sample, limited number of subjects and the methodology in our study. Moreover, our results extend their findings by showing that common-carotid-artery intima—media thickness has a strong correlation with the incidence of stroke. This implies that common carotid artery intima media thickness may be used as the predictor of cerebrovascular events. This study has a few other limitations. The small number of participants, limited data about the characteristics of the patients, and methodology (retrospective), are some of the weaknesses of this study. However, our study can be used as a pilot research in determining the correlation of intima—media thickness and stroke among Asian people especially in the Indonesian population.

References

[1] Touboul J, Labrouche J, Vicaut E, Amarenco P. Carotid intima—media thickness, plaques, and Framingham Risk Score as independent determinants of stroke risk. Stroke 2005;36:1741.

[2] Kitamuro A, Iso H, Imano H, Ohira T. Carotid intima—media thickness and plaque characteristics as a risk factor for stroke in Japanese elderly men. Stroke 2004;35:2788.

[3] Hollander M, Hak AE, Koudstaal PJ, Bots ML, Grobbee DE, Hofman A, et al. Comparison between measures of atherosclerosis and risk of stroke: the Rotterdam Study. Stroke 2003;34:2367—72.

[4] Hunt KJ, Evans GW, Folsom AR, Sharrett AR, Chambless LE, Tegeler CH, et al. Acoustic shadowing on B-mode ultrasound of the carotid artery predicts ischemic stroke: the Atherosclerosis Risk in Communities (ARIC) Study. Stroke 2001;32:1120—6.

[5] Chambless LE, Folsom AR, Clegg LX, Sharrett AR, Shahar E, Nieto FJ, et al. Carotid wall thickness is predictive of incident clinical stroke: the Atherosclerosis Risk in Communities (ARIC) Study. Am J Epidemiol 2000;151:478—87.

[6] O'Leary D, Polak J, Kronmal R, Manolio T, Burke J. Carotid-artery intima and media thickness as a risk factor for myocardial infarction and stroke in older adults. N Engl J Med 1999;340:14—22.

[7] Petty GW, Brown Jr RD, Whisnant JP, Sicks JD, O'Fallon WM, Wiebers DO. Ischemic stroke subtypes: a population-based study of incidence and risk factors. Stroke 1999;30:2513—6.

[8] Bots ML, Hoes AW, Koudstaal PJ, Hofman A, Grobbee DE. Common carotid intima—media thickness and risk of stroke and myocardial infarction: the Rotterdam Study. Circulation 1997;96:1432—7.

[9] Bots ML, Hofman A, Grobbee DE. Increased common carotid intima—media thickness. Adaptive response or a reflection of atherosclerosis? Findings from the Rotterdam Study. Stroke 1997;28:2442—7.

[10] Handa N, Matsumoto M, Maeda H, Hougaku H, Kamada T. Ischemic stroke events and carotid atherosclerosis. Results of the Osaka Follow-up Study for Ultrasonographic Assessment of Carotid Atherosclerosis (the OSACA Study). Stroke 1995;26:1781—6.

Carotid atherosclerosis: Socio-demographic issues, the hidden dimensions

Foad Abd-Allah [a,*], Noha Abo-Krysha [a], Essam Baligh [b]

[a] Department of Neurology, Cairo University, Cairo, Egypt
[b] Department of Cardiovascular Medicine, Cairo University, Cairo, Egypt

KEYWORDS
Carotid atherosclerosis;
Egyptian population;
Socio-demographic

Summary

Background and purpose: The effect of conventional vascular risk factors on carotid atherosclerosis had been reported in many studies. Little is known about social and demographic issues on the development of carotid artery disease among different populations. The aim of our study is to demonstrate the prevalence of carotid atherosclerosis among Egyptians and its difference in relations to other studies from industrialized countries.

Methods: We analyzed the data of 4733 Egyptian subjects who underwent extracranial carotid duplex scanning at the vascular laboratories of the largest tertiary referral hospital in Cairo from January 2003 to January 2008. Demographic and clinical data were correlated with ultrasound findings.

Results: Atherosclerotic carotid artery disease was present in 41% of the study population, significant and high grade disease detected in 2.5% of the study populations. Multivariate stepwise logistic regression analysis selected age, hypertension and diabetes mellitus and dyslipidemia as independent predictors of the presence of carotid atherosclerotic disease.

Conclusion: Hemodynamically significant extracranial atherosclerotic carotid disease is rare in Egyptians. Risk factors for carotid atherosclerosis are the same as in societies where carotid disease is more prevalent.
© 2012 Elsevier GmbH. All rights reserved.

Introduction

Atherosclerosis is a major cause of ischemic stroke and a significant proportion of strokes are thromboembolic in nature, arising from atherosclerotic plaques [1]. Several studies have reported racial differences in the severity and distribution of carotid atherosclerosis [2]. In the United States and Western communities, extracranial carotid artery disease was estimated to be responsible for 20—30% of strokes [3,4]. Little is known about the prevalence and distribution of carotid disease among the populations in the developing countries. This hampers preventive measures and promoted us to analyze extra cranial carotid duplex scans of a large sample of Egyptians.

Aim of the study

This study aims to reveal the effect of social, demographic and geographical factors on the prevalence of carotid atherosclerosis among Egyptians.

* Corresponding author at: Department of Neurology, Cairo University Hospitals, Manial, 11562 Cairo, Egypt. Tel.: +20 110110898; fax: +20 235692363.
E-mail address: foadneuro@hotmail.com (F. Abd-Allah).

2211-968X/$ — see front matter © 2012 Elsevier GmbH. All rights reserved.
doi:10.1016/j.permed.2012.02.054

Materials and methods

We conducted a retrospective study to analyze the clinical and duplex ultrasound data of 4733 subjects who underwent carotid artery duplex scans in the vascular laboratories of Cairo University Hospitals from January 1st, 2003, to January 1st, 2008. Cairo University Hospitals are the largest tertiary care center in Egypt. The following data were collected from each individual prior to ultrasound examination:

Cardiovascular risk factors: Age, Sex, Smoking, Hypertension, Diabetes Mellitus, Dyslipidemia and Obesity.

Clinical presentation: Subjects were classified into two groups

(1) Symptomatic group: 758 (39.1%) with stroke or transient ischemic attacks.
(2) Asymptomatic group: 1182 (60.9%) subjects. The causes of referral were routine check up or prior to coronary by pass graft.

Carotid duplex scan

Carotid duplex scanning was performed by qualified vascular operators using Siemens Elegra and Philips HDI 5000 machine. A high-frequency (7–10 MHz) linear array transducer was employed to scan the carotid from the most proximal common carotid artery (CCA) to the internal carotid artery (ICA) as far as the mandible permitted. We used the examination protocol and interpretation according to the criteria published by Society of Radiologists in Ultrasound 2003 [5].

Statistical analysis

Data were described as mean ± standard deviation (SD), range, frequencies (number of cases) and relative frequencies (percentages). Comparative statistics were performed with Student's t test, Mann–Whitney U or χ^2 test as appropriate. Multivariate regression analysis was performed to detect independent predictors of carotid atherosclerosis and carotid stenosis. A probability value (p value) less than 0.05 was considered statistically significant. All statistical calculations were performed using Microsoft Excel version 7 and SPSS version 15 for MS windows (Statistical Package for the Social Science, SPSS Inc., Chicago, IL, USA).

Results

We studied a total of 4733 subjects (3422 men, 1311 women; mean age 55.96 ± 12.3 years; range 32–79). The carotid duplex findings were classified as normal, atherosclerotic or non atherosclerotic disease. Atherosclerotic carotid disease was present in 1940 subjects (41%) of the study populations (Table 1). Multivariate stepwise logistic regression analysis showed that age (odds ratio, OR 1.079, p value < 0.001), diabetes (OR 2.019, p value < 0.001), hypertension (OR 1.541, p value < 0.001), smoking (OR 1.835, p value < 0.001) and dyslipidemia (OR 2.073, p value < 0.001) were independent predictors of the presence of carotid atherosclerotic disease. Obesity Showed marginal significance but OR was less than one (OR 0.800, p value 0.037). The degree of atherosclerotic carotid artery disease was categorized as intimal thickening only, <50% stenosis, stenosis from 50 to 69%, stenosis ≥70% and occlusion. High grade stenosis ≥50% representing 2.5% of our study populations (Table 2).

Table 1 Results of carotid duplex scans.

Ultrasound finding	Number of subjects (n = 4733)	Percentage
Normal	2784	58.8%
Atherosclerotic	1940	41%
Non atherosclerotic	9	0.2%

Fibromuscular dysplasia, arterial wall dissection, Aneurysm and Takayasu's arteritis.

Table 2 Frequency of different degrees of carotid atherosclerosis among the study population.

Degree of carotid atherosclerosis	Number of subjects (n = 4733)	Percentage
Intimal thickening	835	17.6%
<50%	983	20.8%
50–69%	81	1.7%
≥70%	38	0.8%
Occlusion	3	0.06%

Discussion

Racial differences are important factors in the severity and distribution of carotid atherosclerosis, e.g. people of South Asian origin have higher rates of cardiovascular disease and stroke than people of European origin, a finding that cannot be explained entirely by differences in conventional cardiovascular risk factors [6]. Egypt is the most populated nation in the Middle East and the second most populous on the African continent, with an estimated 80 million people. We conducted a 5-year survey study of 4733 Egyptians from January 2003 to January 2008 using extra-cranial duplex as a screening tool, in Cairo University Hospitals. High grade stenosis ≥50% represented 2.5% of our study populations. This prevalence of significant atherosclerotic Carotid disease found among our Egyptian subjects was much lower than that noticed in studies from developed Countries as America, Asia and Europe. The American Cardiovascular Health Study, examined 5441 community-dwelling people aged ≥65 years. Carotid stenosis >50% was found in 7% of the men and 5% of the women [7]. The Suita Study in Japan detected extracranial carotid stenosis >50% in 7.9% of the men and 1.3% of the women or 4.4% of all the subjects [8]. The German Berlin Aging Study, a population-based study of functionally healthy volunteers from 70 to 100 years of age, found 4% of ≥75% carotid stenosis among both men and women [9]. A recently published study from Pakistan, which is a transitional and developing country like Egypt, reported a frequency of carotid disease in the same order as we found in Egypt [10]. This discrepant prevalence of significant carotid atherosclerosis among Egyptians and residents of developed countries raises a number of questions regarding the cause of this discrepancy. Are there any underlying hidden dimensions or unknown factors, whether nutritional, genetic, environmental or life style? Is the rate of intra-cranial atherosclerosis higher than extra-cranial disease? The true answer is still obscure, and only more studies and surveys, with the additional efforts undertaken by health authorities, can help elucidating and clearing this hidden issues. Obesity was surprisingly marginally significant against carotid atherosclerosis with OR 0.800 and a p value 0.037, which can be explained as a chance finding. We suspect that the Cairene lifestyle and nutrition are the major contributors to the lower prevalence of carotid disease in Egyptians. The geopolitical features of Egypt are a real challenge to researchers. The main dichotomy for Egyptian citizens is the demographical division into those who live in the major urban areas and the farmers in rural villages. Almost the whole population is concentrated along the banks of the Nile (notably Cairo and Alexandria). Many Cairo residents have moved only recently from farming lands to Cairo and few are overweight. However, walking through Cairo one can spot, especially among the younger people, many who are overweight; an emerging risk factor. The possibilities to shift to fast food habits in Cairo are increasing and getting abundant. Atherosclerosis among the next generations of Egyptians might be rising. This is a call for health authorities to perform population-based epidemiological studies, monitor the non-communicable diseases and invest into health education and prevention programs. Our study had some limitations; being not population-based compared to studies from developed countries; moreover, the study sample represents Cairo citizens with higher socio-economic level who have better access to health care facilities than those living in rural areas.

Conclusion

The existence of conventional vascular risk factors among our populations is more or less the same like other industrialized countries, yet the prevalence of carotid atherosclerosis is much lower. This reveals hidden factors which are still not discovered.

References

[1] Yadav JS, Wholey MH, Kuntz E. Protected carotid-artery stenting versus endarterectomy in high-risk patients. N Engl J Med 2004;351:1493—501.
[2] Caplan LR, Gorelick PB, Hier DB. Race, sex and occlusive cerebrovascular disease: a review. Stroke 1986;17:648—55.
[3] Timsit SG, Sacco RL, Mohr JP, Foulkes MA, Tatemichi TK, Wolf PA, et al. Early clinical differentiation of cerebral infarction from severe atherosclerotic stenosis and cardioembolism. Stroke 1992;23:486—91.
[4] Grau AG, Weimar C, Buggle F, Heinrich A, Goertler M, Neumaier S, et al. Risk factors, outcome, and treatment in subtypes of ischemic stroke. The German stroke data bank. Stroke 2001;32:2559—66.
[5] Grant EG, Benson CB, Moneta GL, Alexandrov AV, Baker JD, Bluth EI, et al. Carotid artery stenosis. Gray-scale and Doppler ultrasound diagnosis. Society of Radiologists in Ultrasound Consensus Conference. Radiology 2003;229:340—6.
[6] Heyman A, Fields WS, Keating RD. Joint study of extracranial arterial occlusion. Racial differences in hospitalized patients with ischemic stroke. JAMA 1972;222:285—9.
[7] O'Leary DH, Polak JF, Kronmal RA, Kittner SJ, Bond MG, Wolfson SK, et al. Distribution and correlates of sonographically detected carotid artery disease in the Cardiovascular Health Study. The CHS Collaborative Research Group. Stroke 1992;23:1752—60.
[8] Mannami T, Konishi M, Baba S, Nishi N, Terao A. Prevalence of asymptomatic carotid atherosclerotic lesions detected by high-resolution ultrasonography and its relation to cardiovascular risk factors in the general population of a Japanese city: the Suita Study. Stroke 1997;28:518—25.
[9] Hillen T, Nieczaj R, Munzberg H, Schaub R, Borchelt M, Steinhagen-Thiessen E. Carotid atherosclerosis, vascular risk profile and mortality in a population-based sample of functionally healthy elderly subjects: the Berlin Ageing Study. J Intern Med 2000;247:679—88.
[10] Wasay M, Azeemuddin M, Masroor I, Sajjad Z, Ahmed R, Khealani BA, et al. Frequency and outcome of carotid atheromatous disease in patients with stroke in Pakistan. Stroke 2009;40:708—12.

Comparative *in vivo* and *in vitro* postmortem ultrasound assessment of intima-media thickness with additional histological analysis in human carotid arteries

Szabolcs Farkas [a,*], Sándor Molnár [b], Katalin Nagy [a], Tibor Hortobágyi [a,c,1], László Csiba [a,1]

[a] *Department of Neurology, University of Debrecen Medical and Health Science Center, 98 Nagyerdei Street, Debrecen H-4012, Hungary*
[b] *Department of Neurology, Sopron Elizabeth Hospital, 15 Győri Street, Sopron H-9400, Hungary*
[c] *Department of Pathology, University of Debrecen Medical and Health Science Center, 98 Nagyerdei Street, Debrecen H-4012, Hungary*

KEYWORDS
IMT;
In vitro ultrasonography;
In vivo ultrasonography;
Common carotid artery;
Snap freezing;
Comparative analysis

Summary The present study aims to validate the technique of *in vitro* ultrasonography (US) by comparative analysis of premortem intima—media thickness (IMT), postmortem IMT and average wall thickness. *In vivo* common carotid artery (CCA) IMT was measured bilaterally in 25 patients at 30 mm proximal from the flow divider. After autopsy *in vitro* US was performed and postmortem IMT was measured at the same level. Snap frozen arterial specimens were processed for average wall thickness determination and for histology. High degree of correlation was found between *in vivo* IMT, *in vitro* IMT and average wall thickness. Our results demonstrate: (1) *in vitro* US is a reliable and reproducible tool for the examination of autopsied arterial specimens to obtain valuable information about vascular wall properties and to identify the optimal vascular segment for tissue sampling; (2) snap freezing and cryosectioning of *in toto* excised arterial specimens is recommended for comparative histological—US studies.
© 2012 Elsevier GmbH. All rights reserved.

Introduction

Atherosclerosis is a generalized arterial disease that starts decades before the onset of clinical symptoms, such as angina pectoris, myocardial infarction or stroke [1—3]. Atherosclerosis in main arteries begins with the enlargement of the vascular lumen and size [4—7]. Necropsy studies confirmed the premorbid, age-related increase of intimal and medial thickness [7—9]. It has been suggested that early increase in intima—media thickness (IMT) reflects

* Corresponding author at: University of Debrecen-Medical and Health Science Center, Department of Neurology, Móricz Zsigmond Street, no. 22, H-4032 Debrecen, Hungary.
Tel.: +36 52 411 717x55986; fax: +36 52 453 590.
E-mail address: endreszabi@gmail.com (S. Farkas).
[1] L.C. and T.H. are the 'senior authors'.

adaptation to elevated intravascular shear stress whereas increased IMT with US detectable atherosclerotic plaque is associated with end-organ disease [10—12]. Risk factors, including age, gender, diabetes mellitus, blood pressure, smoking, elevated serum low-density lipoprotein cholesterol, homocystein levels and chlamydia infestation of the arterial wall are also associated with larger diameter and IMT of the extracranial carotid arteries [4,13].

In vivo intima—media thickness (IMT) measured non-invasively by high resolution B-mode ultrasonography is considered as a valid and reliable indicator of the local and generalized expansion of subclinical, later, clinical atherosclerosis [8]. IMT is defined as the distance between blood-intima and media-adventitia interfaces of arterial wall [14]. Most often it is measured at the common carotid artery (CCA), because high measurement precision can be obtained in this artery. These are made over a distance of 1 cm at levels 1—2 cm proximal to the bifurcation; a mean value for the selected area is obtained using automated wall-tracking software [5,15,16]. Nevertheless, *in vivo* carotid IMT determination aims primarily the far arterial wall (the side further to the US transducer) since an accurate measurement of the near wall IMT is extremely difficult and requires a high level of technical expertise [17,18]. Moreover, meta-analysis revealed that circumferential scanning of the carotid artery and calculation of the mean maximum carotid IMT provides a more accurate measurement of carotid atherosclerosis [19]. In addition, anatomy, motion artifacts or ultrasound equipment can also influence *in vivo* IMT determination [20—23]. A variety of non-invasive imaging techniques and softwares have been used to improve *in vivo* IMT determination and to increase the reliability of IMT as marker of atherosclerosis [18,20,22—25]. However, these IMT measuring methods have not been validated yet and a quick and reliable method for initial *in vitro* testing of new techniques and softwares, apart from the widely used *in vivo* US, is also needed. The present study addresses these deficiencies.

It has been suggested that changes in intensity of shear stress influence the arterial wall responses from less to more proliferative phenotypes, which may underlie the differences in genetic effects on CCA IMT and bifurcation IMT [26]. Further research is required to clarify genetic effects and local gene expression patterns, which could influence pathological processes in arterial walls and hence the arterial IMT. Therefore, a better knowledge of gene-IMT associations, *i.e.* taking into consideration US IMT measurements in the context of gene expression profile data could improve the accuracy and reliability in prediction of the progression of atherosclerotic vascular disease.

It is accepted that freezing of excised tissues could result in alteration of microanatomic structure especially because of ice crystal formation [27]. On the other hand, histological preparation of arterial sections affects vascular and plaque dimensions [28—31]. Another aspect of our study was to reveal whether snap freezing of arterial samples influences histological preparation of arterial specimens.

In the present study we compared *in vivo* IMT with *in vitro* US measured IMT and average wall thickness. Finally, histological processing of selected frozen arterial specimens was also performed. We aimed to validate *in vitro* US as alternative method, if *in vivo* US data were not available,

Table 1 Summary of patients' data.

Number of patients	n = 25	—
Age (years)	76.4 ± 11.5	—
Gender (male:female)	9:16	—
Risk factors	Hypertension (No; %)	20 (80%)
	Diabetes mellitus (No; %)	8 (32%)
Diagnosis at admission	Cerebral infarction (No)	14
	Cerebral hemorrhage (No)	3
	Others (No)	8
Cause of death	Raised intracranial pressure (No)	5
	Pneumonia (No)	6
	Pulmonary embolism (No)	5
	Cardiac failure (No)	8
	Sepsis (No)	1

Data are means ± SEM.

for postmortem vascular wall investigation, and to examine the applicability of snap freezing histotechnique on utilized vascular specimens.

Patient selection, materials and methods

Patients

Comparisons between ultrasound and postmortem findings were performed in 25 patients. Table 1 contains general data about patients. The study was approved by the local Ethics Committee and informed consent was obtained from the relatives of each examined individual.

In vivo ultrasonography

SONOS 4500 ultrasound system (Agilent, Andover, MA, USA) with a 3—11-MHz linear transducer was used for *in vivo* and *in vitro* ultrasonography. *In vivo* IMT measurements were performed in a longitudinal B-mode projection while the patient was in a supine position. IMT was determined as the distance from the leading edge of the first echogenic line to the leading edge of the second echogenic line of the double line pattern of the far artery wall (Fig. 2). Three measurements along a 2—3-mm portion of the vessel were performed and were averaged. IMT measurements site on the CCA were localized by the distance of 30 mm from tip of the flow divider. This landmark enabled us to reconstruct the position of the *in vivo* IMT measurement later during the postmortem IMT determination. Wall thickening over 2 mm was determined as plaque and excluded from further evaluation, which resulted in an important screening of the postmortem usable arterial specimens.

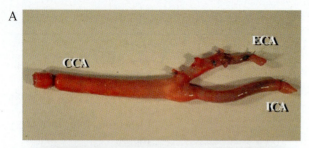

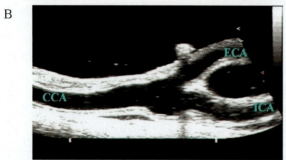

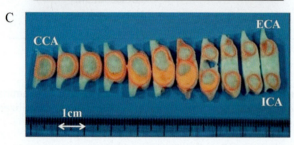

Figure 1 Processing of autopsied arterial specimens. Autopsied carotid arteries were filled with histological embedding material (Cryochrome Blue) (image A) and *in vitro* ultrasonography (US) was performed (image B). This was followed by snap freezing of the filled specimens and, subsequently, 3 mm thick sections were cut (image C) for performing planimetric analysis and histological processing of the samples: CCA, common carotid artery; ICA, internal carotid artery; ECA, external carotid artery.

Preparation of the arteries for *in vitro* IMT and average wall thickness determination

Within 24 h after death, 4 cm of common carotid arteries (CCA) and 4 cm of the proximal segments of internal- and external carotid arteries (ICA and ECA) were removed *in toto* from both sides. The native vessels were filled with histological embedding material (Cryochrome Blue; Thermo Shandon, Pittsburgh, PA, USA) and a constant pressure of 100 mmHg was adjusted (Fig. 1). The presence of ICA and ECA helped us to identify the anatomical position during the insonation to visualize precisely the far and near arterial. Subsequently, *in vitro* IMT was measured in 34 CCAs as described upper using ultrasound gel during the direct contact between transducer and prepared arterial specimens. *In vitro* measurements were compared with *in vivo* IMT values (Fig. 2). A thread has been fixed at 3 cm distance from tip of the flow divider in order to mark the exact location where *in vitro* IMT measurements were performed. Afterwards, filled specimens were frozen at −20 °C

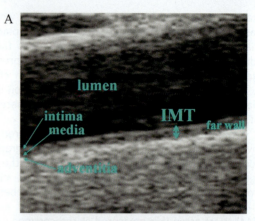

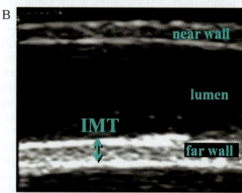

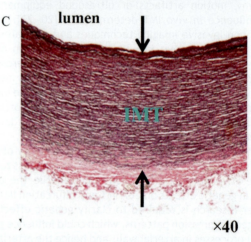

Figure 2 Comparison of common carotid artery (CCA) IMT measured by *in vivo* ultrasonography (US) (image A), *in vitro* US (image B) and histological method (image C). Ultrasonographic IMT is defined as the distance between the leading edge of the first echogenic line and the leading edge of the second echogenic line (A and B) and it was measured at 30 mm distance proximal from the bifurcation of CCA. Histological image (C) shows arterial wall in 40-fold magnification with good tissue preservation. Arrows indicate the lumen-intima and media-adventitia interfaces.

in a box containing embedding material, and subsequently, cut into 3 mm thick slices (Fig. 1) as described previously [31,32]. Consecutive slices were photographed with a high-resolution (3040 × 2016 pixels) digital camera (FinePix S1 Pro; Fuji Photo Film Co., Tokyo, Japan) for digitization and planimetric analysis of the sections. Six to eight slices per vessel were evaluated. A calibration bar was also digitized with each individual sample to determine the magnification of the system and to convert the pixel values into millimeters.

Calculations

The measured parameters (IMT, average wall thickness) were expressed in millimeters. Mean values of the measured *in vivo* IMT, *in vitro* IMT and average wall thickness were calculated.

Mean differences between *in vivo* and *in vitro* IMT were expressed in millimeters and percents according to the following formulas:

IMT difference (mm) = *in vitro* IMT − *in vivo* IMT;
IMT difference(%) = (*in vitro* IMT − *in vivo* IMT)/*in vitro* IMT × 100, respectively

Vessel circumference and lumen circumference on the digitized 3 mm thick arterial sections were measured with free available image analyzer software of the National Institute of Health and mean values were calculated. Subsequently, average wall thickness was determined based on the following formula: average wall thickness (mm) = (vessel circumference − lumen circumference)/2π.

Histological processing

CCA specimens were processed for histology. Three millimeter thick frozen arterial slices prepared as described above and marked by the thread at the level of *in vitro* IMT measurements were used. Afterwards, transverse sections (20 μm) of the marked slices were cut by cryomicrotome (Leica, CM 1850, Stockholm, Sweden) and were stained with hematoxylin & eosin (H&E) and Verhoeff—Van Gieson [33,34]. Sections with artificially damaged intima and/or media at the site of the measurement were excluded.

Statistical analysis

Concordance analysis was performed between *in vivo* IMT and *in vitro* IMT measurements. Furthermore, Bland—Altman plots were applied to illustrate the agreement between *in vitro* and *in vivo* IMT measurements [20]. Linear regression analysis was preformed to correlate *in vivo* IMT, *in vitro* IMT and average wall thickness.

Results

In the present study we have compared postmortem IMT determination with *in vivo* IMT and average wall thickness. Furthermore, histological processing of selected snap frozen arterial specimens was performed.

Table 2 Comparison of IMT measurements on common carotid artery.

IMT	Means ± SD	Range
In vivo (mm)	0.93 ± 0.10	0.67—1.33
In vitro (mm)	0.97 ± 0.14	0.61—1.68
Difference[a] (mm)	0.046	−0.173 to 0.333
Difference[b] (%)	3.8	−20 to 25

Data are means ± SEM, *n* = 34.
[a] Difference (mm) = *in vitro* − *in vivo*.
[b] Difference (%) = (*in vitro* − *in vivo*)/*in vitro* × 100.

In vitro and *in vivo* ultrasonographic IMT measurements, histology

In vivo and *in vitro* IMT measurements were compared in *n* = 34 CCA specimens. Fig. 2 presents *in vivo* and *in vitro* IMT measurements as well as histological image of H&E stained snap frozen arterial section. Results are summarized in Table 2. According to our results the mean IMT was 0.93 ± 0.12 mm by *in vivo* US and 0.97 ± 0.18 mm by *in vitro* ultrasound. The concordance between the two groups was significant: concordance coefficient RC = 0.545, $p < 0.0001$, 95% confidence interval 0.336—0.755. Concordance analysis and Bland—Altman plots for both parameters are shown in Fig. 3.

Ultrasound and gross pathology

Average wall thicknesses were calculated in case of *n* = 34 CCA specimens. Both *in vitro* and *in vivo* IMT values correlated well with average wall thicknesses measured at the corresponding postmortem samples ($r = 0.76$, $R^2 = 0.571$; $r = 0.57$, $R^2 = 0.328$, respectively). Fig. 3 presents the scatter plots and regression equations for average wall thickness related to *in vivo* and *in vitro* US IMT.

Discussion

In this study we analyzed the degree of correlation between *in vivo* IMT, *in vitro* IMT, and the average wall thickness examined in human common carotid arteries. We found significant concordance between *in vivo* and *in vitro* US determined IMT. Both corresponded well with the calculated average wall thickness. Following the *in vitro* tissue processing tissue preservation, shrinkage and overall suitability for microscopic analysis was assessed on stained histological sections from snap-frozen arterial segments. The applicability of *in vitro* US on autopsied vascular specimens has been demonstrated; and confirmed that postmortem IMT measured by *in vitro* US can be used as reliably as *in vivo* IMT.

It is well known the fact that through freezing water expands and forms ice crystals. This process can result in freezing artifacts and tissue damage, which, however, can be prevented by reduced freezing time [27]. Formalin fixation, dehydration in ethanol or other agents and paraffin embedding during processing could result in up to a 30—40% tissue shrinkage, changing vascular dimensions and causing

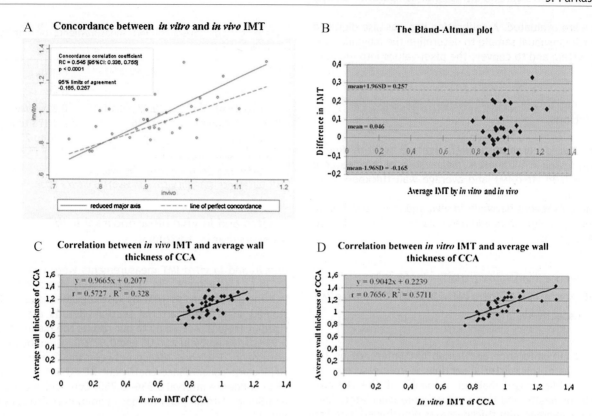

Figure 3 Concordance analysis (A) and Bland—Altman plots (B) of the *in vivo* and *in vitro* ultrasonographic (US) measured CCA IMT; scatter plots of *in vivo* US IMT and average wall thickness at CCA (C) and scatter plots of *in vitro* US IMT and average wall thickness at CCA (D). R^2 and regression equations are included. IMT measurements and average wall thickness values are expressed in millimeters: IMT, intima—media thickness; CCA, common carotid artery.

discrepancy between US and histological IMT measurements [28—31]. CCA IMT values obtained with *in vitro* US and follow-up histological determination showed good agreement (data not shown). However, due to the low number of available specimens for histological processing statistical analysis between *in vitro* and microscopic IMT was not performed. In this study we presented that *in vitro* tissue processing by snap freezing results in low extent of tissue shrinkage and minimal change in vascular wall properties. Therefore frozen postmortem artery sections are comparable with data derived from US methods both *in vivo* and *in vitro* and frozen sections are suitable for histological—US comparative analytical studies.

Despite the fact that carotid IMT is a well established surrogate marker for clinical events, *in vivo* US measured wall thickness has a variability caused by anatomy, ultrasound equipment, angle of insonation, attenuation of US by neck muscles, motion artifacts (swallowing, arterial pulsation and breathing) and examiner skills [20—23]. Furthermore, *in vivo* US investigates mainly the IMT of the far vessel wall, however, atherosclerotical processes and IMT changes are also present in other parts of vascular wall, therefore, a circumferential wall thickness determination is more reliable. In addition, there is a need for new *in vivo* imaging methods providing a detailed view of the arterial tree and vessel wall [17]. Magnetic resonance imaging (MRI) providing detailed cross-sectional images of all sides of carotid artery wall and three-dimensional motion sensitized segmented steady-state black-blood gradient echo technique

(3D MSDS) with rapid artifact-free overview imaging of the carotid wall are very promising techniques [21,24]. Finally, it has been suggested that computer-aided measuring techniques could result in increased accuracy and reduction of operator dependent subjectivity of IMT determination [23]. In our present study we have demonstrated that measuring IMT in postmortem arterial specimens by US is a reliable and reproducible method, which could be used for US standardization in subsequent studies. Hence, *in vitro* US measured IMT could be used to develop, improve, compare or validate new imaging techniques (*e.g.* fast three dimensional imaging techniques), automated IMT measurement algorithms, or new softwares for ultrasound methods.

Carotid IMT is strongly determined by genetic factors acting independently of traditional cardiovascular risk factors [35,36]. A heritability range of 20—40% has been estimated by studies in unselected subjects, twins, and people with type II diabetes [36—40]. Genes related to hemostasis, lipid and lipoprotein levels, extracellular matrix remodeling, antioxidation, renin—angiotensin system, endothelium function, inflammation have been associated with carotid IMT changes [34,41]. On the other hand, laminar flow and oscillatory shear stress trigger diverse local endothelial responses and altered gene expressions and result in an atherogenic phenotype [26,42—44] which may vary in different carotid segments with a possible impact on IMT. Our results implicate that *in vitro* US including IMT provide valuable information about autopsied arterial specimens. These, afterwards, can be stored and made available in tissue banks for a wide range of '-omics' investigations. In addition, *in vitro* US of arterial specimens could serve as a guide to identify the most appropriate region of an intact autopsied vascular tissue for histological sampling.

Furthermore, Liao et al. (2008) applied the gene risk score (GRS) to estimate a cumulative effect of genes significantly associated with IMT and emphasize the importance of future gene-IMT association studies on different populations. The use of the GRS may simplify an assessment of multiple gene effects in complex diseases and may provide a better estimate of individual susceptibility to atherosclerosis [26]. The accuracy and utility of GRS can possibly be improved by including an US artifact free postmortem IMT measurements of different parts of arterial wall (*e.g.* 'far wall, near wall', *etc.*). GRS combined with IMT could improve the precision and reliability of prognosis determination models for a complex disease like atherosclerosis.

In the present study we measured arterial IMT applying *in vitro* US and compared it to *in vivo* determined IMT, histological IMT and average arterial wall thickness. We demonstrate that for microscopic IMT determination purposes cutting and processing frozen arterial sections after *in vitro* US is a suitable histological technique which has advantages compared to use of formalin fixed paraffin embedded (FFPE) slides. Our data confirm that frozen sections from autopsied arteries are suitable for both histological IMT determination and US—histological comparative analysis.

We demonstrate that postmortem *in vitro* US is a reliable and reproducible technique for detection of arterial wall changes as alternative method of its *in vivo* analogue. In addition, validated *in vitro* US is a reliable tool to identify, without plaque manipulation, the vascular segment for tissue sampling. In particular, it is as suitable for IMT determination as *in vivo* US, without the methodological/technical/ethical limitations of *in vivo* human studies. Standardized *in vitro* US measured IMT provides basis for the development and validation of novel non-invasive imaging techniques to study vessel wall abnormalities.

In conclusion, *in vitro* US can be widely used in vascular research with the potential of correlative morphological, genetic, biochemical and imaging to study complex vascular diseases such as arteriosclerosis.

Acknowledgements

Drs László Kardos and Katalin Hegedüs are thankfully acknowledged for statistical and general advice. The authors express their gratitude to Katalin Nagy for the outstanding technical assistance.

References

[1] Neunteufl T, Maurer G. Noninvasive ultrasound techniques for the assessment of atherosclerosis in coronary artery disease. Circ J 2003;67:177—86.
[2] Stary HC. Evolution and progression of atherosclerotic lesions in coronary arteries in children and young adults. Atherosclerosis 1989;99(Suppl. I):19—32.
[3] Tuzcu EM, Kapadia SR, Tutar E, Ziada KM, Hobbs RE, McCarthy PM, et al. High prevalence of coronary atherosclerosis in asymptomatic teenagers and young adults: evidence from intravascular ultrasound. Circulation 2001;103:2705—10.
[4] Crouse JR, Goldbourt U, Evans G, Pinsky J, Sharrett AR, Sorlie P, et al. Arterial enlargement in the atherosclerosis risk in communities (ARIC) cohort. In vivo quantification of carotid arterial enlargement. The ARIC Investigators. Stroke 1994;25:1354—9.
[5] Fernhall B, Agiovlasitis S. Arterial function in youth: window into cardiovascular risk. J Appl Physiol 2008;105:325—33.
[6] Glagov S, Weisenberg E, Zarins CK, Stankunavicius R, Kolettis GJ. Compensatory enlargement of human coronary arteries. N Engl J Med 1987;316:1371—5.
[7] Velican D, Velican C. Comparative study on age-related changes and atherosclerotic involvement of the coronary arteries of male and female subjects up to 40 years of age. Atherosclerosis 1981;38:39—50.
[8] Nissen SE, Gurley JC, Grines CL. Intravascular ultrasound assessment of lumen size and wall morphology in normal subjects and patients with coronary artery disease. Circulation 1991;84:1087—99.
[9] Potkin BN, Bartorelli AL, Gessert JM. Coronary artery imaging with intravascular high-frequency ultrasound. Circulation 1990;81:1575—85.
[10] Bots ML, Hoes AW, Koudstaal PJ. Common carotid intima-media thickness and risk of stroke and myocardial infarction: the Rotterdam study. Circulation 1997;96:1432—7.
[11] Frauchiger B, Schmid HP, Roedel C, Moosmann P, Staub D. Comparison of carotid arterial resistive indices with intima—media thickness as sonographic markers of atherosclerosis. Stroke 2001;32:836—41.
[12] Johnsen SH, Mathiesen EB, Joakimsen O, Stensland E, Wilsgaard T, Løchen ML, et al. Carotid atherosclerosis is a stronger predictor of myocardial infarction in women than in men: a 6-year follow-up study of 6226 persons: the Tromsø Study. Stroke 2007;38:2873—80.
[13] Crouse JR, Furberg CD, Byington RP, Riley W. B-mode ultrasound: a noninvasive method for assessing atherosclerosis. In: Willerson JT, Cohn JN, editors. Cardiovascular medicine. 2nd ed. Philadelphia: Churchill Livingstone; 2000. p. 1446—53.
[14] Amato M, Montorsi P, Ravani A, Oldani E, Galli S, Ravagnani PM, et al. Carotid intima—media thickness by B-mode ultrasound as surrogate of coronary atherosclerosis: correlation with quantitative coronary angiography and coronary intravascular ultrasound findings. Eur Heart J 2007;28:2094—101.
[15] Bots ML, Hoes AW, Hofman A, Witteman JC, Grobbee DE. Cross-sectionally assessed carotid intima—media thickness relates to long-term risk of stroke, coronary heart disease and death as estimated by available risk functions. J Intern Med 1999;245:269—76.
[16] O'Leary DH, Polak JF, Kronmal RA, Manolio TA, Burke GL, Wolfson Jr SK. Carotid-artery intima and media thickness as a risk factor for myocardial infarction and stroke in older adults. Cardiovascular Health Study Collaborative Research Group. N Engl J Med 1999;340:14—22.
[17] Bots ML, De Jong PT, Hofman A, Grobbee DE. Left, right, near or far wall common carotid intima—media thickness measurements: associations with cardiovascular disease and lower extremity arterial atherosclerosis. J Clin Epidemiol 1997;50:801—7.
[18] Lane HA, Smith JC, Davies JS. Noninvasive assessment of preclinical atherosclerosis. Vasc Health Risk Manage 2006;2:19—30.
[19] Bots ML, Evans GW, Riley WA. Carotid intima—media thickness measurements in intervention studies: design options, progression rates, and sample size considerations; a point of view. Stroke 2003;34:2985—94.
[20] Bland JM, Altman DG. Statistical methods for assessing agreement between two methods of clinical measurement. Lancet 1986;1:307—10.

[21] Boussel L, Herigault G, de la Vega A, Nonent M, Douek PC, Serfaty JM. Swallowing, arterial pulsation, and breathing induce motion artifacts in carotid artery MRI. J Magn Reson Imaging 2006;23:413—5.

[22] Lo J, Dolan SE, Kanter JR, Hemphill LC, Connelly JM, Lees RS, et al. Effects of obesity, body composition, and adiponectin on carotid intima—media thickness in healthy women. J Clin Endocrinol Metab 2006;91:1677—82.

[23] Molinari F, Zeng G, Suri JS. A state of the art review on intima—media thickness (IMT) measurement and wall segmentation techniques for carotid ultrasound. Comput Methods Programs Biomed 2010;100:201—21.

[24] Bornstedt A, Burgmaier M, Hombach V, Marx N, Rasche V. Dual stack black blood carotid artery CMR at 3T: application to wall thickness visualization. J Cardiovasc Magn Reson 2009;11:45.

[25] Djaberi R, Beishuizen ED, Pereira AM, Rabelink TJ, Smit JW, Tamsma JT, et al. Non-invasive cardiac imaging techniques and vascular tools for the assessment of cardiovascular disease in type 2 diabetes mellitus. Diabetologia 2008;51:1581—93.

[26] Liao YC, Lin HF, Rundek T, Cheng R, Guo YC, Sacco RL, et al. Segment-specific genetic effects on carotid intima—media thickness: the Northern Manhattan study. Stroke 2008;39:3159—65.

[27] Bridgman PC, Reese TS. The structure of cytoplasm in directly frozen cultured cells. I. Filamentous meshworks and the cytoplasmic ground substance. J Cell Biol 1984;99:1655—68.

[28] Bahr GF, Bloom G, Friberg U. Volume changes of tissues in physiological fluids during fixation in osmium tetroxide or formaldehyde and during subsequent treatment. Exp Cell Res 1957;12:342—3.

[29] Persson J, Formgren J, Israelsson B, Berglund G. Ultrasound-determined intima—media thickness and atherosclerosis. Direct and indirect validation. Arterioscler Thromb 1994;14:261—4.

[30] Pignoli P, Tremoli E, Poli A, Oreste P, Paoletti R. Intimal plus medial thickness of the arterial wall: a direct measurement with ultrasound imaging. Circulation 1986;74:1399—406.

[31] Schulte-Altedorneburg G, Droste DW, Felszeghy S, Kellermann M, Popa V, Hegedüs K, et al. Accuracy of in vivo carotid B-mode ultrasound compared with pathological analysis: intima—media thickening, lumen diameter, and cross-sectional area. Stroke 2001;32:1520—4.

[32] Molnár S, Kerényi L, Ritter MA, Magyar MT, Ida Y, Szöllosi Z, et al. Correlations between the atherosclerotic changes of femoral, carotid and coronary arteries: a post mortem study. J Neurol Sci 2009;287:241—5.

[33] Constantine VS, Mowry RW. Selective staining of human dermal collagen II: the use of picrosirius red F3BA with polarization microscopy. J Invest Dermatol 1968;50:419—23.

[34] Módis L. Organization of the extracellular matrix: a polarization microscopic approach. Boca Raton, FL: CRC Press; 1991.

[35] Zannad F, Benetos A. Genetics of intima—media thickness. Curr Opin Lipidol 2003;14:191—200.

[36] Zannad F, Visvikis S, Gueguen R. Genetics strongly determines the wall thickness of the left and right carotid arteries. Hum Genet 1998;103:183—8.

[37] Jartti L, Ronnemaa T, Kaprio J, Jarvisalo MJ, Toikka JO, Marniemi J, et al. Population-based twin study of the effects of migration from Finland to Sweden on endothelial function and intima—media thickness. Arterioscler Thromb Vasc Biol 2002;22:832—7.

[38] Lange LA, Bowden DW, Langefeld CD, Wagenknecht LE, Carr JJ, Rich SS, et al. Heritability of carotid artery intima—medial thickness in type 2 diabetes. Stroke 2002;33:1876—81.

[39] North KE, MacCluer JW, Devereux RB, Howard BV, Welty TK, Best LG, et al. Heritability of carotid artery structure and function: the Strong Heart Family Study. Arterioscler Thromb Vasc Biol 2002;22:1698—703.

[40] Swan L, Birnie DH, Inglis G, Connell JM, Hillis WS. The determination of carotid intima medial thickness in adults—a population-based twin study. Atherosclerosis 2003;166:137—41.

[41] Zhao J, Cheema FA, Bremner JD, Goldberg J, Su S, Snieder H, et al. Heritability of carotid intima—media thickness: a twin study. Atherosclerosis 2008;197:814—20.

[42] De Keulenaer GW, Chappell DC, Ishizaka N, Nerem RM, Alexander RW, Griendling KK. Oscillatory and steady laminar shear stress differentially affect human endothelial redox state: role of a superoxideproducing NADH oxidase. Circ Res 1998;82:1094—101.

[43] Malek AM, Alper SL, Izumo S. Hemodynamic shear stress and its role in atherosclerosis. JAMA 1999;282:2035—42.

[44] Topper JN, Cai J, Falb D, Gimbrone Jr MA. Identification of vascular endothelial genes differentially responsive to fluid mechanical stimuli: cyclooxygenase-2, manganese superoxide dismutase, and endothelial cell nitric oxide synthase are selectively up-regulated by steady laminar shear stress. Proc Natl Acad Sci U S A 1996;93:10417—22.

5. Cerebral Hemodynamics in Ischemic Stroke

Hemodynamic causes of deterioration in acute ischemic stroke

Georgios Tsivgoulis[a],*, Nicole Apostolidou[a], Sotirios Giannopoulos[b], Vijay K. Sharma[c]

[a] Department of Neurology, Democritus University of Alexandroupolis School of Medicine, Alexandroupolis, Greece
[b] Department of Neurology, University of Ioannina School of Medicine, Ioannina, Greece
[c] Division of Neurology, National University Hospital, Singapore, Singapore

KEYWORDS
Early neurological deterioration;
Acute ischemic stroke;
Hemodynamic;
Transcranial Doppler;
Reocclusion

Summary Neurological deterioration can occur in 13—38% of patients with acute ischemic stroke due to hemodynamic and non-hemodynamic causes. Several non-hemodynamic mechanisms can lead to ischemic lesion extension and subsequent neurological worsening, including infections, cerebral edema, hemorrhagic conversion of infarction and metabolic disorders. The most common hemodynamic causes related to infarct expansion, leading to neurologic deterioration in the setting of acute cerebral ischemia are the following: (i) cardiac complications, (ii) arterial reocclusion, (iii) intracranial arterial steal phenomenon, and (iv) cerebral microembolization. The present review aims to address the underlying mechanisms and potential clinical implications of the hemodynamic causes of neurological deterioration in patients with acute cerebral ischemia. The contribution of neurosonology in detection of changes in cerebral hemodynamics in real-time are also going to be discussed. Finally, potential treatment strategies for specific causes of hemodynamic deterioration in acute ischemic stroke patients are reported.
© 2012 Elsevier GmbH. All rights reserved.

Early neurological deterioration: prevalence and definitions

Early neurological deterioration (END) has been described as worsening in neurological function during the first days of acute cerebral ischemia (ACI) [1]. The prevalence of END varies in different studies according to the definition used for END detection [1]. An Italian study reported that END occurred in 20—26% of non-thrombolysed patients presenting with acute ischemic stroke (AIS) [2]. END was defined

* Corresponding author at: Kapodistriou 3, Nea Xili, Alexandroupolis 68100, Greece. Tel.: +30 6937178635; fax: +30 2551030479.
E-mail address: tsivgoulisgiorg@yahoo.gr (G. Tsivgoulis).

as a decrease of 1 or more points, in the Canadian Neurological Scale (CNS) score from hospital admission to 48 h after stroke onset. The investigators of European Cooperative Acute Stroke Study (ECASS) I identified factors that potentially predicted or were associated with progression of stroke and evaluated the influence of stroke progression on neurologic worsening. Early progressing stroke (EPS) was defined as a decrease of ≥2 points in consciousness or motor power or a decrease of ≥3 points in speech scores in the Scandinavian Neurological Stroke Scale from hospital admission to the 24-h evaluation. END was documented in 37.5% of all patients during the first 24 h after inclusion in the study (37% in the placebo group and 38% in the recombinant tissue plasminogen activator group) [3]. Grotta et al. used the National Institute of Neurological Disorders and Stroke (NINDS) rt-PA Stroke Trial database to document the prevalence of clinical deterioration following improvement (DFI) and of any significant clinical deterioration (CD) even if not preceded by improvement. DFI was defined as any 2-point deterioration on the NIH Stroke Scale (NIHSS) score after an initial 2-point improvement after treatment. CD was defined as any 4-point worsening after treatment compared with baseline. DFI and CD identified in 13% and 16% of all patients, respectively [4]. END was also detected in 19% and 13% of patients hospitalized in general medical wards and acute stroke units, respectively, according to the findings of an Australian [5] and German [6] study, respectively. END was defined as 1-point and 2-point increase in NIHSS (during the first three and five days of ictus respectively) in the Australian and German study, respectively.

Recent studies have shown that END is an independent predictor of poor outcomes in the setting of AIS. More specifically, the investigators of SORCan (Stroke Outcomes Research Canada) registry have reported that END (defined as 1-point decrease in CNS) was an independent predictor of 7-day, 30-day and 1-year case fatality rate in a cohort of 3631 patients [7]. Similarly, END was associated with higher rates of death during hospitalization, longer duration of hospitalization and lower rates of functional independence in an Australian study [5].

Causes of early neurological deterioration

The causes of END can be classified into two major groups: hemodynamic and non hemodynamic [1]. Several non-hemodynamic mechanisms can lead to ischemic lesion extension and subsequent neurological worsening, including infections, cerebral edema/increased intracranial pressure, hemorrhagic conversion of infarction and metabolic disorders (hypoxia, hyperglycemia and fever) [1]. The most common hemodynamic causes related to infarct expansion, leading to END in the setting of ACI are the following: (i) cardiac complications, (ii) arterial reocclusion, (iii) intracranial arterial steal phenomenon and (iv) cerebral microembolization.

Cardiac complications and END

Patients with severe disabling strokes are particularly vulnerable to cardiac complications because stroke can provoke disturbances in autonomic and neurohormonal control and predispose patients to severe cardiac adverse events (SCAEs). It is well-known that acute stroke may lead to a variety of cardiac abnormalities such as myocardial infarction, electrocardiographic changes, cardiac arrhythmias, cardiac arrest, stress cardiomyopathy (tako-tsubo syndrome) and intracardiac thrombus [8]. SCAEs can hinder functional recovery and contribute to cardiac morbidity and mortality [8]. They are common in the acute period after stroke onset (19.0% of all patients experience at least one SCAE) and are responsible for 2–6% of the total mortality three months after acute ischemic stroke [9]. The main predictors of SCAE are outlined below: history of heart failure, diabetes mellitus, baseline creatinine >115 μmol/L, severe stroke, and a long QTc (>450 ms in men and >470 ms in women) or ventricular extrasystoles on ECG, low admission systolic blood pressure (<110 mmHg) and right insular stroke

[8,9]. Right insular region has been shown to moderate the autonomic control of the heart and this may partly explain the potential relationship of right insular stroke with SCAEs. Moreover insular infarction is associated with abnormal cardiac repolarization and increased risk of vascular mortality [9].

The main mechanisms linking SCAEs with END are outlined below: (i) hemodynamic instability/hypotension (which may in turn worsen the impaired cerebral autoregulation and further reduce perfusion in the infracted brain tissue), (ii) increased risk of sudden cardiac death, and (iii) increased risk of recurrent stroke and systemic embolism. There is mounting evidence linking extremely low admission BP levels with adverse early and late functional outcomes in patients presenting with ACI [10,11]. In addition the results of a recent randomized phase III trial showed that acute antihypertensive therapy causing mild BP reductions (3–6 mmHg) during the first 7 days of AIS was not related to better functional outcome or lower rates of cardiovascular events when compared to placebo. In contrast, stroke progression was increased by almost 50% in patients treated with antihypertensive therapy in comparison to the placebo group [12].

Potential therapeutic strategies of END caused by cardiac complications

The following therapeutic measures may be considered in patients with END caused by SCAEs:

1. Avoiding antihypertensive medications during the first 48 h of ACI (unless systolic blood pressure/diastolic blood pressure > 220/120 mmHg).
2. Prolonging cardiac monitoring in patients at high risk for cardiac arrhythmias in order to increase the yield of timely detection of cardiac arrhythmias and early initiation of appropriate medications (e.g. beta-blockers).
3. Avoiding fluid overload in patients with congestive heart failure.
4. Using early anticoagulation (unfractioned heparin) in patients with intracardiac thrombus.
5. Using pressors in patients wih Tako-tsubo syndrome in order to increase the cardiac output.

Arterial reocclusion and END

Early reocclusion may be the most common mechanism of early clinical fluctuation and worsening after thrombolytic therapy and intra-arterial procedures for acute ischemic stroke, leading to poor clinic outcome and higher in-hospital mortality [13,14]. Thrombolytic therapy has been demonstrated to be effective in acute stroke by dissolving the arterial occlusion and reestablishing tissue perfusion. However, the beneficial effect of tissue plasminogen activator (tPA)-induced recanalization may be eventually hampered by the occurrence of reocclusion [13,14].

Early reocclusion occurs in 15–34% of AIS patients treated with iv-tPA achieving any initial recanalization, accounting for up 2/3 of deterioration following improvement [13,14]. Reocclusion can be detected in real-time using transcranial Doppler (TCD) monitoring [13–16]. Reocclusion is observed in 17% of patients, who undergo intra-arterial thrombolysis based on catheter angiographic surveillance [17]. Reocclusion can also occur during or after catheter-based interventions [18]. In particular, the prevalence of reocclusion occurring during and within an hour after intra-arterial reperfusion procedures (mechanical thrombectomy, thromboaspiration, intra-arterial thrombolysis) is 19% and 8%, respectively [18].

Reocclusion in stroke patients appears to occur most in those with partial initial recanalization. These patients may be prone to repeated thrombosis and artery-to-artery reembolization particularly in the setting of a large vessel atherosclerosis [14,19]. Another potential independent predictor of reocclusion is severe stroke given the fact that increased stroke severity as reflected by higher NIHSS-scores represents larger thrombus burden [20]. Interestingly, Rubiera et al. have documented that admission NIHSS-scores higher than 16 points and severe ipsilateral carotid disease were independently associated with reocclusion in multivariate logistic regression models adjusting for potential confounders [14]. Finally, arterial reocclusion was related to lesser neurological improvement during hospitalization and lower rates of three-month functional independence in two stroke registries of systemic thrombolysis [14,19].

Early reocclusion can be detected in real-time with continuous 1-h TCD-monitoring during iv-tPA infusion [13,14] and our pilot study demonstrated that TCD can detect arterial reocclusion during or within an hour after completion of intra-arterial procedures [18]. There is also small anecdotal data indicating that continuous ultrasound surveillance may provide rapid detection of reocclusion (Fig. 1) as well as persistent occlusion and assist in subsequent management decisions including GPIIb-IIIa antagonist administration [21] or direct thrombin inhibitor administration (such as argatroban) [22] in patients with END due to reocclusion.

Potential therapeutic strategies of END caused by arterial reocclusion

The following therapeutic measures may be considered in patients with END caused by arterial reocclusion:

- TCD-monitoring of intracranial vessel patency during the first hours following reperfusion procedures (especially during the first 2 h following tPA-bolus).
- Emergent intra-arterial reperfusion procedures (thrombectomy/thromboaspiration) if reocclusion is detected.
- Continuous 2-h argatroban infusion following standard intravenous thrombolysis may be a future therapeutic option for reducing reocclusion.

Intracranial arterial steal phenomenon and END

The Starling resistor model defines cerebral perfusion pressure as the difference between arterial pressure and venous, intracranial, or tissue pressure (whichever is highest) [23]. Blood flow occurs due to pressure gradient with blood following the path of least resistance and flow diversion being caused by effective outflow differences for the Starling resistors [23]. The concept of blood flow steal in the cerebral circulation is well established [24]. In brain, hemodynamic steal and shunts were documented with angiomas and hypervascularized brain tumors [24,25]. Neurological symptoms were linked to cerebral blood flow reduction with

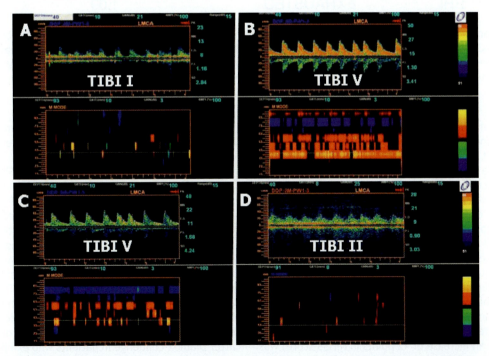

Figure 1 (A) Left M2MCA (middle cerebral artery) occlusion (thrombolysis in brain ischemia TIBI II) before the onset of intravenous thrombolysis (MFV = 13 cm/s, high-resistance flow on M-Mode spectrum). (B) Complete recanalization was achieved 28 min after tPA bolus (TIBI V; MFV = 27 cm/s, low-resistance flow on M-Mode spectrum), (C) Complete recanalization is sustained at 42 min following tPA-bolus (TIBI V) but high-resistance flow signatures appear on M-Mode spectrum, while spectral interrogation reveals an increase in Pulsatility Index (from 1.3 in (B) to 1.7), and (D) re-occlusion occurred at 56 min following tPA-bolus (TIBI II).

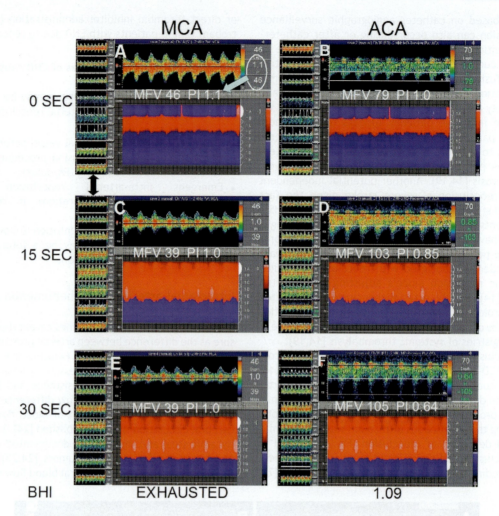

Figure 2 Intracranial arterial steal phenomenon during voluntary breath-holding in a patient with acute cerebral ischemia due to proximal M1MCA occlusion. A decrease in M1MCA MFV (mean flow velocity) is documented during voluntary breath-holding (from 46 cm/s at the beginning to 39 cm/s at the end of breath-holding). A simultaneous substantial flow diversion toward ipsilateral ACA (anterior cerebral artery) is documented during voluntary breath-holding (from 79 cm/s at the beginning to 105 cm/s at the end of breath-holding).

arterio-venous malformations [24] or rare cases of the subclavian steal syndrome [26].

The concept of arterial steal has been evaluated in real-time in the setting of ACI. Alexandrov et al. observed paradoxical decreases in flow velocity during episodes of hypercapnia in vessels supplying ischemic areas of the brain at the time of expected velocity increase in nonaffected vessels [27]. Hypercapnia triggered vasodilation more effectively in normal vessels, thus producing arterial blood flow steal toward the path of least resistance (Fig. 2) [27]. The hemodynamic steal was also documented on CT perfusion before and after challenge with acetazolamide (Diamox). The steal magnitude was linked to severity of neurological worsening in patients with acute stroke [27,28]. This intracranial steal phenomenon when coupled with END (determined as an increase of >2 points in NIHSS-score) was termed ''Reversed Robin Hood Syndrome (RRHS)'' for an analogy with ''rob the poor to feed the rich [27].

Sharma et al. attempted to evaluate RRHS in a prospective series of patients with severe intracranial steno-occlusive disease using bilateral TCD-monitoring with voluntary breath-holding and acetazolamide-challenged ^{99m}Tc-HMPAO (hexamethylpropylene amine oxime) SPECT [29,30]. The magnitude of arterial steal was calculated using changes in mean flow velocities (MFVs) during TCD-monitoring and net deficit in metabolic perfusion after acetazolamide-challenge on HMPAO-SPECT (Fig. 3). Interestingly, identification of intracranial steal phenomenon on TCD had satisfactory agreement with detection of inadequate vasodilatory reserve leading to perfusion deficit on acetazolamide-challenged HMPAO-SPECT. Moreover, a strong linear correlation was identified between intracranial steal magnitude (%) on TCD [calculated as $[(MFVm - MFVb)/MFVb] \times 100$, where m = minimum and b = baseline MFVs during the 15- to 30-s period of a total 30 s of breath-holding] [27] and net perfusion deficit on SPECT after Diamox-challenge in patients who exhibited both steal phenomenon on TCD and failed vasodilatory reserve on SPECT (Fig. 4).

Alexandrov et al. conducted a pilot study to investigate the prevalence of RRHS in a consecutive series of patients with ACI. They showed that among 153 patients admitted

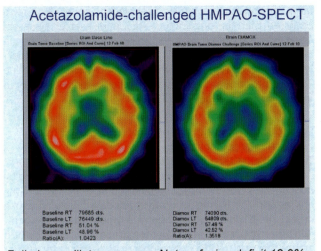

Failed vasodilatory reserve; Net perfusion deficit 12.9%

Figure 3 HMPAO SPECT (single-photon emission computed tomography) imaging after acetazolamide (Diamox) challenge shows a paradoxical reduction in the left MCA territory perfusion (net perfusion deficit 12.9%) resulting from the Reversed Robin Hood Syndrome in a patients with acute cerebral arterial ischemia due to left terminal internal carotid artery occlusion.

within 48 h from ACI onset, 21 (14%) had steal phenomenon (median steal magnitude, 20%; interquartile range, 11%; range, 6—45%), and 11 (7%) had RRHS. RRHS was most frequent in patients with proximal arterial occlusions in the anterior circulation (17% versus 1%; $p < 0.001$). Male gender, younger age, persisting arterial occlusions, and excessive sleepiness (evaluated by the Epworth Sleepiness Scale and Berlin Questionnaire) were independently associated with RRHS on multivariate logistic regression models [31].

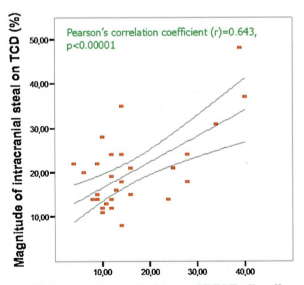

Figure 4 Linear correlation of magnitude of steal phenomenon as quantified on bilateral TCD-monitoring with net perfusion deficit as quantified on SPECT after Diamox-challenge in patients who exhibited both steal phenomenon on TCD and failed vasodilatory reserve on SPECT.

The same group also sought to determine the potential association of RRHS with risk of early recurrent stroke. Their findings indicated that patients with acute anterior circulation ischemic events and RRHS have a significantly higher risk of new ischemic stroke occurrence than acute stroke patients without this condition [32]. This longitudinal association persisted even after adjustment for demographic characteristics, vascular risk factors, and secondary prevention therapies. They also observed that all recurrent strokes in the RRHS subgroup occurred in the anterior circulation vascular territory ipsilateral to the index event [32]. Moreover the risk of recurrent stroke was front-loaded with a four-fold increase being documented during the first 30 days of ictus [30-day stroke risk in RRHS(+) and RRHS(−) patients: 12% and 3%, respectively] [32]. These findings indicate that the hemodynamic compromise caused by the vascular steal phenomenon may be an underlying mechanism linking large vessel atherosclerosis both with neurologic deterioration in the acute stroke setting as well as with recurrent cerebral ischemia during the first month after the index event.

Potential therapeutic strategies of END caused by intracranial arterial steal phenomenon

In the first documented cases of reversed Robin Hood syndrome (RRHS), neurological worsening was also more pronounced in patients with sleep apnea [27] or excessive sleepiness [31]. Hence, patients with persisting arterial occlusions and excessive sleepiness can be particularly vulnerable to the steal. In the first two reports describing RRHS no further END was observed in patients with intracranial arterial steal that were treated with non-invasive ventilatory correction. [27,31] Moreover, early noninvasive ventilatory correction in AIS patients has been shown to be safe and feasible in a recent pilot study [33]. In view of the former considerations, it has been hypothesized that:

(i) RRHS may provide a missing link between the respiratory status and END in ACI with history of obstructive sleep apnea [34]
(ii) and intracranial arterial steal phenomenon and sleep-disordered breathing may represent linked therapeutic targets [34].

Cerebral microembolization and END

TCD can reliably detect in real-time asymptomatic microembolic signals (MESs) in cerebral circulation that are characterized as ''High Intensity Transient Signals'' (HITS) [35—39]. Asymptomatic cerebral embolization can be detected by TCD in 7—71% of patients with ACI (Fig. 5) [35—39]. The prevalence of MES is highest in patients with large-artery atherosclerotic stroke with cardioembolic infarction being the second most common stroke subtype with concomitant asymptomatic microembolization. MES are rarely identified in patients with lacunar stroke. The number of MES detected by TCD negatively correlates to the elapsed time from symptom onset in patients with ACI [35—39]. In other words, the sooner TCD-monitoring is performed from symptom onset the higher the yield of ultrasound detection of MES.

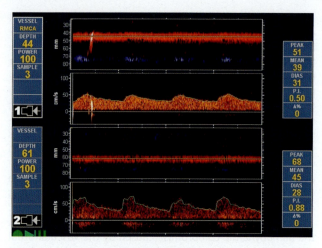

Figure 5 Detection of a microembolic signal in right MCA in a patient with severe (>70%) extracranial carotid artery stenosis during bilateral TCD-monitoring of MCAs. The flow in right MCA displays a characteristic "blunted" waveform appearance that is indicative of a more proximal hemodynamically significant steno-occlusive lesion.

MES have been shown to predict recurrent stroke risk in acute stroke, symptomatic carotid stenosis and postoperatively after CEA (Table 1) [35]. MES may also predict first-ever stroke risk in patients with asymptomatic carotid stenosis (Table 1) [36]. More specifically, MES detection by TCD-monitoring increases the risk of recurrent stroke by almost ten-fold (OR: 9.6; 95%CI: 1.5—59.3) in patients with symptomatic carotid artery stenosis (Table 1). Similarly, MES detection by TCD-monitoring increases the risk of ipsilateral stroke by almost seven-fold (OR: 6.6; 95%CI: 2.9—15.4) in patients with asymptomatic carotid artery stenosis (Table 1). Consequently, MES have been used for risk stratification and assessment of therapeutic efficacy in the former conditions [35—37,39]. Hao et al. have recently shown that MES have been associated with END and worsening of neurological deficit in patients with ACI due to large artery atherosclerosis [38]. Iguchi et al. have also reported that the presence of MES at 48 h after symptom onset was associated with recurrence of cerebral ischemia on diffusion weighted imaging (DWI) independent of underlying stroke subtype, [40] while MES detection on baseline TCD-monitoring has been related to the presence of multiple infarction on baseline DWI [35,38].

Potential therapeutic strategies of END caused by cerebral microembolization

Two small pilot randomized clinical trials have provided preliminary evidence that clopidogrel load (300 mg) followed by dual antiplatelet therapy (combination of clopidogrel 75 mg and aspirin 75—100 mg for up to seven days following stroke onset) may reduce substantially asymptomatic microembolization in patients with symptomatic extracranial carotid artery stenosis [CARESS (clopidogrel and aspirin for reduction of emboli in symptomatic carotid stenosis) trial] [41] or symptomatic stenosis in cerebral or extracranial carotid arteries [CLAIR (clopidogrel plus aspirin versus aspirin alone for reducing embolization in patients with acute symptomatic cerebral or carotid artery stenosis) trial]. [42] Neither CARESS nor CLAIR showed a beneficial effect of dual therapy in reducing the risk of recurrent stroke, but when both studies were combined there was an absolute risk reduction of 6% (95% CI 1—11%) in recurrent stroke with use of dual therapy (combination of aspirin and clopidogrel) compared with aspirin monotherapy. [42] In view of the former considerations, it may be postulated that:

(i) Continuous TCD-monitoring to detect the presence of cerebral microembolization in real-time in patients with large-artery atherosclerotic stroke may be indicated.
(ii) Aggressive antiplatelet therapy (clopidogrel load followed by combination antiplatelet therapy) may be considered during the first days of ictus in patients with ACI due to large-artery atherosclerosis and detection of MES on TCD-monitoring [43].

Table 1 Association of microembolic signals (MESs) detected by TCD and risk of recurrent events in different clinical subgroups.

Patient subgroup	N (studies/patients)	Outcome event	OR (95%CI)	Heterogeneity (I^2)
ACI (AIS/TIA) [35]	8/737	Rec. stroke	2.4 (1.2—5.1)#	12% (NS)
ACI (AIS/TIA) [35]	8/737	Rec. stroke/TIA	3.7 (1.6—8.4)¶	47% (NS)
Sym. Car. Sten. [35]	4/270	Rec. stroke	9.6 (1.5—59.3)#	6% (NS)
Sym. Car. Sten. [35]	4/270	Rec. stroke/TIA	6.4 (2.9—13.4)*	0% (NS)
Asym. Car. Sten. [36]	6/1144	Ips. stroke	6.6 (2.9—15.4)*	13% (NS)
Asym. Car. Sten. [36]	6/1144	Ips. st./TIA	7.6 (2.3—24.7)&	73% ($p=0.002$)
Post-oper. CEA [35]	6/649	Rec. stroke	2.5 (0.8—7.7)$	0% (NS)
Post-oper. CEA [35]	6/649	Rec. stroke/TIA	3.6 (1.4—9.2)@	0% (NS)

ACI, acute cerebral ischemia; AIS, acute ischemic stroke; TIA, transient ischemic attack; Asym., asymptomatic; Sym., symptomatic; Car. Sten., carotid stenosis; Post-Oper. CEA, post-operative carotid endarterectomy; Rec, recurrent; Ips., ipsilateral; St, stroke; Heter/ty, heterogeneity; and NS, non-significant.
$p=0.02$.
¶ $p=0.002$.
* $p<0.00001$.
& $p<0.001$.
$ $p=0.1$.
@ $p=0.009$.

(iii) Urgent carotid revascularization procedure (within 2 weeks from symptom onset) should be performed in patients with symptomatic extracranial carotid artery stenosis independent of the presence of MES on TCD-monitoring [44].

Conclusions

Numerous studies using different definitions have shown that END is common in ACI and is associated with adverse functional outcomes. The causes of END may be stratified in two major groups: hemodynamic and non-hemodynamic. The four main hemodynamic causes of END include: cardiac complications, arterial reocclusion, intracranial arterial steal phenomenon and cerebral microembolization. TCD can reliably detect reocclusion in real-time offering us the opportunity to pursue alternative reperfusion strategies. Intracranial arterial steal/RRHS can also be detected by TCD during voluntary breath-holding or using acetazolamide-challenged perfusion CT or HMPAO SPECT. RRHS and sleep-disordered breathing in ACI may represent linked therapeutic targets that potentially could be managed using non-invasive ventilatory correction. TCD can also reliably detect in real-time MES in cerebral circulation that have been independently associated with higher risk of recurrent stroke in patients with ACI. Aggressive antiplatelet therapy may be considered in patients with symptomatic carotid stenosis and MES on TCD, while urgent carotid revascularization procedure (within 2 weeks from symptom onset) should be performed in patients with symptomatic extracranial carotid artery stenosis independent of the presence of MES on TCD-monitoring.

References

[1] Siegler JE, Martin-Schild S. Early neurological deterioration (END) after stroke: the END depends on the definition. Int J Stroke 2011;6:211–2.

[2] Toni D, Fiorelli M, Zanette EM, Sacchetti ML, Salerno A, Argentino C, et al. Early spontaneous improvement and deterioration of ischemic stroke patients: A serial study with transcranial Doppler ultrasonography. Stroke 1998;29:1144–8.

[3] Davalos A, Toni D, Iweins F, Lesaffre E, Bastianello S, Castillo J, et al. Neurological deterioration in acute ischemic stroke: potential predictors and associated factors in the European Cooperative Acute Stroke Study (ECASS) I. Stroke 1999;30:2631–6.

[4] Grotta JC, Welch KM, Fagan SC, Lu M, Frankel MR, Brott T, et al. Clinical deterioration following improvement in the NINDS rt-PA Stroke Trial. Stroke 2001;32:661–8.

[5] Kwan J, Hand P. Early neurological deterioration in acute stroke: clinical characteristics and impact on outcome. QJM 2006;99:625–33.

[6] Weimar C, Mieck T, Buchthal J, Ehrenfeld CE, Schmid E, Diener HC, et al. Neurologic worsening during the acute phase of ischemic stroke. Arch Neurol 2005;62:393–7.

[7] Saposnik G, Hill MD, O'Donnell M, Fang J, Hachinski V, Kapral MK, et al. Variables associated with 7-day, 30-day, and 1-year fatality after ischemic stroke. Stroke 2008;39:2318–24.

[8] Prosser J, MacGregor L, Lees KR, Diener HC, Hacke W, Davis S. Predictors of early cardiac morbidity and mortality after ischemic stroke. Stroke 2007;38:2295–302.

[9] Kumar S, Selim MH, Caplan LR. Medical complications after stroke. Lancet Neurol 2010;9:105–18.

[10] Vemmos KN, Tsivgoulis G, Spengos K, Zakopoulos N, Synetos A, Manios E, et al. U-shaped relationship between mortality and admission blood pressure in patients with acute stroke. J Intern Med 2004;255:257–65.

[11] Leonardi-Bee J, Bath PM, Phillips SJ, Sandercock PA, IST Collaborative Group. Blood pressure and clinical outcomes in the International Stroke Trial. Stroke 2002;33:1315–20.

[12] Sandset EC, Bath PM, Boysen G, Jatuzis D, Kõrv J, Lüders S, et al. The angiotensin-receptor blocker candesartan for treatment of acute stroke (SCAST): a randomised, placebo-controlled, double-blind trial. Lancet 2011;377:741–70.

[13] Alexandrov AV, Grotta JC. Arterial reocclusion in stroke patients treated with intravenous tissue plasminogen activator. Neurology 2002;59:862–7.

[14] Rubiera M, Alvarez-Sabín J, Ribo M, Montaner J, Santamarina E, Arenillas JF, et al. Predictors of early arterial reocclusion after tissue plasminogen activator-induced recanalization in acute ischemic stroke. Stroke 2005;36:1452–6.

[15] Burgin WS, Alexandrov AV. Deterioration following improvement with tPA therapy: carotid thrombosis and re-occlusion. Neurology 2001;56:568–70.

[16] Baracchini C, Manara R, Ermani M, Meneghetti G. The quest for early predictors of stroke evolution: can TCD be a guiding light? Stroke 2000;31:2942–7.

[17] Qureshi AI, Siddiqui AM, Kim SH, Hanel RA, Xavier AR, Kirmani JF, et al. Reocclusion of recanalized arteries during intra-arterial thrombolysis for acute ischemic stroke. Am J Neuroradiol 2004;25:322–8.

[18] Rubiera M, Cava L, Tsivgoulis G, Patterson DE, Zhao L, Zhang Y, et al. Diagnostic criteria and yield of real-time transcranial Doppler monitoring of intra-arterial reperfusion procedures. Stroke 2010;41:695–9.

[19] Tsivgoulis G, Saqqur M, Demchuk AM, Rubiera M, Sharma VK, Molina CA, et al. Predictors of early arterial reocclusion in patients with acute proximal arterial occlusions treated with intravenous thrombolysis. Stroke 2009;40:e157.

[20] Fischer U, Arnold M, Nedeltchev K, Brekenfeld C, Ballinari P, Remonda L, et al. NIHSS score and arteriographic findings in acute ischemic stroke. Stroke 2005;36:2121–5.

[21] Zhao L, Rubiera M, Harrigan MR, Alexandrov AV. Arterial reocclusion and persistent distal occlusion after thrombus aspiration. J Neuroimaging 2010;10:1552–6569.

[22] Sugg RM, Pary JK, Uchino K, Baraniuk S, Shaltoni HM, Gonzales NR, et al. Argatroban tPA stroke study: study design and results in the first treated cohort. Arch Neurol 2006;63:1057–62.

[23] Pranevicius M, Pranevicius O. Cerebral venous steal: blood flow diversion with increased tissue pressure. Neurosurgery 2002;51:1267–74.

[24] Mosmans PC, Jonkman EJ. The significance of the collateral vascular system of the brain in shunt and steal syndromes. Clin Neurol Neurosurg 1980;82:145–56.

[25] Schwartz A, Hennerici M. Noninvasive transcranial Doppler ultrasound in intracranial angiomas. Neurology 1986;36:626–635.

[26] Tan TY, Schminke U, Chen TY. Hemodynamic effects of subclavian steal phenomenon on contralateral vertebral artery. J Clin Ultrasound 2006;34:77–81.

[27] Alexandrov AV, Sharma VK, Lao AY, Tsivgoulis G, Malkoff MD, Alexandrov AW. Reversed Robin Hood syndrome in acute ischemic stroke patients. Stroke 2007;38:3045–8.

[28] Tsivgoulis G, Sharma VK, Ardelt AA, Brenner D, Taylor M, Robinson A, et al. Reversed Robin Hood Syndrome: correlation of neurological deterioration with intracerebral steal magnitude. Stroke 2008;39:725.

[29] Sharma VK, Tsivgoulis G, Ahmad A, Paliwal PR, Teoh HL, Wong LY, et al. Validation of 'Reversed Robin Hood Syndrome'

by acetazolamide-challenged HMPA-SPECT in patients with severe steno-occlusive disease of intracranial carotid or middle cerebral artery. Stroke 2011;42:e227.

[30] Sharma VK, Teoh HL, Paliwal PR, Chong VF, Chan BPL, Sinha AK. Reversed Robin Hood Syndrome in a patient with luxury perfusion after acute ischemic stroke. Circulation 2011;123: e243—4.

[31] Alexandrov AV, Nguyen HT, Rubiera M, Alexandrov AW, Zhao L, Heliopoulos I, et al. Prevalence and risk factors associated with reversed Robin Hood syndrome in acute ischemic stroke. Stroke 2009;40:2738—42.

[32] Palazzo P, Balucani C, Barlinn K, Tsivgoulis G, Zhang Y, Zhao L, et al. Association of reversed Robin Hood syndrome with risk of stroke recurrence. Neurology 2010;75:2003—8.

[33] Tsivgoulis G, Zhang Y, Alexandrov AW, Harrigan MR, Sisson A, Zhao L, et al. Safety and tolerability of early noninvasive ventilatory correction using bilevel positive airway pressure in acute ischemic stroke. Stroke 2011;42:1030—4.

[34] Barlinn K, Alexandrov AV. Sleep-disordered breathing and arterial blood flow steal represent linked therapeutic targets in cerebral ischaemia. Int J Stroke 2011;6:40—1.

[35] King A, Markus HS. Doppler embolic signals in cerebrovascular disease and prediction of stroke risk: a systematic review and meta-analysis. Stroke 2009;40:3711—7.

[36] Markus HS, King A, Shipley M, Topakian R, Cullinane M, Reihill S, et al. Asymptomatic embolisation predicts stroke in asymptomatic carotid stenosis: the Asymptomatic Carotid Emboli Study (ACES). Lancet Neurol 2010;9:663—71.

[37] Markus HS, MacKinnon A. Asymptomatic embolization detected by Doppler ultrasound predicts stroke risk in symptomatic carotid artery stenosis. Stroke 2005;36:971—5.

[38] Hao Q, Leung WH, Leung C, Mok CT, Leung H, Soo Y, et al. The significance of microembolic signals and new cerebral infarcts on the progression of neurological deficit in acute stroke patients with large artery stenosis. Cerebrovasc Dis 2010;29:424—30.

[39] Tsivgoulis G, Alexandrov AV, Sloan MA. Advances in transcranial Doppler ultrasonography. Curr Neurol Neurosci Rep 2009;9:46—54.

[40] Iguchi Y, Kimura K, Kobayashi K, Ueno Y, Shibazaki K, Inoue T. Microembolic signals at 48 h after stroke onset contribute to new ischaemia within a week. Neurol Neurosurg Psychiatry 2008;79:253—325.

[41] Markus HS, Droste DW, Kaps M, Larrue V, Lees KR, Siebler M, et al. Dual antiplatelet therapy with clopidogrel and aspirin in symptomatic carotid stenosis evaluated using Doppler embolic signal detection: the clopidogrel and aspirin for reduction of emboli in symptomatic carotid stenosis (CARESS) trial. Circulation 2005;111:2233—40.

[42] Wong KS, Chen C, Fu J, Chang HM, Suwanwela NC, Huang YN, et al., CLAIR study investigators. Clopidogrel plus aspirin versus aspirin alone for reducing embolisation in patients with acute symptomatic cerebral or carotid artery stenosis (CLAIR study): a randomised, open-label, blinded-endpoint trial. Lancet Neurol 2010;9:489—97.

[43] Kaste M. Time matters for reducing risk of stroke. Lancet Neurol 2010;9:451—3.

[44] Brott TG, Halperin JL, Abbara S, Bacharach JM, Barr JD, Bush RL, et al. ASA/ACCF/AHA/AANN/AANS/ACR/ASNR/CNS/ SAIP/SCAI/SIR/SNIS/SVM/SVS guideline on the management of patients with extracranial carotid and vertebral artery disease: executive summary: a report of the American College of Cardiology Foundation/American Heart Association Task Force on practice guidelines, and the American Stroke Association, American Association of Neuroscience Nurses, American Association of Neurological Surgeons, American College of Radiology, American Society of Neuroradiology, Congress of Neurological Surgeons, Society of Atherosclerosis Imaging and Prevention, Society for Cardiovascular Angiography and Interventions, Society of Interventional Radiology Society of NeuroInterventional Surgery, Society for Vascular Medicine, and Society for Vascular Surgery. Stroke 2011;42:e420—63.

Transcranial Doppler in acute stroke management — A "real-time" bed-side guide to reperfusion and collateral flow

Christopher Levi [a,b,*], Hossein Zareie [a], Mark Parsons [a]

[a] *Centre for Translational Neuroscience & Mental Health Research, University of Newcastle & Hunter Medical Research Institute, Australia*
[b] *Director, Acute Stroke Services, John Hunter Hospital, Newcastle, NSW, Australia*

KEYWORDS
Transcranial Doppler;
Acute ischemic stroke;
Collateral flow;
Recanalization;
Microembolic signals

Summary

Introduction: Assessment of cerebral hemodynamics with transcranial Doppler (TCD) can provide real-time, bed-side assessment of important prognostic variables in acute stroke such as the status of collateral flow and vessel recanalization status. In acute middle cerebral artery (MCA) occlusion, anterior cerebral artery (ACA) flow diversion (FD) is correlated with leptomeningeal collateral flow and may be a clinically useful prognostic indicator. Continuous TCD monitoring of MCA recanalization may also provide useful prognostic information including changes in flow pattern and the occurrence of microembolic signals (MES). We present studies examining associations between ACA FD, MCA recanalization and MES patterns on the characteristics of ischemia and infarction in acute MCA stroke.

Methods: Patients studied were consecutive sub-6 h from onset internal carotid artery (ICA) territory ischemic stroke cases. A subset of these cases with MCA occlusion were studied with 2 h of continuous MCA monitoring. All patients underwent baseline multimodal computed tomographic (CT) scanning, baseline diagnostic TCD, and 24 h post stroke magnetic resonance (MR) imaging. All MCA occlusion patients studied with continuous monitoring were treated with intravenous thrombolysis. ACA flow diversion was defined as ipsilateral mean velocity of 30% or greater than the contralateral artery. Recanalization status was assessed using the Thrombolysis In Brain ischemic (TIBI) grading system and MES counted "off-line" by experienced observers. Leptomeningeal collateralisation (LMC) was graded on CT angiography. Infarct core and penumbral volumes were defined using CT perfusion thresholds. Infarct volume, reperfusion, and vessel status were measured at 24 h using MR techniques. In patients undergoing recanalization monitoring, comparison was made between those with and without major reperfusion. Multivariable regression analysis was performed to assess for any associations between ACA flow diversion, TIBI grades and MES on infarction controlling for other important clinical variables.

* Corresponding author at: Department of Neurology, John Hunter Hospital, Locked Bag No. 1., Hunter Regional Main Centre, 2310 NSW, Australia. Tel.: +61 249855593; fax: +61 249213488.
  E-mail address: christopher.levi@hnehealth.nsw.gov.au (C. Levi).

Results: Flow diversion: 53 patients qualified for FD analysis. ACA FD was associated with good collateral flow on CT angiography ($p < 0.001$) and was an independent predictor of admission infarct core volume ($p < 0.001$), and 24 h infarct volume ($p < 0.001$). The likelihood of a favourable outcome (modified Rankin score 0–2) was higher (Odds ratio = 27.5, $p < 0.001$) in those with flow diversion.

Recanalization monitoring: 27 patients with MCA occlusion treated with intravenous thrombolysis were included in the analysis of recanalization patterns (16 cases with major reperfusion, 11 cases of non-reperfusion). Major TIBI grade improvement ($\Delta \geq 3$ grades overall) was associated with major reperfusion ($p = 0.04$) excellent 90 day clinical outcome ($p = 0.03$), improvement in clinical outcome at 24 h ($p = 0.049$) and attenuated infarct growth ($p = 0.06$). MES did not associate with reperfusion status or outcome variables.

Conclusions: ACA FD is independently associated with the smaller infarction volumes and more favourable 90 day clinical outcome. Flow diversion may provide enhanced perfusion of ischemic tissue, offering some protection against infarct expansion and ''buying-time'' for effective reperfusion and tissue salvage.

Major TIBI grade improvement associates with major reperfusion, favourable 24 h and 90 day clinical outcomes along with a trend to smaller infarct volumes in patients treated with intravenous thrombolysis.

Acute bedside transcranial Doppler assessment of ACA FD and recanalization aids prognostication and therapeutic decision making in acute stroke.

© 2012 Published by Elsevier GmbH.

Introduction

Reperfusion therapies in acute ischemic stroke are becoming both more widely used and more varied. In routine clinical practice, intravenous thrombolysis is generally regarded as ''first-line'' therapy and is being delivered to over 20% of ischemic stroke patients in many centers [1]. Advances in endovascular therapies, in particular, the various mechanical thrombectomy techniques [2,3], are being increasingly applied and, although generally regarded as ''second-line'' treatment options based on the limited randomised evidence, have significant potential advantages over intravenous thrombolysis. With this increase in therapeutic options comes a need for development of validated methods for both selection of patients for specific therapies and also, the identification of patients not responding to intravenous thrombolysis. Advanced MR and CT imaging are well suited to guide initial patient selection for reperfusion therapy. Both techniques can provide information on the characteristics of vessel occlusion, collateral flow and the extent of both hypoperfusion and established infarction [4,5]. Both techniques have been used in randomised clinical trials and are now commonly used in routine clinical practice to identify likely ''responders'' to reperfusion therapy [6]. However, imaging methods for identifying ''non-responders'' to intravenous thrombolysis have been less well studied and currently no well validated or generally accepted approach exists.

Transcranial Doppler is well suited to the task of identifying both collateralisation and the time course and completeness of recanalization of the arteries of the circle of Willis [7]. Numerous studies [8] have examined characteristics and patterns of recanalization and its association with early neurological improvement. Recent advances in multimodal CT and MR imaging now allow more detailed investigation and understanding of the potential role for TCD in guiding acute stroke therapy, where correlation is possible between important TCD characteristics and important clinical surrogates such as reperfusion and infarct core growth.

Leptomeningeal collateralisation (LMC) is a recognised determinant of tissue fate in patients with acute anterior circulation ischemic stroke [9–14]. The status of LMC as measured on catheter angiography in middle cerebral artery occlusion (MCAO) has been shown to influence brain perfusion and clinical outcomes [12,15]. Collateral flow in MCAO measured using CT angiography (CTA) has been demonstrated to influence the volume of ischemic penumbra measured on CT perfusion (CTP) and clinical outcome [16]. In MCA occlusion, flow is commonly diverted from the distal internal carotid artery (ICA) to the ACA [11,17–20]. This flow diversion (FD) can be detected using TCD, where typically, a higher velocity flow in the ipsilateral ACA can be measured as compared with that of the contralateral ACA [17,20–24]. A retrospective review of data of patients with a proximal MCA occlusion from the CLOTBUST trial demonstrated that ACA FD was associated with earlier and better neurological improvement, supporting the hypothesis that FD may provide nutrient flow to the ischemic brain [23].

To further clarify the potential clinical role for TCD in selecting patients for reperfusion therapies we investigated

1. The relationship between ACA-FD on TCD, LMC status on CTA, and measures of the acute perfusion lesion and extent of infarction.
2. The relationship between TCD features of recanalization and major reperfusion, infarct growth attenuation and clinical outcomes.

Patients and methods

Patients

The overall study population is a prospective cohort of consecutive TCD examinations in acute anterior circulation ischemic stroke patients presenting within 6 h of symptom onset. The cohort was collected between June 2007 and January 2010. Eligibility criteria were presence of a demonstrated occlusion of either MCA or ICA on baseline acute CTA in a patient undergoing assessment for potential suitability for intravenous thrombolytic therapy. A subgroup of patients with MCA occlusion and baseline TIBI grades ≤3 treated with intravenous thrombolysis was used to study recanalization features and MES characteristics. Patients were excluded if a pre-morbid Rankin score (mRS) was greater than 3 or serious co-morbid illness limited the patient's life expectancy, if posterior circulation stroke was suspected, of temporal acoustic windows were inadequate, if unilateral ACA hypoplasia or aplasia was evident on CTA (dominant ACA at least twice the size of the contralateral ACA [25,26]). Stroke severity was measured using the National Institutes of Health Stroke Scale (NIHSS). Patient outcome was determined using the NIHSS at 24 h from stroke onset modified Rankin scale at 90 days blind to imaging data. The study was approved by the institutional ethics committee and individual patient consent was obtained.

Baseline TCD examination

TCD ultrasound was performed using a digital power-motion Doppler unit (PMD 100, Spencer Technologies) with 2-MHz pulsed wave diagnostic transducers. The initial TCD examination was performed immediately prior to commencement of intravenous t-PA, or immediately following CT scanning in the case of those not eligible for thrombolysis. The insonation protocol was as follows: initially the non-affected MCA was insonated from a depth of 60—45 mm as a unidirectional signal towards the probe. This included M1 and M2 segments to determine the depths and velocity ranges and continued to bifurcation, terminal ICA (TICA), ACA and PCA. The proximal ACA waveform was determined from a depth of 60—70 mm as a unidirectional signal away from the probe. Next, the affected MCA waveform was determined and then the bifurcation, TICA, ACA and PCA. Flow measurements for ACA FD were taken at ACA A1 segment (depth 60—70 mm) as a flow away from the probe. The ophthalmic arteries (depths: 40—50 mm) and ICA siphons (55—65 mm) were then checked for flow direction and pulsatility through the transorbital windows bilaterally [27].

Peak systolic, diastolic and mean flow velocities and pulsatility indices were measured off-line. FD was considered present when the ipsilateral ACA mean blood flow velocity was at least 30% greater than that of the contralateral ACA [20,22]. All TCD studies and measurements were attended by an experienced sonographer (DQ) who remained blind to CT and MR imaging data. Baseline measurements and vessel segment insonation were checked where appropriate by another experienced sonographer (CRL).

Middle cerebral artery TCD monitoring and recanalization characteristics

Unilateral TCD monitoring was also performed using the digital power-motion Doppler unit (PMD 100, Spencer Technologies) with a 2-MHz pulsed wave transducer fixed in place using the Spencer Marc series head frame. The monitoring protocol was as follows: after determining TIBI grade of 3 or less, the sample volume length was set at 10 mm and insonation depth set immediately distal at the site of the commencement of attenuation in MCA waveform. Power output was set at the maximum permitted level; monitoring commenced immediately after commencement of intravenous thrombolysis and continued for 2 h. Continuous off-line review of recanalization status was performed by an experienced neurosonologist (HZ) and documentation of TIBI grades made a 5 minutely intervals through the 2 h monitoring period. Sudden major improvement in TIBI grade was defined as increase of ≥3 TIBI grades in <15 min. Full recanalization was defined as achievement of TIBI grades 4 or 5. All TCD analyses were performed blind to CT and MR imaging analyses.

MES were counted at off-line review of the by consensus human expert assessment (HZ and CRL) using standard acoustic and spectral criteria and also using PMD TCD criteria and related embolic signatures [28,29].

Brain imaging

CT scans were obtained with a multidetector scanner (16-slice Philips Mx8000). Whole brain noncontrast CT was performed: 120 kV, 170 mA, 2 s scan time, contiguous 6-mm axial slices. Perfusion CT (CTP) followed, comprising two 60-s series. Each series consisted of one image per slice per second, commencing 5 s after intravenous administration of 40 ml of non-ionic iodinated contrast at a rate of 5 ml/s via a power injector. Each perfusion series covers a 24 mm axial section acquired as two adjacent 12-mm slices. The first section was at the level of the basal ganglia/internal capsule, and the second was placed directly above, towards the vertex. Thus, the two perfusion CT series allows assessment of two adjacent 24 mm cerebral sections [30].

CT angiography

CTA was performed after CTP, using the parameters 120 kV, 125 mA, slice thickness 1.5 mm, pitch 1.5:1, helical scanning mode, intravenous administration of 70 ml of non-ionic contrast at 4 ml/s. Bolus-tracking software was used to maximise image acquisition at peak contrast arrival. Data acquisition was from base of skull to the top of lateral ventricles. Patients were selected if complete occlusion on CTA was present. Contrast within the distal MCA (beyond the occlusion) was presumed secondary to retrograde filling via leptomeningeal collaterals. Collateral status was divided into "good", "moderate" or "poor" based on degree of reconstitution of the MCA up to the distal end of its occlusion on CTA [16]. Moderate flow and poor collateral flow were graded together as "reduced".

MRI

Follow-up imaging used a 1.5 T MRI (Siemens Avanto). The stroke MRI protocol included an axial spin-echo T2-weighted series, an axial isotropic diffusion-weighted echoplanar spin-echo sequence (DWI), time of flight MR angiography

(MRA), and perfusion-weighted imaging (PWI) with an axial T2*-weighted echoplanar sequence [31].

Assessment of perfusion lesions and final infarct volumes

De-identified CTP and perfusion MR data were analysed with MIStar software using an identical deconvolution algorithm to generate both CTP and MR perfusion maps, including mean transit time (MTT) and cerebral blood volume (CBV) [30,31]. A MTT delay of >145% compared with the contra-lateral hemisphere was used to calculate automated CTP MTT lesion volumes [32]. Within the CTP MTT lesion, baseline infarct core volume was determined from CBF maps using an automated threshold of <40% normal tissue [5]. Thus, penumbral volume was determined from the difference between the baseline CTP MTT lesion and CBF lesions, and the "CTP mismatch" ratio was calculated from MTT lesion volume/CBV lesion volume (using the above thresholds for MTT and CBF lesion volumes). The same software was used to measure 24h infarct volume using automated signal intensity thresholds for MR-DWI, or Hounsfield unit thresholds for CT [31]. The follow-up infarct maps were co-registered with baseline CTP maps to obtain volumes from the same spatial position and axis orientation. To determine reperfusion, the automated threshold (MTT delay of >145% compared with contra-lateral hemisphere) was used to calculate 24h MR (or CTP)-MTT lesion volumes. The MR-MTT maps were co-registered with baseline CTP so that MR-MTT volumes were obtained from the same spatial position and axis orientation as the CTP-MTT maps. All lesion volumes were obtained from the average of measurements taken on separate occasions by a stroke neurologist and stroke fellow. Reperfusion was defined as "major" in patients with >80% reduction in baseline-24h MTT lesion volume and/or complete vessel recanalization [30,31]. All imaging analyses were performed blind to TCD data.

During the study a subgroup of patients were included in the randomised Tenecteplase in Stroke trial receiving either intravenous tenecteplase (0.1 mg/kg or 0.25 mg/kg as a bolus dose) or standard alteplase therapy within 6h of symptom onset [33].

Statistical analysis

Statistical analysis was performed using "Stata" (Version 10, College Station, TX 2007). Statistical comparisons between patients with and without FD were performed for the total sample (ICAOs and MCAOs, $n=53$) as well as for the MCAOs alone ($n=42$). Comparisons between patients with major reperfusion and no reperfusion were made in the subgroup pf patients with MCA occlusion treated with intravenous thrombolysis. Differences in continuous measurements were tested using the Mann—Whitney U test and differences in categorical outcomes were tested using the Fisher's exact test with two tailed p values. The impact of FD and TIBI grade on admission and 24h perfusion lesions, infarct volumes and clinical outcome was examined using regression analyses to adjust for potential confounding factors.

Results

Among 90 consecutive patients assessed for intravenous thrombolysis eligibility within 6h of stroke onset, 53 (42 of whom received thrombolytic therapy) were included in the analysis for ACA FD. A subgroup of 27 patients with MCA occlusion treated with intravenous thrombolysis was included in the analysis of recanalization characteristics. Patients were excluded due to lack of evidence of ICA or MCA occlusion on CTA [17], absence of temporal windows [11], incomplete or poor quality CTA [4], PCA occlusion [1] or aplastic or hypoplastic ACA [3], and non-stroke [1]. Occlusion site was determined by CTA and included 42 M1/M2 occlusions and 11 intracranial ICA occlusions. Baseline characteristics of the main sample and MCA thrombolysis subgroup are shown in Tables 1 and 2.

Flow diversion

Significant FD to the ACA was present in 24/53 (45%) patients and to the PCA in 8/38 (21%) patients. Because adequate insonation of both PCAs was not possible in 15/53 (28%) of patients, further analysis of PCA FD was not undertaken. The differences in admission and outcome variables between groups defined by the presence or absence of FD are displayed in Table 3.

The presence of ACA FD was strongly associated with a CTA good collateral flow grade; 18 of 23 (78%) with good CTA collaterals had an ACA ratio greater than 1.3. However, 23 of 26 (88%) with reduced CTA collaterals had an ACA FD ratio less than 1.3 (Odds ratio 27.6, $p<0.001$).

Twenty-four hour core infarct expansion (Δ core >5 ml between baseline and 24h imaging) was also strongly

Table 1 Baseline characteristics of all patients presenting with acute anterior circulation ischemic stroke studied with TCD ($n=53$).

Variables	
Age, years[a]	72 (65—79)
Male gender[b]	30 (56.6)
Admission National Institution Health Stroke Score; mean (SD)	17 (4.9)
History of hypertension[b]	39 (74)
Atrial fibrillation by history or ECG[b]	22 (42)
History of myocardial infarction or ischemic heart disease[b]	23 (43)
History of previous stroke[b]	13 (25)
History of diabetes mellitus[b]	8 (15)
Current smoking[b]	8 (15)
Time from symptom onset to hospital arrival in minutes[a]	79 (60—114)
Time from hospital arrival to CT in minutes[a]	32 (20—50)
Time from CT to transcranial Doppler ultrasound in minutes[a]	44 (27—52)

[a] Median (IQR) values.
[b] Values are n (%); SD, standard deviation.

Table 2 MCAO thrombolysis subgroup — baseline characteristics by 24 h reperfusion status.

Baseline characteristics	Major reperfusion n = 16		Non-reperfusion n = 11		p
Mean age	71 years	SD 18.1	55.7	SD 19.1	p = 0.02
Female	56%		33%		
Mean NIHSS	15.8	SD 5.1	18.2	SD 3.7	p = 0.18
Median infarct core volume	17.6 ml	Range: 0.4—88.8	34.4 ml	Range: 0.4—77 ml	p = 0.15
Median perfusion lesion volume	110.6 ml	Range: 30.3—141.2	144 ml	Range: 59.1—169.8 ml	p = 0.007
Good collateral grade	50%		40%		p = 0.30
ACA flow diversion	44.40%		50%		p = 0.80
Mean systolic BP	152 mmHg	SD 20.5	150.6 mmHg	SD 26.8	
Mean diastolic BP	87 mmHg	SD 11.1	86.7 mmHg	SD 15.4	
Risk factors					
AF	50%		20%		
HT	61%		60%		
DM	11%		20%		
HC	27%		50%		
Current smoking	17%		20%		
Antithrombotic medication (%)					
Antiplatelet	27%		10%		
Warfarin	11%		0%		

associated with ACA FD where only 6 of 22 patients (27%) with an ACA FD ratio of greater than 1.3 had infarct core growth compared with 22 of 28 (78%) with ACA FD ratios of less than 1.3 (Odds ratio 9.7, $p < 0.001$). The presence of ACA FD may indicate a subgroup of patients with better collateral flow and a relatively stable ischemic penumbra.

After adjusting for occlusion site, stroke onset time to CT, age and gender, the two predictors of baseline infarct core volume on linear regression analysis were FD ($p < 0.001$) and acute NIHSS ($p = 0.002$). Predictors of penumbral volume, after adjusting for occlusion site, acute NIHSS, onset time to CT and gender, FD ($p < 0.001$) and younger age ($p = 0.016$) ($r^2 = 0.3707$) remained significant.

Table 3 Differences in admission and outcome variables between groups defined by the presence or absence of TCD detected flow diversion (FD).

	All patients (n = 53)					
	MCAO and ICAO (n = 53)			MCAO only (n = 42)		
	FD+ 24	FD− 29	p	FD+ 23	FD− 19	p
Good collaterals according to CTA[b]	21/24 (87.5)	6/29 (20.7)	<0.001	20/23 (87)	6/19 (32)	<0.001
Admission NIHSS[a]	16 (12—18.5)	18 (16—22)	0.024	16 (12—19)	17 (13—19)	0.454
Admission infarct core volume[a]	6.4 (4—15)	52.2 (26—80)	<0.001	6.2 (4—16)	36.1 (21—58)	0.001
Admission penumbral volume[a]	95.3 (78—113)	65.5 (33—76)	<0.001	93.9 (78—113)	69 (25—79)	0.002
Total perfusion lesion[a]	107.6 (87—130)	118 (85—146)	0.357	104 (86—131)	105 (48—142)	0.859
Mismatch ratio[a]	12.4 (8—27)	1.95 (1.8—3.4)	<0.001	12.3 (7.5—27)	2.7 (1.9—4)	<0.001
Thrombolysis[b]	22/24 (91.7)	20/29 (69)	0.086	21/23 (91)	17/19 (89)	1.000
Major recanalization/reperfusion[b]	16/23 (69.7)	16/29 (55)	0.392	16/22 (73)	12/19 (63)	0.737
Infarct expansion (ml)[a]	2.3 (−0.5 to 15)	38 (9—69)	0.001	1.9 (−0.5 to 5)	23 (3—84)	0.006
Final infarct volume (ml)[a]	14 (7—25)	92 (46—142)	<0.001	14 (7—20)	65 (25—143)	<0.001
24 h NIHSS[a]	4 (1—12)	17 (8—25)	<0.001	3 (1—12)	12 (4—19)	0.016
90 day mRS ≤ 2[b]	18/24 (75.0)	6/29 (21.7)	<0.001	17/23 (74)	6/19 (32)	0.012

FD+, anterior cerebral artery flow diversion positive; FD−, anterior cerebral artery flow diversion negative; CTA, computed tomography angiography; NIHSS, National Institute of Health Stroke Scale; mRS, modified Rankin score; mismatch ratio calculated by dividing mean transit time lesion volume by cerebral blood volume lesion volume.
[a] Median (IQR) values.
[b] Values are n (%).

Table 4 Predictors of favourable clinical outcome in patients following acute anterior circulation ischemic stroke.

Variable	mRS 0—2 n (%)	Unadjusted analysis		Adjusted analysis (stepwise regression)	
		Odds ratio (CI)	p value	Odds ratio (CI)	p value
Recanalization/reperfusion					
No (n = 20)	3 (15.0)	1.00		1.00	
Yes (n = 32)	21 (65.6)	10.3 (2.3—66.7)	<0.001	21.1 (2.0—1208)	0.005
Flow diversion					
No (n = 29)	6 (20.7)	1.00		1.00	
Yes (n = 24)	18 (75.0)	10.8 (2.7—51.3)	<0.001	27.5 (3.0—1451)	<0.001
Age		0.98 (0.94—1.02)	0.385		
Gender					
Female (n = 23)	14 (60.9)	1.00			
Male (n = 30)	10 (33.3)	0.33 (0.09—1.14)	0.085		
Admission National Institute of Health Stroke Scale score		0.78 (0.66—0.90)	<0.001	0.83 (0.67—1.01)	0.061
Stroke onset time to thrombolysis		0.99 (0.98—1.00)	0.136		
Stroke onset time to transcranial Doppler ultrasound		1.00 (0.99—1.00)	0.685		
Thrombolysis					
No (n = 11)	1 (9.1)	1.00			
Yes (n = 42)	23 (54.8)	11.6 (1.4—547.6)	0.014		
Middle cerebral artery occlusion					
No (n = 11)	0 (0.0)	1.00			
Yes (n = 42)	24 (57.1)	18.9 (2.8—∞)	<0.001		

CI, confidence interval (95%); mRS, modified Rankin score.

Predictors of 24 h infarct volume after adjusting for occlusion site, therapy with thrombolytic agent, and stroke onset to thrombolytic treatment time were: FD ($p < 0.001$), major reperfusion ($p < 0.001$) and lower acute NIHSS ($p = 0.02$) ($r^2 = 0.6689$).

Independent predictors of a favourable clinical outcome, as measured by 90 day mRS 0—2, were FD (OR 27.5, $p < 0.001$), major reperfusion (OR 21.1, $p = 0.005$; Table 4). All patients with ICAO as the site of vessel occlusion had a poor outcome.

Recanalization monitoring subgroup

The characteristics of the patients with MCA occlusion treated with intravenous thrombolysis are shown in Table 2. Patients with major reperfusion post-thrombolysis were significantly older than those with non-reperfusion (71 years vs 56 years, $p = 0.02$); however, the major reperfusion patients showed smaller perfusion lesion (111 ml vs 144 ml, $p = 0.007$) and a trend towards smaller infarct core volumes (18 ml vs 34 ml, $p = 0.15$) at baseline. TCD monitoring times were not significantly different between groups (major reperfusion, 103 min; non-reperfusion, 124 min; $p = 0.34$). Consistent with other studies, patients with major reperfusion showed smaller median 24 h infarct core volumes (28 ml vs 46 ml, $p = 0.005$), lower 24 h mean NIHSS score (12.1 vs 16.7, $p = 0.009$), and a higher proportion of patients with favourable 90 day functional outcomes (mRS 0—2, 63% vs 10%, $p = 0.002$).

The TIBI grade profiles for each case is shown in Fig. 1A and B. Major TIBI grade change (improvement by ≥3 grades during the post-thrombolysis monitoring period) was associated with major reperfusion ($p = 0.04$) along with higher odds of attenuation of infarct core growth ($p = 0.06$), improvement in NIHSS score ($p = 0.049$) and excellent 90 day functional outcome (mRS 0—1; $p = 0.03$). Major sudden TIBI grade change (improvement of ≥3 grades over ≤15 min) was associated with a trend towards excellent functional outcome (mRS 0—1; $p = 0.09$).

MES were detected in 36% proportion of cases overall, 37% in the patients with major reperfusion and 33% in patients with non-reperfusion ($p = 0.55$). There was no association between the presence of microemboli and major TIBI grade change, 24 h infarct core volume or clinical outcomes.

Discussion

This is the first description of the relationship between TCD features of leptomeningeal collateralisation and recanalization, hyperacute brain perfusion status, and their relationships to tissue fate and clinical outcomes in acute ischemic stroke. Our data demonstrate that the ACA FD is associated with improved LMC and is independently associated with 24 h infarct volume and 90 day clinical outcome in acute anterior circulation stroke patients with identifiable large artery occlusion. ACA FD may therefore define a group of patients who have a greater tolerance to ICA or MCA occlusion and, potentially, a longer-lived ischemic penumbra. Our data also demonstrate that in MCA occlusion patients treated with intravenous thrombolysis, major improvement in TIBI grade is associated with major reperfusion at 24 h

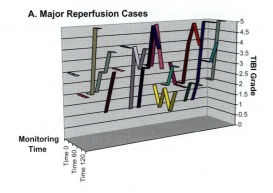
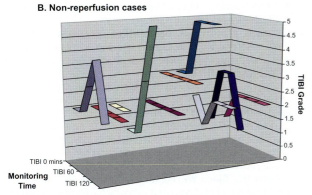

Figure 1 Comparison of TIBI grade change over time post intravenous thrombolysis between patients with major reperfusion (A) and non-reperfusion (B). Reperfusion measured at 24 h post intravenous thrombolysis using MR perfusion. Major reperfusion defined as >80% reperfusion of baseline perfusion lesion volume.

along with improved 24 h and 90 day clinical outcome and a trend towards less infarct core growth.

Flow diversion

Although definitions and indices of ACA flow diversion vary in the literature [17,20—23] the ACA asymmetry index used by Zanette [20], based on comparison between digital cerebral angiography and TCD performed within 6 h of stroke onset, is likely to be the most reliable and easily applicable measure in hyperacute stroke. The same asymmetry index was used to define TCD FD in the retrospective analysis of the CLOT-BUST trial. In this study, FD was observed in 83% of patients with MCAO treated with tissue plasminogen activator therapy. This patient population excluded cases with ICAO and also those cases with early TCD measured recanalization, but noted that FD was associated with early neurological improvement [23]. To date no other published acute stroke studies have correlated TCD FD with CT angiographic measures of collateral flow, nor have examined associations with perfusion lesion volumes and long-term functional outcome.

We did not find any significant association between the presence of FD and the total volume of the perfusion lesion despite the admission NIHSS being lower in patients with ACA FD. In contrast, we demonstrated a strong and independent association between FD and the volume of the CTP defined infarct core. This finding suggests the importance of collateral flow and its TCD correlate in predicting acute infarct volume [34] and clinical outcome.

Patients with ICA occlusion are more likely to have compromised ACA collateral flow. This was demonstrated in the results, where, 55% of patients with combined ICA + MCA occlusion showed no FD as opposed to 42% of patients with MCA occlusion showing no FD (derived from Table 2).

When accompanied by major reperfusion, FD significantly increased the chances of a favourable outcome in keeping with other reports of a potential synergistic effect between LMC and major reperfusion [12,16]. In our study, 43% of FD positive patients who did not undergo major reperfusion had a favourable outcome suggesting that LMCs are capable, in some patients, of perfusing the territory of an occluded artery to a level sufficient to avoid infarction even without complete recanalization [11], ACA FD therefore appears to be a rapid onset internal protection mechanism for the ischemic area, mitigating infarct core expansion.

Recanalization monitoring

TCD is recognised to accurately reflect recanalization status of the MCA when compared to catheter angiography [35] and TCD defined TIBI recanalization grades recognised to correlate with baseline stroke severity and clinical recovery [36]. There is, however, limited data describing recanalization characteristics in the initial hours following acute MCA stroke and no data correlating TCD recanalization characteristics with reperfusion status and the extent of early infarction. Alexandrov et al. [37] described a cohort of 65 patients treated with intravenous tissue plasminogen activator within 3 h of stroke onset and monitored with TCD post-thrombolysis. Similar to our findings, major improvements in TIBI grades (in this study over time periods of less than 30 min) were associated with significantly lower 24 h post-thrombolysis NIHSS. Using transcranial colour coded duplex (TCCD) the Duplex Sonography in Acute Stroke Study group performed TCCD 30 min and 6 h post-thrombolysis in patients with a variety of ICA and MCA occlusion patterns [38]. In this patient group, cases showing recanalization assessed by TIBI grade change also showed significant improvements in 24 h NIHSS when compared to those without TCCD features of recanalization.

Studies examining use of transcranial ultrasound in guiding clinical decision in acute stroke are also limited. In the small sample of patients entered into the Intervention Management of Stroke (IMS) trial, MCA blood flow velocity ratios comparing the affected to unaffected artery accurately identified angiographic lesions amenable to endovascular therapy [39]. The clinical relevance and application of this finding are uncertain.

We have identified only one study evaluating the use of TCCD as a decision-assistance aid in identifying intravenous thrombolysis treated patients who require triage to endovascular reperfusion therapy. Sekoranja et al. [40] examined patients treated with intravenous thrombolysis for MCA occlusion (TIBI grade 0—3 at baseline) monitored with intermittent TCCD. At 30 min post-commencement of intravenous thrombolysis, lack of improvement by at least 1 TIBI grade was used to shift management to endovascular management. Although uncontrolled, the study showed that favourable long-term outcome (mRS 0—2) was achieved in the acceptable proportions of patients (59%) where intravenous therapy alone was continued. This assuming a TIBI grade of at least 3 was achieved at 30 min post-intravenous thrombolysis. For those patients triaged to endovascular therapy on the basis of lack of any TIBI improvement at 30 min, 56% of patients had a favourable long-term outcome.

MES were commonly detected during the process of recanalization; however, in this relatively small sample of patients, the occurrence of MES did not associate with more effective reperfusion, 24 h infarct volumes neither improved early nor improved late clinical outcomes.

Conclusion

The growth in endovascular reperfusion therapy options in acute stroke is driving a need for more sophisticated imaging approaches to gauge both the time-frame of survival of the ischemic penumbra and the effectiveness of "first-line" intravenous thrombolytic therapies. In MCA stroke the use of TCD to gauge the adequacy of collateral flow and the effectiveness of thrombolysis-induced recanalization holds promise as a clinically useful test. Further validation is needed through both observational studies using both clinical and imaging outcome measures and ideally, randomised studies evaluating TCD-guided decision assistance.

Acknowledgements

We would like to thank the patients and family members involved in this study and members of the John Hunter Hospital acute stroke team, in particular Debbie Quain, neurosonologist. This work was supported by: Hunter New England Local Health District, Hunter Medical Research Institute, University of Newcastle, the National Stroke Foundation (Australia) and the National Health & Medical Research Council (Australia).

References

[1] Quain DA, Parsons MW, Loudfoot AR, Spratt NJ, Evans MK, Russell ML, et al. Improving access to acute stroke therapies: a controlled trial of organised pre-hospital and emergency care. Med J Aust 2008;189(October (8)):429—33.

[2] Smith WS, Sung G, Starkman S, Saver JL, Kidwell CS, Gobin YP, et al. Safety and efficacy of mechanical embolectomy in acute ischemic stroke: results of the MERCI trial. Stroke 2005;36(July (7)):1432—8.

[3] The Penumbra Pivotal Stroke Trial Investigators. The Penumbra Pivotal Stroke Trial: safety and effectiveness of a new generation of mechanical devices for clot removal in intracranial large vessel occlusive disease. Stroke 2009;40(August (8)):2761—8.

[4] Parsons MW, Christensen S, McElduff P, Levi CR, Butcher KS, De Silva DA, et al. Pretreatment diffusion- and perfusion-MR lesion volumes have a crucial influence on clinical response to stroke thrombolysis. J Cereb Blood Flow Metab 2010;30(June (6)):214—25.

[5] Bivard A, McElduff P, Spratt N, Levi C, Parsons M. Defining the extent of irreversible brain ischemia using perfusion computed tomography. Cerebrovasc Dis 2011;31(3):238—45.

[6] Davis SM, Donnan GA, Parsons MW, Levi C, Butcher KS, Peeters A, et al. Effects of alteplase beyond 3 h after stroke in the Echoplanar Imaging Thrombolytic Evaluation Trial (EPITHET): a placebo-controlled randomised trial. Lancet Neurol 2008;7(April (4)):299—309.

[7] Alexandrov AV, Demchuk AM, Wein TH, Grotta JC. Yield of transcranial Doppler in acute cerebral ischemia. Stroke 1999;30(August (8)):1604—9.

[8] Zanette EM, Roberti C, Mancini G, Pozzilli C, Bragoni M, Toni D. Spontaneous middle cerebral artery reperfusion in ischemic stroke. A follow-up study with transcranial Doppler. Stroke 1995;26(3):430—3.

[9] Bang OY, Saver JL, Buck BH, Alger JR, Starkman S, Ovbiagele B, et al. Impact of collateral flow on tissue fate in acute ischemic stroke. J Neurol Neurosurg Psychiatry 2008;79(June (6)):625—9.

[10] Bozzao L, Fantozzi LM, Bastianello S, Bozzao A, Fieschi C. Early collateral blood supply and late parenchymal brain damage in patients with middle cerebral artery occlusion. Stroke 1989;20(June (6)):735—40.

[11] Brozici M, van der Zwan A, Hillen B. Anatomy and functionality of leptomeningeal anastomoses: a review. Stroke 2003;34(November (11)):2750—62.

[12] Christoforidis GA, Mohammad Y, Kehagias D, Avutu B, Slivka AP. Angiographic assessment of pial collaterals as a prognostic indicator following intra-arterial thrombolysis for acute ischemic stroke. AJNR Am J Neuroradiol 2005;26(August (7)):1789—97.

[13] Roberts HC, Dillon WP, Furlan AJ, Wechsler LR, Rowley HA, Fischbein NJ, et al. Computed tomographic findings in patients undergoing intra-arterial thrombolysis for acute ischemic stroke due to middle cerebral artery occlusion: results from the PROACT II Trial * editorial comment: results from the PROACT II Trial. Stroke 2002;33(June (6)):1557—65.

[14] Maas MB, Lev MH, Ay H, Singhal AB, Greer DM, Smith WS, et al. Collateral vessels on CT angiography predict outcome in acute ischemic stroke. Stroke 2009;40(September (9)):3001—5.

[15] Kucinski T, Koch C, Eckert B, Becker V, Kromer H, Heesen C, et al. Collateral circulation is an independent radiological predictor of outcome after thrombolysis in acute ischemic stroke. Neuroradiology 2003;45(January (1)):11—8.

[16] Miteff F, Levi CR, Bateman GA, Spratt N, McElduff P, Parsons MW. The independent predictive utility of computed tomography angiographic collateral status in acute ischemic stroke. Brain 2009;132(August (Pt 8)):2231—8.

[17] Brass LM, Duterte DL, Mohr JP. Anterior cerebral artery velocity changes in disease of the middle cerebral artery stem. Stroke 1989;20(December (12)):1737—40.

[18] Ishikawa S, Handa J, Meyer JS, Huber P. Hemodynamics of the circle of Willis and the leptomeningeal anastomoses: an electromagnetic flowmeter study of intracranial arterial occlusion in the monkey. J Neurol Neurosurg Psychiatry 1965;28(April):124—36.

[19] Mattle H, Grolimund P, Huber P, Sturzenegger M, Zurbrugg HR. Transcranial Doppler sonographic findings in middle cerebral artery disease. Arch Neurol 1988;45(March (3)):289—95.

[20] Zanette EM, Fieschi C, Bozzao L, Roberti C, Toni D, Argentino C, et al. Comparison of cerebral angiography and transcranial Doppler sonography in acute stroke. Stroke 1989;20(July (7)):899—903.

[21] Demchuk AM, Christou I, Wein TH, Felberg RA, Malkoff M, Grotta JC, et al. Specific transcranial Doppler flow findings related to the presence and site of arterial occlusion. Stroke 2000;31(January (1)):140—6.

[22] Kim Y, Sin DS, Park HY, Park MS, Cho KH. Relationship between flow diversion on transcranial Doppler sonography and leptomeningeal collateral circulation in patients with middle cerebral artery occlusive disorder. J Neuroimaging 2009;19(January (1)):23—6.

[23] Kim YS, Meyer JS, Garami Z, Molina CA, Pavlovic AM, Alexandrov AV. Flow diversion in transcranial Doppler ultrasound is associated with better improvement in patients with acute middle cerebral artery occlusion. Cerebrovasc Dis 2006;21(1—2):74—8.

[24] Kaps M, Damian M, Teschendorf U, Dorndorf W. Transcranial Doppler ultrasound findings in middle cerebral artery occlusion. Stroke 1990;21:532—7.

[25] Kayembe KN, Hazama SMF. Cerebral aneurysms and variations in the circle of Willis. Stroke 1984;15(5):846—50.

[26] Kwon HMLY. Transcranial Doppler sonography evaluation of anterior cerebral artery hypoplasia or aplasia. J Neurol Sci 2005;231(1—2):67—70.

[27] Demchuk AMA. Acute ischemic stroke. In: Alexandrov, editor. Cerebrovascular ultrasound in stroke prevention and treatment. New York: Blackwell Publishing; 2004. p. 170—80.

[28] Markus HS, Ackerstaff R, Babikian V, Bladin C, Droste D, Grosset D, et al. Intercenter agreement in reading Doppler embolic signals. A multicenter international study. Stroke 1997;28(July (7)):1307—10.

[29] Saqqur M, Dean N, Schebel M, Hill MD, Salam A, Shuaib A, et al. Improved detection of microbubble signals using power M-mode Doppler. Stroke 2004;35(1):e14—7.

[30] Parsons MW, Pepper EM, Chan V, Siddique S, Rajaratnam S, Bateman GA, et al. Perfusion computed tomography: prediction of final infarct extent and stroke outcome. Ann Neurol 2005;58(November (5)):672—9.

[31] Parsons MW, Pepper EM, Bateman GA, Wang Y, Levi CR. Identification of the penumbra and infarct core on hyperacute noncontrast and perfusion CT. Neurology 2007;68(March (10)):730—6.

[32] Wintermark M, Flanders AE, Velthuis B, Meuli R, van Leeuwen M, Goldsher D. Perfusion-CT assessment of infarct core and penumbra: receiver operating characteristic curve analysis in 130 patients suspected of acute hemispheric stroke. Stroke 2006;37(April (4)):979—85.

[33] Parsons MW, Miteff F, Bateman GA, Spratt N, Loiselle A, Attia J, et al. Acute ischemic stroke: imaging-guided tenecteplase treatment in an extended time window. Neurology 2009;72(March (10)):915—21.

[34] Parsons MW, Christensen S, McElduff P, Levi CR, Butcher KS, De Silva DA, et al. Pretreatment diffusion- and perfusion-MR lesion volumes have a crucial influence on clinical response to stroke thrombolysis. J Cereb Blood Flow Metab 2010;30(June (6)):1214—25.

[35] Burgin WS, Malkoff M, Felberg RA, Demchuk AM, Christou I, Grotta JC, et al. Transcranial doppler ultrasound criteria for recanalization after thrombolysis for middle cerebral artery stroke. Stroke 2000;31(5):1128—32.

[36] Demchuk AM, Burgin WS, Christou I, Felberg RA, Barber PA, Hill MD, et al. Thrombolysis in Brain Ischemia (TIBI) transcranial Doppler flow grades predict clinical severity early recovery, and mortality in patients treated with intravenous tissue plasminogen activator. Stroke 2001;32(January (1)):89—93.

[37] Alexandrov AV, Burgin WS, Demchuk AM, El-Mitwalli A, Grotta JC. Speed of intracranial clot lysis with intravenous tissue plasminogen activator therapy: sonographic classification and short-term improvement. Circulation 2001;103(June (24)):2897—902.

[38] Wunderlich MT, Goertler M, Postert T, Schmitt E, Seidel G, Gahn G, et al. Recanalization after intravenous thrombolysis: does a recanalization time window exist? Neurology 2007;68(17):1364—8.

[39] Saqqur M, Shuaib A, Alexandrov AV, Hill MD, Calleja S, Tomsick T, et al. Derivation of transcranial Doppler criteria for rescue intra-arterial thrombolysis: multicenter experience from the Interventional Management of Stroke study. Stroke 2005;36(4):865—8.

[40] Sekoranja L, Loulidi J, Yilmaz H, Lovblad K, Temperli P, Comelli M, et al. Intravenous versus combined (intravenous and intra-arterial) thrombolysis in acute ischemic stroke: a transcranial color-coded duplex sonography — guided pilot study. Stroke 2006;37(7):1805—9.

Cerebral autoregulation in acute ischemic stroke

Matthias Reinhard[a,*], Sebastian Rutsch[a], Andreas Hetzel[a,b]

[a] Department of Neurology, University of Freiburg, Germany
[b] Department of Neurology, Park Klinikum, Bad Krozingen, Germany

KEYWORDS
Cerebral autoregulation;
Acute cerebral ischemia;
Transcranial Doppler sonography

Summary Cerebral autoregulation is particularly challenged in acute ischemic stroke. In this review we summarize the data of our previous studies on autoregulation regarding the effect of rtPA on autoregulation after stroke. A pooled analysis of two studies (45 patients) has shown a worsening of the autoregulatory index Mx between an early (first 48 h) and late (days 5–7) measurement. This increase was more pronounced on affected sides than on unaffected sides. Poor ipsilateral Mx was associated with a greater volume of MCA infarction at a late measurement and related to poor clinical outcome. Overall, autoregulatory impairment tends to increase mainly in large infarction and generalize to the contralateral side during the first days after ischemic stroke. As a limitation, transcranial Doppler sonography does not allow to detect focal areas of dysautoregulation in smaller strokes. To better understand the temporal and spatial dynamics of dysautoregulation in acute stroke in relation to the type and size of infarction, new bedside hemodynamic monitoring techniques (like multi-channel near-infrared spectroscopy) are needed.
© 2012 Elsevier GmbH. All rights reserved.

Introduction

Cerebral autoregulation is particularly challenged during acute ischemic stroke. Working autoregulation is important both during the acute vessel occlusion and during the reperfusion phase. Potential changes in autoregulatory capacity are considered in the treatment of blood pressure in ischemic stroke [1].

Dynamic autoregulation allows to noninvasively assess the autoregulatory capacity in acute stroke. Thereby, spontaneous fluctuations in blood pressure and cerebral blood flow velocity (assessed by transcranial Doppler sonography) are analyzed to extract information about how quickly and appropriately autoregulatory action occurs [2]. A recent systematic review of TCD autoregulation studies in acute ischemic stroke revealed a considerable heterogeneity in autoregulation methodology and time points of measurement [3]. Most of the included studies comprised a small number of patients with various types and locations of ischemic stroke.

In this review we summarize data of our previous studies on autoregulation assessed by TCD in acute ischemic stroke. We focus on the time course of autoregulation in acute stroke and clinical factors associated with autoregulation in acute stroke and will discuss future challenges in the field of autoregulation in acute stroke.

Methods

This review comprises a total of 45 patients from two previous studies [4,5]. Patients were admitted with acute ischemic stroke in the middle cerebral artery (MCA) territory

* Corresponding author at: Department of Neurology, University of Freiburg, Neurocenter, Breisacherstr. 64, D-79106 Freiburg, Germany.
E-mail address: matthias.reinhard@uniklinik-freiburg.de (M. Reinhard).

to our stroke unit and had no relevant obstructive carotid artery disease. The protocol for the studies included an early measurement of autoregulation (within 48 h after stroke onset) and a late measurement around days 5—7.

Flow velocity in both MCA was measured by TCD and blood pressure was recorded noninvasively via finger plethysmography. Cerebral autoregulation was assessed from spontaneously occuring fluctuations in blood pressure during a period of 10 min in each study. In this review we focus on results of the correlation coefficient analysis. With this approach (index Mx), mean values of ABP and CBFV are correlated by Pearson's correlation coefficient. In case of a high correlation, CBFV fluctuations depend on those of ABP. Higher Mx values thus reflect poorer autoregulation [6].

Results

The course of autoregulation during the first week after stroke onset

In a group of 45 patients with acute MCA stroke, the index Mx increased significantly between an early measurement within 48 h after stroke onset and a second (late) measurement around day 6 (late). This increase indicates worsening autoregulation and was larger on the MCA side affected by the stroke, but was also significant on the contralateral side (Fig. 1a). Group mean values did not differ from those of controls. A separate analysis of patients with large MCA stroke, however, showed that Mx is clearly impaired in the MCA ipsilateral to the stroke side around day 6 after stroke onset but not during the first day after stroke (Fig. 1).

The relation between autoregulation and clinical factors

Deteriorating autoregulation (increasing Mx) on ipsi- more than contralateral sides between days 1—2 and days 5—7 was

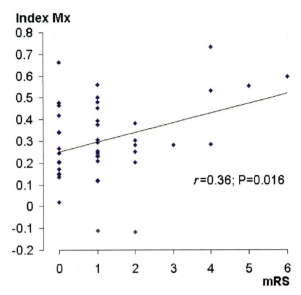

Figure 2 Relation between autoregulation (index Mx) and outcome after stroke. Data sets of 44 eligible patients from previous studies [7]. Pearson correlation between autoregulatory index Mx (higher values mean poorer autoregulation in the middle cerebral artery ipsilateral to the stroke) and outcome. The index Mx was measured around day 6 after stroke onset, outcome assessed after 4 ± 2 months by modified Rankin scale (mRS).

associated with larger infarcts [7]. Furthermore, there was a positive relation between poorer ipsilateral autoregulation and poorer clinical status (NIH stroke scale) at the early and late measurement. On contralateral sides, a similar but non significant trend was observed. Poorer autoregulation (higher Mx) around day 6 was associated with poorer outcome (Fig. 2). In a multivariate model, however, only infarction size remained a significant predictor for clinical

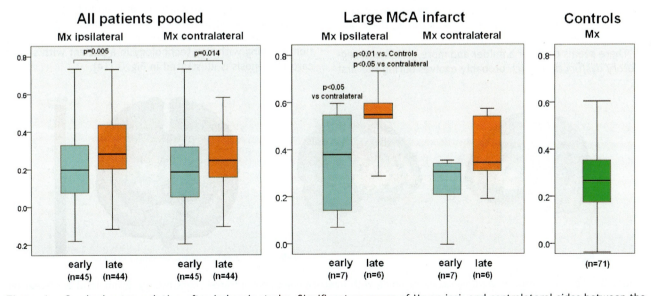

Figure 1 Cerebral autoregulation after ischemic stroke. Significant oncrease of Mx on ipsi- and contralateral sides between the early (first 48 h) and late (days 5—7) measurement after stroke onset [7]. Separate analysis of patients with poor outcome and large infarction ($62 \pm 21\%$ of MCA territory) [5]. Controls refer to 71 age-matched healthy persons (64 ± 9 years).

outcome. A separate detrimental effect of rtPA treatment on autoregulation after stroke was not found [5].

Discussion

The main findings of our studies so far is that dynamic autoregulation in acute stroke detected by TCD worsens over the first days after stroke onset (more on affected than unaffected sides) and that this worsening of autoregulation associates with a larger MCA infarct size and poorer outcome.

Various other studies have generally shown mild to moderate impairment of dynamic autoregulation affecting the MCA ipsi- and contralateral to the ischemic stroke [8,9]. Previous TCD studies on autoregulation in stroke did not consider the actual size of infarction [9,10].

When using TCD for measuring dynamic autoregulation in acute ischemic stroke, two mechanisms need to be considered: 1. *Local dysautoregulation* related to the affected stroke territory. Within the infarction core, cerebral autoregulation is probably severely disturbed in the early stages. Tissue lactate acidosis leads to local vasoparalysis, compromising the autoregulatory mechanism in both the ischemic core and the direct periinfarct region [11]. Such a presumed early impairment is, however, not univocally detected by the index Mx in larger strokes in our studies. The Mx value rather indicated a secondary decline in autoregulation after reperfusion mainly in large infarcts. This means that either autoregulation in the area of large infarction becomes worse, or that additional areas within the territory become involved. Such a pattern of secondary deterioration was also reported in a study using invasive autoregulation monitoring of malignant MCA stroke [11]. A vicious cycle of reperfusion, producing inflammatory vasotoxic substances, dysautoregulation, edema and further ischemia has been discussed [5,11]. Whether such a mechanism also exists for smaller MCA infarctions cannot be determined by transcranial Doppler sonography. However, an impairment within large areas of the MCA territory seems unlikely in this situation, because TCD recordings in the MCA should then have produced clearly pathological results.

There seems to occur a milder and more *global autoregulatory dysfunction* which probably evolves during the first days after ischemic stroke. Studies in which autoregulation in the MCA was measured once within four days of MCA- or non-MCA-territory stroke onset found a bilateral reduction in dynamic autoregulatory capacity independent of infarct type and vascular risk factors [9,10]. Such changes were not detectable for static autoregulation, leading to the assumption that dynamic autoregulatory measures are more sensitive to general vascular dysfunction in acute stroke [10]. The reason for this general impairment, which seems to be limited to dynamic autoregulation, is not clear. Pre-existing endothelial dysfunction may exacerbate within an acute phase response shortly after cortical ischemic stroke [12], when inflammatory or autonomic changes additionally affect the cerebral vasculature. In a further study, we found that secondary impairment of autoregulation in the subacute stage after stroke was associated with alterations in the neurovascular coupling mechanism outside the infarcted area using functional magnetic resonance imaging [13]. This underlines the assumption of a secondary endothelial dysfunction leading to both impaired autoregulation and impaired neurovascular coupling. A general autoregulatory dysfunction could thus potentially interfere with functional restitution and thus affect the clinical outcome [13].

We have indeed found an association between impaired autoregulation after ischemic stroke and clinical outcome. The association between autoregulation and outcome might, however, be linked via the size of MCA infarction. However, the infarction size in the current cohort of patients was mainly derived from demarcated lesions visualized by follow-up imaging. Dysautoregulation could still have contributed to the final size of infarction.

A main methodological problem of the studies reported here is the low spatial resolution of TCD. A small infarct within the MCA territory could also lead to severe focal dysautoregulation without a clear autoregulatory impairment in the main stem of the MCA. To better understand the spatial characteristics of impaired autoregulation in ischemic stroke (focal versus global dysautoregulation) we need new bedside hemodynamic monitoring techniques with a high spatial resolution. One promising but technically demanding method is multi-channel near-infrared spectroscopy. A first example of noninvasive autoregulation mapping with this technology in a patient with severe carotid stenosis is illustrated in Fig. 3 [14].

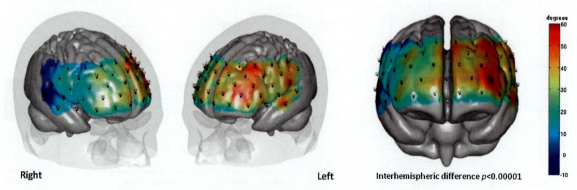

Figure 3 Spatially resolved autoregulation mapping with multi-channel near infrared spectroscopy. Example of a 68-year-old patient with near occlusion of left internal carotid artery [14]. Dynamic autoregulation is graded from the phase shift between respiratory-induced 0.1 Hz oscillations in ABP and oxy-hemoglobin. Autoregulation is impaired on the side ipsilateral to the stenosis and this is most prominent in the borderzone between middle cerebal and anterior cerebral artery.

Conclusions

Impairment of dynamic autoregulation detected by TCD in acute ischemic stroke is associated with larger MCA stroke and a poor clinical status. It tends to worsen and generalize during the initial post-stroke days and associates with poor clinical outcome. To better understand the temporal and spatial dynamics of dysautoregulation in acute stroke in relation to the type and size of infarction, new bedside hemodynamic monitoring techniques (like multi-channel near-infrared spectroscopy) are needed.

References

[1] Guidelines for management of ischaemic stroke and transient ischaemic attack 2008. Cerebrovasc Dis 2008;25(5):457—507.
[2] Panerai RB. Transcranial Doppler for evaluation of cerebral autoregulation. Clin Auton Res 2009;19:197—211.
[3] Aries MJ, Elting JW, De Keyser J, Kremer BP, Vroomen PC. Cerebral autoregulation in stroke. A review of transcranial Doppler studies. Stroke 2010;41(11):2697—704.
[4] Reinhard M, Roth M, Guschlbauer B, Harloff A, Timmer J, Czosnyka M, et al. Dynamic cerebral autoregulation in acute ischemic stroke assessed from spontaneous blood pressure fluctuations. Stroke 2005;36:1684—9.
[5] Reinhard M, Wihler C, Roth M, Harloff A, Niesen WD, Timmer J, et al. Cerebral autoregulation dynamics in acute ischemic stroke after rtPA thrombolysis. Cerebrovasc Dis 2008;26:147—55.
[6] Reinhard M, Roth M, Muller T, Czosnyka M, Timmer J, Hetzel A. Cerebral autoregulation in carotid artery occlusive disease assessed from spontaneous blood pressure fluctuations by the correlation coefficient index. Stroke 2003;34:2138—44.
[7] Reinhard M, Rutsch S, Lambeck J, Wihler C, Czosnyka M, Weiller C, et al. Dynamic cerebral autoregulation associates with infarct size and outcome after ischemic stroke. Acta Neurol Scand 2011:10—0404.
[8] Dawson SL, Panerai RB, Potter JF. Serial changes in static and dynamic cerebral autoregulation after acute ischaemic stroke. Cerebrovasc Dis 2003;16:69—75.
[9] Eames PJ, Blake MJ, Dawson SL, Panerai RB, Potter JF. Dynamic cerebral autoregulation and beat to beat blood pressure control are impaired in acute ischaemic stroke. J Neurol Neurosurg Psychiatry 2002;72:467—72.
[10] Dawson SL, Blake MJ, Panerai RB, Potter JF. Dynamic but not static cerebral autoregulation is impaired in acute ischaemic stroke. Cerebrovasc Dis 2000;10:126—32.
[11] Dohmen C, Bosche B, Graf R, Reithmeier T, Ernestus RI, Brinker G, et al. Identification and clinical impact of impaired cerebrovascular autoregulation in patients with malignant middle cerebral artery infarction. Stroke 2007;38:56—61.
[12] Stevenson SF, Doubal FN, Shuler K, Wardlaw JM. A systematic review of dynamic cerebral and peripheral endothelial function in lacunar stroke versus controls. Stroke 2010;41:e434—42.
[13] Altamura C, Reinhard M, Vry MS, Kaller CP, Hamzei F, Vernieri F, et al. The longitudinal changes of BOLD response and cerebral hemodynamics from acute to subacute stroke. A fMRI and TCD study. BMC Neurosci 2009;10:151.
[14] Rutsch S, Schelter B, Kaller CP, Timmer J, Hetzel A, Reinhard M. Spatial mapping of dynamic cerebral autoregulation with multichannel near infrared spectroscopy. Cerebrovasc Dis 2010;29(Suppl. 1):51.

Vertebral artery hypoplasia and the posterior circulation stroke

Andrea Skultéty Szárazová [a,*], Eva Bartels [b], Peter Turčáni [a]

[a] *University Hospital of Bratislava, 1st Neurological Clinic, Bratislava, Mickiewicziva 13, Slovakia*
[b] *Center for Neurological Vascular Diagnostics, München, Germany*

KEYWORDS
Posterior circulation stroke;
Vertebral artery hypoplasia (VAH);
Ultrasound;
Duplex ultrasonography;
Magnetic resonance angiography (MRA);
Computed tomography angiography (CTA)

Summary The aim of this preliminary study is to evaluate the hypothesis of a possible causal link between the anatomical findings of vertebral artery hypoplasia (VAH) and the incidence of posterior circulation stroke. We used full ultrasonographic examination to evaluate patients with stroke in the vertebrobasilar circulation territory over a period of 1.5 years. The diameter equal or less than 2.5 mm (in V1 and V2 segment of the vertebral artery) was set as a feature of vertebral artery hypoplasia. Magnetic resonance imaging and angiography (MRI and MRA) or computed tomography and angiography (CT and CTA) were performed to confirm the anatomic variation of hypoplasia and the site of the cerebral ischemic territory. In the group of 44 stroke patients, 9 (20%) had a hypoplastic vertebral artery and 35 (80%) were without VAH. Although vertebral artery hypoplasia in previously published literature is seldom shown as a leading risk factor for stroke in vertebrobasilar (posterior) circulation, its occurrence is not negligible and in coexistence with known risk factors of stroke may increase the negative clinical impact. Vertebral artery hypoplasia can be diagnosed non-invasively with duplex ultrasonography. It is therefore a useful method for detection of this anatomic variation and for follow-up examination.
© 2012 Published by Elsevier GmbH.

Introduction

The vertebral artery (VA) as a part of the vertebrobasilar cerebral circulation is one of the main branches of the subclavian artery. The course of the VA is divided into 4 sections [1,2]. It originates as section V0 from the posteromedial part of the arc of the subclavian artery and continues cranially. It is followed by the prevertebral segment (V1), which in 90% enters into the costotransverse foramen of the sixth cervical vertebra (C6). Variations as entrance in the C5 or above the C6 vertebra, coiling or kinking of the vertebral artery can occur. The intervertebral segment (V2) passes through the costotransverse canal of the cervical vertebrae up to the C2 vertebra. The atlas loop segment (V3) is created by a curved course of the artery around the atlas. The intracranial segment V4 is the section of the vertebral artery after penetrating the atlantooccipital membrane, dura mater and arachnoidea. At the clivus the right and left vertebral artery merge to form the basilar artery, which is a part of the intracranial posterior circulation.

The diameter of vertebral arteries varies from 1.5 to 5.0 mm. Identical width of VA occurs in 25% of the population, in 65% the left vertebral artery is wider, whereas in the remaining 10% the right vertebral artery is larger [3]. Khan et al. found dominance of the left vertebral artery in 50%, and of the right vertebral artery in 25% in regard to the diameter of the vessel [4].

* Corresponding author.
  E-mail address: aszarazova@gmail.com (A.S. Szárazová).

The following congenital anatomic variations of the vertebral artery are described in the literature: vertebral artery aplasia and vertebral artery hypoplasia (VAH). Aplasia of VA occurs in about 1% of the population [5].

Vertebral artery hypoplasia (VAH) is classified as a vessel with a diameter in the entire course of less than 2 mm [6], respectively less than 3 mm [7], or with a side difference equal or greater than 1:1.7 [8]. Additionally to the vessel diameter, another criterion contains reduced blood flow velocity and increased resistance index values in the ultrasonographic findings [1,9]. There is a tendency of compensatory increase in the vessel diameter of the contralateral vertebral artery of more than 5 mm [1]. These various definitions of the incidence of VAH are based on subsequent characteristics: a diameter of less than 2 mm was observed by the method of duplex ultrasonography by the authors Delcker and Diener in 1.9% of the population [6], a diameter of less than 3 mm was described by Touboul et al. in 6% of the population [7]. Trattnig et al. set a side asymmetry in the ratio 1:1.7 for more than 10% of patients examined by ultrasonography [8]. Frequency of VAH (diameter equal or less than 2 mm) in the general population is 26.5% in unilateral and 1.6% in bilateral hypoplasia of the vertebral artery [10]. In terms of side difference, the right hypoplastic vertebral artery occurs in 6.2% of the population, while left vertebral hypoplasia is present less frequently in 4.5% [2]. Visualization of vertebral artery is possible by ultrasonographic examination, by invasive or non-invasive angiography (MRA, CTA), and also by autopsy findings. As mentioned previously, a more narrow vessel lumen is present in the ultrasonographic image in vertebral artery hypoplasia, and additionally, blood flow parameters are defined by a reduced diastolic flow velocity associated with higher peripheral resistance. The resistance index (RI) is equal to or greater than 0.75. The peak systolic velocity (PSV) is usually less than 40 cm/s [1,5].

In the literature, morphological variations of the vertebral artery are described as being associated with different clinical symptoms. Nevertheless, vertebral hypoplasia as a possible risk factor for pathology, particularly of stroke in the vertebrobasilar circulation territory, was little emphasized yet.

The aim of this preliminary study is to evaluate a hypothesis of a possible causal link between the anatomical findings of VAH and the incidence of posterior circulation stroke. For this purpose, we assessed the relative frequencies of posterior circulation strokes in patients with VAH as compared to patients without VAH, and also the relative frequencies of the conventional vascular risk factors (hypertension, diabetes, hyperlipidemia and smoking). Additionally, we determined the possible mechanism of stroke in our patients.

Materials and methods

A group of 44 patients (30 men, 14 women; mean age 67 years [range 44–88]) with acute ischemia in the vertebrobasilar territory had a full ultrasonographic examination of the extra- and intracranial arteries between September 2009 and February 2011.

The location of the acute ischemic infarct was judged clinically and confirmed by CT scan or MRI.

We excluded patients with transient ischemic attacks (TIA), patients with other vertebral artery findings (such as atheromatosis, stenosis or occlusion) or other cerebral lesions, as well as those in whom a full ultrasonographic examination of the vertebral arteries was not possible.

We used a 7.5-MHz linear array transducer for the duplex ultrasonographic examination of the vertebral arteries (B-mode and color-coded duplex flow imaging). In the V1 (prevertebral) and V2 (intervertebral) segments of the extracranial vertebral artery the distance between the internal layers of the parallel walls of the vessel (caliber of VA) and the hemodynamic characteristics of blood flow were measured.

The diameter equal or less than 2.5 mm, respectively the side difference equal or greater than 1:1.7 were set as a feature of vertebral artery hypoplasia. Additionally, reduced flow velocities as compared to the contralateral side, and higher peripheral resistance ipsilaterally (RI equal or greater than 0.75) were considered.

MRA, CTA or conventional angiography was performed to confirm the presence or absence of the anatomic variation of hypoplasia.

We also investigated the occurrence of other concomitant vascular risk factors such as hypertension, diabetes, hyperlipidemia and smoking.

Results

In the group of 44 posterior circulation stroke patients, 9 (20%) had a hypoplastic vertebral artery and 35 (80%) were without VAH (Fig. 1A). There was more frequent right-sided VAH in 7 (78%), as compared to left-sided VAH in 2 (22%) cases (Fig. 1B). One patient had bilateral VAH (both vertebral arteries had a diameter of less than 2.5 mm), more significant on the right side. None of the patients had basilar artery hypoplasia. In the group of non-VAH patients were 22 men and 13 women, in the VAH group 8 men and 1 woman (Fig. 1C). There was a slight difference for age between the non-VAH (mean age 68.3 years) and VAH group (mean age 62.3 years).

The distribution of other vascular risk factors in both groups was represented as follows (Fig. 1D): hypertension (n = 40 patients), diabetes mellitus (n = 19), hyperlipidemia (n = 17) and smoking (n = 16).

The frequency of the presence of these risk factors (hypertension: p = 0.99; diabetes mellitus: p = 0.26 and smoking: p = 0.45) in patients with posterior circulation strokes with or without VAH did not differ.

We found that in the group of patients without VAH hyperlipidemia occurred more often than in the VAH group (16:1). There was a statistically significant relationship between finding of non-VAH and hyperlipidemia (p = 0.027).

Possible mechanism of stroke were embolism, especially cardioembolism (n = 10), atherosclerotic changes of vessels (small vessel disease n = 16, or large vessel disease n = 25). In 6 cases, the mechanism of stroke was cryptogenic (unknown mechanism n = 6) (Fig. 1E).

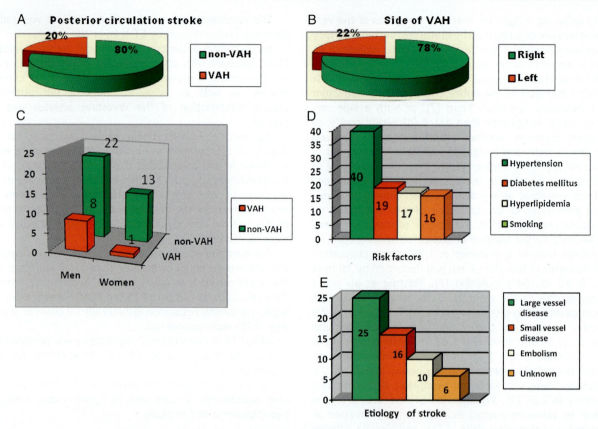

Figure 1 Descriptive statistics of the study data. (A) Percentage of the presence and absence of VAH (vertebral artery hypoplasia) in patients with posterior circulation stroke. (B) Percentage of vertebral artery hypoplasia location in patients with posterior circulation stroke. (C) The presence and absence of VAH (vertebral artery hypoplasia) by gender in the study group in absolute numbers. (D) The presence of risk factors (in absolute numbers) by patients with posterior circulation stroke in the study group (patients with more than one risk factor were present). (E) The representation of stroke etiology (in absolute numbers) by patients with posterior circulation stroke in the study group (a combination of different stroke mechanisms occurred).

The frequency of the presence of the stroke mechanisms (cardioembolism: $p = 0.69$; atherosclerotic changes of large vessels: $p = 0.14$) in non-VAH and VAH groups did not differ.

There was a non-significant tendency ($p = 0.053$) for atherosclerotic changes of small vessels to be more frequent in posterior circulation strokes with VAH than in non-VAH group (6:10).

We found no recurrent strokes of the posterior circulation over the 1.5-year period of this still ongoing study.

Discussion

Ischemic stroke localized in the vertebrobasilar circulation territory accounts for about a quarter of all ischemic strokes [11,12]. Mumenthaler describes the presence of ischemia in this localization in 15% of strokes [13]. The clinical significance of vertebral artery hypoplasia is currently not sufficiently recognized. Perren et al. carried out a study which examined 725 patients with established diagnosis of first ever stroke. Two thirds of ischemic events were localized in the carotid circulation and 247 patients had ischemia in the posterior fossa. Vertebral artery hypoplasia was observed in 13% of ischemic strokes in the posterior fossa, in the other localizations the presence of VAH was 4.6%. Based on these results, the authors conclude that the hypoplastic vertebral artery on one side (predominantly right — in the study group in 70%) is more frequently a possible risk factor for vertebrobasilar ischemia, as compared to other localizations of stroke. According to this, vertebral artery hypoplasia was considered as a risk factor, equivalent to other conventional risk factors such as hypertension, diabetes, smoking and hyperlipidemia [14]. In the article "Arterial occlusion — depending on the size (diameter) of blood vessels?" Caplan declared essential importance of baseline vessel diameter before subsequent obstruction of any etiology occurs [15]. He stated that a restricted artery (in the paired arteries) is more prone to closure, especially when other vascular risk factors are present. It is assumed that if this claim is true for carotid circulation territory [16], it is also highly likely in the vertebrobasilar localization. He based this argument on findings in the New England Medical Center Posterior Circulation Registry from 2004 [17], which proved the occurrence of ischemia in the area supplied by the vertebral artery (brainstem and posterior–inferior territory of cerebellum) located ipsilaterally to the narrower vertebral artery.

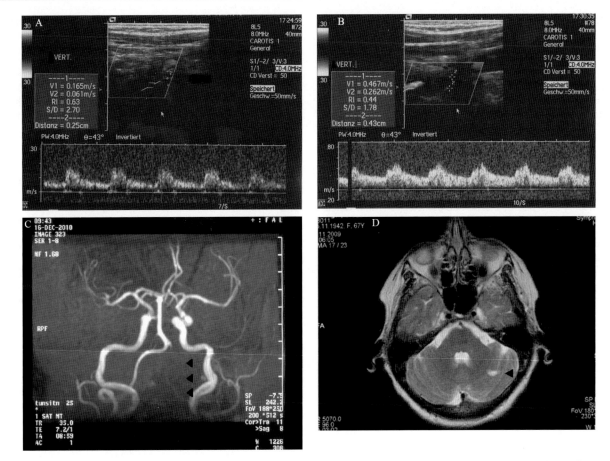

Figure 2 Findings in a 48 years old female patient of our study with a left-sided VAH and an ipsilateral cerebellar ischemia. (A) Ultrasonographic view of a V2 segment of a hypoplastic vertebral artery on the left side with a diameter of 2.5 mm and reduced blood flow velocity (max. syst. velocity 16.5 cm/s). (B) Ultrasonographic view of diameter (4.3 mm) and hemodynamic characteristics of a non-hypoplastic vertebral artery on the right side by the same patient. (C) Magnetic resonance angiography image of vertebral artery hypoplasia (black arrows) on the left side. The black arrows show an inadequate circulation. (D) Magnetic resonance view of ischemic focus in the left cerebellum (black arrow) in a patient with VAH (vertebral artery hypoplasia) on the left side.

Similar to Caplan's findings our results show that posterior circulation strokes occur more often ipsilateral to the VAH (Fig. 2A). The pathomechanism of ischemia in the presence of VAH has not yet been determined precisely. The clinical severity of VAH depends on how well the collateral supply functions, especially via the circle of Willis, and the sufficiency of the anterior circulation and of the cervical collaterals. The compensatory hyperplasia of the contralateral artery plays also an important role in maintaining an adequate blood supply to the brain, particularly in the posterior fossa. However, if the supplemental system fails, the compensatory mechanisms are exhausted and that can lead to stroke [1,5].

In our study we found that the distribution of vascular risk factors, except hyperlipidemia, was equal between the group with and without VAH. Therefore, we assume that VAH contributes as an additional risk factor to ischemic events in the posterior circulation, presumably due to hemodynamic reasons. Nevertheless, the relatively small sample size as a limitation to this study should be considered, when evaluating our results. In summary, the current data on this topic show that there is a tendency of coincidence of posterior circulation stroke and the presence of VAH. Further evidence regarding these findings and profound comprehension of the pathomechanism is needed.

Conclusions

As a result from our study we emphasize the need for increased attention that should be directed to hypoplastic vertebral arteries. It is not negligible, that the vertebral artery hypoplasia in coexistence with known risk factors for stroke may increase their negative clinical impact. Duplex sonography as an important diagnostic method may contribute to detect vertebral artery hypoplasia non-invasively.

Acknowledgments

This work was supported by the Framework Programme for Research and Technology Development, Project: Building of Centre of Excellency for Sudden Cerebral Vascular Events, Comenius University Faculty of Medicine in Bratislava (ITMS:26240120023), cofinanced by European Regional Development Fund.

References

[1] Bartels E. Color-coded duplex ultrasonography of the cerebral vessels. Stuttgart, NY: Schattauer; 1999. p. 43—58, p. 113—55, ISBN:3794517407.

[2] Krayenbühl HA, Yasargil GM. Die vaskulären Erkrankungen im Gebiet der Arteria Basialisqq. III. Variationen der A. Vertebralis, basialis und ihrer Äste. Stuttgart: Thieme; 1957. p. 37—52.

[3] Reurtern G-M, von Büdingen HJ. Ultrasound diagnosis of cerebrovascular disease. Stuttgart, NY: Thieme; 1993. p. 37—52.

[4] Khan S, Cloud GC, Kerry S, Markus HS. Imaging of vertebral artery stenosis: a systematic review. J Neurol Neurosurg Psychiatry 2007;78:1218—25.

[5] Školoudík D, Škoda O, Bar M. Neurosonologie. Praha: Galén; 2003. p. 12—151, ISBN:8072622455.

[6] Delker A, Diener HC. Die verschiedenen Ultraschallmethoden zur ntersuchung der Arteria vertebralis-eine vergleichende Wertung. Ultraschall Med 1992:13213—20.

[7] Touboul P-J, Bousser M-G, La Plane D, Castaigne P. Duplex scanning of normal vertebral arteries. Stroke 1986;17:921—3, 1986.

[8] Trattnig S, Schwaighofer B, Hübsch P, Schuster H, Polzleitner D. Color-coded sonography of vertebral arteries. J Ultrasound Med 1991;10:221—6.

[9] Bartels E. Farbkodierte Dopplersonographie der Vertebralarterien. Vergleich mit der konventionellen Duplexsonographie. Ultraschall Med 1992;13:59—66.

[10] park HJ, Kim JM, Roh JK. Hypoplastic vertebral artery: frequency and associations with ischaemic stroke territory. J Neurol Neurosurg Psychiatry 2007;78(September (9)):954—8.

[11] Bogousslavsky J, van Melle G, Regli F. The Lausanne Stroke Registry: analysis of 1,000 consecutive patients with first stroke. Stroke 1988;19:1083—92.

[12] Bamford J, Sandercock P, Dennis M, Burn J, Warlow C. Classification and natural history of clinically identifiable subtypes of cerebral infarction. Lancet 1991;337:1521—6.

[13] Mumenthaler M, Mattle H. Neurologie. Praha: Grada Publishing; 2001. p. 625.

[14] Perren F, Poglia D, Landis T, Sztajzel R. Vertebral artery hypoplasia: a predisposing factor for posterior circulation stroke? Neurology 2007;68(January (1)):65—7.

[15] Caplan LR. Arterial occlusions: does size matter? J Neurol Neurosurg Psychiatry 2007;78:916.

[16] Caplan LR, Baker R. Extracranial occlusive vascular disease: does size matter. Stroke 1980;11:63—6.

[17] Caplan LR, Wityk RJ, Glass TA, Tapia J, Pazdera L, Chang HM. New England Medical Center Posterior Circulation registry. Ann Neurol 2004:56389—98.

Volume flow rate

Disya Ratanakorn*, Jesada Keandaoungchan

Division of Neurology, Department of Medicine, Faculty of Medicine Ramathibodi Hospital, Mahidol University, Bangkok, Thailand

KEYWORDS
Volume flow rate;
Doppler method;
Color velocity imaging quantification;
Quantitative flow measurement system;
Angle-independent Doppler technique by QuantixND system

Summary Vascular imaging of carotid and vertebral arteries may not be sufficient to evaluate the patients with stroke and other cerebrovascular disorders. Cerebral blood flow measurement can add information to increase the accuracy in diagnosis, assessment, and plan of management in these patients. There are many noninvasive quantitative methods to measure cerebral blood flow including volume flow rate measured by ultrasound. This article addresses mainly the different ultrasound techniques to measure cerebral blood flow. Clinical applications, volume flow rate in normal and abnormal conditions with a case example, and advantage and disadvantage of the ultrasound techniques are also described.
© 2012 Elsevier GmbH. All rights reserved.

Introduction

Vascular imaging of carotid and vertebral arteries may not be sufficient to evaluate the patients with stroke and other cerebrovascular disorders. Cerebral blood flow (CBF) measurement can add information to increase the accuracy in diagnosis, assessment, and plan of management in these patients.

Methods for measurement of cerebral blood flow

There are many noninvasive quantitative methods to measure CBF including stable xenon-enhanced computed tomography, single-photon emission computed tomography, positron-emission tomography, and magnetic resonance imaging. These methods are reliable and accurate for CBF measurement. However, they are rather expensive and requiring to transfer patients to the imaging or radio-nuclei facility which may be a limitation in the critical ill, sedated, or ventilated patients [1].

Volume flow rate measurement by ultrasound

Several ultrasound methods have been used to measure volume flow rate (VFR) of CBF such as Doppler method [2], color velocity imaging quantification (CVIQ) [3], quantitative flow measurement system (QFM) [4,5], and angle-independent Doppler technique by QuantixND system [6]. The common carotid artery (CCA) is quite accessible and reliable to measure VFR, whereas it is more difficult to obtain reliable VFR in the internal carotid artery (ICA) or vertebral artery (VA) due to the deeper vessels. VFR measurements are usually obtained at 1.5–2.0 cm below carotid bifurcation in CCA, 1–2 cm above carotid bifurcation in ICA, and between the 4th and 5th cervical vertebra in the inter-osseous segment of VA using high-resolution linear probe with pulsed Doppler imaging [7].

Doppler method

Doppler method can estimate VFR at a specific point in a vessel by multiplying the flow velocity with cross-sectional lumen diameter at that specific point in time (Fig. 1). However, Doppler method does not provide a profile of instantaneous peak velocities across the entire vessel and

* Corresponding author. Tel.: +66 2 201 2318; fax: +66 2 201 1645.
E-mail address: radrt@mahidol.ac.th (D. Ratanakorn).

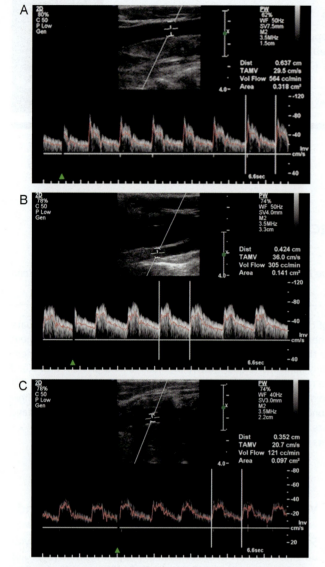

Figure 1 VFR measurements using Doppler method in CCA (A), ICA (B), and VA (C) with large sample volumes across the entire vessel lumens.

cannot adjust for changes in the flow lumen throughout the cardiac cycle.

Color velocity imaging quantification

CVIQ measures VFR by using time-domain processing with color velocity imaging combined with a synchronous M-mode color display to provide an instantaneous profile of the peak velocities across the flow lumen as well as a continuous estimate of the diameter of the flow lumen throughout the cardiac cycle (Fig. 2). By assuming a circular vessel and axial symmetrical flow, CVIQ can be calculated automatically with built-in software.

Quantitative flow measurement system

QFM is comprised of two components. One component uses one transducer with ultrasonic echo tracking to measure

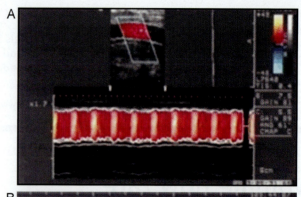

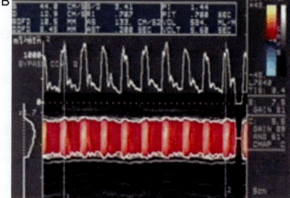

Figure 2 VFR measurement using CVIQ in CCA with the optimal color box across the entire lumen in M-mode display (A) and synchronous instantaneous peak velocities across the flow lumen (B).
With permission from Professor Charles H. Tegeler.

vessel diameter, and the other uses three transducers with continuous Doppler independent of incident angles to measure absolute blood flow velocity. QFM can be calculated using a vessel diameter in cross-sectional area and the absolute blood flow velocity.

Angle-independent Doppler technique by QuantixND system

QuantixND system is an angle-independent Doppler technique which employs dual ultrasound beams within one insonating probe in a defined angle to each other. The real time information is stored automatically and analyzed by the computer.

VFR measured by CVIQ and Doppler method

The mean values of VFR in 50 healthy subjects as measured by CVIQ and Doppler method are 340.9 ± 75.6 and 672.8 ± 152.9 ml/min for CCA, 226.9 ± 65.0 and 316.2 ± 89.1 for ICA, and 92.2 ± 36.7 and 183.5 ± 90.8 for ECA, respectively [2]. VFR is higher in male compared to those in female and decreasing with increasing age. Doppler method tends to overestimate VFR and CVIQ seems to be more accurate than Doppler method to measure the carotid artery VFR. However, CCA VFR measured by CVIQ and Doppler method has no difference in 0-95% ICA stenosis but CCA VFR by

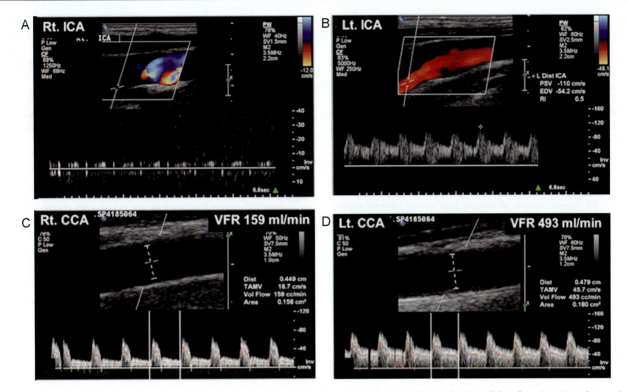

Figure 3 CCA VFR measured by Doppler method in a 46-year-old male with right ICA occlusion. Color flow imaging shows right ICA occlusion (A) and normal left ICA (B) with right CCA VFR of 159 ml/min (C), and left CCA VFR of 493 ml/min (D).

Doppler method is higher than that measured by CVIQ in 95–100% ICA stenosis [8].

Clinical applications

VFR measurement can be useful for grading carotid stenosis especially with coexisting contra-lateral carotid stenosis or occlusion to avoid overestimation of degree stenosis by using only flow velocity criteria, evaluating collateral flow and cerebrovascular reserve, identification of feeders and use as follow-up study in intra-cranial arteriovenous malformation, quantification of hemodynamic changes in subclavian steal syndrome, assessment of vasospasm in subarachnoid hemorrhage, and monitoring of CBF before and after carotid endarterectomy [9,10]. In addition, there is a direct correlation between middle cerebral artery mean flow velocity (MCA Vm), CCA VFR, and end-expiratory CO_2 in normal subjects. The MCA Vm and CCA VFR increase 6.1% and 5.3% per mmHg increase in end-expiratory CO_2, respectively, and the MCA Vm increases 0.3 cm/s for each 1 ml/min increase in CCA VFR [11]. Therefore, measurement of CCA VFR changes during CO_2 inhalation may be an alternative method to measure cerebral vasoreactivity in the patients with inadequate temporal windows.

VFR in carotid stenosis

CCA VFR measured by Doppler method and CVI-Q at different degree of carotid stenosis are 359 ± 130 and 337 ± 96 ml/min, respectively, for the individuals without ICA stenosis, 310 ± 99 and 293 ± 133 ml/min for 50–75% ICA stenosis, 347 ± 80 and 195 ± 131 ml/min for 75–95% ICA stenosis, 152 ± 36 and 63 ± 25 ml/min for 95–99% ICA stenosis, and 125 ± 47 and 58 ± 22 ml/min for ICA occlusion [8]. The reduction of ipsilateral CCA VFR is present in the patients with severe ICA stenosis of 75–99% or ICA occlusion as shown in Fig. 3.

Conclusions

When comparing with other brain perfusion imaging techniques, VFR obtained with ultrasound does not provide values for each brain region, but represents only one value for each supplying vessel [10]. It may be limited by operator dependent, extra examination time, requirement for patient cooperation, extensive plaque formation, turbulent flow, and tortuous and asymmetrical vessels. Nevertheless, VFR measured by ultrasound is still the easiest, feasible, noninvasive, and repeatable bedside examination with no exposure to contrast media or radiation.

Appendix A. Supplementary data

Supplementary data associated with this article can be found, in the online version, at http://dx.doi.org/10.1016/j.permed.2012.03.008.

References

[1] Markus HS. Cerebral perfusion and stroke. J Neurol Neurosurg Psychiatry 2004;75:353–61.

[2] Ho SSY, Metreweli C. Preferred technique for blood volume measurement in cerebrovascular disease. Stroke 2000;31:1342—5.
[3] Eicke BM, Tegeler CH, Howard G, Myers LG. In vitro reliablity of flow volume measurements with color velocity imaging. J Ultrasound Med 1993;12:543.
[4] Furuhata H, Sugano R, Kodaira K, Aoyagi T, Matsumoto H, Hayashi J, et al. An ultrasonic Doppler method designed for the measurement of absolute blood velocity values. Med Elec Bioeng 1978;16:264—8.
[5] Mizukami M, Yamaguchi K, Yunoki K. Evaluation of occlusive cerebrovascular disease using ultrasonic quantitative flow measurement. Stroke 1981;12:793—8.
[6] Schebesch KM, Simka S, Woertgen C, Brawanski A, Rothoerl RD. Normal values of volume flow in the internal carotid artery measured by a new angle-independent Doppler technique for evaluating cerebral perfusion. Acta Neurochir (Wien) 2004;146:983—6.
[7] Peter Scheel MD, Christian Ruge, Uwe R, Petruch MD, Martin Schöning MD. Color Duplex measurement of cerebral blood flow volume in healthy adults. Stroke 2000;31:147—50.
[8] Likittanasombut P, Reynolds P, Meads D, Tegeler C. Volume flow rate of common carotid artery measured by Doppler method and color velocity imaging quantification (CVI-Q). J Neuroimaging 2006;16:34—8.
[9] Tegeler CH, Ratanakorn D, Neurosonology. In: Fisher M, Bogousslavsky J, editors. Textbook of neurology. Newton, MA: Butterworth Heinemann; 1998. p. 101—18.
[10] Wintermark M, Sesay M, Barbier E, Borbély K, Dillon WP, Eastwood JD, et al. Comparative overview of brain perfusion imaging techniques. Stroke 2005;36:e83—99.
[11] Ratanakorn D, Greenberg J, Meads DB, Tegeler CH. Middle cerebral artery flow velocity correlates with common carotid artery volume flow rate after CO_2 inhalation. J Neuroimaging 2001;11:401—5.

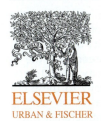
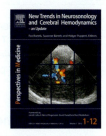

Bartels E, Bartels S, Poppert H (Editors):
New Trends in Neurosonology and Cerebral Hemodynamics — an Update.
Perspectives in Medicine (2012) 1, 207—210

journal homepage: www.elsevier.com/locate/permed

Intra- and extracranial stenoses in TIA — Findings from the Aarhus TIA-study: A prospective population-based study

Paul von Weitzel-Mudersbach [a,*], Soeren Paaske Johnsen [b], Grethe Andersen [a]

[a] The Department of Neurology, Aarhus Hospital, Aarhus University Hospital, Denmark
[b] The Department of Clinical Epidemiology, Aarhus University Hospital, Denmark

KEYWORDS
Transient ischemic attack;
Intracranial atherosclerosis;
Transcranial doppler sonography;
Prevalence

Summary

Background: Atherosclerotic stenoses of the intracranial arteries (ICAS) is associated with high risk of stroke after TIA. The prevalence of intracranial stenoses is considered to be low in Caucasians, however population-based data are lacking and only a minority of patients with acute TIA or stroke is evaluated for ICAS.

Methods: We prospectively examined the prevalence of stenoses of the pre- and intracerebral vessels using transcranial colour coded sonography (TCCS) in a population based cohort of all TIA patients in the community of Aarhus, Denmark in the period 1.3.2007—29.2.2008.

Results: The TIA cohort included 203 patients fulfilling the diagnostic criteria for TIA. We examined 195 patients with extra- and intracranial TCCD.

Any stenoses and symptomatic ICAS was found in 12.3% and 8.2%, respectively. The stenoses were located in the intracranial internal carotid artery in 3.6% and 3.1%, anterior cerebral artery in 0.5% and 0%, middle cerebral artery in 4.6% and 2.6%, intracranial vertebral artery in 2.1% and 1.5%, and in the basilar artery in 1.5% and 1.5%, respectively. In comparison, we found any stenoses and symptomatic stenoses in the extracranial carotid artery in 14.4% and 10.8%, and the extracranial vertebral artery in 5.6% and 2.1% of the patients, respectively. Carotid occlusion was found in 3.6%, combined extra- and intracranial stenoses in 4.9%.

Conclusion: The prevalence of ICAS was in this population-based TIA cohort of Caucasians comparable with the prevalence of carotid stenoses. Systematic evaluation for intracranial stenoses should be considered in all patients with acute ischemic cerebrovascular disease.
© 2012 Elsevier GmbH. All rights reserved.

Introduction

Stenoses in the intracranial vessels (ICAS), caused by atherosclerosis, are associated with a risk of stroke after TIA of 11—23% during the first year [1—3]. The prevalence of ICAS has been reported to be high in east Asian countries including Japan and China, but is supposed to be low in Caucasians

* Corresponding author at: Department of Neurology, Aarhus University Hospital, Aarhus Hospital, Nørrebrogade 44, 8000 Aarhus C, Denmark. Tel.: +45 20952953; fax: +45 89493300.
E-mail address: paulvonw@rm.dk (P. von Weitzel-Mudersbach).

2211-968X/$ — see front matter © 2012 Elsevier GmbH. All rights reserved.
doi:10.1016/j.permed.2012.02.013

[4—6]. However, population-based data on the prevalence of ICAS in Caucasian TIA-patients are not available.

In this study, we examined the prevalence of ICAS in a population based purely Caucasian cohort of TIA-patients by using TCCS.[1]

Material and methods

Study setting and design

We conducted this cohort study within the population served by the Department of Neurology, Aarhus University Hospital. The department serves as the only local stroke unit in the Aarhus area, which is clearly defined and mostly urban. The catchment area had 328,542 inhabitants in 2007. The Danish National Health Service provides tax-supported health care for all inhabitants, guaranteeing free access to general practitioners and hospitals. All acute medical conditions including TIA are exclusively treated at public hospitals, either as in or as outpatients.

Identification of TIA patients

We established an acute TIA-team, which served TIA-patients both on the stroke unit and the TIA-clinic. Patients with TIA symptoms during the preceding 48 h or crescendo TIA were admitted directly to the stroke unit and monitored for 1—2 days. All other patients were seen as outpatients 1—3 days after received referral.

TIA was defined as a sudden focal neurologic deficit of presumed vascular origin lasting less than 24 h.

Inclusion criteria were: TIA according to definition, residence in the Aarhus area, TIA during the last six months, and date of referral 1 March 2007—28 February 2008. Patients with a modified Rankin Score (mRS) >2 were excluded. Informed consent was obtained from all participants. All patients fulfilling the inclusion criteria for TIA were registered prospectively, including those admitted for suspected stroke but ending up as TIA.

Patient characteristics

The TIA diagnosis was made by a specialist. Patients underwent a neurological examination (more than 95% of the TIA patients were examined by the first author), CT or MR of the brain, ECG, laboratory tests and ankle brachial index. Furthermore, we performed duplex sonography of the extra- and intracranial vessels (TCCS). All ultrasound examinations were done by one experienced neurologist, performing at least 500 examinations per year and certified by the European Society of Neurosonoly and Cerebral Haemodynamics (ESNCH). Atherosclerosis of the carotid arteries was considered significant if a stenoses ≥50% was found (NASCET criteria). Intracranial stenoses were defined according to the criteria established by Baumgartner: stenoses in the anterior (ACA), middle (MCA) and posterior (PCA) cerebral artery was defined by peak systolic velocity of ≥120 cm/s, ≥155 cm/s, and ≥100 cm/s respectively, Stenoses in the VA and BA was defined by peak systolic velocity of ≥90 cm/s, and ≥100 cm/s respectively [7]. Additionally to these criteria, stenoses in ICA, and the extracranial VA was defined by systolic peak velocity ≥120 cm/s. All intracranial velocities were measured with an insonation angle of 0° without angle correction. A stenosis was considered symptomatic if a patient had TIA symptoms during the last six months before inclusion, related to the supply area of a carotid artery with a significant stenosis, or an extracranial vertebral or an intracranial stenosis according to the criteria above. Patients with combined extra- and intracranial stenoses e.g. ICA and MCA-stenoses on the symptomatic side were counted both as symptomatic ICA- and MCA-stenoses.

Hypertension was defined as history of hypertension or antihypertensive treatment, blood pressure systolic >140 mm Hg, or diastolic >90 mm Hg. Hypercholesterolemia was defined as total cholesterol >5.0 mmol/l, LDL cholesterol >3.0 mmol/l, or cholesterol lowering treatment. Diabetes was defined as history or treatment for diabetes, fasting glucose >6.9 mmol/l, or any glucose >10.9 mmol/l. Peripheral artery disease was defined as history of claudication, or ankle-brachial index <0.9.

Our study was approved by the local ethics committee (protocol number 20060188).

Results

We identified 203 patients fulfilling the diagnostic criteria for TIA. The characteristics of the patients are shown in

Table 1 Patient characteristics.

	TIA N = 203
Age	66.3 (range 19—93)
Male	109 (53.7%)
Smoking (active)	30.5%
High alcohol consumption	8.9%
Hypertension	71.9%
Diabetes	15.3%
Hypercholesterolaemia (>5 mmol/l)	82%
Atrial fibrillation	8.9%
All cardioembolic causes[a]	15.8%
PAD[b] (history or symptoms)	5.9%
PAD, incl. ABI[c] measurement	19.2%
History of MI[d]	7.4%
History of ischaemic heart disease including MI	12.3%
History of stroke	11.8%
History of TIA	10.4%

[a] Atrial fibrillation, dilated cardiomyopathy, mitral valve prolapse, patent oval foramen.
[b] PAD: peripheral arterial disease.
[c] ABI: Ankel brachial index.
[d] MI: myocardial infarction.

[1] Abbreviations: ICAS: stenosis in the intracranial vessels transcranial; TCCS: colour coded sonography; ACA: anterior cerebral artery; MCA: middle cerebral artery; PCA: posterior cerebral artery; VA: vertebral artery; BA: basilar artery; ICA: internal carotid artery.

Table 2 Frequencies of precerebral and intracranial stenoses in 195 TIA patients.

	All stenoses/occlusions (%)	Symptomatic stenoses (%)	Symptomatic occlusions (%)
All extra- and intracranial stenoses (N = 195)	27.2% (n = 53)	19.5% (n = 38)	3.1% (n = 6)
Extracranial common/internal carotid artery	16.4 (32)	10.8 (21)	3.1 (6)
Extracranial vertebral artery	5.6 [a] (11)	2.1 [a] (4)	
Intracranial carotid artery	3.6 (7)	3.1 (6)	
Anterior cerebral artery	0.5 (1)	0 (0)	
Middle cerebral artery	4.6 (9)	2.6 (5)	
Posterior cerebral artery	1.5 (3)	0 (0)	
Intracranial vertebral artery	2.1 (4)	1.5 (3)	
Basilar artery	1.5 (3)	1.5 (3)	
All intracranial stenoses	12.3 (24)	8.2 (16)	
Combined extra- and intracranial stenoses	4.9 (10)		

[a] Including one patient with vertebral artery dissection.

Table 1. In 195 patients we conducted TCCS of the pre- or intracranial vessels. In 39 patients the transcranial part of the examination was partly inconclusive due to insufficient bone window. Ultrasound contrast agents were not used in this study. Any stenoses or occlusion and symptomatic stenoses or occlusion was found in 27.2% and 22.6%, respectively. We found extracranial carotid artery stenoses in 14.4% and 10.4%, carotid occlusion in 4.1% and 3.1%, extracranial vertebral artery stenoses in 5.6% and 2.1% (including one dissection), and intracranial artery stenoses in 12.3% and 8.2%, respectively (Table 2).

Discussion

In our population-based TIA study, the prevalence of symptomatic ICAS diagnosed according to TCCS criteria was only slightly lower than the prevalence of symptomatic carotid stenosis. Furthermore, the estimated prevalence of ICAS may even be conservative due to the incomplete intracranial vascular assessment in 20% of the patients.

To the best of our knowledge, no other population-based data on the prevalence of ICAS are available. In the French SOS-TIA study, 1.823 unselected consecutive patients admitted at an acute TIA-clinic were examined with transcranial Doppler, and a prevalence of 8.8% for any ICAS or intracranial occlusion was found. Restricting the analysis in that study to patients defined as with definite TIA or minor stroke, the prevalence of ICAS increased to 11.5%, and about half of them were symptomatic [7].

In Denmark only a minority of patients with acute TIA or stroke is currently evaluated for ICAS. This may be explained by the assumption that intracranial atherosclerotic disease in Caucasians is rare, and by the lack of evidence for a specific treatment. Recently published data provides some evidence for the efficacy of dual platelet inhibition [8], and preliminary data on rapid and aggressive treatment seem to show a reduction of the risk of stroke in patients with TIA and intracranial stenoses [9]. Moreover, intra-arterial stenting may be an option in unstable ICAS not responding to medical treatment, even if this cannot be recommended as standard procedure [10].

Conclusion

The prevalence of ICAS in TIA-patients was substantial in a population-based cohort of Caucasians. The prevalence of symptomatic stenoses or occlusion was almost similar in the precerebral and intracerebral arteries, including a minor number of tandem stenoses in the pre- and intracerebral vessels. We suggest that a systematic screening with ultrasound examination for intracranial stenoses should be considered in all patients with acute ischaemic cerebrovascular disease.

Sources of funding

This study was supported by the Danish Heart Foundation and the Research Council in the former Aarhus County. None of the sponsors influenced the study design.

References

[1] Chimowitz MI, Lynn MJ, Howlett-Smith H, Stern BJ, Hertzberg VS, Frankel MR, et al. Comparison of warfarin and aspirin for symptomatic intracranial arterial stenosis. N Engl J Med 2005;352(March (13)):1305—16.
[2] Mazighi M, Tanasescu R, Ducrocq X, Vicaut E, Bracard S, Houdart E, et al. Prospective study of symptomatic atherothrombotic intra- cranial stenoses: the GESICA study. Neurology 2006;66(April (8)):1187—91.
[3] Kasner SE, Chimowitz MI, Lynn MJ, Howlett-Smith H, Stern BJ, Hertzberg V, et al. Predictors of ischemic stroke in the territory of a symptomatic intracranial arterial stenosis. Circulation 2006;113:555—63.
[4] Wong KS, Huang YN, Gao S, Lam WW, Chan YL, Kay R. Intracranial stenosis in Chinese patients with acute stroke. Neurology 1998;50(March (3)):812—3.
[5] Feldmann E, Daneault N, Kwan E, Ho KJ, Pessins MS, Langenberg F, et al. Chinese-white differences in the distribution of occlusive cerebrovascular disease. Neurology 1990;40(October (10)):1541—5.
[6] Mak W, Cheng TS, Chan KH, Cheung RTF, Ho SL. A possible explanation for the racial difference in distribution of large-arterial cerebrovascular disease: ancestral European settlers evolved genetic resistance to atherosclerosis, but confined to the intracranial arteries. Med Hypotheses 2005;65: 637—48.

[7] Baumgartner RW, Mattle HP, Schroth G. Assessment of ≥50% and <50% intracranial stenoses by transcranial color-coded duplex sonography. Stroke 1999;30(January (1)):87—92.

[8] Wong KS, Chen C, Fu J, Chang HM, Suwanwela NC, Huang YN, et al. Clopidogrel plus aspirin versus aspirin alone for reducing embolization in patients with acute symptomatic cerebral or carotid artery stenosis (CLAIR study): a randomised, open-label, blinded-endpoint trial CLAIR study investigators. Lancet Neurol 2010;9(May (5)):489—97.

[9] Meseguer E, Lavallée PC, Mazighi M, Labreuche J, Cabrejo L, Olivot JM, et al. Yield of systematic transcranial Doppler in patients with transient ischemic attacks. Ann Neurol 2010;68(July (1)):9—17.

[10] Chimowitz MI, Lynn MJ, Derdeyn CP, Turan TN, Fiorella D, Lane BF, et al. Stenting versus aggressive medical therapy for intracranial arterial stenosis. N Engl J Med 2011;365(September (11)):993—1003. Epub 2011 Sep 7.

Symptomatic intracranial stenosis: A university hospital-based ultrasound study

Federica Viaro*, Filippo Maria Farina, Angelo Onofri, Giorgio Meneghetti, Claudio Baracchini

Department of Neuroscience, University of Padua, Italy

KEYWORDS
Ischemic stroke;
Intracranial stenosis;
Atherosclerosis

Summary

Introduction: Stenosis of intracranial arteries are responsible for 30–50% of strokes in Orientals, 11% in Hispanics, 6% in Blacks and only 1% in Caucasians. However, the clinical importance of intracranial stenosis in Whites may have been underestimated.

Subjects and methods: We examined our database registry of all TIA/ischemic stroke Caucasian patients over a two-year period, from January 1st 2009 to December 31st 2010. All patients underwent a complete cervical and intracranial ultrasound assessment, MRA and/or CTA and/or DSA.

Results: Among 292 patients (males 79.7%; mean age, 71.0 ± 12.8 years), we found 59 (20.2%) subjects harboring at least one intracranial stenosis and 20 (33.9%) patients with 2 stenosis; the total number of intracranial stenosis was 95. Regarding risk factors, hypertension was present in 67.8% of patients, diabetes in 27.1%, smoking in 30.5%, obesity in 10.2%, hypercholesterolemia in 37.3%, previous TIA/stroke in 23.7%, heart disease in 18.6%. Forty-six (77.9%) patients presented with stroke, while 13 (22.1%) with TIA. Concerning the site of stenosis, 50 (52.6%) were located in the anterior circulation [MCA 46 (48.4%), ACA 4 (4.2%)], 45 (47.4%) in the posterior circulation: [PCA 28 (29.5%), BA 11(11.6%), VA 6(6.5%)]; 46 (54.8%) on the right hemisphere, 38 (45.2%) on the left hemisphere.

Conclusions: In this university hospital-based study among Caucasian patients with acute cerebral ischemia, ultrasound disclosed a higher prevalence of intracranial stenosis than previously thought, suggesting the clinical importance of this condition in White European TIA/stroke patients.

© 2012 Elsevier GmbH. All rights reserved.

Introduction

Intracranial atherosclerotic disease (ICAD) is characterized by the development and progression of atherosclerotic lesions affecting large intracranial arteries. According to the international literature ICAD is a common cause of ischemic stroke worldwide [1,2], with a high recurrence stroke rate [3], representing the cause of 30–50% strokes in Orientals, 11% in Hispanics, 6% in Blacks but only 1% in Caucasians [4]. However, the clinical importance of intracranial stenosis in Caucasians may have been underestimated. A French autoptic series of 339 patients who died from ischemic or hemorrhagic stroke showed a strikingly high prevalence of intracranial stenosis (43.2%) [5]. For these reasons, we

* Corresponding author at: Department of Neuroscience, University of Padua, School of Medicine, Via N. Giustiniani 5, 35128 Padua, Italy. Tel.: +39 0498213600; fax: +39 0498214366.
E-mail address: federica.viaro@gmail.com (F. Viaro).

2211-968X/$ — see front matter © 2012 Elsevier GmbH. All rights reserved.
doi:10.1016/j.permed.2012.02.004

Table 1 Risk factors in patients with intracranial stenosis.

Risk factor	Number of patients	%
Hypertension	40	67.8%
Hypercholesterolemia	21	37.3%
Smoking	18	30.5%
Diabetes	16	27.1%
Previous stroke/TIA	13	23.7%
Heart disease	11	18.6%
Diffuse arterial disease	9	15.3%
Obesity	6	10.2%
Alcohol abuse	2	3.4%
≥1 risk factor	45	76.3%

conducted a University Hospital-based study to assess the prevalence of ICAD in our Caucasian patients with TIA or ischemic stroke.

Subjects and methods

A prospectively compiled, computerized database of all Caucasian patients with TIA/ischemic stroke who were admitted to our Clinic over a two-year period, from January 1st 2009 to December 31st 2010, was analyzed. All patients underwent a complete cervical and intracranial ultrasound assessment with a high-resolution color-coded duplex sonography scanner (Philips iU22) using a high frequency (5–10 MHz) linear probe for the cervical arteries and a low frequency (1–3 MHz) phased-array probe for the intracranial arteries. The examination was performed by an experienced neurosonographer in the same room, in a quiet atmosphere, with the subjects lying in a supine position. Only patients with the following characteristics entered the final analysis: (1) >50% intracranial stenosis [6] in any major intracranial artery at TCCD. (2) Diagnostic confirmation by Magnetic Resonance Angiography/CT Angiography/Digital Subtraction Angiography. (3) Persistent >50% intracranial stenosis at 6-month follow-up TCCD assessment, in order to exclude a "stenosis" of cardioembolic origin.

Results

Among 292 patients included into our study, 59 (20.2%) subjects harbored at least one intracranial stenosis, while 20 (33.9%) patients had 2 stenosis; the total number of intracranial stenosis was 95. The patients were mainly males (79.7%) and their mean age was 71.0 ± 12.8 years, with an age range between 33 and 96; mean age in women was 75.0, in men 69.7 years. The most frequent risk factor was hypertension, present in 40 (67.8%) patients. Hypercholesterolemia was present in 21 (37.3%), diabetes in 16 (27.1%), smoking in 18 (30.5%), obesity in 6 (10.2%), previous TIA/stroke in 13 (23.7%), and heart disease in 11 (18.6%) (Table 1). Forty-six (77.9%) patients presented with ischemic stroke, while 13 (22.1%) with TIA. Concerning the site of stenosis, 50 (52.6%) were located in the anterior circulation [MCA 46 (48.4%), ACA 4 (4.2%)], 45 (47.4%) in the posterior circulation [PCA 28 (29.5%), BA 11 (11.6%), VA 6 (6.5%)] (Table 2); 46 (54.8%) on the right hemisphere, 38 (45.2%) on the left one.

Table 2 Intracranial stenosis: frequency by site.

Site of stenosis	Number of patients (%)
MCA	46 (48.4%)
ACA	4 (4.2%)
PCA	28 (29.5%)
BA	11 (11.6%)
VA	6 (6.5%)

Discussion and conclusions

In this university hospital-based study among Caucasian patients with acute cerebral ischemia, ultrasound revealed intracranial stenosis in 20.2% of patients, a higher prevalence than expected on the basis of previous reports [2]. Furthermore, more than one third of these patients were found to harbor at least two intracranial stenoses, suggesting the clinical importance of this condition in white Italian patients with TIA or acute ischemic stroke.

In our opinion, ICAD might be relatively neglected in Caucasian patients, because the main focus is maintained on a more accessible disorder, such as extracranial carotid artery occlusive disease [7] and in many cases the diagnosis is not actively sought, because of the "a priori" assumption that the condition is relatively rare.

Moreover, compared to cervical artery stenosis, atherosclerotic lesions of intracranial vessels cannot be directly visualized by ultrasound and therefore it is not possible to collect information on the characteristics of the plaque. They are detected at a late stage, when they alter blood flow and are more susceptible to embolize.

In our population, ICAD was more frequent in males, who were also younger than females, confirming previous data on atherosclerotic disease [8]. The most relevant risk factor for ICAD in our study resulted to be hypertension, followed by hypercholesterolemia; previous reports have shown similar results and aggressive treatment of these risk factors has been shown to reduce the recurrence of ischemic stroke in patients with intracranial stenosis [9,10].

Our data do not show a significant difference in the location of stenosis (anterior circulation compared to posterior circulation) suggesting that intracranial atherosclerotic disease is part of a widespread pathology, so that an accurate examination of the entire Circle of Willis is advisable in all patients with stroke or TIA, considering also the high risk of stroke recurrence in ICAD patients.

In conclusion, according to this study ICAD must enter into the differential diagnosis of Caucasians patients with acute cerebral ischemia, because it is a more frequent cause of stroke than previously reported.

References

[1] Wong KS, Huang YN, Gao S, Lam WW, Chan YL, Kay R. Intracranial stenosis in Chinese patients with acute stroke. Neurology 1998;50:812–3.
[2] Arenillas JF. Intracranial atherosclerosis current concepts. Stroke 2011;42:S20–3.
[3] Chimowitz MI, Lynn MJ, Howlett-Smith H, Stern BJ, Hertzberg VS, Frankel MR, et al., for the Warfarin-Aspirin Symptomatic

Intracranial Disease Trial Investigators. Comparison of warfarin and aspirin for symptomatic intracranial arterial stenosis. N Engl J Med 2005;352:1305—16.

[4] Sacco RL, Kargman DE, Gu Q, Zamanillo MC. Race-ethnicity and determinants of intracranial atherosclerotic cerebral infarction. The Northern Manhattan study. Stroke 1995;26: 14—20.

[5] Mazighi M, Labreuche J, Gongora-Rivera F, Duyckaerts C, Hauw JJ, Amarenco P. Autopsy prevalence of intracranial atherosclerosis in patients with fatal stroke. Stroke 2008;39:1142—7.

[6] Baumgartner RW, Mattle HP, Schroth G. Assessment of $\geq 50\%$ and <50% intracranial stenosis by transcranial color-coded duplex sonography. Stroke 1999;30(January (1)):87—92.

[7] Gorelick PB, Wong KSMD, Bae HJ, Pandey DK. Large artery intracranial occlusive disease a large worldwide burden but a relatively neglected frontier. Stroke 2008;39(8):2396—9.

[8] De Weerd M, Greving JP, de Jong AWF, Buskens E, Bots LM. Prevalence of asymptomatic carotid artery stenosis according to age and sex: systematic review and metaregression analysis. Stroke 2009;40:1105—13.

[9] Turan TN, Makki AA, Tsappidi S, Cotsonis G, Lynn MJ, Cloft HJ, et al. Risk factors associated with severity and location of intracranial arterial stenosis. Stroke 2010;41(8):1636—40.

[10] Turan TN, Derdeyn CP, Fiorella D, Chimowitz MI. Treatment of atherosclerotic intracranial arterial stenosis. Stroke 2009;40:2257—61.

6. Detection of Microembolic Signals, Right-to-Left Shunt (Patent Foramen Ovale)

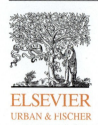
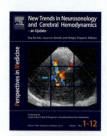

The contribution of microembolic signals (MES) detection in cardioembolic stroke

Martin A. Ritter*

Department of Neurology, University Hospital of Münster, Münster, Germany

KEYWORDS
Microembolic signals;
Atrial fibrillation;
Left ventricular assist devices;
Cardioembolic stroke

Summary

Background: Cardioembolic stroke accounts for about one third of all strokes. Microembolic signals (MES) are frequently found in patients with acute stroke. The role of MES in cardioembolic stroke is less well investigated.
Methods: Medline based literature review of clinical trials linking MES and stroke with cardiac sources of various risks.
Results: MES are a rare finding in patients with cardioembolic stroke as well as in sources of potential cardiac embolism (e.g. myocardial infarction, atrial fibrillation, left ventricular thrombus). The low number of patients with MES and the low number of MES during the investigation times leads to a limited statistical power of positive and negative findings. MES in patients with artificial heart valves and the DeBakey left ventricular assist device (LVAD) are predominantly gaseous and do not correlate with stroke risk. In patients with the Novacor LVAD, MES strongly correlate with stroke risk.
Conclusion: Currently, the role of MES in cardioembolic stroke is only limited due to both, the low prevalence of MES and the number of MES per investigation. Larger studies would be needed to strengthen this role.
© 2012 Published by Elsevier GmbH.

Background

Cardioembolic stroke accounts for about one third of all strokes. In some registries, percentages even reach 40%. The diagnosis of cardioembolic stroke requires that alternative stroke etiologies have been ruled out comprehensively. Diagnosis of cardiac embolism thus usually requires the presence of a structural abnormality of the heart or the diagnosis of rhythm disturbances with high embolic risk such as atrial fibrillation (AF) [1].

According to general consensus, cardiac lesions can be divided into ''high risk'' and ''low or uncertain risk'' of subsequent embolism [2]. The differentiation is of considerable importance, as the therapeutic regimen to prevent future embolism varies between different embolic risks. Table 1 gives an overview of ''high'' and ''low'' risk lesions.

Even without proving a cardiac source, some features of an acute stroke give clues to a cardiac source of stroke. For example, patients with cardioembolic stroke frequently have clinically more severe stroke than others, frequently decreased level of consciousness, and severe cortical symptoms such as neglect or aphasia [2]. On cerebral imaging especially multiple lesions in different arterial territories

* Correspondence address: Department of Neurology, University of Münster, Albert-Schweitzer-Campus 1, Gebäude A1, D-48149 Münster, Germany. Tel.: +49 251 8345536; fax: +49 251 8348181.
E-mail address: Martin.Ritter@ukmuenster.de

2211-968X/$ — see front matter © 2012 Published by Elsevier GmbH.
doi:10.1016/j.permed.2012.02.031

Table 1 High and low risk lesions for cardiac embolism [2].

High risk	Low risk
Atrial	Atrial
Atrial fibrillation	Patent foramen ovale
Atrial flutter	Atrial aneurysm
Sick sinus syndrome	Spontaneous echo contrast
Left atrial thrombus	
Left atrial myxoma	
Ventricular	Ventricular
Left ventricular thrombus	Dyskinetic wall segments
Left ventricular myxoma	Hypertrophic cardiomyopathy
Recent myocardial infarction	Congestive heart failure
Dilated cardiomyopathy	
Valvular	Valvular
Mitral stenosis	Lambl's excrescences
Prosthetic valves	Fibroelastoma
Infective/non-infective endocarditis	Mitral-valve prolapse

Table 2 Prevalence of MES in various stroke etiologies.

Author, year	Large artery embolism n/N, %	Cardioembolic stroke n/N %	Small vessel disease n/N %
Idicula, 2010 [4]	4/13, 30%	4/7, 36%	0/2, 0%
Poppert, 2006 [5]	20/103, 20%	5/143, 3.5%	0/147, 0%
Serena, 2000 [6]	8/39, 20%	6/35, 17%	0/64, 0%
Kaposzta, 1999 [7]	10/20, 50%	1/22, 4%	0/20, 0%
Daffertshofer, 1996 [8]	18/105, 17.1%	4/65, 6.2%	3/67, 4.5%
Sum	60/280, 21%	20/272, 5%	3/300, 1%

strongly favours a cardiac source of embolism. Furthermore, microembolic signals (MES) detected in both middle cerebral arteries make a proximal source of embolism, mainly the heart, very likely [2].

Microembolic signals (MES) are frequently found in patients with acute stroke and especially in those with symptomatic carotid stenosis [3]. The role of MES in cardioembolic stroke is less well investigated. The following overview will highlight the current role of MES detection in the diagnosis and therapy of various sources of cardiac embolism.

Methods

Medline listed studies were identified by the following search terms: ''MES'' OR ''ES'' OR ''HITS'' AND ''Cardia*'' OR ''heart'' OR ''atri*'' OR ''ventri*''. Studies were selected upon relevance to the subtitles of the following overview. If appropriate, data from different studies were grouped in tables and commented in context.

Prevalence of MES in patients with cardioembolic stroke

There are a number of studies investigating the prevalence of MES in unselected stroke cohorts. An overview on the studies comparing the prevalence of MES in detailed stroke etiologies according to TOAST criteria is given in Table 2.

In a recent study, Idicula found quite a high prevalence of MES in patients with cardiac embolism that even topped the prevalence found in patients with symptomatic carotid stenosis [4]. However, in this study, only 40 patients had been included in total and MES were found in four of eleven patients with cardiac embolism. In the larger studies the prevalence of MES was generally low. The lowest percentage was found in the largest study of Poppert and colleagues, finding MES in only five of 143 (3.5%) patients with cardiac embolism [5]. The overall prevalence of MES in patients with cardio-embolic stroke is about 5%. No study found MES to be predictive of recurrent cardioembolic stroke, which could also be the effect of the low case numbers with MES and the restricted observation times.

Ferro commented in his paper that cardioembolic stroke should be assumed in case MES are found bilaterally [2]. However although this assumption is quite plausible, its clinical relevance is very low. First, as mentioned above, only a minority of patients with cardioembolic stroke will have MES at all. Second, the number of MES per investigation is very low (about 1 or 2 MES per hour). Finding larger numbers of MES is rare. However, bilateralism cannot be assumed in case of only one MES per session and even with two signals during the session there is still a 50% chance that these two signals occur on the same side of the brain.

Furthermore, bilateral MES can also be found in cases with artery to artery embolism. Poppert et al. found in his study bilateral MES in 3 of 20 patients with this stroke etiology [5]. In one patient, contralateral carotid occlusion may have accounted for this finding, but no obvious reason was depicted in two cases. In summary, MES are an infrequent finding in cardioembolic stroke, MES detection does thus not contribute to the work-up of unselected stroke patients to determine stroke etiology.

MES in cardiac disease with a risk of stroke

This paragraph will look at cardiac embolism from the other side of the medal. What does MES detection contribute to the patients' work-up in case there are known cardiac lesions and the investigator wants to address the risk of future stroke.

MES after myocardial infarction

Stroke is a possible complication of acute myocardial infarction and affects 2—3% of patients with acute coronary syndromes (ACS) [9]. The risk to suffer stroke within the

Table 3 Prevalence of MES in various sources of cardiac embolism [12].

Cardiac pathology	n	Prevalence of MES
Infective endocarditis	7	43%
Left ventricular aneurysm	38	34%
Intracardiac thrombus	23	26%
Dilated cardiomyopathy	39	26%
Non-valvular atrial fibrillation	24	21%
Valvular disease	80	15%
Prosthetic heart valves	89	55%
Overall		23% (without prosthetic heart valves)

30 days after myocardial infarction is about 10 times higher than before and thereafter. It is therefore reasonable to use MES detection as a predictor of future stroke in this setting.

Nadareishvili et al. found MES in 17 of 100 patients within 72 h from onset of an acute coronary syndrome [10]. MES were more frequently found in patients with LV thrombus, akinetic left ventricle and decreased ejection fraction on echocardiography. They also found that during the following days 3 patients suffered stroke, all of which had MES at baseline [10].

Unfortunately, these results could not be reproduced in a recent study from Spain, in which 209 patients with ACS had been investigated with a very similar protocol [11]. The authors found MES in only 7 patients (prevalence of 3.4%) and patients were followed for 14 months. In the follow-up period, only 3 patients had a subsequent stroke, none of them had MES at baseline. Apart from stroke, no other vascular event could be predicted by the presence of MES.

Overall, the data are thus inconclusive, again in part due to the low prevalence of MES in this cohort and the low overall case number in the studies. From a practical point of view, MES detection does not seem to be very helpful in predicting stroke after ACS.

MES in other cardiac sources of embolism

Georgiadis et al. reported in his milestone paper on this subject the prevalence of MES in 300 patients with various cardiac sources of embolism [12]. The detailed numbers are given in Table 3. The highest prevalence was found for patients with infective endocarditis, the lowest for chronic valvular disease. No associations could be found for MES and patients' age or sex or actual medication. Only "high risk lesions" according to Table 1 were investigated. Although the study was quite large, no data on patient outcome and the risk of future stroke for patients with and without MES are given. Thus, for most of the sources prospective studies would be needed to determine the role of MES detection to predict future cardioembolic stroke.

MES in atrial fibrillation

Atrial fibrillation is the single most frequent cause of cardioembolic stroke. No wonder MES detection has been used in a number of studies in this entity. Studies have tried to determine the prevalence of MES, the risk of patients with MES to suffer subsequent stroke and to correlate the presence of MES with anticoagulation therapy.

In the paper of Georgiadis et al., 5 of 24 patients (21%) with atrial fibrillation (AF) had MES [12]. Nabavi et al. found MES in 11 of 26 patients (42%) with valvular AF compared with 3 of 21 patients (21%) with non-valvular AF [13]. MES were also more frequently found in patients with a history of thromboembolism. Cullinane et al. found MES in 13 of 86 patients with non-valvular AF (15%) [14]. There was no difference in the prevalence between symptomatic (16%) and asymptomatic (13%) patients. Furthermore, there was no correlation between MES and the use of aspirin or left atrial thrombus. There was also no correlation between MES and echocardiographic risk markers (such as left atrial enlargement). One study investigated, whether MES were more frequent in 37 patients with stroke due to AF compared with 10 patients with AF but without stroke and 92 controls [15]. MES were detected in 11 (29%) of the symptomatic patients and only in one without a history of stroke. The MES count was quite high in this study with ~15 events per hour which sheds some doubt on the credibility of the data. Over a follow-up period of 18 months one patient with MES at baseline had a recurrent stroke; however this occurred 1 year from study inclusion.

Overall, studies were too small to address the question of stroke risk and studies are too heterogeneous to perform a meta-analysis of studies performed. Until larger studies report otherwise, there seems to be no added value of MES detection to address clinical questions in patients with AF.

MES and left ventricular assist devices

MES detection is a well-established method to monitor cardiac or vascular procedures. Currently, a well-established procedure is the implantation of cardiac left ventricular assist devices (LVAD) that allow "bridging" of patients with very severe left ventricular cardiac failure to heart transplantation or until the heart has recovered from a temporary disease. These patients are constantly endangered by the occurrence of systemic and frequently cerebral embolism although antiplatelet and anticoagulation strategies are both used to decrease this risk. These patients are well characterised and an attractive group of patients to test whether silent microembolism is associated with clinical events. In one study, 20 patients with the Novacor N100 LVAD were investigated [16]. MES detections were performed once weekly for 30 min, and thromboembolic events were recorded. 44 events occurred in 3876 LVAD days resulting in an incidence of 1.1% events per day (400%/year). The overall MES prevalence was 35.3% with a median MES number of 2.3/h. There was a strong correlation between MES activity and incidence of thromboembolism and times with events were predicted by MES activity with a moderate positive predictive value (0.37—0.7) and a high negative predictive value (0.82—1.0). Concerning therapy, patients on both medications, oral anticoagulants and antiplatelets, had less events (0.7% vs. 2.8%) and a lower MES prevalence (18.3% vs. 65.4%) than patients on anticoagulation alone. Therefore, MES detection seems very useful in patients with the Novacor device as it correlates with therapy and clinical events. In another study patients with the DeBakey were investigated [17]. 23 patients were monitored twice weekly with and without oxygen inhalation. Therapy and documentation of clinical events was identical to the first study. In these patients the embolic risk of 0.24%/per day was 80% less than for patients with the Novacor LVAD, although the prevalence of MES (35.1%) was the same as in Novacor patients and the number of MES was much higher (mean 81 ± 443/h) than in the Novacor device. The authors found no correlation between MES activity and incidence of thromboembolism or hemostatic treatment for patients with the DeBakey device. The authors also found that the number of MES with the DeBakey device decreased significantly after oxygen inhalation suggesting a gaseous nature of most of the MES in patients with the DeBakey device. Gaseous MES have been shown to not correlate with stroke risk, something that has been observed with artificial heart valves in the past.

Sliwka and Georgiadis retrospectively evaluated 369 patients with various types of artificial heart valves >3 months concerning the risk of stroke and the presence and number of MES [18]. They found significant differences in MES prevalence and counts depending on valve type. Although the prevalence of MES ranged from 9% (biological valves) to 92% (Björk Shiley) and the average MES numbers from 0 to 133 per hour there was no association between MES counts and INR, age, cardiac rhythm, and implant duration. There was also no predictive value of MES for a history of neurological symptoms which were prevalent in 42 patients.

In summary, MES detection seems useful in patients with Novacor LVAD to guide therapy and to predict clinical events. However this does not hold true for patients with the DeBakey LVAD and not for patients with artificial heart valves as most MES in these patients are from gaseous nature.

Conclusion

MES are an infrequent finding in most cardiac sources of embolism and due to the low case numbers in most studies and the low absolute number of MES any conclusion is premature. Much larger studies would be needed with homogeneous study populations to address most questions covered in this review, especially to monitor therapeutic effects or to predict future strokes. From a pragmatic point of view, there is currently no established role of MES detection in cardiac embolism.

References

[1] Low molecular weight heparinoid, ORG 10172 (danaparoid), and outcome after acute ischemic stroke: a randomized controlled trial. The Publications Committee for the Trial of ORG 10172 in Acute Stroke Treatment (TOAST) Investigators. JAMA 1998;279:1265—72.

[2] José MF. Cardioembolic stroke: an update. Lancet Neurol 2003;2:177—88.

[3] Ritter MA, Dittrich R, Thoenissen N, Ringelstein EB, Nabavi DG. Prevalence and prognostic impact of microembolic signals in arterial sources of embolism. A systematic review of the literature. J Neurol 2008;255:953—61.

[4] Idicula T, Naess H, Thomassen L. Microemboli-monitoring during the acute phase of ischemic stroke: is it worth the time? BMC Neurol 2010;10:79.

[5] Poppert H, Sadikovic S, Sander K, Wolf O, Sander D. Embolic signals in unselected stroke patients. Stroke 2006;37: 2039—43.

[6] Serena J, Segura T, Castellanos M, Davalos A. Microembolic signal monitoring in hemispheric acute ischemic stroke: a prospective study. Cerebrovasc Dis 2000;10: 278—82.

[7] Kaposzta Z, Young E, Bath PMW, Markus HS. Clinical application of asymptomatic embolic signal detection in acute stroke: a prospective study. Stroke 1999;30:1814—8.

[8] Daffertshofer M, Ries S, Schminke U, Hennerici M. High-intensity transient signals in patients with cerebral ischemia. Stroke 1996;27:1844—9.

[9] Witt BJ, Brown RD, Jacobsen SJ, Weston SA, Yawn BP, Roger VL. A community-based study of stroke incidence after myocardial infarction. Ann Intern Med 2005;143:785—92.

[10] Nadareishvili ZG, Choudary Z, Joyner C, Brodie D, Norris JW. Cerebral microembolism in acute myocardial infarction. Stroke 1999;30:2679—82.

[11] Meseguer E, Labreuche J, Durdilly C, Echeverría A, Lavallee PC, Ducrocq G, et al. Prevalence of embolic signals in acute coronary syndromes. Stroke 2010;41:261—6.

[12] Georgiadis D, Lindner A, Manz M, Sonntag M, Zunker P, Zerkowski HR, et al. Intracranial microembolic signals in 500 patients with potential cardiac or carotid embolic source and in normal controls. Stroke 1997;28:1203—7.

[13] Nabavi DG, Arato S, Droste DW, Schulte-Altedorneburg G, Kemeny V, Reinecke H, et al. Microembolic load in asymptomatic patients with cardiac aneurysm, severe ventricular dysfunction, and atrial fibrillation. Clinical and hemorheological correlates. Cerebrovasc Dis 1998;8:214—21.

[14] Cullinane M, Wainwright R, Brown A, Monaghan M, Markus HS. Asymptomatic embolization in subjects with atrial fibrillation not taking anticoagulants: a prospective study. Stroke 1998;29:1810—5.

[15] Kumral E, Balkir K, Uzuner N, Evyapan D, Nalbantgil S. Microembolic signal detection in patients with symptomatic and asymptomatic lone atrial fibrillation. Cerebrovasc Dis 2001;12:192—6.

[16] Nabavi DG, Stockmann J, Schmid C, Schneider M, Hammel D, Scheld HH, et al. Doppler microembolic load predicts risk of thromboembolic complications in Novacor patients. J Thorac Cardiovasc Surg 2003;126:160—7.

[17] Thoennissen NH, Schneider M, Allroggen A, Ritter M, Dittrich R, Schmid C, et al. High level of cerebral microembolization in patients supported with the DeBakey left ventricular assist device. J Thorac Cardiovasc Surg 2005;130: 1159—66.

[18] Sliwka U, Georgiadis D. Clinical correlations of Doppler microembolic signals in patients with prosthetic cardiac valves: analysis of 580 cases. Stroke 1998;29:140—3.

Exploration of a zero-tolerance regime on cerebral embolism in symptomatic carotid artery disease

Ruud W.M. Keunen [a,*], Agnes van Sonderen [a], Maayke Hunfeld [a], Michael Remmers [b], D.L. Tavy [a], S.F.T.M. de Bruijn [a], A. Mosch [a]

[a] Department of Neurology and Clinical Neurophysiology, Haga Teaching Hospitals, The Hague, The Netherlands
[b] Department of Neurology, Amphia Hospital, Breda, The Netherlands

KEYWORDS
TCD;
Embolus;
Stroke;
TIA;
Carotid;
Artery

Summary

Background: Current protocols stress the importance of short-term diagnosis and treatment in recent TIA or minor stroke. The risk of a recurrent event can be predicted with embolus detection. Studies have shown that the presence of micro-emboli is associated with an increased risk of recurrent events. We explored in our patient population the effect of a zero-tolerance regime for cerebral embolism on outcome.

Methods: Patients with a recent TIA or minor stroke were assigned to a study group or control group. Both groups were treated according to European Stroke guidelines, including prompt start of anti-thrombotic therapy, statins and short-term carotid arteries duplex scanning. The study group was subjected to TCD (Delica 9 series, Shenzen Delicate Electronics Co., LTD., China) embolus detection as soon as possible (EDS, SMT Medical, Wuerzburg, Germany). If emboli were detected, treatment was started immediately to stop cerebral embolization. This was achieved by either an altered drug regimen (clopidogrel) or angioplasty or carotid endarterectomy within one or two days. If carotid intervention was indicated in the control group, it was performed within two weeks, according to European guidelines.

Results: 133 patients were enrolled in the study with three months follow-up. 61 patients were subjected to the control group, 72 patients were enrolled in the study group. Recurrent events occurred in 10.2% and 3.0%, respectively ($p = 0.145$).

Conclusion: The current study shows a non-significant reduction in recurrent events in the study group. Probably sample size in this pilot study was insufficient to detect a significant decline. Nevertheless, the results show that embolus detection is feasible and the zero-tolerance regime may enhance the outcome of TIA and minor stroke patients. The findings support the start of a multicenter randomized trial to assess the clinical value of emboli detection in TIA and stroke care.

© 2012 Elsevier GmbH. All rights reserved.

Introduction

The primary goals of the TIA and stroke services are two-fold: first to promote full recovery of patients with neurological deficits and secondly prevention of stroke

* Corresponding author.
E-mail address: r.keunen@hagaziekenhuis.nl (R.W.M. Keunen).

recurrence. Stroke recurrence can be divided in early and late stroke recurrence. Recent literature has shown that early stroke recurrence is seen especially within the first two weeks after the ischemic event. Age, blood pressure, clinical presentation and duration of symptoms are known predictors of stroke recurrence in this patient group. Diagnostic procedures such as duplex of the carotid arteries and transcranial Doppler (TCD) of the middle cerebral artery may enhance the prediction of early stroke risk recurrence as high grade carotid artery stenosis in combination with ongoing cerebral embolism is a strong independent risk factor of stroke recurrence [1,2]. Although duplex examinations have been implemented in current stroke protocol for screening high-risk individuals, TCD embolus detection has till date not gained a prominent place in screening TIA and stroke patients to evaluate the stroke risk recurrence. Nevertheless there are a number of potential advantages of embolus detection in stroke care. First it may reassure embolus negative patients. Secondly it may speed up the process of source location and treatment in embolus positive patients and finally it may refine indications for carotid artery surgery. To evaluate the efficacy to prevent stroke recurrence of embolus detection in a clinical setting we designed this pilot study. Basically we explored the effect of a zero-tolerance regime for cerebral embolism on outcome. The gathered data may be used for future design of clinical trials that will prove or disapprove the value of embolus detection in TIA and stroke care.

Methods

Study design

To study the outcome patients with a recent (>6 weeks) carotid artery TIA or minor stroke were subjected to either a conventional duplex-guided protocol (control group) or a TCD embolus detection guided protocol (study group). Minor stroke was defined as a modified Rankin disability score between 0 and 2 [3]. The randomization of patients was not determined by chance but by availability of vascular technologist which could perform the TCD embolus detection (pseudo-randomization). Both groups followed the internationally accepted guidelines of the European Stroke Organisation [4]. This included a prompt start of an anti-thrombotic drug regime in every patient and a rapid (<48 h) duplex scanning.

Patients in the study group were subjected to a 30 min TCD embolus detection of the symptomatic middle cerebral artery to detect micro-embolic signals (MES). If patients showed positive embolism in relation to an unstable carotid artery stenosis, the carotid surgery or angioplasty was performed within 48 h. In case of positive embolism without a known embolic source clopidogrel was administered. If patients within the control group exhibit a symptomatic carotid stenosis or if patients in the control group exhibited a symptomatic carotid stenosis without MES, surgery or angioplasty was performed at the time interval advised by the guidelines of the European Stroke Organisation (within two weeks).

Patients contacted the hospital either by an admission at the emergency department or were referred by their house physician at the outpatient TIA and stroke clinic. Patients with an ischemic event of more than six weeks ago were excluded for this study. All patients were followed up for three months.

Treatment protocol

The protocol included a prompt start of an anti-thrombotic drug regime in every patient (300 mg acetylsalicylic acid for 14 days in case of a minor stroke or an initial dose of 300 mg acetylsalicylic acid on day 1 followed by a prescription of 100 mg daily in TIA patients). All patients underwent laboratory examinations, ECG, duplex examination of the carotid and vertebral arteries and a CT and/or MR of the brain. If duplex revealed a stenosis of more than 50% or the TCD embolus detection revealed active cerebral embolism a CT angiography was performed from the aortic arc including the basal arteries of the brain.

Therapeutic drug interventions included the prescription of anti-thrombotic drug such as acetylsalicylic acid in combination with dipyridamole acid (in case of atrial fibrillation: anti-coagulants), statines and anti-hypertensive treatment. Patients used clopidogrel for six months; in case of persistent cerebral embolization (for instance after carotid surgery or when cerebral embolism was still present after the administration of acetylsalicylic acid) the drug regimes were switched to a combination of anti-thrombotic drugs that more effectively reduced the level of cerebral embolism.

Carotid interventions

In case of a symptomatic carotid stenosis patients were asked to participate in the International Carotid Stenting Study (ICSS). The ICSS is an international multicenter trial which compares the efficacy of stenting versus surgery in the treatment of symptomatic carotid artery stenosis [5]. Patients scheduled for stent were treated with clopidogrel for at least six months, after carotid surgery they received acetylsalicylic acid and dipyridamole acid. Patients scheduled for surgery and stenting were observed for two days at the stroke unit.

Monitoring during stent procedure was done in awake patients by a neurologist. During carotid surgery the patients were exposed to general anesthesia and monitored by a clinical neurophysiologist. Monitoring techniques during surgery included both TCD and electro-encephalography. Based on monitoring results patients were electively shunted during the carotid endarterectomy. TCD monitoring was performed in all patients in the first hours after surgery and stenting procedures to detect persistent cerebral embolism or malignant cerebral hyperperfusion. All patients underwent a full neurological exam on regular time intervals after the stent or surgery until they were discharged from the stroke unit.

Data sampling

The following information on patient history was obtained: TIA and minor strokes we classified into the following categories: retinal TIA, cerebral TIA or stroke. Documented were the nature of the events such as visual, pure motor, pure sensory, dysarthria, dysphasia, ataxia, apraxia or combination of events. ABCD2 scores were obtained in all patients [6]. MRI findings were classified into cortical infarcts, subcortical infarcts and leucoaraiosis. Infarcts were further subdivided into recent or non-recent and left or right sided. The side, severity of the stenosis and presence of plaque ulceration on duplex and CTA were documented as well. Furthermore, blood pressure was documented as well as the current use of anti-thrombotic drugs or anti-coagulants. Documentation of the TCD embolus detection included: the side of insonation, the peak systolic-, mean and end-diastolic velocity, the duration of the measurement and the presence or absence of cerebral embolism by human experts. If experts found cerebral embolism the following parameters of that embolus were noted: velocity, phase of cardiac cycle (systolic/diastolic) in which the events occurred, intensity, duration and a parameter related to the musical characteristics of the embolus (the zero-crossing index) [7].

Data of stent procedures and surgery were prospectively documented including the occurrence of neurological or non-neurological complications. The follow-up at three month included a neurological visit at the outpatient clinic. Documented were the TIA and stroke recurrence rate. If complications had occurred in the post-operative phase of angioplasty or surgery they were evaluated including the occurrence of new medical events in the last three months.

All data were stored in a downloadable Internet based electronic management system which allowed online statistical analysis of all included case records. This data management system has been developed by Mediwebdesign© The Netherlands (http://www.mediwebdesign.nl/spi/stroke/loginreal.php).

Embolus detection by TCD

A TCD Delica 9 series (Delicate/Shenzen/China) equipped with a 2 MHz TCD transducer and a notebook PC (Acer®, Aspire 1800 Series) were used for this study. A special Delicate headband was used to hold the 2 MHz transducer, which allowed hands-off monitoring. The insonated artery was the middle cerebral artery at its origin, just lateral of the terminal internal carotid artery, on the ipsilateral side of the symptomatic carotid artery territory. Patients were monitored for 30 min. In case of positive embolism the other contra-lateral middle cerebral artery was examined to estimate whether the cerebral embolism was a uni-lateral or bilateral phenomenon. Insonation depth varied between 45 mm and 55 mm. Patients were asked to not speak or move their head during the monitoring session because angular or lateral probe movements may induce false positive embolic events.

To facilitate reliable embolus detection at the Haga Teaching Hospitals we developed an embolus detection system (EDS, SMT Medical, Wuerzburg, Germany) specially designed to detect the low intensity micro-embolic signal

Table 1 Inclusion data of all patients.

Numbers	Study group 72	Control group 61
General aspects		
Age (yrs)	71.3	70.4
Ratio (female: male)	0.21	0.47
Modified Rankin score	0.59	0.61
Risk factors		
ABCD2 score	4.6	4.3
Clinical presentation		
Retinal events	17%	15%
Cortical events (aphasia)	30%	21%
Subcortical events (motor/sensory)	53%	64%
Duplex/CTA findings		
Carotid stenosis < 70% or no stenosis	72%	76%
Carotid stenosis > 70% or occlusion	28%	24%
Intervention		
Surgery or angioplasty	23%	30%

seen in TIA and stroke patients [7]. The EDS is a universal software package that can be used on every ultrasound system. On the basis of a neural network technology it classifies every intensity increase into MES or artefacts. The EDS allows full verification of the whole time series and has an export function which for instance allows consultation of a fellow colleague over the Internet. The final classification of the outcome of the EDS was done by two human experts which evaluated every event in both the embolus and artefact list. Human experts now decided whether the embolus in the embolus list was a true embolus or a false positive one. The same has been done for the artefact event list. In this list they searched for the presence of so called false negative embolus (which is an embolus in the artefact event list that has not been correctly classified by the EDS). On the basis of these examinations they finally decided: 'active cerebral embolism' or 'no active embolism'.

Statistical analysis

Categorical values were presented as numbers (percentages). Because of the limited number of observations statistical analysis were not supplied for Tables 1—4. Independent t-test was used to evaluate stroke and TIA recurrence for the control and the study group (whose distributions approximate normality). Statistical significance was considered at $P < 0.05$. SPSS (v 17.0) statistical software was used for statistical analysis.

Ethical aspects

Informed consent was given by all patients. They were explained about the observational nature of the study and were informed about the rapid and regular treatment regimes. They gave also consent for the three months follow-up monitoring. The study has been submitted to the Central Committee on Research involving Human Subjects but according to their guidelines ethical approval was not

Table 2 Epidemiological data of the study group.

Numbers	11	61
General aspects		
Age (yrs)	73	76
Male sex	55%	85%
Female sex	45%	15%
Modified Rankin score (mean)	0.36	0.45
Risk factors		
ABCD2 score (mean)	4.6	5.5
Clinical presentation		
Retinal events	27.3%	14.7%
Cortical events (aphasia)	27.3%	24.5%
Subcortical events	45.4%	63.8%
Duplex/CTA findings.		
Carotid stenosis > 70% or occlusion	72.7%	31.1%
CT/MRI findings		
Recent ipsilateral infarcts (%)	18.8%	22.9%

Table 3 Epidemiological aspects of the cerebral MES.

Embolic frequency TIA and stroke patients	Mean 3.4 (range 1—12)/30 min
Embolus characteristics	
Total number of MES	36
Mean intensity (dB)	3.8 (range 3.1—6.3)
Mean duration (ms)	35.7 (range 11.0—57.6)
Mean zero-crossing index	13.2 (range 2.6—40.2)
Mean velocity and (cm/s)	35.4 (range 10—53)
Ratio embolus in systolic and diastolic phase	1:12
Embolic sources	
Internal carotid artery origo stenosis	9 out of 11 patients
Carotid siphon stenosis	2 out of 11 patients
Cardiac source	0 out of 11 patients
Embolic activity 2—5 days after treatment	
Drug switch from Aspirin to Clopidogrel: complete disappearance in	2 out of 2 patients
Carotid surgery complete disappearance in	2 out of 2 patients
Carotid angioplasty complete disappearance in	7 out of 7 patients

Table 4 Outcome of the study group.

Embolic activity	Pos	Neg
Numbers	11	61
Timing of therapeutical intervention after EDS (days)	1.6[a]	14.0
Outcome at three month		
TIA recurrence rate	0%	1.6%
Stroke recurrence rate	0%	1.6%
Sum TIA and stroke rate	0%	3.2%

[a] Calculated for nine patients; two patients could not be treated within the time of 48 h.

required for this study because the patients were not randomized into different treatment regimes. Merely patients were given the opportunity to participate in a new diagnostic procedure which was implemented at the Haga Teaching Hospitals. Both rapid and regular treatment protocols follow the current stroke guidelines of the European Stroke Organisation [4].

Results

Baseline data

Patient inclusion started on 1.8.2008 to 31.12.2009, the follow up was finished on 1.4.2010. 133 patients enrolled in the study with three months follow-up. 61 patients were subjected to the control group, 72 patients enrolled in the study group. All patients could be evaluated to establish outcome. Table 1 shows the data of both patient groups. The table shows that both groups have more or less similar basic demographic parameters. In the control group there is a preponderance of women compared to the study group. Age, modified Rankin scores, ABCD2 scores, clinical presentation, duplex findings and frequency of carotid surgery and/or angioplasty showed similar distributions.

Epidemiology of cerebral embolism

Table 2 gives specific data of the study group and shows the relationship between clinical data and the presence or absence of cerebral embolism. Table 2 shows that cerebral embolism in this patient cohort was associated with a high-grade internal carotid artery stenosis. Retinal events and aphasia were more frequently seen in patients who experienced cerebral embolism.

Table 3 shows the epidemiology of cerebral embolism. It showed a wide range of frequencies of emboli during the 30 min monitoring. Most emboli were short lasting, low intensity events that occurred in the diastolic phase of the cardiac cycle. The emboli had a very prominent musical sound expressed by the low zero-crossing index. The most prominent source of the embolus was an internal carotid artery stenosis. In most patients the internal carotid artery stenosis was located at the origin of the vessel. In two out of eleven patients the stenosis was located at the level of the carotid syphon. The embolic activity decreased after therapeutical interventions such as carotid surgery, angioplasty and a drug switch from aspirin to clopidogrel.

Outcome

Table 4 shows the outcome of the study protocol in relation to positive and negative embolism. Table 5 shows the outcome of both the control and study group. Table 4 shows

Table 5 Outcome for all patients.

Number	Study group 72	Control group 61	p-Value
Timing of therapeutical intervention after event (days)	24	22	
Angioplasty	11.2%	13.1%	
Carotid surgery	11.2%	14.8%	
Total number	22.4%	27.9%	
Outcome at three months			
Modified Rankin score (mean)	0.39	0.25	n.s.
TIA recurrence rate	1.4%	6.3%	
Stroke recurrence rate	1.6%	4.9%	
Sum TIA and stroke recurrence	3.0%	10.2%	0.145

that the diagnosis and treatment of patients with positive cerebral embolism was performed much faster than the diagnosis and treatment of patients without cerebral embolism. Stroke and TIA recurrence rate in both groups were very low (respectively 0.0% and 3.2%). In the study group, one patient experienced a stroke recurrence in the ipsilateral posterior cerebral artery resulting in a permanent hemi-anopsia. In the control group four recurrent strokes were observed. All these events occurred in the ipsilateral middle cerebral artery territory; two of these events occurred in the post-operative phase of carotid surgery. One of these events was classified as a possible cerebral hyperperfusion syndrome.

Discussion

Spencer was the first investigator who showed that detection of cerebral embolism was possible with TCD [8]. His initial study describes the ongoing cerebral embolism in patients scheduled for carotid surgery. Soon after his publication the first reports appeared about MES signals in TIA and stroke patients. In the last ten years a number of studies showed unequivocal that ongoing cerebral embolism in carotid artery disease is a strong independent predictor of stroke [1,2]. The current clinical study tried to explore the potential of embolus detection to enhance the outcome of patients with symptomatic carotid artery disease. Briefly summarized this study revealed a non-significant reduction in recurrent events in the study group. Probably sample size in this pilot study was insufficient to detect a significant decline. Nevertheless, the results show that embolus detection is feasible and the zero-tolerance regime may enhance the outcome of TIA and minor stroke patients. The findings support the start of a multicenter randomized trial to assess the clinical value of embolus detection in TIA and stroke care.

During this study we observed that some patients with a low ABCD2 score may exhibit ongoing cerebral embolism and other patients with high score ABCD2 scores did not always show cerebral embolism and vice versa. It seems that both methods could in a way be complementary as the EDS results are more indicative for plaque *stability* while some of the ABCD2 score components are more indicative for plaque *formation* (such as age, blood pressure and diabetes).

This study showed that EDS monitoring can be used for diagnosis and monitoring unstable carotid artery disease and gave insight in the epidemiology of cerebral embolism. MES were seen during the diastolic phase of the cardiac cycle and disappeared by anti-thrombotic drugs or plaques removal. The aforementioned aspects of the MES could best be explained by the hypothesis that these MES were generated by small solid particles that were disloged into the circulation by unstable carotid artery stenosis [9]. In some patients we noted >12 MES in 30 min which means that hundreds of these small particles must go to the brain within a 24 h timeframe. Only a minority of these micro emboli resulted in TIA's or minor strokes. It seemed that the normal brain has the capacity to clear these of tiny micro-emboli.

An important aspect is the duration of monitoring that is needed to detect emboli. Previous studies showed that embolism is non-continuous phenomenon so it might be that very short observation times result in false negative monitoring results. The present study however shows that 30 min of monitoring gives relevant clinical information which, in combination with a zero-tolerance regime can, reduce the stroke recurrence rate. If the frequency of embolism is high the observation time might be limited less than 30 min. We feel that the time that is needed to document at least two MES is the minimum time for embolus detection. Future studies with ambulatory TCD systems will focus on the value of extended embolus detection beyond the 30 min [10].

This study showed that therapeutical interventions could arrest ongoing cerebral embolism. This was observed after angioplasty, carotid stenting or after a drug switch to clopidogrel. The latter is in accordance with the CARESS trial [11] which showed that in patients with recently symptomatic carotid stenosis, combination therapy with clopidogrel and aspirin is more effective in reducing asymptomatic embolism.

Although the number of observation are small in the present study Table 4 indicates a trend that patients who experienced cerebral embolism have a different vascular profile than those who do not exhibit cerebral embolism. Embolus positive patients showed in contrast to embolus negative patients more retinal and cortical TIA in combination with a symptomatic high-grade carotid artery stenosis. Patients without cerebral embolism presented often a subcortical type of stroke or TIA and that these events are less often associated with a high-grade carotid artery stenosis. Therefore, it seems that embolus negative patients suffer more from a local thrombosis in relation to cerebral micro-angiopathy than carotid artery macro-angiopathy. However, micro-embolism may still play a role in genesis of microangiopathy in embolus negative patients. It is important to realize that TCD cannot detect very tiny embolic particles. The lower limit of TCD embolus detection is approximately about 0.3 mm [12]. The diameter of the origin of the perforating arteries of the brain is around 0.2—0.8 mm [13]. Thus lacunar strokes could be the result of sub 0.3 mm particles which cannot be detected by TCD. The second reason why embolus negative patients may experience an embolic stroke is that the source of the embolus is located more distal to the TCD sample volume. In this study the sample volume was located around the origin of the MCA, while in lacunar stroke the emboli may for instance arise from unstable microvascular lesions of the perforating arteries which are located both distal and perpendicular to the sample volume. Therefore, the current TCD equipment will not answer the question whether very small emboli can cause lacunar and/or subcortical infarcts.

In summary at the HAGA Teaching Hospitals an embolus detection system (EDS) has been developed with a special focus to detect the short lasting, low intensity emboli which can be observed in TIA and stroke patients. The EDS can detect embolic activity in patients with a symptomatic carotid stenosis and can be used as a monitor to guard the safety and measure the efficacy of treatment. Reduction of cerebral embolism can be done by a number of interventions. Early prescription of anti-thrombotic drugs, carotid surgery or angioplasty is established means to arrest cerebral embolism. The outcome of the present study shows that with the EDS approach very low recurrence rate can be within range. The stroke recurrence rate at three months for TIA and minor stroke has decreased over the past ten years below the 5% level by the introduction of TIA and stroke services; however, much effort will be needed to achieve a further decrease. To achieve very low stroke recurrence rates (between 0% and 1%), patients need to be seen early after the event, high-risk individuals should be identified rapidly and delivery of anti-thrombotic drug regimes, surgery and angioplasty should be implemented without delay. Randomized clinical studies are needed to evaluate the clinical value of embolus detection in reducing the stroke recurrence rate in TIA and stroke patients.

References

[1] Ritter MA, Dittrich R, Thoenissen N, Ringelstein EB, Navabi DG. Prevalence and prognostic impact of microembolic signals in arterial sources of embolism. A systematic review of the literature. J Neurol 2008;255:953—61.

[2] King A, Markus HS. Doppler embolic signals in cerebrovascular disease and prediction of stroke risk: a systematic review and meta-analysis. Stroke 2009;40:3711—7.

[3] Rankin J. Cerebral vascular accidents in patients over the age of 60. II. Prognosis. Scott Med J 1957;2:200—15.

[4] European Stroke Organisation (ESO) Executive Committee, ESO Writing Committee. Guidelines of management of ischaemic stroke and transient ischaemic attack 2008. Cerebrovasc Dis 2008;25:457—507.

[5] Ederle J, Dobson J, Featherstone RL, Bonati LH, van der Worp HB, de Borst GJ, et al. Carotid artery stenting compared with endarterectomy in patients with symptomatic carotid stenosis (International Carotid Stenting Study): an interim analysis of a randomised controlled trial. Lancet 2010;375:985—97.

[6] Rothwell MP, Gilles MF, Flossmann E, Lovelock CE, Redgrave JN, Warlow CP, et al. A simple score (ABCD) to identify individuals at high early risk of stroke after transient ischaemic attack. Lancet 2005;366(July):29—36.

[7] Keunen RW, Hoogenboezem R, Wijnands R, Van den Hengel AC, Ackerstaff RG. Introduction of an embolus detection system based on analysis of the transcranial Doppler audio-signal. J Med Eng Technol 2008;32:296—304.

[8] Spencer MP. Transcranial Doppler monitoring and causes of stroke from carotid endarterectomy. Stroke 1997;28:685—91.

[9] Chung EM, Fan L, Naylor AR, Evans DH. Characteristics of Doppler embolic signals observed following carotid endarterectomy. Ultrasound Med Biol 2006;32:1011—23.

[10] Mackinnon AD, Aaslid R, Markus HS. Long-term ambulatory monitoring for cerebral emboli using transcranial Doppler ultrasound. Stroke 2004;35:73—8.

[11] Markus HS, Droste DW, Kaps M, Larrue V, Lees KR, Siebler M, et al. Dual antiplatelet therapy with clopidogrel and aspirin in symptomatic carotid stenosis evaluated using Doppler embolic signal detection: the Clopidogrel and Aspirin for Reduction of Emboli in Symptomatic Carotid Stenosis (CARESS) trial. Circulation 2005;111:2233—40.

[12] Martin MJ, Chung EM, Ramnarine KV, Goodall AH, Naylor AR, Evans DH. Thrombus size and Doppler embolic load. Cerebrovasc Dis 2009;28:397—405.

[13] Fisher CM. The arterial lesions underlying lacunes. Acta Neuropathol 1968;12:1—15.

Late septic encephalopathy and septic shock are not associated with ongoing cerebral embolism

Maayke Hunfeld[a], Michael Remmers[a], Remco Hoogenboezem[b], Michael Frank[c], Marianne van der Mee[d], H.S. Moeniralam Hazra[e], Selma C. Tromp[d], Eduard H. Boezeman[d], Denes L. Tavy[b], Ruud W. Keunen[a,*]

[a] Department of Neurology, Haga Teaching Hospitals, Leyweg 275 2545 CH, The Hague, The Netherlands
[b] Department of Clinical Neurophysiology, Haga Teaching Hospitals, Leyweg 275 2545 CH, The Hague, The Netherlands
[c] Intensive Care, Haga Teaching Hospitals, Leyweg 275 2545 CH, The Hague, The Netherlands
[d] Department of Clinical Neurophysiology, Antonius Hospital, Koekkoekslaan 1 3430 EM, Nieuwegein/Utrecht, The Netherlands
[e] Intensive Care, Antonius Hospital, Koekkoekslaan 1 3430 EM, Nieuwegein/Utrecht, The Netherlands

KEYWORDS
Embolus;
Septic;
Shock;
Sepsis;
Encephalopathy;
TCD

Summary

Background: The hypothesis that cerebral embolism plays no role in late septic encephalopathy and septic shock is based on indirect clinical evidence in the literature. The goal of this study was to prove the hypothesis that cerebral embolism plays no role in the pathophysiology of sepsis by direct evidence.

Methods: To examine this hypothesis, 20 patients with a late septic encephalopathy and septic shock were examined for direct evidence of ongoing cerebral embolism with transcranial Doppler for 30 min. Clinical data analysis included age, gender, cause of sepsis (gram-positive or -negative microorganisms), an index of severity of illness (the APACHE II score) and outcome (survivor/non survivor). Cerebral embolism was quantified by embolus detection software.

Findings: The study revealed no ongoing cerebral embolism during sepsis.

Conclusion: Cerebral micro-embolism plays no role in cerebral dysfunction during sepsis. This negative finding has an important clinical repercussion, because if transcranial Doppler exams should reveal ongoing cerebral embolism in septic shock, the embolism cannot be attributed to the septic shock itself rather it would indicate for a vigorous search for an embolic source.
© 2012 Elsevier GmbH. All rights reserved.

Abbreviations: APACHE II, Acute Physiology and Chronic Health Evaluation II; dB, Decibel; EDS, embolus detection system; ICU, Intensive Care Unit; MCA, middle cerebral artery; MES, micro-embolic signal; SPSS, Statistical Package for the Social Sciences; TCD, transcranial Doppler.
* Corresponding author.
E-mail addresses: r.keunen@hagaziekenhuis.nl, keunenrwm@tiscali.nl (R.W. Keunen).

Introduction

The mortality rate of patients who experience a septic shock and subsequent multi-organ failure is high [1]. Encephalopathy is often the first manifestation of sepsis and septic patients with encephalopathy have a higher mortality than those without encephalopathy. These findings suggest that encephalopathy may be a cause of death in septic patients. The encephalopathy of sepsis can be classified as either "early or septic encephalopathy," that presents before multiple organ failure occurs or "late encephalopathy" that is accompanied by multiple organ failure, hypotension, and other systemic phenomena. Early reports suggested that septic encephalopathy may be caused by disseminated cerebral micro-abscesses caused by septic micro-emboli but postmortem studies failed to find micro-abscesses in the brains of patients with septic encephalopathy [2—4]. Similar proportions of septic patients with gram-negative bacteremia, gram-positive bacteremia, fungemia or patients without an identified causative organism develop septic encephalopathy [5]. Another argument not in favour of cerebral embolism as a causative factor of septic encephalopathy is the fact that it is not associated with an increased stroke risk. These findings, together with the fact that encephalopathy occurs in noninfectious conditions such as pancreatitis, suggest that infecting organisms and/or their toxins do not directly cause encephalopathy [6]. Instead of septic micro-embolism recent studies showed that the etiology of septic encephalopathy involves a complex of factors which includes reduced cerebral blood flow and oxygen extraction by the brain, cerebral edema, and disruption of the blood brain barrier that may arise from the action of inflammatory mediators on the cerebrovascular endothelium, abnormal neurotransmitter composition of the reticular activating system, impaired astrocyte function, and neuronal degeneration [7].

Until recently no techniques were available to measure ongoing cerebral embolism in septic patients. Therefore there are no reports in the literature available that test the hypothesis that ongoing cerebral embolisation plays no role in patients who experience a septic encephalopathy during septic shock. Due to the high temporal resolution of transcranial Doppler ultrasound (TCD) it is possible to determine accurately ongoing cerebral embolism [8]. Recently reliable automatic algorithms have been developed which facilitate embolus detection [9]. The present study has been designed to study the relation between sepsis and cerebral embolism based on the presumption that late septic encephalopathy and septic shock are not associated.

Methods

To determine the incidence of ongoing cerebral embolism during a late septic encephalopathy and septic shock patients were monitored by transcranial Doppler ultrasound. The Doppler audiosignal was analysed by a recently developed and validated embolus detection system (EDS), which allows automatic detection of micro-embolic signals (MES) [10]. The final classification of the presence of cerebral embolism was done by two human experts. To rule out the presence of pre-existent active embolic sources, patients with known embolic sources were excluded.

Study design

This was an observational study at two intensive care units of both the Haga Teaching Hospital (The Hague) and Antonius Hospital (Nieuwegein/Utrecht) in the Netherlands. Patients met the following inclusion criteria: they are over 18 years old and they suffered from a septic shock according to Bone's criteria [11]. As late septic encephalopathy is always present in patients who have a septic shock, the late septic encephalopathy itself was not further specified in the inclusion criteria.

Exclusion criteria were absent temporal windows (which do not allow a TCD examination). Moreover patients with pre-existing sources of cerebral embolism (such as an infective endocarditis, biological and/or mechanical heart valves and/or symptomatic carotid artery stenosis were excluded.

Clinical variables included age, gender, type of sepsis (gram-positive or -negative microorganisms), an index of severity of illness (the APACHE II score) and outcome (survivor/non survivor). TCD data included the number of micro-embolic signals observed during 30 min.

Population

20 patients were included in the study.

Embolus detection

Each patient, the left or right middle cerebral artery (MCA) was insonated for 30 min with a 2 MHz transcranial Doppler (EMS-9U/DelicaSystem/Shenzen Delicate Electronics Co. Ltd./China). If small emboli are circulating towards the brain, the middle cerebral artery Doppler velocity waveform will show MES, which can be quantified by automatic software algorithms (see Fig. 1).

Video 1 shows a solid single MES. This video can be also be downloaded at http://goo.gl/Nsl1F.

Off-line analysis of the audio signal was performed by two human experts (RH and RK) who used software that had been developed and validated to detect intensity transients of short duration indicative for micro-embolism (embolus detection system distributed by SMT Medical/Wuerzburg/Germany) [10]. The MES must be differentiated from other short intensity increases not caused by emboli. These intensity increases are called by definition 'artefacts' (see Fig. 2).

The EDS has a neural network that classifies an intensity increase in either a MES or artefact. According to an International Consensus Committee, the following three main criteria were used to define a MES signal. First, the MES should have an unidirectional velocity, second the MES sound should have a musical aspect and third, the intensity should increase the 3 dB level [12]. All other transients above the 3 dB which do not fulfill MES criteria are labelled as artefacts. For viewing a so-called TCD probe movement artefact look at video 2. This video 2 can also be downloaded at: http://goo.gl/T7uEY.

Statistics

Data were entered and analysed in SPSS, version 16.0 (SPSS Inc., Chicago, Illinois). Baseline characteristics included descriptive statistics of the patients. According to the hypothesis no embolism is expected. However if embolism would be present Student t-two-tests with cerebral embolism (present/not present) as grouping parameter will be applied to determine whether cerebral embolism

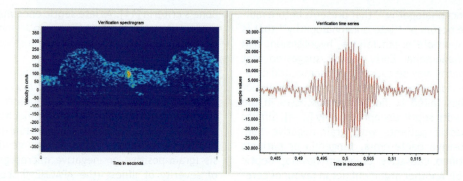

Figure 1 Normal blood flow velocity waveforms of the middle cerebral artery on the left with a high intensity transient indicative for an embolus that flows through this artery towards the brain. On the right side the TCD audio signal that shows a very rapid oscillation indicative for a so-called micro-embolic signal (MES).

were related to certain patient parameters such as age, gender, gram type of sepsis, APACHE II score and outcome. To evaluate the contribution of these parameter and cerebral embolism 2 × 2 matrixes are used. A significant value of $p < 0.05$ is employed.

Publishing ethics

Ethical and legal aspects of this study were approved by the Medical Research Committee Zuid Holland (#07-030). All representatives of the ICU patients signed an informed consent.

Results

Epidemiology

13 male and 7 female patients were investigated, with a mean age of 61.3 years (range 23—79 years). Mean pulse rate of these patients was 106 beats/min with a range between 60 and 170 beats/min. APACHE II score varied between 11 and 47 (mean value 28.8). In 3 patients the bacterial cultures were not conclusive, 11 patients experienced a gram-negative sepsis, 6 patients a gram-positive sepsis. Sixty five percent of the patients did not survive.

TCD embolism

None of the patients showed cerebral embolism.

Discussion

The present study shows that none of the patients showed signs of ongoing cerebral embolism. Cerebral embolism seems at least an infrequent finding during septic shock. This study proves direct evidence that (late) septic encephalopathy and septic shock are not related to cerebral micro-embolisation [7]. One should realize that in the current study we excluded patients with known embolic sources. It is for instance well known that patient with septic endocarditis and patients with unstable carotid artery lesions do show ongoing embolism and that these embolism are predictors of an increased stroke risk [13,14]. However, neither embolism nor strokes seems to play a role in septic encephalopathy and septic shock.

Strong aspects of this study are that TCD, due to its high special resolution, is extremely sensitive to pick up MES and secondly that to our best knowledge no earlier studies are published which addressed ongoing cerebral embolism during septic shock.

There are, however, also some critical points to make regarding the duration of monitoring, the intensity threshold

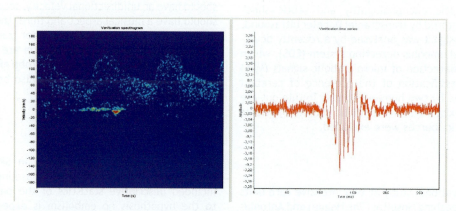

Figure 2 Normal blood flow velocity waveforms of the middle cerebral artery on the left with a high intensity transient around the baseline indicative for a movement artefact. On the right side the audio signal. Due to the probe movement the audio signal starts to oscillate at a very low frequency.

and the timing of monitoring. The current study was performed in patients with a late encephalopathy already treated with antibiotics. Therefore the current observations cannot be extended to the early septic encephalopathy which precedes the multi-organ failure and hypotension. Secondly the duration of the monitoring was limited to 30 min. This time-window seems reasonable to detect MES in patients with septic endocarditis and symptomatic carotid artery stenosis however longer periods of monitoring might be needed in case embolism during septic shock is an infrequent event. Long term monitoring by for instance robotic TCD probes built into a head band could easily increase the monitoring time for 24 h or more [15]. Finally according to established criteria in the literature human experts use the 3 dB intensity. However, very small embolic particles which generate sub 3 dB intensity MES signals might escape detection. These so-called low intensity emboli are observed in patients with symptomatic carotid artery stenosis and are related to the high intensity MES [16].

In conclusion this study proved direct evidence that ongoing cerebral embolism plays no role in the development of late septic encephalopathy. This observation has an important clinical repercussion, because if TCD exams reveals ongoing embolism in septic shock patients, these events cannot be attributed to the septic shock itself rather it would indicate for a vigorous search for an embolic source.

Competing interest

Keunen declares that he develops and distributes medical software in order to prevent cerebral ischemia. The products include an embolus detection system and electronical patient data management systems. These stroke prevention initiatives are promoted on a sponsored website (www.strokeprevention.nl).

The other authors declare that they have no competing interests.

Authors contribution

Maayke Hunfeld	Performed TCD registrations at Haga.
Michael Remmers	Performed TCD registrations at Haga.
Remco Hoogenboezem	Software engineer of EDS.
Michael Frank	Included ICU patients at Haga, reviewed manuscript.
Marianne van der Mee	Performed TCD registrations at Antonius.
H.S. Moeniralam	Included patients at Antonius, reviewed manuscript.
Selma C. Tromp	Reviewed manuscript.
Eduard H. Boezeman	Designed protocol, wrote manuscript.
Denes L. Tavy	Database management, reviewed manuscript.
Ruud W. Keunen	Designed EDS, protocol and wrote manuscript.

Appendix A. Supplementary data

Supplementary data associated with this article can be found, in the online version, at http://dx.doi.org/10.1016/j.permed.2012.03.011.

References

[1] Alberti C, Brun-Buisson C, Burchardi H, Martin C, Goodman S, Artigas A, et al. Epidemiology of sepsis and infection in ICU patients from an international multicenter cohort study. Intensive Care Med 2002;28:108—21.
[2] Jackson AC, Gilber JJ, Young GB, Bolton CF. The encephalopathy of sepsis. Can J Neurol Sci 1985;12:30—7.
[3] Pendlebury WW, Perl DP, Munoz DG. Multiple microabcesses in the central nervous system. J Neuropathol Exp Neurol 1989;48:290—300.
[4] Bleck TP, Smith MC, Pierre-Louis SJ-C, Jares JJ, Murray J, Hansen CA. Neurological complications of critical medical illnesses. Crit Care Med 1993;21:98—103.
[5] Sprung CL, Peduzzi PN, Shatney CH, Schein RM, Wilson MF, Sheagren JN, et al. Impact of encephalopathy on mortality in the sepsis syndrome. Crit Care Med 1990;18:801—6.
[6] Estrada RV, Moreno J, Martinez E, Hernandez MC, Gilsanz G, Gilsanz V. Pancreatic encephalopathy. Acta Neurol Scand 1979;59:135—9.
[7] Papadopoulos MC, Davies DC, Moss RF, Tighe D, Bennett ED. Pathophysiology of septic encephalopathy: a review. Crit Care Med 2000;28:3019—24.
[8] Spencer MP. Transcranial Doppler monitoring and causes of stroke from carotid endarterectomy. Stroke 1997;28:685—91.
[9] VanZuilen E, Mess WH, Jansen C, van der Tweel T, van Gijn J, Ackerstaff RGA. Automatic embolus detection compared with human experts. Stroke 1996;27:1840—3.
[10] Keunen RW, Hoogenboezem R, Wijnands R, Van den Hengel AC, Ackerstaff RG. Introduction of an embolus detection system based on analysis of the transcranial Doppler audio-signal. J Med Eng Technol 2008;32:296—304.
[11] Bone RC, Fisher CJ, Clemmer TP, Slotman GJ, Metz CA, Balk RA. Sepsis syndrome: a valid clinical entity. Crit Care Med 1989;17:389—93.
[12] Ringelstein EB, Droste DW, Babikian VL, Evans DH, Grosset DG, Kaps M, et al. Consensus on microembolus detection by TCD: International Consensus Group on Microembolus Detection. Stroke 1998;29:725—9.
[13] Lepur D, Barsić B. Incidence of neurological complications in patient with native valve infective endocarditis and cerebral microembolisation: an open cohort study. Scand J Infect Dis 2009;(10):708—13.
[14] King A, Markus HS. Doppler embolic signals in cerebrovascular disease and prediction of stroke risk: a systematic review and meta-analysis. Stroke 2009;40:3711—7.
[15] Mackinnon AD, Aaslid R, Markus HS. Long-term ambulatory monitoring for cerebral emboli using transcranial Doppler ultrasound. Stroke 2004;35:73—8.
[16] Telman G, Sprecher E, Kouperberg E. Potential relevance of low-intensity micro-embolic signal by TCD monitoring. Neurol Sci 2011;32:107—11.

Patent foramen ovale

Susanna Horner*, Kurt Niederkorn, Franz Fazekas

Department of Neurology, Medical University of Graz, Austria

KEYWORDS
Patent foramen ovale;
Right-to-left shunt;
Transcranial Doppler sonography;
Ultrasound contrast agent;
Transesophageal echocardiography;
Cryptogenic stroke

Summary Paradoxical embolism is a possible cause of ischemic stroke, particularly in younger patients without any other cause, i.e. cryptogenic stroke, and a patent foramen ovale is the most frequently assumed cause. The contrast transcranial Doppler monitoring mode has a sensitivity that is comparable to contrast transesophageal echocardiography for detection of a right-to-left shunt, however, the contrast transesophageal echocardiography remains the "golden standard" for the detection of a patent foramen ovale. Diagnostic studies that can identify a patent foramen ovale may be considered for prognostic purposes. In most cases, however, it is difficult to establish a firm etiological association and the debate about medical or interventional management is ongoing. Other possible causes of right-to-left shunting leading to cerebral complications like pulmonary arteriovenous malformations have also been noted but are rarely discussed.
© 2012 Elsevier GmbH. All rights reserved.

Introduction

Patients with cryptogenic stroke should be screened for possible paradoxical cerebral embolism via a cardiac or pulmonary right-to-left shunt (RLS).

There is evidence for an increased prevalence of patent foramen ovale (PFO) in cryptogenic stroke, in both younger [1—5] and elderly patients [6]. An atrial septal aneurysm (ASA) may increase the stroke risk as well, whether occurring alone or combined with a PFO [2,5]. Diagnostic studies that can identify PFO with RLS or ASA may be considered for prognostic purposes [7]. Echocardiography is recommended in selected stroke and TIA patients and is particularly required in patients with suspected paradoxical embolism and no other identifiable causes of stroke [8]. Transesophageal echocardiography (TEE) is superior to transthoracic echocardiography for evaluation of the aortic arch, left atrium, and atrial septum [9] and represents the "golden standard" to establish the presence of a RLS and a PFO. The contrast transcranial Doppler (cTCD) monitoring mode has a sensitivity that is comparable to contrast TEE (cTEE) for detection of a PFO with RLS. Its diagnostic sensitivity ranges from 70% to 100% and the specificity is more than 95% [10,11].

Although positive cTCD studies in pulmonary RLS have been described, only cTEE allows localization of the RLS to the cardiac or pulmonary level [12—15]. The distinction between cardiac and pulmonary shunts based on the time window of contrast appearance and contrast amount shunted is unreliable by cTCD [13,16].

cTCD allows estimation of the shunt size by quantification and categorization of the contrast shunted. The results are comparable with shunt quantification using cTEE [3,11,17—21]. Large RLS assessed by cTCD have been reported to be associated with a higher risk of first and recurrent stroke, particularly with cryptogenic stroke [17,22]. In contrast, results of a study showed that massive RLS sized with TCD were not an independent risk factor for recurrent stroke [18]. Therefore, the clinical significance of cTCD shunt sizing remains unclear.

* Corresponding author at: Department of Neurology, Medical University of Graz, Auenbruggerplatz 22, 8036 Graz, Austria. Tel.: +43 0316 385 83617; fax: +43 0316 385 3512.
E-mail address: susanna.horner@medunigraz.at (S. Horner).

Table 1 Summary of test procedures for detection of right-to-left shunt with ultrasound contrast agent and transcranial Doppler sonography ([16], modified).

Preparation of the patient and TCD recording
Supine position. Insert 18-gauge needle — preferred over a 20-gauge needle to increase the sensitivity [56] — into (right) cubital vein. A higher sensitivity is reported by using the femoral vein as injection site [43] which is, however, more uncomfortable for the patient. Insonate (if possible both) middle cerebral arteries (MCA), bilateral recordings increase the sensitivity compared with unilateral insonation [12,34]. In case of insufficient acoustic bone window, transforaminal insonation of the basilar artery might be an alternative approach [57].

Preparation of contrast agent and injection
Syringe I: 9 ml saline; syringe II: 1 ml air. Connect both syringes with three-way stopcock connected with a short flexible line to an intravenous line of 18-gauge with the patient. Exchange air/saline mixture vigorously between the syringes at least ten times. Inject immediately as a bolus. In case of little or no detection of microembolic signals, repeat the examination with Valsalva maneuver. Commercially traded contrast agents should be prepared according to the manufacturer's instructions.

Application of Valsalva maneuver
The patient should start with Valsalva maneuver on examiner's command 5 s after injection of the contrast agent; the control of an adequate Valsalva maneuver will be performed by assessment of the reduction of peak flow velocity of the TCD curve. Overall Valsalva maneuver duration should be 10 s.

Evaluation of test results
Categorization (for unilateral testing, values for bilateral monitoring in parentheses): (1) 0 microembolic signals (negative result); (2) 1—10 (1—20) microembolic signals; (3) >10 (>20) microembolic signals, but no curtain; (4) curtain or shower of microembolic signals, where a single signal cannot be discriminated within the TCD spectra. The microembolic signal count must be documented and evaluated separately for baseline condition and Valsalva maneuver.

The impact of cTCD in RLS detection has been studied in a number of conditions other than cerebrovascular disease; however, the grade of evidence from these studies is low to moderate: a significant association was reported between the degree of cTCD sized shunting and the number of signal abnormalities on MRI in asymptomatic sport divers [23]. Divers with RLS show a higher risk of decompression sickness [24]. There is evidence of an increased prevalence of PFO in patients with migraine with aura [25], supported by cTCD studies [26,27]. Furthermore, cTCD has been described to be useful to detect residual shunting following transcatheter closure of a PFO [28].

Depending on methodological factors, cTCD results vary considerably. Therefore, criteria of the examination technique were established by an International Consensus Meeting. The goal was a standardized approach and minimal variability for RLS detection by cTCD [16]. The examination technique recommended by this Consensus Meeting is summarized in Table 1.

Fig. 1 shows a video demonstration of a positive contrast study in a patient with large PFO. Additional data are available also from publications summarizing the impact and technique of cTCD for diagnosis of PFO [29,30].

cTCD uses air-containing echo contrast agents (CAs) which normally are unable to pass the pulmonary capillary bed. The diagnosis of a RLS by cTCD is established if TCD observes microembolic signals after contrast injection. However, the minimal amount of microembolic signals suggestive of a clinically relevant RLS is not established [16]. Different authors require different numbers of microembolic signals for the diagnosis of a PFO. They range from a minimum of one microembolus to more than five microemboli. In addition, the time from contrast injection to signal detection ranges from 6 to 10 cardiac cycles or from 4 s to 24 s [31—33]. Most authors used agitated saline solution as contrast agent [4,18,33—39] or D-galactose Mb solution (Echovist®) [12,32,34,40—46]. Only few authors used other agents such as Oxypolygelatine (Gelifundol®, Gelofusin®) [3,31,39]. A sensitivity up to 100% was achieved by both Echovist® [42,47] and agitated saline solution [4,35,38]. The Consensus Meeting recommended using the saline/air mixture. Saline/air mixture is not subject to local approval rules and has proven as effective as Echovist® in numerous studies. However, Echovist® is out of use in most countries because this CA is not longer commercially available.

Recommendations

In younger stroke patients, studies that can identify PFO or ASA may be considered for prognostic purposes (class II, level C). Echocardiography is recommended in selected stroke and TIA patients, and particularly in cryptogenic stroke and when paradoxical embolism is suspected (class III, level B). TCD is probably useful to detect cerebral microembolic signals in a wide variety of cardio- and cerebrovascular disorders or procedures (classes II—IV, level B). Standardized technique cTCD has a sensitivity similar to cTEE for detection of a PFO with RLS (class II, level A) but does not provide information of the anatomic location of the shunt or the presence of an ASA. The examination should be performed according to the instructions of the International Consensus Conference [16] (class II, level A). Although cTCD provides information about the size of the shunt, the clinical usefulness remains to be determined (level C). cTEE remains the "golden standard" for the detection of PFO. However, cTCD can be used as a minimally invasive screening test before cTEE or as an alternative method if cTEE is not available (classes III—IV, level C).

Uncertainties exist regarding optimal treatment of paradoxical cerebral embolism and therapeutic considerations have focussed primarily on the management of

PFO. Although international guidelines [48,49] recommend antiplatelet therapy as first line strategy for treating stroke patients with PFO, transcatheter closure has become common practice in many centres and is one of the most frequent interventional procedures performed in adult congenital heart disease [50]. Unfortunately, results from large randomized trials [51—54] that compare interventional closure of a PFO with medical therapy regarding the prevention of further cerebral ischemic events do not yet exist or have just been reported at meetings [55]. Therefore individual counselling is variable and the benefit of either strategy largely unknown.

Appendix A. Supplementary data

Supplementary data associated with this article can be found, in the online version, at http://dx.doi.org/10.1016/j.permed.2012.03.003.

References

[1] Overell JR, Bone I, Lees KR. Interatrial septal abnormalities and stroke: a meta-analysis of case—control studies. Neurology 2000;55:1172—9.

[2] Mas JL, Arquizan C, Lamy C, Zuber M, Cabanes L, Derumeaux G, et al. Recurrent cerebrovascular events associated with patent foramen ovale, atrial septal aneurysm, or both. New England Journal of Medicine 2001;345:1740—6.

[3] Job FP, Ringelstein EB, Grafen Y, Flachskampf FA, Doherty C, Stockmanns A, et al. Comparison of transcranial contrast Doppler sonography and transesophageal contrast echocardiography for the detection of patent foramen ovale in young stroke patients. American Journal of Cardiology 1994;74:381—4.

[4] Nemec JJ, Marwick TH, Lorig RJ, Davison MB, Chimowitz MI, Litowitz H, et al. Comparison of transcranial Doppler ultrasound and transesophageal contrast echocardiography in the detection of interatrial right-to-left shunts. American Journal of Cardiology 1991;68:1498—502.

[5] Cabanes L, Mas JL, Cohen A, Amarenco P, Cabanes PA, Oubary P, et al. Atrial septal aneurysm and patent foramen ovale as risk factors for cryptogenic stroke in patients less than 55 years of age: a study using transesophageal echocardiography. Stroke 1993;24:1865—73.

[6] Handke M, Harloff A, Olschschewski M, Hetzel A, Geibel A. Patent foramen ovale and cryptogenic stroke in older patients. New England Journal of Medicine 2007;357:2262—8.

[7] Messe S, Siverman I, Kizer J, Homma S, Zahn C, Gronseth G, et al. Practice parameter: recurrent stroke with patent foramen ovale and atrial septal aneurysm: report of the Quality Standards Subcommittee of the American Academy of Neurology. Neurology 2004;62:1042—50.

[8] Guidelines for management of ischaemic stroke and transient ischaemic attack 2008. The European Stroke Organization (ESO) Executive Committee and the ESO Writing Committee. http://www.eso-stroke.org/pdf/ESO08_Guidelines_Original_english.pdf.

[9] Lerakis S, Nicholson WJ. Part I: use of echocardiography in the evaluation of patients with suspected cardioembolic stroke. American Journal of the Medical Sciences 2005;329:310—6.

[10] Masdeu JC, Irimia P, Asenbaum S, Bogousslavsky J, Brainin M, Chabriat H, et al. EFNS guideline on neuroimaging in acute stroke. Report of an EFNS task force. European Journal of Neurology 2006;13:1271—83.

[11] Sloan MA, Alexandrov AV, Tegeler CH, Spencer MP, Caplan LR, Feldmann E, et al. Transcranial Doppler ultrasonography in 2004: a comprehensive evidence-based update. Background paper to the Official AAN Assessment of TCD: transcranial Doppler ultrasonography. Neurology 2004;62(9):1468—81.

[12] Horner S, Ni XS, Weihs W, Harb S, Augustin M, Duft M, et al. Simultaneous bilateral contrast transcranial Doppler monitoring in patients with intracardiac and intrapulmonary shunts. Journal of the Neurological Sciences 1997;150:49—57.

[13] Horner S, Schuchlenz S, Harb S, Weihs W, Ni XS, Fazekas F, et al. Contrast transcranial Doppler monitoring in stroke patients with pulmonary right-to-left shunts (abstract). Cerebrovascular Diseases 1998;8(Suppl. 3):7.

[14] Shibazaki K, Iguchi Y, Inoue T, Yuji UenoY, Kimura K. Serial contrast saline transcranial Doppler examination in a patient with paradoxical brain embolism associated with pulmonary embolism. Journal of Clinical Neuroscience 2007;14(8):788—91.

[15] Yeung M, Khan KA, Antecol DH, Walker DR, Shuaib A. Transcranial Doppler ultrasonography and transesophageal echocardiography in the investigation of pulmonary arteriovenous malformation in a patient with hereditary hemorrhagic telangiectasia presenting with stroke. Stroke 1995;26:1941—4.

[16] Jauss M, Zanette EM, for the Consensus Conference. Detection of right-to-left shunt with ultrasound contrast agent and transcranial Doppler sonography. Cerebrovascular Diseases 2000;10:490—6.

[17] Serena J, Segura T, Perez-Ayuso MJ, Bassaganyas J, Molina A, Davalos A. The need to quantify right-to-left shunt in acute ischemic stroke. A case control study. Stroke 1998;29:1322—8.

[18] Serena J, Marti-Fàbregas J, Santamarina E, Rodríguez JJ, Perez-Ayuso MJ, Masjuan J, et al. Recurrent stroke and massive right-to-left shunt: results from the prospective Spanish multicenter (CODICIA) study. Stroke 2008;39(12):3131—6.

[19] Kobayashi K, Iguchi Y, Kimura K, Okada Y, Terasawa Y, Matsumoto N, et al. Contrast transcranial Doppler can diagnose large patent foramen ovale. Cerebrovascular Diseases 2009;27:230—4.

[20] Telman G, Yalonetsky S, Kouperberg E, Sprecher E, Lorber, Yarnitsky D. Size of PFO and amount of microembolic signals in patients with ischaemic stroke or TIA. European Journal of Neurology 2008;15(9):969—72.

[21] Belvis R, Leta RG, Marti-Fabregas J, Cocho D, Carreras F, Pons-Llado G, et al. Almost perfect concordance between simultaneous transcranial Doppler and transesophageal echocardiography in the quantification of right-to-left shunts. Journal of Neuroimaging 2006;16:133—8.

[22] Anzola GP, Zavarize P, Morandi E, Rozzini L, Parrinello G. Transcranial Doppler and risk of recurrence in patients with stroke and patent foramen ovale. European Journal of Neurology 2003;10(2):129—35.

[23] Knauth M, Ries S, Pohlmann S, Kerby T, Forsting M, Daffertshofer M, et al. Cohort study of multiple brain lesions in sport divers: role of a patent foramen ovale. BMJ 1997;314:701.

[24] Gempp E, Blatteau JE, Stephant E, Louge P. Relation between right-to-left shunts and spinal cord decompression sickness in divers. International Journal of Sports Medicine 2009;30(2):150—3.

[25] Schwedt TJ, Demaerschalk BM, Dodick DW. Patent foramen ovale and migraine: a quantitative systematic review. Cephalalgia 2008;28(5):531—40.

[26] Anzola GP, Magoni M, Guindani M, Rozzini L, Dalla Volta G. Potential source of cerebral embolism in migraine with aura: a transcranial Doppler study. Neurology 1999;52:1622—5.

[27] Del Sette M, Angeli S, Leandri M, Ferriero G, Brunzone GL, Finocchi C, et al. Migraine with aura and right-to-left shunt on transcranial Doppler: a case—control study. Cerebrovascular Diseases 1998;8:327—30.

[28] Van de Wyngaert F, Kefer J, Hermans C, Ovaert C, Pasquet A, Beguin C, et al. Absence of recurrent stroke after percutaneous

closure of patent foramen ovale despite residual right-to-left cardiac shunt assessed by trancranial Doppler. Archives of Cardiovascular Diseases 2008;101(7–8):435–41.
[29] Nedeltchev K, Mattle HP. Contrast-enhanced transcranial Doppler ultrasound for diagnosis of patent foramen ovale. In: Baumgartner RW, editor. Handbook on neurovascular ultrasound, vol. 21. Basel: Karger; 2006. p. 206–15 [Front Neurol Neurosci.].
[30] Anzola GP. Clinical impact of patent foramen ovale diagnosis with transcranial Doppler. European Journal of Ultrasound 2002;16:11–20.
[31] Karnik R, Stollberger C, Valentin A, Winkler WB, Slany J. Detection of patent foramen ovale by transcranial contrast Doppler ultrasound. American Journal of Cardiology 1992;69:560–2.
[32] Jauss M, Kaps M, Keberle M, Haberbosch W, Dorndorf W. A comparison of transesophageal echocardiography and transcranial Doppler sonography with contrast medium for detection of patent foramen ovale. Stroke 1994;25:1265–7.
[33] Zanette EM, Mancini G, De Castro S, Solaro M, Cartoni D, Chiarotti F. Patent foramen ovale and transcranial Doppler: comparison of different procedures. Stroke 1996;27:2251–5.
[34] Droste DW, Reisener M, Kemeny V, Dittrich R, Schulte-Altedorneburg G, Stypmann J, et al. Contrast transcranial Doppler ultrasound in the detection of right-to-left shunts: reproducibility, comparison of two agents, and distribution of microemboli. Stroke 1999;30:1014–8.
[35] Devuyst G, Despland PA, Bogousslavsky J, Jeanrenaud X. Complementarity of contrast transcranial Doppler and contrast transesophageal echocardiography for the detection of patent foramen ovale in stroke patients. European Neurology 1997;38:21–5.
[36] Anzola GP, Renaldini E, Magoni M, Costa A, Cobelli M, Guindani M. Validation of transcranial Doppler sonography in the assessment of patent foramen ovale. Cerebrovascular Diseases 1995;5:194–8.
[37] Di Tullio M, Sacco RL, Venketasubramanian N, Sherman D, Mohr JP, Homma S. Comparison of diagnostic techniques for the detection of a patent foramen ovale in stroke patients. Stroke 1993;24:1020–4.
[38] Teague SM, Sharma MK. Detection of paradoxical cerebral echo contrast embolization by transcranial Doppler ultrasound. Stroke 1991;22:740–5.
[39] Chimowitz MI, Nemec JJ, Marwick TH, Lorig RJ, Furlan AJ, Salcedo EE. Transcranial Doppler ultrasound identifies patients with right-to-left cardiac or pulmonary shunts. Neurology 1991;41:1902–4.
[40] Blersch WK, Draganski BM, Holmer SR, Koch HJ, Schlachetzki F, Bogdahn U, et al. Transcranial duplex sonography in the detection of patent foramen ovale. Radiology 2002;225:693–9.
[41] Droste DW, Kriete JU, Stypmann J, Castrucci M, Wichter T, Tietje R, et al. Contrast transcranial Doppler ultrasound in the detection of right-to left shunts: comparison of different procedures and different contrast agents. Stroke 1999;30:1827–32.
[42] Schwarze JJ, Sander D, Kukla C, Wittich I, Babikian VL, Klingelhöfer J. Methodological parameters influence the detection of right-left shunts by contrast transcranial Doppler ultrasonography. Stroke 1999;30(6):1234–9.
[43] Hamann GF, Schätzer-Klotz D, Fröhlig G, Strittmatter M, Jost V, Berg G, et al. Femoral injection of echo contrast medium may increase the sensitivity of testing for a patent foramen ovale. Neurology 1998;50:1423–8.
[44] Klötzsch C, Janssen G, Berlit P. Transesophageal echocardiography and contrast-TCD in the detection of a patent foramen ovale: experiences with 111 patients. Neurology 1994;44:1603–6.
[45] Schminke U, Ries S, Daffertshofer M, Staedt U, Hennerici M. Patent foramen ovale: a potential source of cerebral embolism. Cerebrovascular Diseases 1995;5:133–8.
[46] Droste DW, Jekentaite R, Stypmann J, Grude M, Hansberg T, Ritter M, et al. Contrast transcranial Doppler ultrasound in the detection of right-to-left shunts: comparison of Echovist®-200 and Echovist®-300, timing of the Valsalva maneuver, and general recommendations for the performance of the test. Cerebrovascular Diseases 2002;13:235–41.
[47] Uzuner N, Horner S, Pichler G, Svetina D, Niederkorn K. Right-to-left shunt assessed by contrast transcranial Doppler sonography. Journal of Ultrasound in Medicine 2004;23:1475–82.
[48] European Stroke Organisation (ESO) Executive Committee, ESO Writing Committee. Guidelines for management of ischaemic stroke and transient ischaemic attack 2008. Cerebrovascular Diseases 2008;25(5):457–507 [Epub 2008 May 6].
[49] Furie KL, Kasner SE, Adams RJ, Albers GW, Bush RL, Fagan SC, et al. Guidelines for the prevention of stroke in patients with stroke or transient ischemic attack: a guideline for healthcare professionals from the American Heart Association/American Stroke Association. Stroke 2011;42(January (1)):227–76.
[50] Kenny D, Turner M, Martin R. When to close a patent foramen ovale. Archives of Disease in Childhood 2008;93(March (3)):255–9.
[51] PC-Trial. Patent foramen ovale and cryptogenic embolism. http://clinicaltrials.gov/ct2/show/NCT00166257?term=Patent+foramen+ovale+and+Cryptogenic+embolism&rank=1.
[52] RESPECT. Randomized evaluation of recurrent stroke comparing PFO closure to established current standard of care treatment. http://www.amplatzer.com/clinical_trials/tabid/94/default.aspx.
[53] CLOSE. Patent foramen ovale closure or anticoagulants versus antiplatelet therapy to prevent stroke recurrence. ClinicalTrials.gov. http://clinicaltrials.gov/ct2/show/NCT00562289?term=NCT00562289&rank=1.
[54] CARDIA STAR™ Trial: A United States Randomized Clinical Trial of the CARDIA STAR™ Patent Foramen Ovale Closure System (The CARDIA STAR™ Trial). http://www.mplsheart.com/Publications/Research/InterventionalCardiologyResearch/CARDIASTAR.aspx.
[55] Furlan AMJ, Mauri L, Adams H, Albers G, Felberg R, Herrmann H, et al. Late breaking clinical trial and science abstracts from the American Heart Association's scientific session 2010; abstract 21752: CLOSURE I: A prospective, multicenter, randomized, controlled trial to evaluate the safety and efficacy of the Starflex septal closure system versus best medical therapy in patients with a stroke or transient ischemic attack due to presumed paradoxical embolism through a patent foramen ovale. Circulation 2010;122:2218.
[56] Khan KA, Yeung M, Shuaib A. Comparative study of 18 gauge and 20 gauge intravenous catheters during transcranial Doppler ultrasonography with saline solution contrast. Journal of Ultrasound in Medicine 1997;16:341–4.
[57] Perren F, Savva E, Landis T. Transforaminal Doppler: an alternative to transtemporal approach for right-to-left cardiac shunt assessment. Journal of the Neurological Sciences 2008;273(1–2):49–50.

Microbubble signal properties from PFO tests using transcranial Doppler ultrasound

Caroline Banahan[a,*], Rizwan Patel[b], Vikram Jeyagopal[b], Amit Mistri[a,b], James P. Hague[c], David H. Evans[b], Emma M.L. Chung[b]

[a] Medical Physics Department, University Hospitals of Leicester NHS Trust, UK
[b] Department of Cardiovascular Sciences, University of Leicester, UK
[c] Department of Physical Sciences, Open University, Milton Keynes, UK

KEYWORDS
Embolus detection;
Transcranial Doppler ultrasound;
Gaseous emboli

Summary

Background: A limitation of transcranial Doppler (TCD) ultrasound is the inability to distinguish tiny benign bubbles from potentially hazardous particulate emboli based on analysis of the intensity of backscattered ultrasound. This study examines the Doppler characteristics of small microbubbles detected during screening of patients for a patent foramen ovale (PFO). The aim of this study was to identify unique microbubble properties that could differentiate between solid and gaseous emboli.

Methods: Bilateral TCD monitoring of the middle cerebral arteries (MCA) was performed for 34 patients during PFO screening using agitated saline. Patients were injected up to three times and asked to perform a valsalva manoeuvre. The raw audio data was recorded onto an external laptop for subsequent analysis.

Results: Eleven patients tested positive for a PFO, yielding 331 embolic signals with intensities <35 dB. The median peak measured-embolus-blood-ratio (MEBR) was 25.7 dB and the median duration was 33.0 ms. The majority of signals lasted between 12 and 92 ms, which are much longer than previously reported for particulate thrombus where the majority of signal durations are between 6 and 41 ms. Pearson correlation tests revealed a weak positive correlation between estimated microbubble velocity and signal duration (0.26, $p < 0.0001$).

Conclusions: Doppler signal properties were analysed for over 300 microbubbles recorded in vivo. Microbubble signal duration was found to be higher than measured for solid emboli. Further work to develop a clinically useful model based on microembolus properties to differentiate solid and gaseous is ongoing.

© 2012 Elsevier GmbH. All rights reserved.

Introduction

Although transcranial Doppler ultrasound (TCD) is a sensitive tool for detecting emboli as they pass through the cerebral circulation, the challenge remains to characterise emboli by size and composition using the backscattered Doppler signal.

* Corresponding author.
E-mail address: Caroline.Banahan@uhl-tr.nhs.uk (C. Banahan).

It is believed that embolus composition (solid emboli) and size (larger emboli) are important in predicting clinically significant complications. For example, patients on bypass for open-heart surgery are known to receive multiple showers of predominantly gaseous emboli but may also have some solid emboli due to pre-existing cardiovascular disease. These emboli have been linked to post-operative neurocognitive decline and stroke [1]. Most studies estimate the risk to these patients by counting the number of emboli detected during surgery without considering how size and composition may influence the outcome; a small microbubble is likely to be insignificant compared to a larger macrobubble or solid embolus [2,3].

Studying the backscattered intensity alone does not provide enough information to determine embolus composition; calculations using scattering theory reveal that a small microbubble will backscatter with a comparable intensity to a larger solid embolus: assuming a vessel radius of 1.25 mm and a sample volume length of 10 mm, a 4 μm gaseous embolus is predicted to backscatter with a similar intensity to a 130 μm solid (thrombus) embolus [4]. Different signal properties therefore need to be explored to determine embolus composition. One such property is the frequency modulation. Previous studies have shown that the embolic signatures of gaseous emboli have a high frequency modulation index compared to solid emboli [5,6]. Souchon et al. suggested that this high frequency modulation index was due to a radiation force effect, which alters the trajectory of gas bubbles in the artery [7]. Promising results were shown in their in vitro study but as discussed by the authors, due to natural complications in vivo, one could expect to see a low frequency modulation from a gas bubble if it crosses a small part of the sample volume. Thus the technique may produce a high false positive when identifying solid emboli.

Another avenue explored has been the dual-frequency method [8]. It is based on the frequency dependent nature of backscattering from different emboli types. For a 2.0 and 2.5 MHz probe, the ratio of the backscattered intensity from the embolus compared to the backscattered signal from blood (MEBR) from gas bubbles will be lower at 2.5 MHz compared to 2.0 MHz. For small solid particles the MEBR value from both frequencies will be approximately the same until the particle size approaches the ultrasound wavelength, at which point the MEBR at 2.5 MHz will be greater than for 2.0 MHz. In theory this technique sounds plausible, but Evans and Gittins [9] found that in practice differences in the beam shapes for 2.0 and 2.5 MHz led to uncertainties in the measurements of the ratios of MEBR at both frequencies. This, in turn, limits the accuracy of the technique with a significant percentage of emboli misclassified.

Other studies have tried to determine embolus composition by analysing the signal properties from 'pure' sources of either solid or gaseous emboli. Darbellay et al. studied 3428 high intensity transient signals (HITS) recorded from stroke patients with carotid stenosis and patients undergoing a patent foramen ovale (PFO) test [10]. They used three types of statistical classifiers: binary decision trees, artificial neural networks and support vector machines to try and distinguish between gas and solid particles. They drew up a list of features from these signals and found that MEBR and SDSE (standard deviation of the slope of the envelope) produced the most stable binary decision tree to differentiate between the two types (with a sensitivity and specificity of 81%). The best classification was achieved using 20 features from recorded emboli and the support vector machines (86% sensitivity and specificity). However, for such an increase in complexity the improvement was marginal when at least 95% specificity and sensitivity is needed to make the classifier valuable in a clinical environment.

Chung et al. studied the characteristics of Doppler embolic signal properties from solid emboli detected following carotid endarterectomy [11]. Characteristic distributions were observed for embolic velocities, implying that solid emboli had a preferred trajectory through the middle cerebral artery (MCA). A signature peak was also observed when the MEBR was combined with embolic signal duration. In this study, a similar analysis is carried out using the Doppler signal properties from microbubbles detected using TCD during screening tests for a PFO. Thus a comparison can be made between the signal properties of solid and gaseous emboli to determine if any unique property or set of properties exists for microbubbles that may allow us to distinguish between solid and gaseous emboli.

Materials and methods

Transcranial Doppler ultrasound signals were recorded from patients being screened for a PFO after paradoxical stroke. These patients had no significant carotid artery abnormalities and transesophageal echocardiography showed no thrombus lodged in the heart. A Nicolet Biomedical Companion III TCD machine was used and bilateral monitoring of the MCAs was performed using 2 MHz transducers. The contrast consisted of 0.5 ml of air and 0.5 ml of blood vigorously mixed with 8.5 ml of saline solution and injected into the anticubital vein via a three-way stopcock immediately after contrast preparation. If no microbubbles were detected after the first injection, then a further two injections were made with a valsalva manoeuvre. The analogue signal from the Companion III was recorded onto a Dell Precision laptop (1.995 GHz, 2 MB L2 cache) using a Sony EX-UT10 data acquisition system. The data were analysed offline using an in-house program developed in Matlab.

Data analysis

Due to the limited dynamic range of the Companion III, many Doppler signals recorded from the gaseous emboli were saturated; therefore only signals that were not clipped were used for further analysis. Raw audio data were extracted and analysed using an in-house program developed in Matlab (Mathworks Inc., Natick, MA, USA). Embolus and background windows were manually selected by the operator to ensure no artefacts were present. The background window was integrated and normalised with respect to time to estimate an average background value, for comparison with the average intensity of backscatter from the embolus to give a measured embolus-to-blood ratio (MEBR):

$$\text{MEBR} = 10 \log_{10} \left(\frac{I_{E+B}}{I_B} \right) \text{dB} \qquad (1)$$

where I_E is the average intensity of the embolic signal and I_B is the intensity of the average background audio signal. The

Table 1 Signal properties from 331 microbubbles recorded during a screening test for a PFO using transcranial Doppler ultrasound.

Microbubble signal properties

	Median	5th centile	95th centile
MEBR (dB)	15.6	7.9	21.7
Peak MEBR (dB)	25.7	17.4	31.3
Duration (ms)	33.3	12.3	91.6
ZCF (Hz)	520.8	244.3	1025.9
Estimated velocity (cm s^{-1})	23.0	10.9	45.6

Table 2 Pearson correlation tests for the various embolic signal properties.

Pearson correlation test ($p < 0.01$) (331 bubbles)

	MEBR (dB)		Duration (ms)
	Peak	Average	
Velocity (cm s^{-1})	0.16	0.17	−0.23
Duration (ms)	n/a	−0.16	

peak MEBR was calculated by replacing I_E with I_{EP} in Eq. (1) where I_{EP} is the maximum intensity of backscatter from the embolus. The duration of the embolus was also extracted in milliseconds and the zero-crossing frequency (ZCF) in Hertz. The latter was then used to calculate embolus velocity via the Doppler equation. Velocities are angle-corrected based on a Doppler angle of 30°. Pearson correlation tests were then used to discern if any correlation exists between these properties.

Results

Eleven patients tested positive for a PFO yielding 331 embolic signals with intensities less than 35 dB. Table 1 displays the average values for various signal properties along with median values and 5% and 95% percentiles due to the non-normal distribution of these properties. 90% of gaseous emboli possess MEBR values between 7.9 and 21.7 dB and peak MEBR values between 17.4 and 31.3 dB. The majority of microbubble signals lasted between 12.3 and 91.6 ms with a median signal duration of 33.3 ms. Combining the above information a characteristic peak for microbubble signals was observed with a peak at ∼15.6 dB and duration of ∼33.3 ms (see Fig. 1). The median ZCF of 520 Hz corresponds to an estimated velocity of 23.2 cm s^{-1} and 90% of the signals had velocities between approximately 10.9 and 45.6 cm s^{-1}. Table 2 lists the Pearson correlation coefficients for various pairs of embolic signal parameters. Pearson correlation tests showed a weak positive correlation between estimated velocity and duration (0.24, $p < 0.0001$). A weak negative correlation was also found for the average MEBR and embolic signal duration (−0.16, $p < 0.01$).

Discussion

The signal properties from 331 microbubbles have revealed some interesting distinguishing features that differ from the same signal properties previously analysed for solid emboli [11]. The majority of solid emboli in [11] had signal durations between 6.2 and 40.5 ms which are much shorter than the range observed for gaseous emboli in this study (12.3—91.6 ms). Solid emboli had a distinctive peak at ∼7 dB with a duration of ∼12.5 ms which contrasts with that observed for gaseous emboli (peak at ∼15.6 dB, duration ∼33.3 ms). This indicates that gaseous emboli tend to have higher MEBR values with longer durations compared to solid emboli.

A weak negative correlation was observed between MEBR and embolic signal duration for microbubbles (−0.16, $p < 0.01$) compared to the positive correlation found for solid emboli (0.57, $p < 0.0001$). This positive correlation was also noted by Martin et al. who where studying the relationship between thrombus size and MEBR [12]. They found that larger solid emboli generated signals of longer duration. The weak negative correlation between MEBR and signal duration for microbubbles may relate to a preferred trajectory through the insonated vessel. The velocity distribution shown in Fig. 2 demonstrates that velocities of emboli have a broad distribution over a wide range of speeds, but these speeds are relatively low compared to typical speeds at the centre of the MCA (1 m s^{-1}). This is consistent with gas emboli floating to the top of the MCA where the speed at the edge of a vessel is lower, rather than the more even distribution expected for neutrally buoyant small particles.

Due to the low dynamic range of the TCD machine only microbubbles with peak MEBRs below 35 dB, corresponding to estimated diameters between 2 and 4 μm, were analysed. The embolic signal properties in this study therefore represent a very small distribution of bubble sizes and these properties may differ for larger bubbles. However, Chung et al. observed disruptions in blood flow for solid emboli with backscattered intensities of ∼35 dB indicating that the

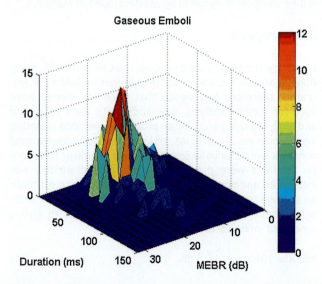

Figure 1 The characteristic peak for 331 microbubble signals (peak ∼15.6 dB and duration ∼33.3 ms).

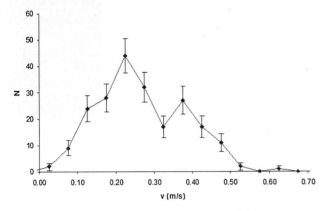

Figure 2 Velocity distribution for 331 microbubbles.

diameter of the embolus may have been close to the diameter of the MCA [11]. They set an upper limit on the maximum MEBR that can be observed from large solid (thrombus) emboli of 35 dB. Thus studying microbubbles with MEBR values equal to or below this threshold provides an excellent opportunity to determine what signal properties may help in differentiating between potentially harmful solid emboli and benign gaseous emboli.

Conclusions

Gaseous embolus properties from 331 microemboli recorded in vivo during TCD screening for a PFO were significantly different from those previously reported for solid emboli. In particular, gaseous embolus signal duration was found to be higher than that reported for solid emboli. There was a weak negative correlation between MEBR and embolus duration in this study, contrasting with the positive correlation between MEBR and solid embolus signal duration reported previously. These distinct properties hold potential in the future development of a model, which will enable differentiation of gaseous from solid emboli using TCD.

References

[1] Newman MF, Kirchner JL, Phillips-Bute B, Gaver V, Grocott H, Jones RH, et al. Longitudinal assessment of neurocognitive function after coronary—artery bypass surgery. N Engl J Med 2001;344(February (6)):395—402.

[2] Martin KK, Wigginton JB, Babikian VL, Pochay VE, Crittenden MD, Rudolph JL. Intraoperative cerebral high-intensity transient signals and postoperative cognitive function: a systematic review. Am J Surg 2009;197(January (1)):55—63.

[3] Stump DA, Rogers AT, Hammon JW, Newman SP. Cerebral emboli and cognitive outcome after cardiac surgery. J Cardiothorac Vasc Anesth 1996;10(January (1)):113—8.

[4] Lubbers J, Van Den Berg JW. An ultrasonic detector for microgasemboli in a bloodflow line. Ultrasound Med Biol 1977;2(4):301—10.

[5] Smith JL, Evans DH, Bell PR, Naylor AR. A comparison of four methods for distinguishing Doppler signals from gaseous and particulate emboli. Stroke 1998;29(June (6)):1133—8.

[6] Girault JM, Kouame D, Menigot S, Souchon G, Tranquart F. Analysis of index modulation in microembolic Doppler signals. Part I. Radiation force as a new hypothesis-simulations. Ultrasound Med Biol 2011;37(January (1)):87—101.

[7] Souchon G, Girault JM, Biard M, Kouame D, Tranquart F. Gaseous and solid emboli differentiation using radiation force. IEEE Ultrason Symp 2005;(September):2070—3.

[8] Moehring MA, Klepper JR. Pulse Doppler ultrasound detection, characterization and size estimation of emboli in flowing blood. IEEE Trans Biomed Eng 1994;41(January (1)):35—44.

[9] Evans DH, Gittins J. Limits of uncertainty in measured values of embolus-to-blood ratios in dual-frequency TCD recordings due to nonidentical sample volume shapes. Ultrasound Med Biol 2005;31(February (2)):233—42.

[10] Darbellay GA, Duff R, Vesin JM, Despland PA, Droste DW, Molina C, et al. Solid or gaseous circulating brain emboli: are they separable by transcranial ultrasound? J Cereb Blood Flow Metab 2004;24(August (8)):860—8.

[11] Chung EM, Fan L, Naylor AR, Evans DH. Characteristics of Doppler embolic signals observed following carotid endarterectomy. Ultrasound Med Biol 2006;32(July (7)):1011—23.

[12] Martin MJ, Chung EM, Ramnarine KV, Goodall AH, Naylor AR, Evans DH. Thrombus size and Doppler embolic signal intensity. Cerebrovasc Dis 2009;28(4):397—405.

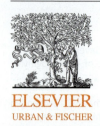
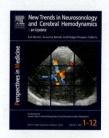

Bartels E, Bartels S, Poppert H (Editors):
New Trends in Neurosonology and Cerebral Hemodynamics — an Update.
Perspectives in Medicine (2012) 1, 236—240

journal homepage: www.elsevier.com/locate/permed

Italian patent foramen ovale survey (I.P.O.S.): Early results

Luigi Caputi [a,*], Gianfranco Butera [b], Eugenio Parati [a], Giuseppe Sangiorgi [c], Eustaquio Onorato [d,1], Gian Paolo Anzola [d], Massimo Chessa [b], Mario Carminati [b], Gian Paolo Ussia [e], Isabella Spadoni [f], Gennaro Santoro [g], on behalf of IPOS investigators [2]

[a] Fondazione IRCCS Neurological Institute C. Besta. Department of Cerebrovascular Diseases, Via Celoria 11, 20133 Milan, Italy
[b] Policlinico San Donato, Via Morandi 30, San Donato Milanese, Italy
[c] Modena University, Modena, Italy
[d] Ospedale S. Orsola, Unita' Operativa di Cardiologia — Fatebenefratelli, Service of Neurology, Via Vittorio Emanuele II 27, Brescia, Italy
[e] Ospedale Ferrarotto, Laboratorio di Emodinamica Divisione Clinicizzata di Cardiologia, Azienda Policlinico Vittorio Emanuele, Via Salvatore Citelli 1, Catania, Italy
[f] Ospedale ''G: Pasquinucci'' U.O. Cardiologia Pediatrica e GUCH, Via Aurelia Sud Loc. Montepepe, Massa, Italy
[g] S.O.D. ''Diagnostica ed Interventistica Cardiovascolare, AOU Careggi, Viale Pieraccini, 17, Florence, Italy

KEYWORDS
Patent foramen ovale;
Percutaneous PFO closure;
Stroke;
Survey;
Transcranial Doppler;
Echocardiography

Summary

Background: Percutaneous patent foramen ovale (PFO) closure is gaining wide acceptance. Aims of the study were to analyse clinical practice regarding PFO closure in Italy, to study indications, devices, results, and the follow-up of large series of patients treated by percutaneous PFO closure.

Methods and patients: Italian patent foramen ovale survey (IPOS) is a prospective, observational, multi-centric survey that uses a web-based database. The survey lasted 12 months, (November 2007—October 2008). 50 centres participated. Ongoing follow-up will continue up to 36 months. 1035 patients (m.a. 46 years, 60% females) were included in the registry. Most subjects were treated due to a previous history of TIA/ischemic stroke (~80% of patients). PFO diagnosis and right-to-left shunt (RLS) were assessed by contrast-enhanced transesophageal (cTEE) and/or transthoracic echocardiography and/or transcranial doppler. An aneurysm of the

* Corresponding author. Tel.: +39 02 23941; fax: +39 02 70631911.
E-mail addresses: luigi_caputi@yahoo.it (L. Caputi), gianfra.but@lycos.com (G. Butera), parati@istituto-besta.it (E. Parati), gsangiorgi@gmail.com (G. Sangiorgi), eonorato@libero.it (E. Onorato), gpanzola@numerica.it (G.P. Anzola), massimo.chessa@grupposandonato.it (M. Chessa), mario.carminati@grupposandonato.it (M. Carminati), gian.paolo.ussia@gmail.com (G.P. Ussia), ispadoni@ifc.cnr.it (I. Spadoni), santorog@aou-careggi.toscana.it (G. Santoro).

[1] Present address: Visiting Professor at ''Cardiologia Interventistica, Policlinico Universitario Tor Vergata, Rome, Italy'' and expert Consultant at ''Cardiologia Interventistica, Humanitas Gavazzeni, Bergamo, Italy and Clinica Montevergine, Mercogliano, Italy''.
[2] IPOS investigators (see Appendix A).

2211-968X/$ — see front matter © 2012 Elsevier GmbH. All rights reserved.
doi:10.1016/j.permed.2012.02.010

interatrial septum was associated in 41% of patients. Intraprocedural monitoring was assessed by using cTEE and fluoroscopy in 70% and intracardiac echocardiography in 30% of subjects. Procedures were performed under general anesthesia and local anesthesia/conscious sedation in 54% and 46% of patients respectively. The most used device for PFO closure was Amplatzer (~70% of cases).

Results: The procedure was successful in all patients. Early complications occurred in 24/1035 patients (2.3%): 12/24 (50%) of them had cardiac arrhythmias, 1 subject had a TIA. Data regarding both clinical and cardio-neurosonological follow-up were assessed in 444/1035 (43%) subjects. The rate of neurological events and cardiac and extra-cardiac complications were around 3% and 9% up to the 24-month follow-up respectively. A large permanent residual RLS and no RLS were observed in less than 1% and in ~82% of patients at the 1-year follow-up, respectively.

Conclusions: Our data confirm that percutaneous PFO closure is a safe procedure. Early complications and those during follow-up are mostly related to arrhythmias. Longer follow-up is under way.

© 2012 Elsevier GmbH. All rights reserved.

Introduction

During the last years, percutaneous patent foramen ovale (PFO) closure has gained wide acceptance with a huge number of patients successfully undergoing this procedure. Few large databanks exist with mid-long term follow-up after PFO closure [1–8]. Moreover, the rate of peri- and post-procedural clinical complications was differently characterized in many studies all over the world.

The aim of our study was, therefore, to analyse clinical practice regarding PFO closure in Italy, to study indications, devices used, results of percutaneous PFO closure and to evaluate a 36-month follow-up of a large series of patients treated by percutaneous closure.

Waiting for the final results, this paper describes early results concerning crucial aspects related to PFO closure up to the 24-month follow-up.

Methods and patients

Study design

IPOS is a prospective, observational, multi-centric survey that uses a web-based database. An independent neurological evaluation of all cases included in the registry was assessed. Doubtful or inconsistent reports regarding a neurological recurrence were ruled out.

Study period

The survey lasted 12 months and the patients were enrolled between November 2007 and October 2008. Ongoing follow-up will continue up to 36 months.

Flow-chart

Patients' screening consisted with demographic characteristics, current medical treatment, neurological evaluation, indication for PFO closure and RLS evaluation.

Imaging with cardiomorphological data, different devices and possible complications were indicated during the procedures.

In the post-procedural phase early complications, length of hospitalization and treatment at discharge were described.

Follow-ups were within the 6th, 12th, 24th and 36th month. Data regarding cardiac imaging, residual RLS, neurological recurrences and/or cardiac extra-cardiac complications were specified.

Indications

Most subjects who underwent PFO closure had a previous history of TIA/cryptogenic ischemic stroke (~80% of patients). The remaining indications were consistent with migraine with aura, other events of paradoxical embolism as myocardial or retinal ischemia, residual PFO after a previous procedure, platypnea–orthodeoxia syndrome, neurosurgical procedures in sitting/semisitting position, diving, thrombophilic status and asymptomatic patients with neuroradiological ischemic lesions.

Baseline data and PFO diagnosis

Fifty Italian cardiology departments accepted to participate. Forty of them enrolled at least one patient in the registry. 1035 patients (mean age 46 years [range 5–75], 619/1035 [60%] females) were included in the registry.

PFO diagnosis and right-to-left shunt (RLS) were assessed by contrast-enhanced transesophageal (cTEE) and/or transthoracic echocardiography (cTTE) and/or transcranial Doppler (cTCD).

RLS was assessed in a visual semi-quantitative method by cTEE and cTTE: RLS was diagnosed if at least 1 microbubble (MB) appeared early in the left atrium either spontaneously or after provocative manoeuvres, thus indicating no shunt if no MB were revealed up to a severe shunt if >20 MB occurred.

cTCD methods regarding RLS diagnosis were previously described [9]. cTCD was performed according to the standardized procedure agreed on in the Consensus Conference of Venice [10]. Briefly, the total MB count consisted of all MB detected during a time interval of 20 s or less after the appearance of the first MB. The proposed classification is as follows: small (0–10 MB), moderate (>10 MB, without shower or curtain pattern), and large (shower or curtain pattern)

RLS. All our patients who exhibited RLS of 5 or more MB were considered to have a positive test result [11].

Aneurysm of the interatrial septum (ASA) was diagnosed in the presence of atrial septal excursion greater than 10 mm beyond the plane of the interatrial septum in the presence of a base width greater than 15 mm. ASA was associated in 423/1035 (41%) patients.

Cardiac monitoring

Intraprocedural monitoring was assessed by using TEE and fluoroscopy in 70% and intracardiac echocardiography in 30% of subjects. Procedures were performed under general anesthesia and local anesthesia/conscious sedation in 58% and 42% of patients, respectively. The most used device for PFO closure was Amplatzer (~70% of cases).

Results

The procedure was successful in all patients.

Early complications

They occurred in 24/1035 (2.3%) patients in the peri-procedural phase. 12/24 (50%) subjects experienced cardiac arrhythmia: 5 patients had transient atrial fibrillation (AF), one patient a transient bradycardia, one patient a I° atrioventricular block, 4 had AF and 1 had a wide QRS tachycardia, before starting the procedure, and needed electrical cardioversion. 2/24 (8.3%) patients had a femoral arteriovenous fistula, thus needing vascular surgery. 4/24 (16.6%) subjects had respiratory problems after general anesthesia. One patient experienced a device embolization, retrieved percutaneously. One patient had a transient visual loss and 4 patients had a vagal reaction, allergy to antibiotics, right coronary spasm and mild pericardial effusion.

Follow-up

Both clinical and cardio-neurosonological follow-ups were assessed in 444/1035 (43%), 243/1035 (23.5%) and in 31/1035 (3%) subjects, at the 6- 12- 24-month follow-up, respectively. Up to the 12-month follow-up, fourteen neurological recurrences were observed in 12/444 (2.7%) patients: 8 TIA and 2 hemorrhagic and 4 ischemic strokes. 10/14 (71.5%) neurological recurrences occurred within the 6-month follow-up. 41 cardiac and extra-cardiac complications occurred in 40/444 (9%) subjects, up to the 12th month. 34/41 (83%) complications were related to arrhythmias, 16 of them had AF, one atrial flutter, 10 supraventricular paroxysmal tachycardia and the remaining 7 patients non specific arrhythmic patterns. 7/41 (17%) complications were related to myocardial ischemia, atrial erosion, device malposition, gluteal hematoma, apical thrombus, pericardial effusion and dyspnoea. Most cardiac complications (34/41, 83%) occurred within the 6-month follow-up. Neither neurological recurrences nor cardiac-extra-cardiac complications were observed at the 24-month follow-up.

Data concerning residual RLS were available in 401/444 (90.3%) and in 198/243 (81.5%) subjects, at the 6- and 12-month follow-up, respectively. A large permanent residual RLS was observed in 1/401 (0.25%) and 1/198 (0.5%) patient at the 6- and 12-month follow-up, respectively.

cTTE was the most utilized diagnostic technique during the follow-up (47.1%, 42.4% and 74.2% at the 6- 12- 24-month follow-up, respectively); successively, in a lesser extent, were the data obtained by cTTE plus cTCD (23.2%, 24.3% and 16.1% at the 6- 12- 24-month follow-up, respectively).

Discussion

The aim of our study was to analyse the clinical practice regarding PFO closure in Italy by a prospective, observational and multi-centric survey using a web-based database.

The number of the entire population that underwent PFO closure was, to our knowledge, one of the highest among similar studies. Although there was a considerable drop in number of patients at the follow-up, the absolute amount is still worthy of note, mostly at the 6- and 12-month. This could be explained by the fact that the study was conducted by cardiologists whose aims were, first, to evaluate the success of the procedure and possible early complications and, second, to assess neurological recurrence and residual RLS.

Nowadays, the only neurological indication for PFO closure is a cryptogenic stroke or TIA. In our study ~20% of the subjects underwent the procedure with other clinical indications. The "enlargement" of indications might be due to a greater effort in primary prevention. The question at issue was, therefore, whether all indications were assessed by neurologists or by other specialists. A closer collaboration between neurologists and cardiologists or other specialists who work together in the patient's management is desirable.

Our study showed an absolute technical procedural success, comparable to previous reports [4,8—11]. The occurrence of early complications are mostly related to cardiac arrhythmias as described in previous reports [12—15].

We observed that a 2.7% of patients had neurological recurrences with major complications (i.e. ischemic and hemorrhagic stroke), and up to the 1.3% at the 12-month follow-up. It is noteworthy that about 70% of these patients had neurological recurrences within the 6-month follow-up. This would indicate that the medical therapy should be carefully monitored, mostly during the critical process of endothelization. Previous reports described similar incidence of recurrent thromboembolic events ranging from 0 to 4% per year [16—21].

Cardiac and extra-cardiac complications were around 9% up to 12-month follow-up, with 83% of them within the 6th month. Major, even transient, complications (i.e. AF, atrial flutter, myocardial ischemia, apical thrombus) were observed in 19/40 (47.5%) patients. Our data, in line with previous studies [13,22, Furlan A. CLOSURE I trial. Presented at the AHA 2010 meeting], draw attention to these critical adverse events, mostly related to cardiac arrhythmias, thus indicating the need to improve the peri- and postprocedural safety and prevention both with technical advances and medical therapy.

Finally, given the low rate of large permanent residual RLS at the 6- and 12-month follow-up (<1%), considered crucial for increased risk of paradoxical embolism, we would substantially rule out that the re-occurrence of neurological events in our patients be correlated with the patent foramen ovale, as sole cause. Remarkably, Mono et al. recently described that concurrent etiologies, apart from PFO, were observed in more than one third of recurrent ischemic events in 308 patients with cryptogenic ischemic stroke who received medical therapy or underwent percutaneous PFO closure [4].

Conclusions

Our data regard early results from Italian Patent Foramen Ovale Survey and we need a longer follow-up in order to assess a comprehensive and conclusive evaluation of all clinical and technical characteristics correlated with a population who underwent percutaneous PFO closure.

Our study would confirm that percutaneous PFO closure is a safe procedure, pointing out that early complications and those during follow-up are not uncommon and are mostly related to cardiac arrhythmias.

Acknowledgment

We thank Dr. Andrea Smith for help with English version.

Appendix A.

IPOS investigators: Tommaso Langialonga (E.E. Ospedale Generale Regionale "F. Miulli", Acquaviva delle Fonti, Italy); Alessandro Santo Bortone (Emodinamica Interventistica — Sezione di Cardiochirurgia — DETO — Università degli Studi di Bari — Policlinico, Bari, Italy); Francesco De Luca (Cardiologia Pediatrica Ospedale Ferrarotto, Catania, Italy); Corrado Tamburino (Divisione Clinica di Cardiologia Ospedale Ferrarotto, Catania, Italy); Mario Zanchetta (Dipartimento di Malattie Cardiovascolari, Ospedale Civile, Cittadella, Italy); Mario De Martini (A.O. Ospedale Civile di Vimercate, Desio, Italy); Felice Achilli (Dipartimento Cardiovascolare Ospedale di Lecco, Lecco, Italy); Roberto Zanini (Ospedale "Carlo Poma", Mantova, Italy); Sandra Giusti (Ospedale "G: Pasquinucci" U.O. Cardiologia Pediatrica e GUCH, Massa, Italy); Antonio Colombo (Ospedale San Raffaele, Milan, Italy); Francesco Bedogni (Istituto Clinico Sant'Ambrogio, Milan, Italy); Maurizio Viecca (Laboratorio di Emodinamica "Bruno Scolari" c/o Ospedale L. Sacco, Milan, Italy); Gabriele Vignati (Cardiologia Pediatrica Ospedale Niguarda, Milan, Italy); Alberto Margonato (IRCCS San Raffaele, Milan, Italy); Bernhard Reimers (Divisione di cardiologia — Ospedale Civile, Mirano, Italy); Alberto Benassi (Hesperia Hospital Ospedale Privato, Modena, Italy); Giulietto Romeo Zennaro (U.O. Cardiologia/Nocsae, Modena, Italy); Raffaele Calabrò (U.O.C. CARDIOLOGIA, S.U.N. — A.O. "Monaldi" — Azienda Ospedaliera "Monaldi — II Università di Napoli", Naples, Italy); Diego Ardissino (Azienda Ospedaliero-Universitaria di Parma Unità Operativa di Cardiologia, Parma, Italy); Claudio Cavallini (Struttura Complessa Di Cardiologia — Laboratorio di Emodinamica e Cardiologia Interventistica, Perugia, Italy); Alessandro Capucci (Ospedale polichirurgico - U.O. di Cardiologia, Piacenza, Italy); Francesco Chiarella (Struttura semplice di emodinamica e interventistica cardiovascolare. UC Cardiologia O Santa Corona, Pietra Ligure, Italy); Ugo Vairo (Cardiologia Pediatrica — Azienda Ospedaliera San Carlo, Potenza); Antonino Nicosia Azienda Ospedaliera Civile — M.p. Arezzo — Emodinamica, Ragusa, Italy); Paolo Pantaleo (Villa Azzurra Hospital, Rapallo, Italy); Alberto Cremonesi (Villa Maria Cecilia Hospital, Ravenna, Italy); Danilo Manari (Salus Hospital — Gruppo Villa Maria Cecilia, Reggio Emilia, Italy); Andrea Berni (U.O.S. di Emodinamica e Cardiologia Interventistica, U.O.C. di Cardiologia Ospedale Sant'Andrea, Rome, Italy); Paolo Cardaioli (Servizio di Diagnostica Cardiovascolare ed Interventistica Endoluminale, Ospedale Civile di Rovigo, Rovigo, Italy); Patrizia Presbitero (Istituto Clinico Humanitas, Rozzano, Italy); Luigi Inglese (Policlinico San Donato IRCCS, San Donato Milanese, Italy); Raffaele Fanelli (Ospedale Casa Sollievo della Sofferenza IRCCS, San Giovanni Rotondo, Italy); Carlo Pierli (Azienda Ospedaliera Universitaria Senese — Le Scotte, Siena, Italy); Sebastiano Marra (Cardiologia Ospedaliera. Azienda Ospedaliera San Giovanni Battista, Molinette di Torino, Turin, Italy); Zoran Olivari (Emodinamica — Cardiologia Ospedale Ca' Fondello, Treviso, Italy); Jorge Salerno Uriarte (Ospedale di circolo fondazione Macchi — Cardiologia I, Varese, Italy); Alessandro Fontanelli (U.O. Complessa di Cardiologia, Vicenza, Italy).

References

[1] Wahl A, Praz F, Findling O, Nedeltchev K, Schwerzmann M, Tai T, et al. Percutaneous closure of patent foramen ovale for migraine headaches refractory to medical treatment. Catheter Cardiovasc Interv 2009;74:124—9.
[2] Paciaroni M, Agnelli G, Bertolini A, Pezzini A, Padovani A, Caso V, et al. Risk of recurrent cerebrovascular events in patients with cryptogenic stroke or transient ischemic attack and patent foramen ovale: the FORI (Foramen Ovale Registro Italiano) study. Cerebrovasc Dis 2011;31:109—16.
[3] Becker M, Frings D, Schröder J, Ocklenburg C, Mühler E, Hoffmann R, et al. Impact of occluder device type on success of percutaneous closure of atrial septal defects — a medium-term follow-up study. J Interv Cardiol 2009;22:503—10.
[4] Mono ML, Geister L, Galimanis A, Jung S, Praz F, Arnold M, et al. patent foramen ovale may be causal for the first stroke but unrelated to subsequent ischemic events. Stroke 2011;42:2891—5.
[5] Patel A, Lopez K, Banerjee A, Joseph A, Cao Qi-Ling, Hijazi ZM. Transcatheter closure of atrial septal defects in adults >40 years of age: Immediate and follow-up results. J Interven Cardiol 2007;20:82—8.
[6] Chessa M, Carminati M, Butera G, Bini RM, Drago M, Rosti L, et al. Early and late complications associated with transcatheter occlusion of secundum atrial septal defect. J Am Coll Cardiol 2002;39:1061—5.
[7] Egred M, Andrn M, Albouaini K, Alahmar A, Grainger R, Morrison W. Percutaneous closure of patent foramen ovale and atrial septal defect: procedure outcome and medium-term follow-up. J Interven Cardiol 2007;20:395—401.
[8] Kefer J, Sluysmans T, Hermans C, Khoury RE, Lambert C, Van de Wyngaert F, et al. Percutaneous transcatheter closure of interatrial septal defect in adults: procedural outcome and long-term results. Catheter Cardiovasc Interv 2011;April.
[9] Caputi L, Carriero MR, Falcone C, Parati E, Piotti P, Materazzo C, et al. Transcranial Doppler and transesophageal echocardiography: comparison of both techniques and prospective clinical

relevance of transcranial Doppler in patent foramen ovale detection. J Stroke Cerebrovasc Dis 2009;18:343—8.

[10] Jauss M, Zanette E. Detection of right-to-left shunt with ultrasound contrast agent and transcranial Doppler sonography. Cerebrovasc Dis 2000;10:490—6.

[11] Schwarze JJ, Sander D, Kukla C, Wittich I, Babikian VL, Klingelhöfer J. Methodological parameters influence the detection of right-to-left shunts by contrast transcranial Doppler ultrasonography. Stroke 1999;30:1234—9.

[12] Scacciatella P, Butera G, Meynet I, Giorgi M, D'Amico M, Pennone M, et al. Percutaneous closure of patent foramen ovale in patients with anatomical and clinical high-risk characteristics: long-term efficacy and safety. J Interv Cardiol 2011;24: 477—84.

[13] Anzola GP, Morandi E, Casilli F, Onorato E. Does transcatheter closure of patent foramen ovale really ''shut the door?'' A prospective study with transcranial Doppler. Stroke 2004;35:2140—4.

[14] Spies C, Reissmann U, Timmermanns I, Schräder R. Comparison of contemporary devices used for transcatheter patent foramen ovale closure. J Invasive Cardiol 2008;20:442—7.

[15] Spies C, Khandelwal A, Timmermanns I, Schräder R. Incidence of atrial fibrillation following transcatheter closure of atrial septal defects in adults. Am J Cardiol 2008;102:902—6.

[16] Bridges N, Hellenbrand W, Latson L, Filiano J, Newburger J, Lock J. Transcatheter closure of patent foramen ovale after presumed paradoxical embolism. Circulation 1992;86: 1902—8.

[17] Braun M, Gliech V, Boscheri A, Schoen S, Gahn G, Reichmann H, et al. Transcatheter closure of patent foramen ovale (PFO) in patients with paradoxical embolism. Periprocedural safety and mid-term follow-up results of three different device occluder systems. Eur Heart J 2004;25:424—30.

[18] Windecker S, Wahl A, Chatterjee T, Garachemani A, Eberli FR, Seiler C, et al. Percutaneous closure of patent foramen ovale in patients with paradoxical embolism. Circulation 2000;101:893—8.

[19] Wahl A, Tai T, Praz F, Schwerzmann M, Seiler C, Nedeltchev K, et al. Late results after percutaneous closure of patent foramen ovale for secondary prevention of paradoxical embolism using the amplatzer PFO occluder without intraprocedural echocardiography. J Am Coll Cardiol Interv 2009;2:116—23.

[20] von Bardeleben RS, Richter C, Otto J, Himmrich L, Schnabel R, Kampmann C, et al. Long term follow up after percutaneous closure of PFO in 357 patients with paradoxical embolism: Difference in occlusion systems and influence of atrial septum aneurysm. Int J Cardiol 2009;134:33—41.

[21] Fischer D, Haentjes J, Klein G, Schieffer B, Drexler H, Meyer GP, et al. Transcatheter closure of patent foramen ovale (PFO) in patients with paradoxical embolism: procedural and follow-up results after implantation of the Amplatzer®-occluder device. J Interv Cardiol 2011;24:85—91.

[22] Luermans JG, Post MC, Plokker HW, Ten Berg JM, Suttorp MJ. Complications and mid-term outcome after percutaneous patent foramen ovale closure in patients with cryptogenic stroke. Neth Heart J 2008;16:332—6.

An increased frequency of right-to-left shunt in patients with chronic hyperventilation syndrome

Jacek Staszewski[a,*], Kazimierz Tomczykiewicz[a], Bogdan Brodacki[a], Renata Anna Piusińska-Macoch[a], Adam Stępień[a], Z. Podgajny[b], P. Smużyński[c], Maciej Zarębiński[d]

[a] Clinic of Neurology, Military Medical Institute, Szaserow 128, 04-141 Warsaw, Poland
[b] Clinic of Endocrinology, Military Medical Institute, Szaserow 128, 04-141 Warsaw, Poland
[c] Clinic of Cardiology, Military Medical Institute, Szaserow 128, 04-141 Warsaw, Poland
[d] Department of Invasive Cardiology, SPS Szpital Zachodni, Daleka 11, 05-825 Grodzisk Mazowiecki, Poland

KEYWORDS
Chronic hyperventilation syndrome;
Tetania;
Spasmophilia;
Right to left shunt;
Patent foramen ovale;
Transcranial Doppler

Summary Relation of right-to-left shunt (RLS) with chronic hyperventilation syndrome (CHVS) has not been previously reported. We evaluated the prevalence of RLS in patients with CHVS. Patients with CHVS and 25 healthy controls (CG) were recruited into the study. Vascular RLS was diagnosed using contrast TCD. Of 25 subjects with CHVS, 16 (64%) had RLS vs 3 from CG (12%). TEE confirmed PFO in 10 patients with CHVS (40%) vs 2 from CG (8%). Pulmonary AVM was found in chest CT in 2 patients (10%) with CHVS and none from CG. The prevalence of RLS and PFO in patients with CHVS was significantly higher than in healthy subjects.
© 2012 Elsevier GmbH. All rights reserved.

Introduction

Chronic hyperventilation syndrome (CHVS, tetania and spasmophilia) represents a relatively common but poorly understood clinical entity. Approximately 10% of patients in a general internal medicine practice are reported to have CHVS. Chronic hyperventilation syndrome typically present with recurrent and different respiratory, neurological, cardiac or dysphoric symptoms, however, the underlying pathophysiology has not been clearly elucidated so far [1]. Patients with CHVS usually undergo extensive and expensive investigations but in majority of them no organic causes are discovered. Chronic hyperventilation syndrome is thought to result from hypocapnia, hypocalcemia or alcalosis due to psychogenic hyperventilation but although CHVS and psychiatric disorders may overlap, only quarter of patients with hyperventilation syndrome manifest panic disorder. Different stressors such as emotional distress but also sodium lactate, caffeine, isoproterenol can provoke an exaggerated respiratory response. We hypothesized that various endogenic trigger substances might enter the systemic circulation through cardiac or pulmonary right-to-left shunt (RLS) instead of being trapped in the pulmonary capillaries and contribute with development of CHVS.

Aim

The aim of this single center study was to evaluate the incidence of RLS in patients with CHVS.

* Corresponding author at: Clinic of Neurology, Military Medical Institute, Szaserow 128, 04-141 Warsaw, Poland.
Tel.: +48 607871754; fax: +48 228106100.
E-mail address: jstaszewski@wim.mil.pl (J. Staszewski).

2211-968X/$ — see front matter © 2012 Elsevier GmbH. All rights reserved.
doi:10.1016/j.permed.2012.02.027

Materials and methods

Twenty-eight patients with previously diagnosed CHVS and 25 healthy subjects (control group, CG) were prospectively recruited to the study and admitted to Clinic of Neurology, Military Medical Institute, Warsaw, Poland. Chronic hyperventilation syndrome was diagnosed basing on typical recurrent clinical symptoms (dizziness, numbness, paresthesias or near syncope), which could be reproduced by voluntary hyperventilation. The diagnosis was confirmed with presence of spontaneous electromyographic (EMG) activity with 2 or more multiplets during provocative ischemia and hyperventilation [2]. All patients with CHVS had undergone brain neuroimaging (MRI), EEG, carotid duplex ultrasonography and transcranial Doppler (TCD) ultrasonography to exclude organic causes of the symptoms before entering the study. Total and ionized calcium was within the normal reference range levels in all examined subjects. Patients were consulted with neuropsychologist and endocrinologist. Three patients in whom diagnosis of panic disorder ($n=1$), agoraphobia ($n=1$) or endocrine disturbance ($n=1$) had been established were not included into the trial. Vascular RLS was diagnosed using contrast TCD (c-TCD, Nicolet Companion III) of the middle cerebral artery (MCA) to detect the presence of microbubble emboli (MB) following the standardized protocol [3]. All patients had adequate temporal window to perform TCD examination. Appearance of at least 1 contrast induced MB signal on the c-TCD trace was regarded pathognomonic for RLS. Patients were prepared with an 18-gauge needle inserted into the cubital vein and were examined in the supine position. Insonation of one MCA using TCD was performed. The contrast agent was prepared using 9 ml isotonic saline solution and 1 ml air mixed with a three-way stopcock by exchange of saline/air mixture between the syringes and injected as a bolus. The MB were recorded with TCD at rest and in case of little or no detection of MB in the MCA under basal conditions the examination was repeated 5 s post injection following Valsalva maneuver (VM) with controlled duration (10 s) and pressure (forced expiration against a manometer to 40 mmHg). All examinations were done by a single experienced operator (J.S.). Grading or RLS was performed by counting the number of embolic tracks on the power M-mode and Doppler spectrogram in real time and offline. A four-level categorization according to the MB count was applied: (1) 0 MB (negative result); (2) 1—10 MB (low-grade shunt); (3) >10 MB + no curtain (medium-grade); (4) curtain (large-grade). Patients with c-TCD diagnosed RLS underwent transoesophagal echocardiography (TEE) to detect cardiac causes of the shunt. The echocardiographers were blinded as to the status of the individual patients. In the case of negative TEE contrast-enhanced chest CT for the presence of pulmonary arteriovenous malformations (AVM) was performed. The protocol of the study has been accepted by the local Ethics Committee. Written informed consent was obtained from each patient.

Results

Fifty patients (mean age 38 years; females 76%), 25 with CHVS and 25 from CG were included to analysis. The groups

Table 1 Baseline characteristics of studied group.

Group	CHVS	Control	p
N (%)	25	25	
Mean age (±SD) years	37 (8)	39 (6)	NS
Females	21 (82%)	18 (70%)	NS
Vertigo	4 (16%)	0	—
Dizziness	5 (20%)	0	—
Numbness	15 (60%)	0	—
Dysesthesias	21 (85%)	0	—
Near syncope	5 (20%)	0	—
Migraine with aura	4 (16%)	0	—
Migraine w/h aura	2 (8%)	0	—

CHVS: chronic hyperventilation syndrome; NS: not significant.

Table 2 Right-to-left shunt in studied groups.

Group	CHVS	Control	p
N (%)	25	25	
RLS in c-TCD	16 (64%)	3 (12%)	<0.05
TEE: PFO	10 (40%)	2 (8%)	<0.05
CT: pulmonary AVM	2 (10%)	0	
Grade of RLS in c-TCD			
1) None	9 (36%)	22 (88%)	<0.05
2) 1—10 MB	8 (32%)	3 (12%)	<0.05
3) >10 MB no curtain	5 (20%)	0	
4) Curtain	3 (12%)	0	

CHVS: chronic hyperventilation syndrome; AVM: arteriovenous malformation; RLS: right-to-left shunt; TEE: transesophageal echocardiography; PFO: patent foramen ovale.

did not differ with regard to mean age and sex. Table 1 represents demographic data and baseline neurological characteristics of the analyzed population. Six patients with CHVS (24%) and none from CG had concomitant migraine. Sixteen (64%) patients with CHVD had documented RLS basing on c-TCD examination compared with 3 subjects from CG (12%, $p<0.05$) (Table 2). All patients with RLS from CG had low-grade shunt compared with CHVD group in which 50% of subjects with shunt had medium- or large-grade shunts. Ten of 16 patients with CHVS and RLS (63%) had spontaneous shunt with MB detected at rest compared with 1 of 3 from CG (33%), the rest subjects had provocative RLS detected only after VM. Transoesophagal echocardiography confirmed patent foramen ovale (PFO) in 10 patients with CHVS (40%) and 2 from CG (8%, $p<0.05$). PFO was a major cause of RLS in CHVS and CG patients (63% vs 67%, respectively). Basing on chest CT examination, pulmonary AVM was found in 2 patients (10%) with CHVS (13% of patients with RLS and CHVS) and none from CG. Overall, TEE and chest CT examinations revealed the source of RLS in 12 patients with CHVS (48%) and 2 from CG (8%, $p<0.05$). Four of six patients with CHVS and migraine (67%) had RLS due to PFO, the rest 2 subjects had normal c-TCD.

Discussion

The underlying mechanism by which some patients develop hyperventilation syndrome is unknown. It often represents a simple manifestation of anxiety, rarely endocrine and respiratory diseases (i.e. hypoparathyroidism, asthma and pulmonary embolism) or central nervous system disorders (i.e. brainstem lesions). In many patients the cause of CHVS remains, however, unclear [4]. The pathogenetic role of RLS is unknown and as far as we know the link between RLS and CHVS has not been reported so far. Patent foramen ovale represents a main cause of cardiac RLS. According to different studies PFO is a common and generally benign finding present on autopsy in approximately 17—29% of population [5]. Direct PFO visualization by TEE is considered the golden standard for PFO diagnosis but contrast TCD of the MCA has similar and high sensitivity (70—100%) [6]. Data from population-based studies showed that prevalence of PFO in the general population is ranging from 11% to 25% by TEE. PFO has been linked with paradoxical embolization of thrombi and other microparticles or vasoactive chemicals leading to cryptogenic stroke and also broad spectrum of neurological diseases (migraine or migraine with aura, transient global amnesia, decompression sickness in sport divers) [7,8]. Anzola et al. reported in TCD study that RLS was present in 48% of individuals with migraine with aura, compared with 20% of healthy controls and 23% of patients with migraine without aura [9].

The present study demonstrated higher prevalence of RLS in CHVS group (64%) than in CG (12%). In over half of all studied patients RLS had been related to PFO, but we also found that AVM was the cause of RLS in 2 patients with CHVS. The prevalence of PFO in all studied CHVS patients (40%) was significantly higher than in CG and expected in the general population ($\approx$25%). The prevalence of extracardiac shunting via pulmonary AVM in the general population is not well studied but its presence is believed to be uncommon. In an autopsy study, only three cases of pulmonary AVM were detected in 15,000 consecutive autopsies [10]. High frequency of PFO and AVM in CHVS suggests a possible link with RLS regardless of its cause, however, causal relationship between these conditions is unknown. As postulated in previous reports, RLS may allow venous-circulating, vasoactive chemicals to bypass the pulmonary filter and reach the cerebral circulation to induce a migraine and possibly hyperventilation attack [11]. This concept is, however, not supported by the observation that inducing a drop in arterial pCO_2 through forced voluntary hyperventilation may provoke CHVS in some but not all patients [12]. Obviously CHVS is related to a variety of mechanisms, which may not be associated with hyperventilation alone. Migraine was a frequent concomitant disease in CHVS group (24%) and majority of these patients (67%) had RLS. This finding suggests that migraine and CHVS may share similar etiology in selected patients with RLS. This observation is in line with some previous reports showing typical picture of CHVS in several patients with migraine at a headache phase [13,14]. Reported association between CHVS and RLS is novel and difficult to explain but whether functional or etiologic it may improve the understanding of these conditions.

Conclusions

The prevalence of RLS and PFO in patients with CHVS was significantly higher than in healthy subjects from control group. The clinical implications of our findings need to be determined.

References

[1] Kern B, Rosh AJ. Hyperventilation syndrome. In: Brenner BE, et al., editors. eMedicine. Medscape; 2010. September 01, 2011, http://emedicine.com/emerg/topic270.htm.
[2] Valls-Solé J, Montero J. Role of EMG evaluation in muscle hyperactivity syndromes. J Neurol 2004;251:251—60.
[3] Jauss M, Zanette E. Detection of right-to-left shunt with ultrasound contrast agent and transcranial Doppler sonography. Cerebrovasc Dis 2000;10:490—6.
[4] Gardner WN. The pathophysiology of hyperventilation disorders. Chest 1996;109:516—34.
[5] Movsowitz C, Podolsky LA, Meyerowitz CB. Patent foramen ovale: a nonfunctional embryological remnant or a potential cause of significant pathology? J Am Soc Echocardiogr 1992;5:259—69.
[6] Blersch W, Draganski B, Holmer SR, Koch HJ, Schlachetzki F, Bogdahn U, et al. Transcranial duplex sonography in the detection of patent foramen ovale. Radiology 2002;225:693—9.
[7] Homma S, Sacco RL. Patent foramen ovale and stroke. Circulation 2005;112:1063—72.
[8] Del Sette M, Angeli S, Leandri M, Ferriero G, Bruzzone GL, Finocchi C, et al. Migraine with aura and right-to-left shunt on transcranial Doppler: a case—control study. Cerebrovasc Dis 1998;8:327—30.
[9] Anzola GP, Magoni M, Guindani M, Rozzini L, Dalla VG. Potential source of cerebral embolism in migraine with aura. A transcranial Doppler study. Neurology 1999;52:1622—5.
[10] Sloan RD, Cooley RN. Congenital pulmonary arteriovenous aneurysm. AJR 1953;70:183—210.
[11] Wilmshurst PT, Nightingale S, Walsh KP, Morrison WL. Effect on migraine of closure of cardiac right-to-left shunts to prevent recurrence of decompression illness or stroke or for hemodynamic reasons. Lancet 2000;356:1648—51.
[12] Hornsveld HK, Garssen B, Dop MJ, van Spiegel PI, de Haes JC. Double-blind placebo-controlled study of the hyperventilation provocation test and the validity of the hyperventilation syndrome. Lancet 1996;348:154—8.
[13] Blau JN, Dexter SL. Hyperventilation during migraine attacks. Br Med J 1980;280(6226):1254.
[14] Razavi M, Razavi B, Fattal D, Afifi A, Adams HP. Hemiplegic migraine induced by exercise. Arch Neurol 2000;57:1363—5.

7. Non Atherosclerotic Stroke Etiology

Diagnosis of non-atherosclerotic carotid disease

Arijana Lovrencic-Huzjan*

Sestre milosrdnice University Hospital Centre, University Department of Neurology, Vinogradska 29, 10000 Zagreb, Croatia

KEYWORDS
Non-atherosclerotic;
Dissection;
Stroke;
Color Doppler imaging;
Transcranial Doppler sonography

Summary Non-atherosclerotic carotid disease in an uncommon group of angiographic defects. It includes the entities: Takayasu's arteritis, giant cell arteritis, fibromuscular disease, moyamoya syndrome, arterial dissection and extracranial carotid aneurysms. Due to advance in imaging techniques, they are being increasingly identified. Growing awareness of diverse clinical picture along with advances in imaging technologies enables early diagnosis. Although catheter angiography is a gold standard in diagnosing most of these diseases, neurosonological tests serve as an excellent screening tool, and are suitable for monitoring. Brain MR and MRA are sometimes essential for confirmation of the diagnosis. Mortality rates are low and functional outcome is generally good if the disease is diagnosed early.
© 2012 Elsevier GmbH. All rights reserved.

Takayasu's arteritis

Takayasu's arteritis is a granulomatous arteritis affecting the aorta and its branches [1]. Its incidence is estimated at 2.6 cases per million per year, more common in Southeast Asia. It is more prevalent in young woman (9 females:1 male). It has three stages. During the systemic stage symptoms and signs of an active inflammatory illness dominate, like e.g. malaise, fever, night sweats, arthralgia, weight loss, anemia and elevated erythrocyte sedimentation rate. The systemic phase is succeeded by the vascular inflammatory stage, when stenosis, aneurysms, and vascular pain (carotidynia) tend to occur. During this phase patients begin to develop symptoms caused by the narrowing of affected arteries. Symptoms are caused by the narrowing of affected arteries like stroke, transitory ischemic attack (TIA), claudication, dizziness, headache, visual symptoms and hypertension as a result of stenosed renal arteries. This stage sometimes overlaps with the systemic stage. At the end a burned-out stage develops when fibrosis sets in, and this stage is usually associated with remission. According to the American College of Rheumatology [2] the criteria for assessing the diagnosis are: angiographic criteria displaying narrowing or occlusion of the entire aorta, its primary branches, or large arteries in the proximal upper or lower extremities. These changes are not due to arteriosclerosis, fibromuscular dysplasia, or similar causes; changes are usually focal or segmental; the lesions can include stenosis, occlusion, or aneurysms. Angiogram is a gold standard, but sonography assesses both vessel anatomy and luminal status in accessible areas and can detect early vessel wall alterations before lumen changes on angiography [3—6]. Its advantage is limited cost, short time required, and there is no radiation. Due to noninvasiveness, it is suitable for monitoring. Direct or indirect signs can be visualized. Color Doppler flow imaging enables visualization of the mural thickening of the common carotid arteries (Fig. 1), hypoechoic in the early, vascular inflammatory stage [7]. With the development of fibrosis, pronounced echogenicity of the lesions develop in the burned-out stage. Due to inflammation, stenosis occurs. If advanced stenosis affects the brachiocephalic trunk or origin of the left common carotid artery, changed hemodynamic spectra like

* Corresponding author. Tel.: +38513768282; fax: +38513768282.
E-mail address: arijana.lovrencic-huzjan@zg.htnet.hr

2211-968X/$ — see front matter © 2012 Elsevier GmbH. All rights reserved.
http://dx.doi.org/10.1016/j.permed.2012.03.004

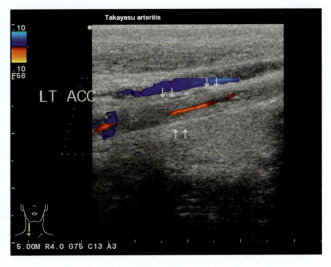

Figure 1 Takayasu arteritis showing advanced mural thickening of the common carotid artery to the level of tight stenosis.

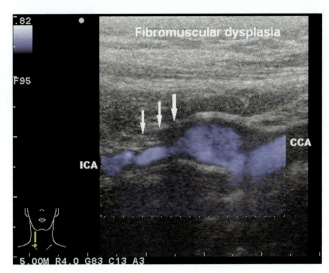

Figure 2 Segmental narrowing and widening or the color coded flow in internal carotid artery showing characteristic "ring of beads" appearance in medial type of fibromuscular dysplasia.

dampened flow in carotid artery, distal from the stenosis, can be recorded. If the stenosis affects subclavian artery, changed hemodynamic spectra suggesting subclavian steal syndrome are recorded (Fig. S1 supplementary file). When occlusion of the subclavian artery sets in, in ipsilateral vertebral artery hemodynamic spectra are completely inverse (Fig. S2 supplementary file), and in the contralateral one it is accelerated. Transcranial Doppler of the Willis circle and vertebrobasilar system shows redistribution of the hemodynamics.

Giant cell arteritis — GCA

GCA, is also known as temporal arteritis or cranial arteritis, is the most common form of vasculitis that occurs in adults [8]. Almost all patients who develop GCA are over the age of 50. It is a granulomas arteritis affecting large or medium-sized artery, usually temporal or ophthalmic artery. It has an acute or subacute start. Symptoms are headache, jaw pain, blurred or double vision. If the disease is undiagnosed complications like blindness and, less often, stroke may occur. Standard test for diagnosing GCA is biopsy of the temporal artery. More samples are needed because the inflammation may not occur in all parts of the artery. Prompt treatment with corticosteroids relieves symptoms and prevents loss of vision. Ultrasound finding will show swelling of the arterial wall presenting as a hypoechoic dark halo around the color coded flow in the temporal, ophthalmic artery or external carotid artery [7,9]. The disease is segmental, therefore, its visualization is suitable for localization of the biopsy. Due to noninvasiveness it is suitable for monitoring the disease. During healing regression of the dark halo will be visible parallel with the restitution of the color coded flow.

Fibromuscular dysplasia

Fibromuscular dysplasia (FMD) is a fibrous thickening of the arterial wall, causing segmental narrowing of arteries in the kidneys (in 75% of patients), carotid or vertebral arteries and the arteries of the abdomen [10]. It is an autosomal dominant disorder, affecting up to 5% of the population, in 2/3 the internal carotid artery (ICA), usually the C2 segment. It is usually asymptomatic, but if dissection occurs, it causes aneurysm and occlusion and becomes symptomatic. There are three types of fibromuscular dysplasia: intimal, medial, and subadventitial (perimedial) of the arterial wall. These three types of FMD are not easily differentiated by findings on angiography. The medial type of FMD is by far the most common (about 80—85%) and it is classically diagnosed on the basis of a "string of beads" appearance on angiography. This appearance is explained by the presence of luminal stenosis alternating with aneurysmal dilatation. Classically, the intimal form of FMD is associated with smooth focal stenoses on angiography. Type 1 is the most common form. In 6—12% of patients with arterial fibroplasia, a long tubular stenosis may be seen. This form is most commonly seen with the intimal form. The unusual form (seen in 4—6% of patients) is characterized by involvement of only one side of an artery. Such involvement leads to diverticularizations of the arterial wall. These lesions may be difficult to distinguish from atherosclerotic ulceration and pseudoaneurysm. Ultrasound findings correlate with the angiographic findings, and may show segmental narrowing and widening or the color coded flow in carotid or vertebral arteries, with the characteristic string of beads appearance in medial type of FMD, long tubular stenosis, usually distally from a widened carotid bulb in intimal type of FMD, or irregular local widening of the arterial wall in subadventitial type of FMD. Fig. 2 shows "string of beads" appearance in medial type, and Fig. S3 supplementary file shows occlusion of the internal carotid artery after the carotid bulb as a result of dissection in intimal type (Fig. S3 supplementary file).

Moyamoya disease

Moyamoya disease is an inherited genetic abnormality causing intimal thickening in the walls of the terminal portions of the internal carotid vessels bilaterally and stenosis

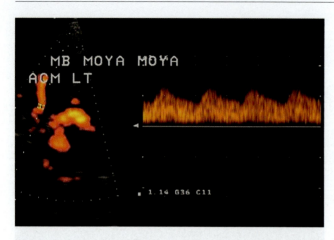

Figure 3 Dampened flow in middle cerebral artery due to advanced stenosis of internal carotid artery in carotid siphon.

[11–13]. Moyamoya means ''puff of smoke'' in Japanese, and describes the look of the tangle of tiny vessels formed to compensate for the blockage — rete mirabile. The disease has two peaks of incidence, first is in the first decade, and second is in the fourth decade. While clinical presentation in children is usually stroke due to occlusion of internal carotid artery or one of the branches of the Willis' circle, in adults subarachnoid hemorrhage is a dominant symptom as a result of hemorrhage of tiny, fragile vessels. Headache is a frequent presenting symptom in patients with moyamoya. A review suggested that dilatation of meningeal and leptomeningeal collateral vessels may stimulate dural nociceptors.

Moyamoya syndrome has a similar angiographic appearance of rete mirabile. It is an acquired syndrome with, usually unilateral, stenosis or occlusion of the proximal parts of the Willis' circle due to neurofibromatosis, Down syndrome, syphilis, acquired immunodeficiency syndrome, juvenile atherosclerosis or sickle cell disease.

Moyamoya disease has six angiographic stages ranging from mild stenosis to occlusion [14–16]. Because the disease is located intracranially, transcranial (Fig. S4 supplementary file) or transcranial color coded Doppler sonography (Fig. 3) will be used for assessing the diagnosis.

Craniocervical artery dissection

Craniocervical artery dissection (CCAD) is a major cause of ischemic symptoms in young adults and can lead to various clinical symptoms [17,18]. In a North American population-based study its incidence was reported to be about 2.6 (95% CI 1.9–3.3) per 100,000 inhabitants per year [17]. This number is probably underestimated, since the clinical picture with mild symptoms including only headache and local signs remain undiagnosed. Vertebral artery dissections are less common than carotid artery dissections, but with the advance in imaging techniques, asymptomatic multiple vessel involvement can be detected.

Genetic factors such as constitutional weakness of the arterial wall might have a role in the pathophysiology of CCAD, and environmental factors such as minor trauma acts as a trigger [17,18]. The presence of an underlying vasculopathy is suggested by commonly present concomitant arterial anomalies such as FMD, monogenic connective tissue disease, mainly Ehlers-Danlos syndrome or Marfan's syndrome. There are several reports of familial cases of CCAD in the absence of known connective tissue disorders. In older patients hypertension plays a role, but despite ample work-up in most patients, the cause is never found [17].

Arterial dissections begin with a tear in the intima or media resulting in bleeding within the arterial wall [18]. Intramural blood dissects longitudinally and spreads along the vessel proximally and distally. Dissections can tear through the intima, permitting partially coagulated intramural blood to enter the lumen of the artery. Expansion of the arterial wall by intramural blood causes compression of the lumen. Narrowing of the lumen by the intramural blood compromises the blood flow stream and perturbation of the vascular endothelium causes release of endothelins and tissue factor, activation of platelets and the coagulation cascade. All these changes contribute to formation of an intraluminal thrombus. The intramural hematoma can create a false lumen that might reconnect with the true lumen and forms parallel flow. The true and false lumen are separated by an elongated intimal flap. If the dissection lies between the media and the adventitia, an aneurysmal dilatation of the arterial wall may extrude. Intracranial rupture through the adventitia causes subarachnoid bleeding.

The most dominant symptom is pain in head and neck, in the region of the dissection, usually developing after minor trauma. Some patients present only with headache, or a combination of headache and local signs. Clinical presentations result from bleeding in subintimal and subadventitial wall [17]. If the dissections compromise the arterial lumen or cause thrombus formation in the lumen, clinical symptoms are the result of luminal compromise and the presence of luminal clot. Ischemic symptoms and infarction in the brain are caused by both reduced perfusion in the brain artery supplying territory or embolism. Neurological symptoms related to hypoperfusion are usually multiple brief transient ischemic attacks (TIAs) during a period of several hours to a few days. Hypoperfusion may decrease washout of emboli and contributes to the development of brain infarction.

Bleeding in the subadventitial wall results in compression of the adjacent structures to the outer arterial wall like lower cranial nerves (IX–XII) that exit near the skull base, or causes bleeding into adjacent tissues. Patients with subadventitial intracranial dissections often present with subarachnoid bleeding, because intracranial arteries have no external elastic envelope and have a thinner media and adventitia. Therefore the intracranial arteries are more prone to rupture.

In general, the closer the dissection to the brain is, the higher probability of brain infarction is present [19]. If the dissection is more extracranial, the higher is the probability of the local symptoms from space occupying lesions. Also, pain is stronger, and may even lead to syncope. This statement is true for arterial occlusive lesions of any cause—the closer the occlusion is to the brain, the more likely that infarction will develop [18].

CCAD can also be asymptomatic and discovered through routine examination. Several cases of asymptomatic or oligosymptomatic CCAD probably remain undiagnosed [17].

Recurrence rate is relatively low, mortality rate is low and functional outcome is generally good.

Imaging of the dissection

The traditional method for visualization of CCAD is catheter angiography that may show: smooth or slightly irregular luminal narrowing (Fig. 4), tapered, flame-like, occlusion, pseudoaneurysm, intimal flap or double lumen (specific, but only in <10%) or distal branch occlusion [20,21]. MR images of the eccentric or circumferential periarterial rim of intramural hematoma typically show hyper intense signal on T1 and T2 weighted images [22—24]. MR angiography has limited value, imaging the same pathomorphologic findings as angiography [3]. MR and MRA showed sensitivity (SE) of 50—100%, and specificity (SP) of 29—100%. Computerized tomography (CT) and CT angiography (CTA) revealed SE of 51—100%, and SP of 67—100% [25]. Doppler and duplex sonography was underrated. Although color Doppler flow imaging (CDFI) showed good results in visualization of the dissection [26—36], the main limitation is visualization of the intracranial dissection, which appears to be the most common site of localization. While CDFI provides visualization of the direct and some indirect findings of CCAD, TCD enables assessment of the intracranial hemodynamic and monitoring of the embolic signals [37,38]. The most important issue is that neurosonological evaluation enables noninvasive daily monitoring of the course of the dissection [37,39].

The reported sensitivity of neurovascular ultrasound for detecting spontaneous CCAD varies from 80 to 96%. It

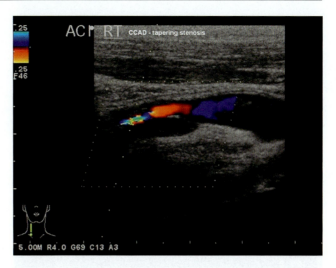

Figure 5 Tapering stenosis as a result of internal carotid dissection.

may show direct or indirect signs [36]. Direct signs are: echolucent intramural hematoma, string sign (Figs. S5 and S6 supplementary file); double lumen, or stenosis and/or occlusion of an arterial segment usually not affected by atherosclerosis (Fig. S7 supplementary file). Indirect signs are: increased or decreased pulsatility index upstream (Fig. S8 supplementary file) or downstream of the suspected lesion; more than 50% difference in blood flow velocity (BFV) compared to the unaffected side, or detection of intracranial collateral flow. Intramural hematoma is echolucent, compromising the color coded flow in the string sign (Fig. S5 supplementary file) with increased pulsatility in the residual flow (Fig. S6 supplementary file), or tapering stenosis (Fig. 5). During follow up, the regression of the hematoma will develop, and restitution of color coded filling of the arterial lumen will be visible (Fig. S9 supplementary file). Resolution of the hematoma is the most specific sign for CCAD [34,39]. Double lumen (Figs. 6 and 7), an irregular membrane crossing the lumen, is usually found in arteries originating from the aortic arch, and multivessel involvement if present. If the dissection spreads to the subclavian artery, typical hemodynamic spectra in vertebral

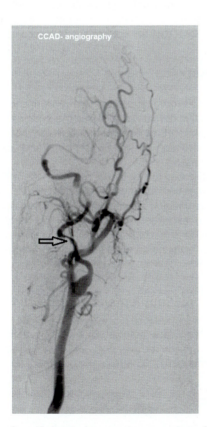

Figure 4 Smooth luminal narrowing as a sign of dissection (arrow).

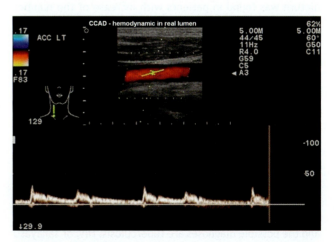

Figure 6 Hemodynamic in real lumen in common carotid artery dissection.

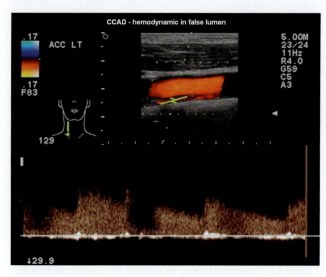

Figure 7 Hemodynamic in false lumen in common carotid artery dissection.

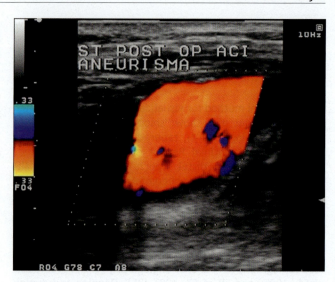

Figure 8 Postoperative aneurysm of the internal carotid artery.

artery suggesting subclavian steal syndrome are found. In the real and false lumen different hemodynamic spectra are found (Figs. 6 and 7). Stenosis and/or occlusion of an arterial segment not affected by atherosclerosis involve distal part of the ICA 2.0 cm or more downstream of the carotid bifurcation (Fig. S7 supplementary file) or V2—V4 segment of the vertebral artery. Increased or decreased pulsatility upstream or downstream of the suspected arterial lesion (Fig. S8 supplementary file) will suggest the presence of CCAD, as well as >50% difference in the BFV compared to the same segment of the artery on the unaffected side. If the hematoma compromises the flow, intracranial redistribution of hemodynamics will be detected by means of TCD or TCCD. It often shows diminished intracranial velocities in the ICA siphon and the MCA. Usually anterior collateral pathway is detected, and in most instances the posterior collateral pathway. Neurosonology enables noninvasive monitoring of the course of dissection, since resolution of the hematoma is the most specific finding. It enables also monitoring the microembolic signals (MES) in correlation with the clinical picture. Amelioration of the clinical finding is found in correlation with reduction of MES, and worsening of the clinical picture was found in patients with increase of the number of MES. Therefore neurosonology offers the possibility of monitoring the therapeutic effect.

Extracranial internal carotid artery aneurysm

Aneurysms of the extracranial internal carotid artery are extremely rare [40]. They are divided in two categories: true and pseudoaneurysm. In order to talk about true aneurysms, the diameter of the vessel expands at least 50% that is possible even with a tiny dilation of internal carotid artery. Most common etiological factor is atherosclerosis, and hypertension is frequently found. They are typically fusiform in shape although saccular aneurysms are also seen. Patients are usually younger if the underlying cause is not atherosclerosis, and the possible diagnoses are tuberculosis, HIV, or Takayasu arteritis. Salmonella and syphilis are the main causes of mycotic aneurysms. Fibromuscular dysplasia, collagen tissue disorders and irradiation are among the rare causes. They can be also be iatrogenic as a result of intervention like puncture or carotid endarterectomy (Fig. 8). Most of these aneurysms are asymptomatic, but atherosclerotic carry the high risk for thromboembolic stroke while located at proximal ICA. Mycotic aneurysms tend to grow and rupture. In diagnosing and characterizing the aneurysms, DSA is the gold standard imaging method, but color Doppler of the carotid arteries may serve as an excellent screening tool. It allows assessment of vessel wall and possible thrombotic material. If the aneurysm is operated, color Doppler imaging will serve as a noninvasive tool for assessment of the control finding.

Conclusion

Non-atherosclerotic carotid disease is an uncommon group of angiographic defects. It includes the entities: Takayasu's arteritis, giant cell arteritis, fibromuscular dysplasia, moyamoya syndrome, arterial dissection and extracranial carotid aneurysms.

These diseases are being increasingly identified due to growing awareness of diverse clinical picture along with advances in imaging technologies. Neurosonological tests serve as an excellent screening tool for most of these diseases, with a perfect monitoring capacity, but neuroradiological imaging is essential for confirmation of the diagnosis.

Appendix A. Supplementary data

Supplementary data associated with this article can be found, in the online version, at http://dx.doi.org/10.1016/j.permed.2012.03.004.

References

[1] Jennette JC, Falk RJ, Andrassy K, Bacon PA, Churg J, Gross WL. Nomenclature of systemic vasculitides proposal of an

international consensus conference. Arthritis and Rheumatism 1994;37:187—92.
[2] Cantu C, Pineda C, Barinagarrementeria F, Salgado P, Gurza A, Paola de Pablo, et al. Noninvasive cerebrovascular assessment of Takayasu arteritis. Stroke 2000;31:2197—202.
[3] Schmidt WA, Blockmans D. Use of ultrasonography and positron emission tomography in the diagnosis and assessment of large-vessel vasculitis. Current Opinion in Rheumatology 2005;17:9—15.
[4] Park JH, Han MC, Kim SH. Takayasu arteritis: angiographic findings and results of angioplasty. American Journal of Roentgenology 1989;153:1069—74.
[5] Pipitone N, Versari A, Salvarani C. Role of imaging studies in the diagnosis and follow-up of large-vessel vasculitis: an update. Rheumatology 2008;47:403—8.
[6] Gotway MB, Araoz PA, Macedo TA, Stanson AW, Higgins CB, Ring EJ, et al. Imaging findings in Takayasu's arteritis. American Journal of Roentgenology 2005;184:1945—50.
[7] Lovrencic-Huzjan A. The role of ultrasound in diagnosing nonatherosclerotic vasculopathies of the nervous system. Acta Clinica Croatica 1998;37(Suppl. 1):68—72.
[8] Salvarani C, Cantini F, Boiardi L, Hunder GG. Polymyalgia rheumatica and giant-cell arteritis. New England Journal of Medicine 2002;347:261—71.
[9] Schmidt WA, Kraft HE, Vorpahl K, Volker L, Gromnica-Ihle EJ. Color duplex ultrasonography in the diagnosis of temporal arteritis. New England Journal of Medicine 1997;337:1336—42.
[10] Slovut DP, Olin JW. Fibromuscular dysplasia. New England Journal of Medicine 2004;350:1862—71.
[11] Kuroda S, Houkin K. Moyamoya disease: current concepts and future perspectives. Lancet Neurology 2008;7.
[12] Kuriyama S, Kusaka Y, Fujimura M, Wakai K, Tamakoshi A, Hashimoto S, et al. Prevalence and clinicoepidemiological features of moyamoya disease in Japan: findings from a nationwide epidemiological survey. Stroke 2008;39:42—7.
[13] Scott R, Smith ER. Moyamoya disease and moyamoya syndrome. New England Journal of Medicine 2009;360:1226—37.
[14] Ruan LT, Duan YY, Cao TS, Zhuang L, Huang L. Color and power Doppler sonography of extracranial and intracranial arteries in Moyamoya disease. Journal of Clinical Ultrasound 2006;4:60—9.
[15] Perren F, Horn P, Vajkoczy P, Schmiedek P, Meairs S. Power Doppler imaging in detection of surgically induced indirect neoangiogenesis in adult moyamoya disease. Journal of Neurosurgery 2005;103:869—72.
[16] Perren F, Meairs S, Schmiedek P, Hennerici M, Horn P. Power Doppler evaluation of revascularization in childhood moyamoya. Neurology 2005;64:558—60.
[17] Debette S, Leys D. Cervical-artery dissections: predisposing factors, diagnosis, and outcome. Lancet Neurology 2009;8:668—78.
[18] Caplan LR. Dissections of brain-supplying arteries. Nature Clinical Practice Neurology 2008;4:34—42.
[19] Lovrencic-Huzjan A, Vukovic V, Azman D, Bene R, Demarin V. Pain and ischemic symptoms in craniocervical artery dissection. Acta Medica Croatica 2008;62:223—7.
[20] Debette, Provenzale JM. MRI and MRA for evaluation of dissection of craniocerebral arteries: lessons from the medical literature. Emergency Radiology 2009;16:185—93.
[21] Houser OW, Mokri B, Sundt TM, Baker HL, Reese DF. Spontaneous cervical cephalic arterial dissection and its residuum: angiographic spectrum. American Journal of Neuroradiology 1984;5:27—34.
[22] Provenzale, Sue DE, Brant-Zawadzki MN, Chance J. Dissection of cranial arteries in the neck: correlation of MRI and arteriography. Neuroradiology 34:273—8.
[23] Hoffmann M, Sacco RL, Chan S, Mohr JP. Noninvasive detection of vertebral artery dissection. Stroke 1993;24:815—9.
[24] Auer A, Felber S, Schmidauer C, Waldenberger P, Aichner F. Magnetic resonance angiographic and clinical features of extracranial vertebral artery dissection. Journal of Neurology, Neurosurgery and Psychiatry 1998;64:474—81.
[25] Provenzale JM, Sarikaya B. Comparison of test performance characteristic of MRI MR angiography and CT angiography in the diagnosis of carotid and vertebral artery dissection: a review of the medical literature. American Journal of Roentgenology 2009;193:1167—74.
[26] Sturzenegger M, Mattle HP, Rivoir A, Rihs F, Schmid C. Ultrasound findings in spontaneous extracranial vertebral artery dissection. Stroke 1993;24:1910—21.
[27] Steinke W, Rautenberg W, Schwartz A, Hennerici M. Noninvasive monitoring of internal carotid artery dissection. Stroke 1994;25:998—1005.
[28] Trattnig S, Rand T, Thurnher M, Breitenseher M, Daha K. Colour-coded Doppler sonography of common carotid artery dissection. Neuroradiology 1995;37:124—6.
[29] de Bray JM, Lhoste P, Dubas F, Emile J, Saumet JL. Ultrasonic features of extracranial carotid dissections: 47 cases studied by angiography. Journal of Ultrasound in Medicine 1994;13:59—64.
[30] Bartels E, Flugel KA. Evaluation of extracranial vertebral artery dissection with duplex color-flow imaging. Stroke 1996;27:290—5.
[31] Lovrencic-Huzjan A, Jurasic MJ, Lovrencic-Prpic G, Vukovic V, Demarin V. Aortic arch dissection presenting with hemodynamic spectrum of aortic regurgitation on transcranial Doppler. Ultraschall in der Medizin 2006;27:280—3.
[32] Lovrencic-Huzjan A, Bosnar-Puretic M, Vukovic V, Demarin V. Sonographic features of craniocervical artery dissection. Acta Clinica Croatica 2002;41:307—12.
[33] Cerimagic D, Glavic J, Lovrencic-Huzjan A, Demarin V. Occlusion of vertebral artery, cerebellar infarction and obstructive hydrocephalus following cervical spine manipulation. European Neurology 2007;58:248—50.
[34] Arning C. Ultrasonographic criteria for diagnosing a dissection of the internal carotid artery. European Journal of Ultrasound 2005;26:24—8.
[35] Nedeltchev K, Bickel S, Arnold M, Sarikaya H, Sturzenegger M, Mattle HP, et al. Recanalization for spontaneous carotid artery dissection. Stroke 2009;40:499—504.
[36] Nedbelsieck J, Sengelhoff C, Nassenstein I, Maintz D, Kuhlebaumer G, Nabavi DG, et al. Sensitivity of neurovascular ultrasound for the detection of spontaneous cervical artery dissection. Journal of Clinical Neuroscience 2009;16:79—82.
[37] Lovrencic-Huzjan A, Klanfar Z, Bosnar-Puretic M, Demarin V. Embolic stroke due to internal carotid dissection: non-invasive monitoring of recanalisation by color Doppler flow imaging and transcranial Doppler. Acta Clinica Croatica 2002;42:201—5.
[38] Molina CA, Alvarez-Sabin J, Schonewille W, Montaner J, Rovira A, Abilleira S, et al. Cerebral microembolism in acute spontaneous internal carotid artery dissection. Neurology 2000;55:1738—41.
[39] Baracchini C, Tonello S, Menaghetti G, Ballotta E. Neurosonographic monitoring of 105 spontaneous cervical artery dissections: a prospective study. Neurology 2010;75:1864—70.
[40] Longo GM, Kibbe MR. Aneurysms of the carotid artery. Seminars in Vascular Surgery 2005;18:178—83.

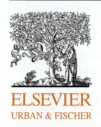

Ultrasound in spontaneous cervical artery dissection

Ralf Dittrich*, Martin A. Ritter, Erich B. Ringelstein

Department of Neurology, University Hospital of Muenster, Albert Schweitzer Campus 1, Building A1, 48149 Muenster, Germany

KEYWORDS
Cervical artery dissection;
Ultrasound;
Spontaneous

Summary Spontaneous cervical artery dissection is caused by a hematoma in the arterial wall. Recent research revealed that the most likely pathophysiological key mechanism is rupture of a vas vasorum resulting in a bleeding into the medio-adventitial borderzone [1]. The expansion of the hematoma into the arterial lumen can secondarily lead to a rupture of the tunica intima with a high risk of thrombus formation and embolic cerebral infarction [2]. Moreover the expansion of the hematoma causes an arterial stenosis or arterial occlusion with the risk of hemodynamic impairment. The risk of an ischemic stroke in the course of a dissection is thought to be about 70% for dissections of the internal carotid artery (ICA) [3] and about 80% for dissections of the vertebral artery (VA) [4]. The annual incidence of dissections of the ICA has been estimated to be 2.5—3/100,000 and for the VA 0.97—1.5/100,000 [5,6]. Although dissections as such are rare they are a frequent etiology of stroke in children and young adults. Approximately 25% of the strokes in patients younger than 50 are caused by dissections with a peak age between 40 and 45 years [7—16].
© 2012 Elsevier GmbH. All rights reserved.

Introduction

Spontaneous cervical artery dissection is caused by a hematoma in the arterial wall. Recent research revealed that the most likely pathophysiological key mechanism is rupture of a vas vasorum resulting in a bleeding into the medio-adventitial borderzone [1]. The expansion of the hematoma into the arterial lumen can secondarily lead to a rupture of the tunica intima with a high risk of thrombus formation and embolic cerebral infarction [2]. Moreover the expansion of the hematoma causes an arterial stenosis or arterial occlusion with the risk of hemodynamic impairment. The risk of an ischemic stroke in the course of a dissection is thought to be about 70% for dissections of the internal carotid artery (ICA) [3] and about 80% for dissections of the vertebral artery (VA) [4]. The annual incidence of dissections of the ICA has been estimated to be 2.5—3/100,000 and for the VA 0.97—1.5/100,000 [5,6]. Although dissections as such are rare they are a frequent etiology of stroke in children and young adults. Approximately 25% of the strokes in patients younger than 50 are caused by dissections with a peak age between 40 and 45 years [7—16].

Due to the technical improvement of the ultrasound devices the investigation of the brain supplying arteries is nowadays an established and indispensable diagnostic tool in the detection and monitoring of spontaneous dissection.

Ultrasound in spontaneous dissection of the internal carotid artery

The ultrasound investigation should include the complete anterior circulation, i.e. both common carotid arteries (CCA), both external carotid arteries (ECA) and both ICA. Moreover, the flow velocities and flow properties of the intracranial portion of the ICA, the anterior (ACA), and

* Corresponding author. Tel.: +49 2518344407.
E-mail address: Ralf.Dittrich@ukmuenster.de (R. Dittrich).

2211-968X/$ — see front matter © 2012 Elsevier GmbH. All rights reserved.
doi:10.1016/j.permed.2012.02.024

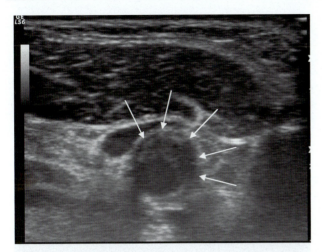

Figure 1 Cross sectional B-mode ultrasound of the ICA with typical half moon shaped echolucent wall thickening, marked with arrows.

middle cerebral arteries (MCA) should be documented and the collateral flow pathways including the periorbital arteries if present. For the extracranial parts of the arteries, a high frequency linear transducer (≥ 7.5 MHz) should be used. The use of a sector probe for the distal portion of the ICA is strongly recommended, as the stenosis is frequently located much further distally to atherothrombotic disease [17,18]. For the intracranial arteries, a phased array transducer (≥ 2 MHz) is recommended.

The ultrasound investigation usually reveals absent or only mild atherosclerosis due to the fact that dissections occur in middle aged people [3,19—22]. A higher incidence of kinking or coiling of arteries has been reported in patients with cervical artery dissection [23]. However, other investigators could not confirm this arterial elongation as a regular finding in this patient group [24]. In patients with fibromuscular dysplasia, a known risk factor for cervical artery dissection [25], irregular wall thickening, multisegmental stenosis or an aberrant course of the ICA are frequently found [26,27].

The typical angiographic signs of an ICA dissection have first been described at first in conventional transfemoral angiography restricted to intraluminal pathologies [28]

- Smooth or slightly irregular tapered stenosis
- Various types of ICA occlusion
  - Rattail-shaped tapered occlusion
  - Flame-like occlusion
- False or double lumen
- Saccular or fusiform aneurysmal dilatation (pseudoaneurysm)
- Irregular dilatation
- Intimal flap

B-mode ultrasound investigation also visualizes the arterial wall and the surrounding tissue. The typical direct finding of a dissection of the ICA is the detection of a wall thickening of low echogenicity caused by the intramural hematoma with adjacent thrombotic material leading to a stenosis of this artery [17,22,29] (see Fig. 1).

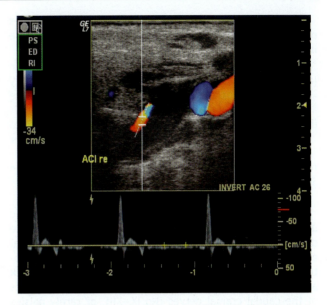

Figure 2 Duplex sonography of the ICA with detection of a high graded stenosis and increased pulsatility of the blood flow due to an echolucent hematoma.

In contrast to atherosclerotic stenosis which is predominantly located at the proximal part of the ICA, the stenosis due to dissection is found primarily in the distal part of the ICA [21,30]. Therefore it is often helpful to examine the distal part of the ICA with a sector probe especially in patients with a short neck, a prominent mandibular angle or a high bifurcation of the carotid artery. The detection rate of an intramural hematoma in the ICA by ultrasound is about 15—25% [17,22,29,31] (Fig. 2).

Another direct ultrasound sign of spontaneous cervical artery dissection is a ''double lumen'' which is found very rarely in the ICA. It is a result of a ruptured Tunica intima due to the space occupying intramural hematoma. The sonographic detection rate varies between 0 and 2% [17,31].

More diagnostic sensitivity is achieved when performing a duplex sonography with measurement of the blood flow velocity and with graduation of stenosis. Due to the fact that a stenosis caused by a dissection is located at the more distal part of the ICA this arterial segment has to be investigated with a sector probe more often. The sector probe has a lower spatial resolution with a lower chance to detect the intramural hematoma directly. In summary the detection of a stenosis in an arterial segment usually not affected by atherosclerosis is the most frequent finding. On the basis of the European Carotid Surgery Trial (ESCT) criteria which considered the percentage of local diameter reduction, a focal increase of the blood flow velocity of more than 120 cm/s is the cut-off for a 50% stenosis. Most of the published ultrasound studies have used the ESCT criteria and therefore it has to be kept in mind that the actual most widely accepted North American Symptomatic Carotid Endarterectomy Trial (NASCET) classification refers to the distal diameter reduction which leads to lower degrees of stenosis [3,18,32]. In one of the largest patient series on 181 patients and 200 dissections of the ICA, stenoses of the ICA have been found according to the ESCT criteria in 88% of the patients (stenosis $\leq 50\%$ in 8%, stenosis 51—80% in 9%, stenosis >80% or occlusion in 71% of the cases) [17].

Due to the distal location of ICA dissection sometimes only indirect signs are detectable with ultrasound. These indirect signs comprise:

(a) increased pulsatility upstream or decreased pulsatility downstream to the suspected lesion. This is detectable in about 77% of cases
(b) >50% difference in the blood flow velocity compared to the corresponding arterial segments of the artery under study, detectable in about 73%
(c) detection of intracranial collateral flow, detectable in about 38% [31].

Taken the indirect and direct signs together, pathologic ultrasound findings suggestive for ICA dissection can be detected in 80—96% of all cases [18,31,33]. However, clinical aspects are also very important. In patients with local symptoms only (new onset of so far unknown head and or neck ache (painful) Horner's syndrome, pulsatile tinnitus, palsies of the caudal cranial nerves (No IX—XII), or rarely palsies of the Nerves Nos. III, IV, VI), the ultrasound investigation is much less sensitive [3]. The initial duplex sonographical investigation in patients with isolated Horner's syndrome can be normal in up to 31% [34].

In summary the ultrasound investigation has a high sensitivity in detecting pathologic findings in patients with ICA dissection. However, it is not the sole investigation to verify the diagnosis of dissection especially in patients with local symptoms only.

Ultrasound in spontaneous dissection of the vertebral artery

The ultrasound investigation of the vertebral artery (VA) should include all segments, the origin and pre-vertebral part of the artery (V0/V1 segment), the part between the foramina of the transverse processes (V2 segment), the atlas loop (V3 segment) and the intracranial part (V4 segment). The V1 and V2 segment is normally investigated with a linear probe. The origin of the VA is sometimes not accessible with the linear probe especially in obese patients, and an investigation with a sector probe is superior. This is also the case when the V3 segment with its curved course is investigated. The V4 segment should be investigated via the transnuchal approach with a phased array transducer.

In analogy to the ICA dissection, the intramural hematoma of a VA dissection can cause an echolucent wall thickening and sometimes a double lumen. These signs can be found in 10—20% [31] (see Fig. 3).

A stenosis or occlusion can be more often diagnosed by detecting a focal increase of the blood flow velocity especially in the V3 segment where it is nearly impossible to visualize the arterial wall with the B mode ultrasound. Comparable to the findings in ICA dissection, a stenosis or occlusion due to dissection occurs in nearly 80% [31]. The corresponding indirect signs such as increased or decreased pulsatility or a blood flow velocity difference of >50%, are more difficult to interpret since the VA can be hyoplastic or is ending in the posterior inferior cerebellar artery [35]. A proximal arterial occlusion may be overlooked when the V4 segment is filled with an orthograde flow via cervical

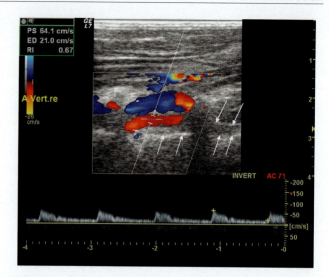

Figure 3 Duplex sonography of the vertebral artery with an echolucent wall thickening due to an intramural hematoma (marked by arrows) without a hemodynamic relevant stenosis.

collaterals [36]. Comparable to ICA dissections, the predilection site for VA dissection is different from atherosclerotic lesions. The dissections occur primarily in the V2 and V3 segment [4] whereas the atherosclerotic disease is mostly found in the V0 or V4 Segments [37]. The overall sensitivity of the ultrasound investigation in detecting pathologies suggestive of a VA dissection varies from 70 to 92% [18,31,38].

In 8—13% the ultrasound investigation reveals normal findings despite MRI proven ICA or VA cervical artery dissection. The reason for this is usually a dissection in the distal part of the ICA especially at the base of the skull where the resolution of the B-mode is not high enough to detect the intramural hematoma directly. Another reason for failure found in ICA and VA dissection is a mild stenosis of <50% without hemodynamic flow changes [18,31].

Recanalization of dissected arteries

Hemodynamic relevant stenosis and arterial occlusion are frequently found in cervical artery dissection. The recanalization rate of ICA or VA occlusion can be easily monitored by ultrasound and varies between 42 and 72% and occurs within 6 weeks to 18 months [20,39—41]. The improvement rate of stenotic or occluded arteries is about 69% within the first 6 months after dissection. Afterwards, the improvement rate is much lower (19%). A complete recanalization without any stenosis after 6 months is achieved in 39% [40]. Beyond 9 months, further recanalization is only rarely seen (1%) [41].

Recurrence of dissection

So far, a recurrence of dissection between 2 days and 8.6 years has been reported and frequencies vary between 0 and 8% [3,6,10,11,42—44]. In a recent study with repetitive MR-investigations in a group of 36 patients, a much higher recurrence rate could be found. A new dissection in a formerly unaffected artery was diagnosed in 19% between 1 and 4 weeks, and in another 6% of patients within 5—7 months

[26,27]. This remarkable finding has been reproduced in a much larger cohort of 76 patients with 105 dissections. The patients have been investigated with repetitive ultrasound daily during the hospitalization, then every month during the first 6 months and afterwards every 6 months with a mean follow-up of 58 months. A recurrent dissection in a formerly unaffected artery has been detected in 20 arteries (26.3%) during the stay in hospital. Afterwards a recurrence was found only in 2 (2.7%) previously affected arteries [41]. Therefore, the recurrence rate is much higher than previously thought and varies from 19 to 26% in the acute phase of the disease.

Summary

Due to the high sensitivity in detecting pathologic findings, ultrasound is an essential investigation method for both the ICA dissection and VA dissection because it can be quickly performed, it has a high availability and it is non-invasive. However, the diagnosis should be confirmed by MR-imaging because this is the method of choice to detect the intramural hematoma [45,46]. We recommend using both methods complementarily. Ultrasound is the most practical method for monitoring of hemodynamics in dissection and follow-up investigations to detect recurrent dissections which are more than twofold more frequent than previously thought.

Authors' contributions

All authors have contributed substantially to the manuscript. They drafted and revised it together and gave final approval to its submission.

Conflict of interests

Dr. Dittrich and Dr. Ritter have no conflict of interest.

Prof. E.B. Ringelstein has received travel expenses and honorariums from Boehringer Ingelheim, Sygnis, Neurobiological Technologies, Novartis, Novo-Nordisc, Sanofi-Aventis, Solvay, Bayer Vital, M's Science, Servier, UCB, Trommsdorff for serving as a member of Steering Committees, Safety Committees in clinical trials, and as a speaker and consultant. Prof. Ringelstein has no ownership interest and does not own stocks of any pharmaceutical company. He has no proprietary or commercial interest in any materials discussed in this article.

References

[1] Völker W, Dittrich R, Grewe S, Nassenstein I, Csiba L, Herczeg L, et al. The outer arterial wall layers are primarily affected in spontaneous cervical artery dissection. Neurology 2011;76:1463—71.

[2] Benninger DH, Georgiadis D, Kremer C, Studer A, Nedeltchev K, Baumgartner RW. Mechanism of ischemic infarct in spontaneous carotid dissection. Stroke 2004;35:482—5.

[3] Baumgartner RW, Arnold M, Baumgartner I, Mosso M, Gönner F, Studer A, et al. Carotid dissection with and without ischemic events: local symptoms and cerebral artery findings. Neurology 2001;57:827—32.

[4] Arnold M, Bousser MG, Fahrni G, Fischer U, Georgiadis D, Gandjour J, et al. Vertebral artery dissection: presenting findings and predictors of outcome. Stroke 2006;37:2499—503.

[5] Schievink WI. Spontaneous dissection of the carotid and vertebral arteries. N Engl J Med 2001;344:898—906.

[6] Lee VH, Brown Jr RD, Mandrekar JN, Mokri B. Incidence and outcome of cervical artery dissection: a population-based study. Neurology 2006;67:1809—12.

[7] Bevan H, Sharma K, Bradley W. Stroke in young adults. Stroke 1990;21:382—6.

[8] Lisovoski F, Rousseaux P. Cerebral infarction in young people. A study of 148 patients with early cerebral angiography. J Neurol Neurosurg Psychiatry 1991;54:576—9.

[9] Bogousslavsky J, Pierre P. Ischemic stroke in patients under age 45. Neurol Clin 1992;10:113—24.

[10] Schievink WI, Mokri B, Piepgras DG. Spontaneous dissection of cervicocephalic arteries in childhood and adolescence. Neurology 1994;44:1607—12.

[11] Schievink WI, Mokri B, O'Fallon WM. Recurrent spontaneous cervical-artery dissection. N Engl J Med 1994;330:393—7.

[12] Dziewas R, Konrad C, Dräger B, Evers S, Besselmann M, Lüdemann P, et al. Cervical artery dissection—clinical features, risk factors, therapy and outcome in 126 patients. J Neurol 2003;250:1179—84.

[13] Nedeltchev K, der Maur TA, Georgiadis D, Arnold M, Caso V, Mattle HP, et al. Ischaemic stroke in young adults: predictors of outcome and recurrence. J Neurol Neurosurg Psychiatry 2005;76:191—5.

[14] Arauz A, Hoyos L, Espinoza C, Cantu C, Barinagarrementeria F, Roman G. Dissection of cervical arteries: long-term follow-up study of 130 consecutive cases. Cerebrovasc Dis 2006;22:150—4.

[15] Arnold M, Pannier B, Chabriat H, Nedeltchev K, Stapf C, Buffon F, et al. Vascular risk factors and morphometric data in cervical artery dissection: a case—control study. J Neurol Neurosurg Psychiatry 2009;80:232—4.

[16] Arnold M, Kurmann R, Galimanis A, Sarikaya H, Stapf C, Gralla J, et al. Differences in demographic characteristics and risk factors in patients with spontaneous vertebral artery dissections with and without ischemic events. Stroke 2010;41:802—4.

[17] Benninger DH, Baumgartner RW. Ultrasound diagnosis of cervical artery dissection. Front Neurol Neurosci 2006;21:70—84.

[18] Dittrich R, Dziewas R, Ritter MA, Kloska SP, Bachmann R, Nassenstein I, et al. Negative ultrasound findings in patients with cervical artery dissection. Negative ultrasound in CAD. J Neurol 2006;253:424—33.

[19] Müllges W, Ringelstein EB, Leibold M. Non-invasive diagnosis of internal carotid artery dissections. J Neurol Neurosurg Psychiatry 1992;55:98—104.

[20] Steinke W, Rautenberg W, Schwartz A, Hennerici M. Noninvasive monitoring of internal carotid artery dissection. Stroke 1994;25:998—1005.

[21] Sturzenegger M, Mattle HP, Rivoir A, Baumgartner RW. Ultrasound findings in carotid artery dissection: analysis of 43 patients. Neurology 1995;45:691—8.

[22] Logason K, Hardemark HG, Barlin T, Bergqvist D, Ahlstom H, Karacagil S. Duplex scan findings in patients with spontaneous cervical artery dissections. Eur J Vasc Endovasc Surg 2002;23:295—8.

[23] Barbour PJ, Castaldo JE, Rae-Grant AD, Gee W, Reed III JF, Jenny D, et al. Internal carotid artery redundancy is significantly associated with dissection. Stroke 1994;25:1201—6.

[24] Dittrich R, Nassenstein I, Harms S, Maintz D, Heindel W, Kuhlenbäumer G, et al. Arterial elongation (''redundancy'') is not a feature of spontaneous cervical artery dissection. J Neurol 2011 February;258:250—4.

[25] de Bray JM, Marc G, Pautot V, Vielle B, Pasco A, Lhoste P, et al. Fibromuscular dysplasia may herald symptomatic recurrence of cervical artery dissection. Cerebrovasc Dis 2007;23:448—52.

[26] Dittrich R, Nassenstein I, Ringelstein EB, Kuhlenbaumer G, Nabavi DG. A distinctive case of fibromuscular dysplasia. Neurol Res 2007;29:551—2.

[27] Dittrich R, Nassenstein I, Bachmann R, Maintz D, Nabavi DG, Heindel W, et al. Polyarterial clustered recurrence of cervical artery dissection seems to be the rule. Neurology 2007;69:180—6.

[28] Paciaroni M, Caso V, Agnelli G. Magnetic resonance imaging, magnetic resonance and catheter angiography for diagnosis of cervical artery dissection. Front Neurol Neurosci 2005;20:102—18.

[29] de Bray JM, Lhoste P, Dubas F, Emile J, Saumet JL. Ultrasonic features of extracranial carotid dissections: 47 cases studied by angiography. J Ultrasound Med 1994;13:659—64.

[30] Benninger DH, Caso V, Baumgartner RW. Ultrasound assessment of cervical artery dissection. Front Neurol Neurosci 2005;20:87—101.

[31] Nebelsieck J, Sengelhoff C, Nassenstein I, Maintz D, Kuhlenbäumer G, Nabavi DG, et al. Sensitivity of neurovascular ultrasound for the detection of spontaneous cervical artery dissection. J Clin Neurosci 2009;16:79—82.

[32] Arning C, Widder B, von Reutern GM, Stiegler H, Görtler M. Revision of DEGUM ultrasound criteria for grading internal carotid artery stenoses and transfer to NASCET measurement. Ultraschall Med 2010;31:251—7 [Article in German].

[33] Benninger DH, Georgiadis D, Gandjour J, Baumgartner RW. Accuracy of color duplex ultrasound diagnosis of spontaneous carotid dissection causing ischemia. Stroke 2006;37:377—81.

[34] Arnold M, Baumgartner RW, Stapf C, Nedeltchev K, Buffon F, Benninger D, et al. Ultrasound diagnosis of spontaneous carotid dissection with isolated Horner syndrome. Stroke 2008;39:82—6.

[35] Baumgartner RW, Siebler M. Ultraschalldiagnostik beim Schlaganfall. München: Ecomed-Verlag; 2002.

[36] Ringelstein EB, Zeumer H, Poeck K. Non-invasive diagnosis of intracranial lesions in the vertebrobasilar system—a comparison of Doppler sonographic and angiographic findings. Stroke 1985;16:848—55.

[37] Compter A, van der Worp HB, Algra A, Kappelle LJ, Second Manifestations of ARTerial disease (SMART) Study Group. Prevalence and prognosis of asymptomatic vertebral artery origin stenosis in patients with clinically manifest arterial disease. Stroke 2011;42:2795—800.

[38] Sturzenegger M, Mattle HP, Rivoir A, Rihs F, Schmid C. Ultrasound findings in spontaneous extracranial vertebral artery dissection. Stroke 1993;24:1910—21.

[39] Caso V, Paciaroni M, Corea F, Hamam M, Milia P, Pelliccioli GP, et al. Recanalization of cervical artery dissection: influencing factors and role in neurological outcome. Cerebrovasc Dis 2004;17:93—7.

[40] Sengelhoff C, Nebelsieck J, Nassenstein I, Maintz D, Nabavi DG, Kuhlenbaeumer G, et al. Neurosonographical follow-up in patients with spontaneous cervical artery dissection. Neurol Res 2008;30:687—9.

[41] Baracchini C, Tonello S, Meneghetti G, Ballotta E. Neurosonographic monitoring of 105 spontaneous cervical artery dissections: a prospective study. Neurology 2010;75:1864—70.

[42] Bassetti C, Carruzzo A, Sturzenegger M, Tuncdogan E. Recurrence of cervical artery dissection. A prospective study of 81 patients. Stroke 1996;27:1804—7.

[43] Pelkonen O, Tikkakoksi T, Leinonen S, Pyhtinen J, Lepojarvi M, Sotaniemi K. Extracranial internal carotid and vertebral artery dissections: angiographic spectrum, course and prognosis. Neuroradiology 2003;45:71—7.

[44] Touzé E, Gauvit JY, Moulin T, Meder JF, Bracrad S, Mas JL. Multicenter survey on Natural History of Cervical Artery Dissection. Neurology 2003;61:1347—51.

[45] Zuber M, Meary E, Meder J, Mas JL. Magnetic resonance imaging and dynamic CT scan in cervical artery dissections. Stroke 1994;25:576—81.

[46] Lévy C, Laissy J, Raveau V, Amarenco P, Servois V, Bousser MG, et al. Carotid and vertebral artery dissections: three-dimensional time-of-flight MR angiography and MR imaging versus conventional angiography. Radiology 1994;190:97—103.

Diagnosis and management of Takayasu arteritis

Narayanaswamy Venketasubramanian*

Division of Neurology, University Medicine Cluster, Level 10, NUHS Tower Block 1E Kent Ridge Road, Singapore 119228, Singapore

KEYWORDS
Takayasu;
Arteritis;
Aortitis;
Ultrasonography;
Diagnosis;
Management

Summary Takayasu arteritis is a panaortitis, more frequent in Japan, South-East Asia India and Mexico, that presents in the 2nd or 3rd decade of life with a non-specific inflammatory phase, then vascular stenosis with 'pulselessness' with collateral development. Clinical features include reduced/absent pulses, bruits, hypertension, aortic regurgitation, neurological symptoms from ischemia. While the gold standard for diagnosis is arteriography, magnetic resonance angiography and ultrasonography are now widely used due to their non-invasive nature. Steroids are the cornerstone of medical therapy; cytotoxics may be used for failures. Surgery or angioplasty may be needed for severe vascular stenosis.
© 2012 Elsevier GmbH. All rights reserved.

History

The earliest description of this ailment was probably made in 1930 by Yamamoto in Japan of a 45-year old man with impalpable carotid and upper limb pulses. The first presentation to a scientific audience of the disease was by Japanese ophthalmologist Mikito Takayasu in 1905 when he described a 21-year old female with coronary anastomosis in her ocular fundus. At that same 12th Annual Meeting of the Japan Ophthalmology Society in Fukuoka, Drs. Kagoshima and Ohnishi each presented a similar case that also had no radial pulse. The disease was thus subsequently called Takayasu Arteritis to honour the first presenter. Ohta attributed the ocular abnormalities to occlusion of the cervical arteries, while Shimizu and Sano coined the now widely phrase 'pulseless disease' for this entity. Another occasionally-used term is Martorell syndrome.

* Corresponding author. Tel.: +65 92380283.
E-mail address: drnvramani@gmail.com

Epidemiology

The frequency of the disease appears to be higher in Japan, South-East Asia, India and Mexico compared to other parts of the world. In North America, the incidence was found to be 2.6/million/year.

Pathology

Takayasu arteritis is pathologically a panaortitis. The adventitia is thickened and filled with inflammatory T-cells and monocytes. It is believed that these cells enter via the vaso vasorum, attracted by adhesion molecules such as ICAM-1 and VCAM-1 expressed in these vessels. It has been found that infection may trigger the disease in mice — no clear consistent relationship as been found in humans; tuberculosis has also been implicated. The aorta later becomes fibrotic, with lumen narrowed patchily in multiple areas.

Genetics

Familial cases have been reported from a number of countries, including among twins. Human Leucocyte Antigen

Table 1 Clinical manifestations of Takayasu arteritis (Ref. [1]).

Clinical feature	Frequency (%)
Reduced/absent pulses	84—96
Bruits	80—94
Hypertension	33—83
Renal artery stenosis	28—75
Aortic regurgitation	20—24
Pulmonary artery involvement	14—100

Table 2 Classification of Takayasu arteritis.

Type	Arterial involvement
I	Branches of aortic arch
IIa	Ascending aorta, aortic arch and its branches
IIb	Ascending aorta, aortic arch and its branches and thoracic descending aorta
III	Thoracic descending aorta, abdominal aorta and/or renal arteries
IV	Only abdominal aorta and/or renal arteries
V	Combined types IIb and IV

(HLA) gene analyses have found increased frequency of HLA B52, B39.2, D12 and A24 among Japanese. The gene may lie between the MIC gene and HLA B locus on chromosome 6. HLA B52 patients may have more severe inflammation while those with HLA B39 may have more renal artery involvement.

Clinical manifestations

The illness ranges from being asymptomatic to a catastrophic illness. It often presents in the 2nd or 3rd decade of life. It may begin with a non-specific inflammatory "pre-pulseless" phase characterised by fever, night sweats, lethargy, loss of weight, pains in the muscles and joints and even a mild anaemia. The erythrocyte sedimentation rate (ESR) tends to be elevated. With progression of the inflammation, vascular stenoses, usually bilateral, occur with resulting development of collateral circulation. Notably, not all patients go through these various stages.

Clinical features are shown in Table 1. Others include neurological involvement leading to transient ischemic attacks or stroke, giddiness, headache or rarely seizures, while cardiac features include congestive cardiac failure.

The 1990 American College of Rheumatology criteria require 3 or 6 features of age of onset ≤40 years, limb claudication, reduced pulsation in at least 1 brachial artery, a >10 mmHg difference in systolic blood pressure between the arms, bruits audible over the subclavian artery or abdominal aorta, and abnormalities on arteriography of the aorta or its principal branches.

Japanese patient are mostly female, while Indian patients are more male. Japanese patients tend to have reduced upper limb pulses due to involvement of the ascending aorta and aortic arch, while those of Indian, Thai, Korean and Chinese origin tend to have renovascular hypertension due to abdominal aorta and renal artery involvement.

Diagnosis

The gold standard for clinical diagnosis is arteriography. The International Conference on Takayasu Arteritis in 1994 classified the disease based on the angiogram (Table 2). Histology is conceivably the most diagnostic. In view of the invasive nature of angiography and impracticality of biopsy, ultrasonography is now widely used to make the diagnosis in a clinically suspected patient.

Ultrasound reveals thickened vessel walls (macaroni sign), including the carotid artery. Magnetic resonance angiography may reveal a better understanding of wall edema, and inflammation if contrast is used. These may be used to monitor response to treatment.

Treatment

Steroids remain the cornerstone of medical therapy. While early studies showed poor benefit, later studies have shown better response rates of about 50%, with reduction of symptoms of inflammation and even return of pulses in some patients. Among non-responders, a further 50% may respond to methotrexate. Other agents that have been tried include azathioprine, cyclophosphamide and mycophenolate mofetil. Hypertension needs to be well-managed, with careful use of angiotensin converting enzyme inhibitors.

Surgery may be needed if there is severe renal artery stenosis, activity-limiting limb ischemia, critical cerebral vessel stenosis, moderately severe aortic incompetence. It is best performed when the disease is 'quiet'. Angioplasty with or without stenting may be used for severe stenosis.

Further reading

[1] Johnston SL, Lock RJ, Gompels MM. Takayasu arteritis: a review. J Clin Pathol 2002;55:481—6.
[2] Numano F, Kobayashi Y. Takayasu arteritis—beyond pulselessness. Int Med 1999;38:226—32.
[3] Andrews J, Mason JC. Takayasu arteriotis—recent advances in imaging offer promise. Rheumatology 2007;46:6—15.

Moyamoya like arteriopathy: Neurosonological suspicion and prognosis in adult asymptomatic patients

Giovanni Malferrari[a], Marialuisa Zedde[a,*], Gianni De Berti[b], Massimo Maggi[b], Norina Marcello[a]

[a] *Neurology Unit, Department of Neuromotor Physiology, Azienda Ospedaliera ASMN, Istituto di Ricovero e Cura a Carattere Scientifico, Viale Risorgimento 80, 42100 Reggio Emilia, Italy*
[b] *Neuroradiology Unit, Department of Radiology, Azienda Ospedaliera ASMN, Istituto di Ricovero e Cura a Carattere Scientifico, Viale Risorgimento 80, 42100 Reggio Emilia, Italy*

KEYWORDS
Moyamoya;
Transcranial;
TCCS;
Intracranial stenosis;
MCA;
Asymptomatic

Summary

Introduction: The epidemiology and the prognosis of asymptomatic moyamoya arteriopathy is virtually unknown, mainly in white western population, while symptomatic moyamoya arteriopathy is a more known disease, both in children and in adult people. We are presenting a single centre case series of six asymptomatic adult people with a neurosonological (Transcranial Colour Coded Sonography — TCCS) suspicion of this type of cerebral arteriopathy, confirmed by Digital Subtraction Angiography (DSA).

Patients and methods: During a time period of three years we collected a series of six patients (5 female and 1 male, mean age 29.16 + 8.45 years) with a neurosonological suspicion and a neuroradiological diagnostic confirmation of moyamoya type arteriopathy. All patients underwent TCCS, brain magnetic resonance imaging (MRI) and magnetic resonance angiography (MRA) and DSA, besides the differential diagnosis of immunological or infectious etiology. The mean follow-up was 1.8 years.

Results and discussion: All patients but one had a bilateral internal carotid artery (ICA) stenosis at terminus and M1 middle cerebral artery (MCA) multiple stenoses. There is only one young patient with an atypical unilateral pathway and narrowing of extracranial ICA with prominent posterior cerebral artery (PCA) compensation. No clinical events occurred during the follow-up and also brain MRI failed to find new ischemic lesions, compared with the baseline examination.

Conclusions: Asymptomatic cerebral moyamoya arteriopathy is an infrequent but underestimated condition in young white people. More prognostic informations are needed in order to define the natural course and propose the treatment.
© 2012 Elsevier GmbH. All rights reserved.

Abbreviations: DSA, Digital Subtraction Angiography; ECA, external carotid artery; ICA, internal carotid artery; MCA, middle cerebral artery; MRI, magnetic resonance imaging; MRA, magnetic resonance angiography; PCA, posterior cerebral artery; TCCS, Transcranial Color Coded Sonography; TCD, TransCranial Doppler.
* Corresponding author. Tel.: +39 0522 296494.
  E-mail addresses: zedde.marialuisa@asmn.re.it, marialuisa.zedde@tiscali.it (M. Zedde).

Introduction

Moyamoya syndrome is a cerebrovascular disease that is associated to a predisposition to stroke because of the presence of multiple progressive stenosis of the intracranial ICAs and their proximal branches. It is a distinguishing feature of the disease the compensatory development of collateral circulation, determining the growth of a widespread network of small vessels at the terminus of the ICA, on the cortical surface, leptomeninges, and anastomotic branches of the ECA. The *moyamoya syndrome* includes patients with the characteristic moyamoya vasculopathy and well recognized associated conditions, whereas *moyamoya disease* concerns patients without known associated risk factors. The pathognomonic arteriographic findings are bilateral in moyamoya disease, with a variable severity between sides. Unilateral findings are indicative of the moyamoya syndrome, even without other associated risk factors [1].

It is more frequent in Asian populations and in children, mainly in Japan, where it is the most common pediatric cerebrovascular disease with a prevalence of about 3 cases per 100,000 children [2], but an adult form is also known and few cases are described in white population. In Europe the incidence of moyamoya among all ages is about 1/10th of that observed in Japan [3]. Therefore several data about the natural history of moyamoya disease concern Asian children [1]. The disease tends to be progressive, both in children and in adult patients. The progression of the vascular involvement usually means the increasing severity of stenosis to occlusion of large intracranial arteries and the increasing number of involved vessel segments, with a parallel development of the collateral circulation. It is believed that the rate of disease progression is high, even among asymptomatic patients, and that medical therapy alone is not sufficient to stop or slow it [4]. Current estimation is similar to the previous one that up to two thirds of patients with moyamoya have symptomatic progression over a 5-year period, and the outcome is reported poor without treatment [4–6].

The natural course of the moyamoya disease in European adult asymptomatic people is not so clear in the literature, because of the small sample of the available studies, and also in neurosurgical studies the subgroup of asymptomatic people is not numerous. Therefore it is not automatically right that in this subpopulation the outcome of surgically untreated patients is poor.

Therefore several data are lacking for *asymptomatic* vs symptomatic patients, *European* vs Asian patients and *adults* vs children patients. The lesser-known group concerns the asymptomatic European adult patient. We are presenting a single center case series of 6 European adult people with asymptomatic moyamoya disease, suspected through TCCS and confirmed by DSA, followed-up in medical treatment.

Materials and methods

During a time period of three years we collected a series of six patients (5 female and 1 male, mean age 29.16 + 8.45 years) with a neurosonological suspicion and a neuroradiological diagnostic confirmation of moyamoya type arteriopathy. All patients underwent to neurosonological examination for episodic not related symptoms, like dizziness, or for a screening purpose in a family history of cerebrovascular atherosclerotic accidents. Besides the neurosonological examination with ultrasound study of the cerebroafferent vessels and of the intracranial arteries by TCCS, all patients underwent brain MRI and MRA and DSA and blood sampling and other investigations for differential diagnosis of immunological or infectious etiology.

Diagnosis was made according to the approved criteria [Research Committee on Spontaneous Occlusion of the Circle of Willis (moyamoya disease) in Japan] [7].

TCCS was performed as a basal evaluation and with contrast agents for the evaluation of intracranial vessels in Power Modulation or Pulse Inversion. Ultrasound perfusional study was also performed but the data were not analyzed, because of the bilateral involvement in most patients and the lesser reliability of PCA territory for a comparison, due to the collateral circulation.

MRI and DSA were analyzed according to the Ministry of Health and Wellness of Japan criteria [7].

The mean follow-up was 1.8 years and it was both clinical and neurosonological–neuroradiological (with MRI). All patients were followed-up in at least 3 control visits, at 3 months from the diagnosis, at 6 months and at 12–18 months.

Results

The main features of the six patients are illustrated in Table 1.

All patients had a bilateral involvement in the intracranial circulation and all but one had a diagnosis of moyamoya disease/phenomenon, because of the absence of the well-known risk factors and associated conditions; one patient had a unilateral involvement, and therefore the diagnosis was a moyamoya syndrome. There is an evident prevalence of the female sex (female to male ratio 5). TCCS study was performed by an experienced neurosonologist both without and with ultrasound contrast agents (SonoVue®) in all patients and no side effects from the procedure were reported.

Neuroradiological examination, first brain MRI and intracranial MRA, and second DSA, were performed because of the suspicion of moyamoya arteriopathy and confirmed it. There was not any brain tissue abnormality suggesting acute cerebrovascular event in all examined patients, nor in basal MRI study and in control examinations. Both neurosonological findings and MRI findings did not change in the follow-up examination, therefore a control DSA was not performed.

TCCS studies were analyzed mainly considering the Doppler waveform, because of the existing classification of the MCA flow patterns (see Appendix A), made to classify TCD findings [8]. All patients with bilateral involvement but one had the same flow pattern in the MCA on both sides and a similar situation was reported for the DSA classification [9] (see Appendix B) but not in the same patients.

Both neurosonological and MRA findings were unchanged in the follow up examinations and no patients reported focal neurological events of vascular origin during the follow-up.

In Fig. 1 it is showed an example of the findings from the three techniques (TCCS, MRA, DSA) in two patients of our series.

Table 1 Main features of followed-up patients.

Subjects	Sex[a]	Age at the diagnosis (years)	Affected side	TCCS right side[b]	TCCS left side[b]	DSA stage right side[c]	DSA stage left side[c]	Cerebrovascular events	Length of follow-up (years)
1	F	18	Left	—	High—high flow pattern	—	Stage 4	None	4
2	F	41	Both	High—low flow pattern	High—low flow pattern	Stage 3	Stage 3	None	2
3	F	31	Both	High—high flow pattern	High—high flow pattern	Stage 3	Stage 3	None	1
4	F	28	Both	High—low flow pattern	High—low flow pattern	Stage 4	Stage 4	None	3
5	F	25	Both	High—low flow pattern	High—low flow pattern	Stage 3	Stage 3	None	2
6	M	32	Both	High—low flow pattern	High—low flow pattern	Stage 4	Stage 5	None	2

[a] F is for female sex and M is for male sex.
[b] TCCS data were presented according to the flow patterns detailed in Appendix A; only Doppler waveforms were used for this classification.
[c] TCCS data were presented according to the flow patterns detailed in Appendix B.

Discussion

For the reasons detailed in the introduction, there are few data about the natural course of the moyamoya disease in asymptomatic patients, mainly in adult people, both in Asian and particularly in European population. The lack of reliable informations is even more evident for asymptomatic patients, particularly for the adult form of the disease, because the introduction of noninvasive diagnostic tools made possible the sporadical identification of asymptomatic subjects. In a Japanese questionnaire survey, made in 88 neurosurgical institutes in 1994, to define clinical features and outcome of asymptomatic moyamoya disease [10], only thirty three asymptomatic moyamoya disease patients were collected (11 male, 22 female) and divided into 2 groups: patients without any symptoms (group 1, mainly adult people), and patients without any symptoms except headache (group 2). In this survey the natural course of asymptomatic moyamoya disease seemed benign and the need of a dedicated prospective study about this item was proposed.

But in the next years the non-invasive screening led to a change in the known epidemiological data, also in the Japanese population, as shown in a more recent all-inclusive survey of moyamoya disease in Hokkaido island

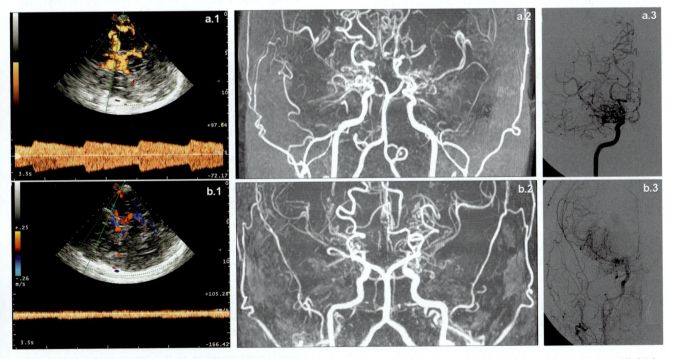

Figure 1 Example of diagnostic results for two patients of our series (1 TCCS, 2 MRA, 3 DSA). In the row 'a' patients with high low flow condition is illustrated; in the row 'b' a patient with low low flow condition is showed.

(population 5.63 million) [11], that analyzed data from 267 newly registered patients with moyamoya disease from 2002 to 2006. Overall the prevalence of the disease and the age at onset were reported higher than those previously known. The highest peak of onset age was older than those reported previously. In addition, 17.8% of patients were asymptomatic at onset in all decades.

In European population the moyamoya disease has also a lesser prevalence, therefore large epidemiological data are lacking, mainly about asymptomatic people. The limited existing European studies mostly deal with a mixed cohort of MMD and angiographic syndromes caused by other conditions, as in Khan's study [12] about surgical revascularization (15 of 23 patients with moyamoya angiopathy had idiopathic moyamoya disease). One of the largest European cohort was recently published, but all 21 adult patients were symptomatic for ischemic cerebrovascular events at the time of diagnosis [13]. There are few data in the literature also about the natural course of the disease in the white American population, and mainly in symptomatic people. In a retrospective study about the moyamoya phenomenon in these adult population, by review of angiographic records, only 3 of 34 patients were asymptomatic [14]. It is interesting to note that these three patients were free of events at the follow-up (5–8 years), but in symptomatic patients the recurrences of ischemic and hemorrhagic events was very high with the medical treatment.

Conclusions

Moyamoya disease is a condition lesser rare than otherwise thought, and it is present also in adult caucasian people with both symptomatic and asymptomatic form. The subgroup of asymptomatic adult caucasian people is very small in the literature, because the diagnostic suspicion is casual, therefore few informations are available on the natural course of this disorder. The smallest series in the literature raised the question about the especially benign course of this form and our series seems to confirm this impression.

Appendix A. Transcranial Doppler evaluation

Takase et al. [8] classified the CBF velocity patterns into 3 types:

1) the *high–high flow pattern*, commonly seen in younger patients, in whom high flow velocities exist with high flow, but with moderate grade stenosis in the ICA or MCA, in the absence of proper collateralization;
2) the *high–low flow pattern*, in which higher-grade stenoses are associated with high velocity but lower overall flow;
3) the *low–low flow pattern*, in which velocity and flow are low secondary to the highest degree of stenosis.

Appendix B. DSA

Suzuki and Takaku [9] have described 6 stages of moyamoya progression:

1) narrowing of the CA termination;

2) dilation of the proximal portions of the ACA and MCA with initial basal moyamoya blush;
3) proximal portions of the ACA and MCA are no longer visualized; distal branches are still present due to collateral vessels from the PCA and intensification of the moyamoya blush;
4) minimization of the basal moyamoya network together with progressive occlusion of the ICA, which reaches the origin of the PCA;
5) further reduction of moyamoya vessels, with complete disappearance of the main arteries arising from the CA, continuous decrease of moyamoya collateral vessels that are more limited to the siphon area, and increased collateral supply from the ECA; and
6) disappearance of the moyamoya blush together with the blood supply from the ICA.

References

[1] Scott RM, Smith ER. Moyamoya disease and moyamoya syndrome. N Engl J Med 2009;360:1226–37.
[2] Wakai K, Tamakoshi A, Ikezaki K, Fukui M, Kawamura T, Aoki R, et al. Epidemiological features of moyamoya disease in Japan: findings from a nationwide survey. Clin Neurol Neurosurg 1997;99(Suppl. 2):S1–5.
[3] Yonekawa Y, Ogata N, Kaku Y, Taub E, Imhof HG. Moyamoya disease in Europe, past and present status. Clin Neurol Neurosurg 1997;99(Suppl. 2):S58–60.
[4] Kuroda S, Ishikawa T, Houkin K, Nanba R, Hokari M, Iwasaki. Incidence and clinical features of disease progression in adult moyamoya disease. Stroke 2005;36:2148–53.
[5] Kurokawa T, Chen YJ, Tomita S. Cerebrovascular occlusive disease with and without moyamoya vascular network in children. Neuropediatrics 1985;16:29–32.
[6] Choi JU, Kim DS, Kim EY, Lee KC. Natural history of moyamoya disease: comparison of activity of daily living in surgery and non surgery groups. Clin Neurol Neurosurg 1997;99(Suppl. 2):S11–8.
[7] Fukui M. Guidelines for the diagnosis and treatment of spontaneous occlusion of the circle of Willis ('moyamoya' disease). Research Committee on Spontaneous Occlusion of the Circle of Willis (Moyamoya Disease) of the Ministry of Health and Welfare, Japan. Clin Neurol Neurosurg 1997;99(Suppl. 2):S238–40.
[8] Takase K, Kashihara M, Hashimoto T. Transcranial Doppler ultrasonography in patients with moyamoya disease. Clin Neurol Neurosurg 1997;99(Suppl. 2):S101–5.
[9] Suzuki J, Takaku A. Cerebrovascular "moyamoya" disease showing abnormal net-like vessels in base of brain. Arch Neurol 1969;20:288–99.
[10] Yamada M, Fujii K, Fukui M. Clinical features and outcomes in patients with asymptomatic moyamoya disease-from the results of nation-wide questionnaire survey. No Shinkei Geka 2005;33:337–42.
[11] Baba T, Houkin K, Kuroda S. Novel epidemiological features of moyamoya disease. J Neurol Neurosurg Psychiatry 2008;79:900–4.
[12] Khan N, Schuknecht B, Boltshauser E, Capone A, Buck A, Imhof HG, et al. Moyamoya disease and moyamoya syndrome: experience in Europe; choice of revascularisation procedures. Acta Neurochir 2003;145:1061–71.
[13] Kraemer M, Heienbrok W, Berlit P. Moyamoya disease in Europeans. Stroke 2008;39:3193–200.
[14] Hallemeier CL, Rich KM, Grubb RL. Clinical features and outcome in North American adults with moyamoya phenomenon. Stroke 2006;37:1490–6.

Posttraumatic vasospasm and intracranial hypertension after wartime traumatic brain injury

Rocco A. Armonda [a], Teodoro A. Tigno [b], Sven M. Hochheimer [a],
Fred L. Stephens [a], Randy S. Bell [a], Alexander H. Vo [b], Meryl A. Severson [a],
Scott A. Marshall [c], Stephen M. Oppenheimer [e], Robert Ecker [e],
Alexander Razumovsky [d],*

[a] *Walter Reed National Military Medical Center, Bethesda, MD, USA*
[b] *The University of Texas Medical Branch, Galveston, TX, USA*
[c] *Department of Neurology, Uniformed Services University of the Health Sciences, Bethesda, MD 20814, USA*
[d] *Sentient NeuroCare Services, Inc., Hunt Valley, MD, USA*
[e] *Maine Medical Center, Portland, ME, USA*

KEYWORDS
Combat associated wartime traumatic brain injury;
Wartime traumatic brain injury;
Transcranial Doppler ultrasonography;
Cerebral blood flow velocity;
Vasospasm;
Intracranial pressure

Summary Traumatic brain injury (TBI) is associated with the severest casualties from Operation Iraqi Freedom (OIF) and Operation Enduring Freedom (OEF). From October 1, 2008 the US Army Medical Department initiated a transcranial Doppler (TCD) ultrasound service for TBI patients; included patients were retrospectively evaluated for TCD-determined incidence of posttraumatic cerebral vasospasm and intracranial hypertension after wartime TBI. Ninety patients were investigated with daily TCD studies and comprehensive TCD protocol and published diagnostic criteria for vasospasm and raised intracranial pressure (ICP) were applied. TCD signs of mild, moderate and severe vasospasms were observed in 37%, 22% and 12% of patients, respectively. TCD signs of intracranial hypertension were recorded in 62.2%, five patients (4.5%) underwent transluminal angioplasty for post-traumatic clinical vasospasm treatment and 16 (14.4%) had cranioplasty. These findings demonstrate that cerebral arterial spasm and intracranial hypertension are frequent and significant complications of combat TBI, therefore daily TCD monitoring is recommended for their recognition and subsequent management.
© 2012 Elsevier GmbH. All rights reserved.

Introduction

Cerebral vasospasm (VSP) is a frequent complication after aneurysmal and traumatic subarachnoid hemorrhage (SAH) and carries significant morbidity and mortality [1—4]. Armonda and co-authors indicated that VSP occurred in a substantial number of patients with war-time TBI and clinical outcomes were worse in such patients [5]. Cerebral angiography remains the standard diagnostic test in

* Corresponding author at: 11011 McCormick Rd, Suite 200, Hunt Valley, MD 21031, USA. Tel.: +1 410 666 2588x123; fax: +1 443 927 7315.
  E-mail address: arazumovsky@sentientmedical.com (A. Razumovsky).

this setting; however, this procedure is invasive, expensive, not always available, and not without risk [6]. In contrast, transcranial Doppler (TCD) ultrasonography has been increasingly used over the past few years for diagnosis and monitoring cerebral VSP and implementing therapeutic interventions [7]. TBI and cerebrovascular injury are associated with the severest casualties from Operation Enduring Freedom (OEF) and Operation Iraqi Freedom (OIF) [8]. From October 1, 2008 the US Army Medical Department TBI program initiated a TCD protocol for examination of head injured patients who were evacuated from the combat theater to receive care at the National Naval Medical Center, the San Antonio Military Medical Center and at the Walter Reed Army Medical Center. The purpose of this retrospective analysis was to evaluate the TCD determined incidence of posttraumatic cerebral VSP and intracranial hypertension after wartime TBI in these patients.

Materials and methods

TCD data were retrospectively analyzed in ninety patients (2 females) aged 18—50 years (mean 25.9 years) who had suffered wartime TBI (with Glasgow Coma Scale scores ranging from 3 to 15). The patients were categorized according to injury: 18 patients with closed head injury (CHI), 19 patients with CHI due to improvised explosive device (CHI/IED), 33 patients with penetrating head injury (PHI) and 20 patients with PHI due to IED (PHI/IED). A total of 567 TCD studies were made after admission. Patients were identified using a computerized registry and a prospective TCD database maintained in the Sentient NeuroCare Services. TCD recordings of mean cerebral blood flow velocities (CBFV in cm/sec) and Pulsatility Indices (PI) of the anterior and posterior circulation vessels were recorded using a 2-MHz transducer (Doppler Box, DWL/Compumedics, USA, Germany, Australia). Comprehensive TCD protocol was applied in all cases [9]: if mean CBFV equaled or exceeded 100 cm/s, 140 cm/s and 200 cm/s the TCD signs of mild VSP, moderate VSP and severe VSP respectively were considered present [10]. Lindegaard ratio was measured when the CBFV exceeded 100 cm/s [11]. On average, patients received 6.4 TCD examinations each (range 1—30). The primary purpose of TCD methodology is to determine the CBFV by quantitative interpretation of Doppler spectrum waveforms. Although the qualitative contour of the TCD waveform during intracranial pressure (ICP) elevation falls into a recognizable pattern, their interpretation depends on the experience and expertise of the TCD examiner/interpreter. Objective, reproducible and verifiable measures of TCD waveform changes are necessary for TCD findings to be used with certainty for evaluation of intracranial hypertension. One method of quantifying these changes is the utilization of the PI [12] which is a reflection of downstream resistance. The PI takes into account the peak systolic CBFV (pCBFV) and the end-diastolic CBFV (edCBFV) and compares changes in these variables against the change in the standard measure of the entire waveform, such as mean CBFV. Changes in arterial pulsatility, especially occurring during intracranial hypertension, will affect both pCBFV and edCBFV, which are easily identified in TCD waveform, and are reflected by the equation PI = pCBFV − edCBFV/mean CBFV. SAS statistical package was used for data analysis (SAS/STAT® 9.3 Software, SAS Institute, Inc., USA). All data was tested for normal distribution using Shapiro Wilk test: non-parametric statistics were used where determined appropriate. All data was described using median and interquartile range (25th and 75th percentiles). Spearman rank correlations of MAP, Hct, ICP, and $PaCO_2$ with measures of the CBFV were calculated. Anterior and posterior CBFV data was compared between groups defined by severity of VSP (mild, moderate, and severe) using Wilcoxon rank sum test for each diagnostic group. General linear models were employed to test between diagnostic group differences, adjusting for severity of VSP. Statistical significance was assumed on the 5% level. Study and analysis of the data was done according to the IRBNet protocol No. 363439-4.

Results

TCD signs of VSP were observed in 57 cases (63.3%): 13 (14.4%) in CHI, 12 (13.3%) in CHI/IED, 21 (23.3%) in PHI and 11 (12.3%) in PHI/IED groups ($p = 0.732$). In PHI patients there were 75%, 35.7% and 14.3% TCD signs of mild, moderate and severe VSP, respectively. In the PHI/IED group there were 36.8%, 5.2% and 5.2% TCD signs of mild, moderate and severe VSP, respectively. In the CHI group there were 68.4%, 31.5% and 15.7% TCD signs of mild, moderate and severe VSP, respectively. Lastly, in the CHI/IED group there were 29%, 23.5% and 17.6% TCD signs of mild, moderate and severe VSP, respectively. TCD evidence of intracranial hypertension was seen in 57.1% PHI patients, in 63% of PHI/IED patients, in 63.1% of CHI patients and in 50% of CHI/IED patients. While there were no overall differences in the presence of VSP, there were statistical significant differences between frequency of degrees of TCD signs of VSP between different TBI groups ($p < 0.001$). Post hoc analysis revealed that PHI and CHI groups had higher frequency of mild VSP compared to both CHI/IED and PHI/IED ($p < 0.05$). The PHI/IED group had higher frequency of moderate VSP compared the CHI, PHI, and CHI/IED groups ($p < 0.05$) (Table 1).

Discussion

These results suggest that abnormal TCD findings are frequent in patients with wartime TBI and indicate posttraumatic VSP and intracranial hypertension in a significant number of patients. Additionally, delayed cerebral arterial spasm is a frequent complication of combat TBI and severity of cerebral VSP is comparable to that seen in aneurysmal SAH. This confirms earlier data that traumatic SAH is associated with a high incidence of cerebral VSP with a higher probability in patients with severe TBI [1,4,5]. Another cause of abnormally high CBFV's could be reactive hyperemia after TBI; however literature suggests that global post-trauma malignant hyperemia is present primarily in acute stage of TBI [13]. Though, more recent data showed that post-TBI focal hyperemia can be present up to 3 weeks [14]. In our study utilization of Lindegaard ratio and qualitative evaluation of Doppler spectrum were helpful to differentiate between hyperemia and VSP. Of interests is the finding that the PHI/IED TBI group had higher frequency of TCD signs of moderate VSP when compared to other TBI

Table 1 Different degree of TCD signs of vasospasm in wartime TBI patients. Numbers represent median CBFV in cm/s (interquartile range, 25th and 75th percentile).

TCD signs of vasospasm	TBI groups			
	PHI	PHI/IED	CHI	CHI/IED
Mild vasospasm				
Anterior circulation	114 (106, 124)	112 (105, 121)	114 (106, 124)	116 (107, 129)
Posterior circulation	66 (63, 71)	(63.5, 71)	68 (63, 74.5)	67 (62, 72)
Moderate vasospasm				
Anterior circulation	159 (149, 172)	162 (148, 181)	154 (146, 173)	150 (146, 164)
Posterior circulation	86 (83.5, 90)	85.5 (83, 89)	9 (85, 97)	87 (85, 92)
Severe vasospasm				
Anterior circulation	220.5 (210, 234)	216 (206, 248)	214 (210, 225)	214 (209, 237)
Posterior circulation	114 (108, 124)	124 (104.5, 161)	115 (107, 132.5)	113 (106.5, 124)

groups. This result emphasizes the point that explosive blast TBI is one of the more serious wounds suffered by United States service members injured in the current conflicts in Iraq and Afghanistan. Observations suggest that the mechanism by which explosive blast injures the central nervous system may be more complex than initially assumed [15].

The purpose of monitoring patients with TBI is to detect treatable and reversible causes of neurological deterioration. There are numerous causes of such deterioration after TBI and frequent neurological examinations, and the availability of urgent neuroimaging and EEG are standards in the management of patients with traumatic SAH. Physiological monitoring modalities include TCD, electroencephalography, brain tissue oxygen monitoring, cerebral microdialysis and near-infrared spectroscopy. TCD has long been used for monitoring patients with SAH, but studies of diagnostic accuracy for detection of vasospasm and cerebral angiography vary widely with regard to sensitivity and specificity of TCD. TCD ability to predict clinical deterioration and infarction from delayed cerebral ischemia is still not yet validated in a prospective trial. In spite of this, TCD examination is non-invasive, inexpensive and the pattern of CBFV's observed in patients after SAH of different etiology is very distinctive, enabling immediate detection of abnormally high CBFV's and appears to be predictive of VSP [16,17].

Recent evidence suggests TCD holds promise for the detection of critical elevations of ICP and decreases in cerebral perfusion pressure (CPP). Using the PI, Bellner et al. [12] have demonstrated that ICP of 20 mm Hg can be determined with a sensitivity of 0.89 and specificity of 0.92. They concluded that the PI may provide guidance in those patients with suspected intracranial hypertension and that repeated measurements may be of use in the neurocritical care unit. There is significant evidence that independent of the type of intracranial pathology, a strong correlation between PI and ICP exists [12,18—20]. A recent study indicated that TCD had 94% of sensitivity to identify high ICP/low CPP at admission and a negative predictive value of 95% to identify normal ICP at admission; the sensitivity to predict abnormal cerebral perfusion pressure was 80% [20]. In 2011 Bouzat and co-authors showed that in patients with mild to moderate TBI, the TCD test on admission, together with brain CT scan, could accurately screen patients at risk for secondary neurological damage [21]. At the same time, to the best of our knowledge, no one as yet has suggested using the PI as an accurate method to quantitatively assess ICP. Nevertheless, even at this juncture, quantitative and qualitative changes in CBFV values and TCD waveform morphologies may persuade physicians to undertake other diagnostic steps and/or change medical treatment that will improve care of these patients and their outcomes. At the moment TCD appears to be useful for following PI's trends and it is a practical ancillary technique for estimating the direction of CBFV changes in response to increasing ICP or falling CPP, and it may also reveal whether there is a response to therapeutic interventions. Though, further sophistication of TCD data analysis is essential before it may be used with confidence to measure ICP and CPP in the ICU. This study has some limitations. First, we were not able to correlate clinical VSP with angiographic VSP and combine TCD data with other neuroimaging methods which help to identify VSP and impaired CPP in patients with traumatic SAH. Secondary, current data should be validated prospectively. Additionally, the lack of established TCD criteria for VSP in younger patients presents interpretative issues. The high sensitivity of TCD to identify abnormally high CBFV's and PI's due to the onset on of VSP and intracranial hypertension, respectively, demonstrates that TCD is an excellent first-line examination to determine those patients who may need urgent aggressive treatment and continuous invasive ICP monitoring. Because VSP and intracranial hypertension represent significant events in a high proportion of patients after wartime TBI, daily TCD monitoring is recommended for the management of such patients.

Acknowledgements

This paper was supported in part by the US Army Medical Research and Material Command's Telemedicine and Advanced Technology Research Center (Fort Detrick, MD, USA). In addition, we would like to express our gratitude to Richard L. Skolasky, Jr., Sc.D., Assistant Professor, Director of the Spine Outcomes Research Center at the Johns Hopkins University for his statistical assistance and guidance (Baltimore, MD, USA). Also we need to thank neurosonographers Dr. A. Dzhanashvili, M.D., RVS and Mirkko Galdo who have been responsible for data collection.

References

[1] Diringer MN, Axelrod Y. Hemodynamic manipulation in the neuro-intensive care unit: cerebral perfusion pressure therapy in head injury and hemodynamic augmentation for cerebral vasospasm. Curr Opin Crit Care 2007;13:156—62.

[2] Dorsch N. A clinical review of cerebral vasospasm and delayed ischaemia following aneurysm rupture. Acta Neurochir Suppl 2011;110(Pt 1):5—6.

[3] Kassell NF, Peerless SJ, Durward QJ, Beck DW, Drake CG, Adams HP. Treatment of ischemic deficits from vasospasm with intravascular volume expansion and induced arterial hypertension. Neurosurgery 1982;11:337—43.

[4] Oertel M, Boscardin WJ, Obrist WD, Glenn TC, McArthur DL, Gravori T, et al. Posttraumatic vasospasm: the epidemiology, severity, and time course of an underestimated phenomenon: a prospective study performed in 299 patients. J Neurosurg 2005;103:812—24.

[5] Armonda RA, Bell R, Vo A, Ling G, DeGraba T, Ecklund J, et al. Wartime traumatic cerebral vasospasm: recent review of combat casualties. Neurosurgery 2006;59:1215—25.

[6] Cloft HJ, Joseph GJ, Dion JE. Risk of cerebral angiography in patients with subarachnoid hemorrhage, cerebral aneurysm, and arteriovenous malformation: a meta-analysis. Stroke 1999;30:317—20.

[7] Washington CW, Zipfel GJ. The participants in the international multi-disciplinary consensus conference on the critical care management of subarachnoid hemorrhage. Detection and monitoring of vasospasm and delayed cerebral ischemia: a review and assessment of the literature. Neurocrit Care 2011;15:312—7.

[8] Bell RS, Ecker RD, Severson III MA, Wanebo JE, Crandall B, Armonda RA. The evolution of the treatment of traumatic cerebrovascular injury during wartime. A review. Neurosurg Focus 2010;28(5):E5.

[9] Alexandrov AV, Sloan MA, Wong LKS, Douville C, Razumovsky AY, Koroshetz W, Tegeler CH, et al. For the American society of neuroimaging practice guidelines committee. Practice standards for Transcranial Doppler (TCD) Ultrasound. Part I. Test performance. J Neuroimaging 2007;17:11—8.

[10] Wozniak MA, Sloan MA, Rothman MI, Burch CM, Rigamonti D, Permutt T, et al. Detection of vasospasm by transcranial Doppler sonography. The challenges of the anterior and posterior cerebral arteries. J Neuroimaging 1996;6:87—93.

[11] Lindegaard KF, Nornes H, Bakke SJ, Sorteberg W, Nakstad P. Cerebral vasospasm after subarachnoid haemorrhage investigated by means of transcranial Doppler ultrasound. Acta Neurochir Suppl 1988;42:81—4.

[12] Bellner J, Romner B, Reinstrup P, Kristiansson KA, Ryding E, Brandt L. Transcranial Doppler sonography pulsatility index (PI) reflects intracranial pressure (ICP). Surg Neurol 2004;62:45—51.

[13] Obrist WD, Langfitt TW, Jaqqi JL, Cruz J, Gennarelli T. Cerebral blood flow and metabolism in comatose patients with acute head injury. Relationship to intracranial hypertension. J Neurosurg 1984;61:241—53.

[14] Bullock PM, Patterson J, Hadley P, Wiper DJ, Teasdale GM. Focal cerebral hyperemia after focal head injury: a benign phenomenon? J Neurosurg 1996;83:277—84.

[15] Ling G, Bandak F, Armonda R, Grant G, Ecklund J. Explosive blast neurotrauma. J Neurotrauma 2009;26:815—25.

[16] Diringer MN, Bleck TP, Hemphill III JC, Menon D, Shutter L, Vespa P, et al. Critical care management of patients following aneurysmal subarachnoid hemorrhage: recommendations from the neurocritical care society's multidisciplinary consensus conference. Neurocrit Care 2011;15:211—40.

[17] Kincaid MS, Souter MJ, Treggiari MM, David Yanez N, Anne Moore ND, Lam AAM. Accuracy of transcranial Doppler ultrasonography and single-photon emission computed tomography in the diagnosis of angiographically demonstrated cerebral vasospasm. J Neurosurg 2009;110:67—72.

[18] Bor-Seng-Shu E, Hirsch R, Teixeira MJ, De Andrade AF, Marino Jr R. Cerebral hemodynamic changes gauged by transcranial Doppler ultrasonography in patients with posttraumatic brain swelling treated by surgical decompression. J Neurosurg 2006;104:93—100.

[19] Gura M, Elmaci I, Sari R, Coskun N. Correlation of pulsatility index with intracranial pressure in traumatic brain injury. Turk Neurosurg 2011;21:210—5.

[20] Melo JR, Di Rocco F, Blanot S, Cuttaree H, Sainte-Rose C, Oliveira-Filho J, et al. Transcranial Doppler can predict intracranial hypertension in children with severe traumatic brain injuries. Childs Nerv Syst 2011;27:979—84.

[21] Bouzat P, Francony G, Declety P, Genty C, Kaddour A, Bessou P, et al. Transcranial Doppler to screen on admission patients with mild to moderate traumatic brain injury. Neurosurgery 2011;68:1603—9.

Role of TCD in sickle cell disease: A review

Viviane Flumignan Zétola

Hospital de Clínicas, Rua General Carneiro 181, Serviço de Neurologia, 80060-150 Curitiba, Brazil

KEYWORDS
Transcranial Doppler;
Stroke;
Sickle cell disease;
Brasilian Guideline

Summary Stroke is an important complication of sickle cell disease. Approximately twenty-four percent of patients have a stroke by the age of 45. Blood transfusions decrease stroke risk in patients deemed at high risk by transcranial Doppler (TCD) by evidence of elevated intracranial internal carotid or middle cerebral artery velocity. This review describes the practical procedure of patient evaluation and illustrates, through Brazilian guidelines, the importance of uniform methodology in a setting with high prevalence of this disease.
© 2012 Elsevier GmbH. All rights reserved.

Sickle cell disease (SCD) is a genetic disorder caused by homozygosity for a single β-globin gene mutation (β6GAG → GTG), in which glutamic acid has been substituted for valine at the sixth codon of the β-globin chain. Although the incidence of strokes is higher in patients with the Hb SS and Hb S/ß0 thalassemia genotype, it should be noted that strokes also occur in patients with other genotypes. The clinical course of patients suffering from SCD is extremely variable and the severity of manifestations ranging from asymptomatic to a very severe course [1]. SCD is characterized by chronic hemolytic anemia and intermittent vaso-occlusive events. These events result in tissue ischemia, which leads to acute and chronic pain as well as damage to any organ in the body. Acute complications include ischemic and hemorrhagic stroke, acute chest syndrome, painful vaso-occlusive crises, splenic sequestration, aplastic crises, and bacterial sepsis due to hyposplenia. Chronic morbidities include cerebrovascular disease, pulmonary hypertension, osteonecrosis, nephropathy and organ failure [2]. The vaso-occlusive process in SCD is of a complex nature mediated by red cell and leukocyte adhesion, inflammation, oxidative stress, and a hypercoagulable state, all resulting in endothelial injury and dysfunction [3]. In addition, by reducing the nitric oxide bioavailability and by damaging the endothelium through catalyzation of oxidative reactions in endothelial cells, chronic hemolysis leads to vascular complications [4–6]. Although stroke can occur at any age, the most vulnerable group for ischemic stroke is between the age of 2 and 20 years (0.30–0.75 acute events/100 patients/year) [7]. Stenotic lesions involve primarily large vessels in the intracranial internal carotid, middle, and anterior cerebral circulation and can progress for months and even years before symptoms develop [8,9]. There is also evidence that sickle cell anemia (SCA) and other chronic hemolytic anemia are characterized by a hypercoagulable state with an increased generation of thrombin and fibrin as well as platelet activation thus increasing the risk for thromboembolic complications [10].

Transfusion therapy has been shown to prevent the development of stroke, but unfortunately this procedure has important side effects such as iron overload and alloimmunization. Identifying these patients at high risk is crucial in the selection of patients that would most benefit from this intervention. Based on two large studies [11,12] we can now detect patients developing cerebral vasculopathy using transcranial Doppler ultrasonography (TCD). Adams et al. first showed the effectiveness of nonimaging Doppler in screening for cerebrovascular disease in SCD. Using the transtemporal and suboccipital approach, they screened 190 asymptomatic sickle cell patients and found in the clinical follow-up that a time-averaged mean of the maximum velocity

E-mail address: viviane.zetola@gmail.com

Table 1 Recommendations for the frequency of TCD according to the result of the examination.

Result of TCD	CBFV (cm/s)	Frequency of exam
Absence of window	—	Use other image resource to analyze the cerebrovascular event
Technical difficulty due to lack of cooperation	—	Repeat every three months. We recommend evaluation by another examiner
Low CBFV	70	Repeat after 1 month
Normal CBFV	<170	Repeat annually
Low conditional*	Between 170 and 184	Repeat at three-month intervals. In the case of normal subsequent results, we should adopt the normal conduct for the group
High conditional*	Between 185 and 199	Repeat after 1 month. In cases of unchanged examinations, it is recommended to repeat every three months. In cases of two consecutive abnormal results, it is recommended to discuss the risk of strokes and consider a chronic transfusion regimen
Abnormal	Between 200 and 219	Repeat after 1 month. If the value remains ≥200, it is recommended to discuss the risk of strokes and consider chronic transfusion regimen. If the result decreases to 170—199, it is recommended to repeat it one month if high conditional (between 185 and 199); or 6 months if conditional low (between 170 and 184). If the result is normalized (<170), it is recommended to repeat in 1 year
	More than 220	Discuss imminent risk of strokes and consider chronic transfusion regime

TCD = transcranial Doppler and CBFV = cerebral blood flow velocity.
* TCD denotes transcranial Doppler and CBFV cerebral blood flow velocity.

(TAMMX) in the middle cerebral artery (MCA) > 170 cm/s was an indicator of a patient at risk for development of stroke [13]. They then compared TCD to cerebral angiography in 33 neurologically symptomatic patients and identified five criteria for cerebrovascular disease:

1. TAMMX of 190 cm/s
2. Low velocity in the MCA <70 cm/s
3. Right/Left MCA ratio <0.5
4. Anterior cerebral artery (ACA)/MCA ratio >1.2 on the same side
5. Inability to detect an MCA in the presence of a demonstrated ultrasound window

A follow-up of neurologically symptomatic and asymptomatic sickle cell patients presented other factors that were significant in the identification of patients at risk: Velocity in the ophthalmic artery > velocity of the ipsilateral MCA, maximum velocity in the posterior cerebral (PCA), vertebral, or basilar arteries > maximum velocity in the MCA, turbulence, PCA visualized without the MCA [13].

The STOP (Stroke Prevention Trial in Sickle Cell Anemia) study confirmed that TCD could reliably identify those at the highest risk for stroke [12]. STOP screened more than 2000 sickle cell children using the nonimaging TCD technique for signs of cerebrovascular disease. TCD results were classified to indicate degree of risk for stroke as normal, conditional, abnormal, or inadequate. In this series, Adams demonstrated that children with TAMMX of >200 cm/s in the distal internal carotid artery or proximal MCA had a stroke risk that was 10—20 times that of the general sickle cell population of the same age. Children with a TAMMX of the MCA >200 cm/s on two separate readings were randomly assigned to two groups. Sixty-seven children received standard supportive care with symptomatic treatment. Sixty-three children received periodic blood transfusions to maintain hemoglobin S levels at 30% or less. After 1 year, ten children in the standard care group had a stroke, while only one child in the transfusion group had a stroke. This presents a 90% relative decline in stroke rate. We must emphasize that the STOP velocity criteria apply only to children with SCD who have not had a stroke. Those with abnormal velocity should undergo repeated screening within the next few weeks and if the second study is also abnormal should be offered transfusion therapy. Those with conditional velocity should be rescreened within 3—6 months, while those with normal studies can be rescreened yearly [15]. Based on these studies and considering that SCD is the most common monogenic hereditary disease in Brazil, occurring predominantly among African descendents, we have decided to publish Brazilian guidelines for transcranial Doppler in children and adolescents with sickle cell disease with the intent to expand health policy and to contribute in reducing morbidity and mortality resulting from this pathology in our setting [16] (Table 1).

For this review we will consider only the nonimaging pulsed Doppler TCD technique used in the STOP trial [12]. We do not currently recommend that centers use an imaging TCD. The use of different machines and different US techniques could result in velocities of up to 10% lower than STOP velocities and the angle correction could result in velocities higher than those obtained using the STOP protocol. At present, there is no consensus regarding the actual velocity that should be considered as a cutoff value for TCD imaging.

The most important methodology: vessels should be examined carefully by obtaining sample volumes throughout the MCA at intervals of 2 mm while gain settings should be optimized to measure the peak-systolic velocity. The angle of insonation is assumed to be 0°. The examination should include manual measurement of the velocity to confirm the findings. Blood flow velocities from the major cerebral arteries are measured through transtemporal and transforaminal windows with the use of a 2-MHz probe. The mean time-averaged maximum velocity (TAMMX) of the terminal portion of the internal carotid artery (ICA), M1 segment of the middle cerebral artery (MCA), A1 of the anterior cerebral artery (ACA), P1 or P2 of the posterior cerebral artery (PCA), V4 segments of the vertebral arteries bilaterally, and basilar artery (BA) were measured in the STOP study for at least 3 complete cardiac cycles. Wave spectral information was not used and the submandibular and transorbital windows were not evaluated. It should be noted that very low speeds (<70 cm/s) may be indicative of severe stenosis. Although a complete exam is recommended when possible, currently, the terminal ICA and proximal MCA are the most essential elements for analysis. All TCD studies should be classified based on the highest time-averaged mean blood flow velocity in the ICA or MCA based on STOP criteria [12]. The cutoff values and considerations about the re-examination are shown in Table 1 [16].

The procedure, as well as the need to remain awake and cooperative during the examination, should be explained to the patient. Some centers allow children to watch a movie during the examination. When the patient becomes sleepy, the CO_2 levels increase which elevates the mean flow velocity and could give a false-positive result. Hypoxia, fever, hypoglycemia and worsening anemia can also increase cerebral blood flow and flow velocity. Thus, if a child has sickle chest syndrome, sequestration, and hemolytic crisis, TCD velocity will appear higher than the true baseline. Although it is tempting to perform TCD examinations while a patient is in the hospital for a medical illness, the results may not be valid if velocities drop to an abnormal or conditional range. These results, therefore, should not be used to determine stroke risk, and repeated examinations should be performed when the patient is stable. It is essential to use educational intervention to target parents and caregivers as well as children about the importance of conducting systematic TCD examinations.

The use of criteria other than ICA/MCA was analyzed in some studies; however, there is no consensus that allows us to recommend chronic transfusion. Nevertheless, we suggest attentiveness to changes in other arteries and a thorough understanding of "individual risk" thereby reducing the need for numerous exam repetitions. Children with abnormal ICA/MCA velocities and elevated anterior cerebral artery (ACA) velocities presented a risk of stroke more than twice that of those with abnormal ICA/MCA but normal ACA velocity [19]. There are similar findings with the basilar artery, vertebral, PCA and OA when compared with the ICA/MCA, however, the recommendations must be more uniform.

Although in the majority of cases, velocities could go back to a normal range (MCA TAMMX < 170 cm/s) after a period of 30 months or longer, discontinuation can result in a high rate of reversion to abnormal blood-flow velocities on the TCD or even in stroke. The STOP II study concluded that we must maintain chronic transfusion indefinitely [17,18]. Other treatment regimens are now being tested [20].

TCD screening rates in children with SCD have increased after the publication of the STOP trial, and medical providers may be targeting those children at the highest stroke risk. Prospective follow-up of a larger sample will be required to assess the impact of this screening on stroke rates. TCD screening itself only stratifies stroke risk, but does not prevent stroke; stroke prevention depends on the implementation of chronic transfusion therapy. However, access to vascular laboratories appears to be a barrier to the implementation of this highly effective stroke prevention strategy, even among children with comprehensive health insurance. The main problems are difficulties in performing the examination, differences in imaging and nonimaging techniques, and interpretation of guidelines.

The identification of sickle cell vasculopathy by MRI, MRA, and MR diffusion imaging has increased our understanding of sickle cell lesions. Silent infarction incidence could be as high as 17% and carries a risk of future infarctions as well [21]. The etiology of silent infarctions, however, remains unresolved, and the implications for preventive therapy continue to be studied. At present, we should attempt to increase the availability of TCD screening by physician training and TCD machine access in the locations of disease prevalence. We have employed a task force in Brazil through publication of guidelines and establishment of medical services training in order to improve the performance of TCD [16].

References

[1] Platt OS, Brambilla DJ, Rosse WF, Milner PF, Castro O, Steinberg MH, et al. Mortality in sickle cell disease. Life expectancy and risk factors for early death. New England Journal of Medicine 1994;330(23):1639—44.
[2] Lottenberg R, Hassel KL. An evidence based approach to the treatment of adults with sickle cell disease. Hematology American Society of Hematology, Educational Programme 2005:58—65.
[3] Frenette PS. Sickle cell vaso-occlusion: multistep and multicellular paradigm. Current Opinion in Hematology 2002;9(2):101—6.
[4] Reiter CD, Wang X, Tanus-Santos JE, Hogg N, Cannon RO, Schechter AN, et al. Cellfree hemoglobin limits nitric oxide bioavailability in sickle-cell disease. Nature Medicine 2002;8(12):1383—9.
[5] Morris CR, Kato GJ, Poljakovic M, Wang X, Blackwelder WC, Sachdev V, et al. Dysregulated arginine metabolism, hemolysis-associated pulmonary hypertension, and mortality in sickle cell disease. JAMA 2005;294(1):81—90.
[6] Jeney V, Balla J, Yachie A, Varga Z, Vercellotti GM, Eaton JW, et al. Pro-oxidant and cytotoxic effects of circulating heme. Blood 2002;100(3):879—87.
[7] Ohene-Frempong K, Weiner SJ, Sleeper LA, Miller ST, Embury S, Moohr JW, et al. Cerebrovascular accidents in sickle cell disease: rates and risk factors. Blood 1998;91(1):288—94.
[8] Steinberg MH, Adewoye AH. Modifier genes and sickle cell anemia. Current Opinion in Hematology 2006;13:131—6.
[9] Adams GT, Snieder H, McKie VC, Clair B, Brambilla D, Adams RJ, et al. Genetic risk factors for cerebrovascular disease in children with sickle cell disease: design of a case—control

association study and genome wide screen. BMC Medical Genetics 2003;4:6.
[10] Ataga KI, Orringer EP. Hypercoagulability in sickle cell disease: a curious paradox. American Journal of Medicine 2003;115:721—8.
[11] Adams R, McKie V, Nichols F, Carl E, Zhang DL, McKie K, et al. The use of transcranial ultrasonography to predict stroke in sickle cell disease. New England Journal of Medicine 1992;326:605—10.
[12] Adams RJ, McKie VC, Hsu L, Files B, Vichinsky E, Pegelow C, et al. Prevention of a first stroke by transfusions in children with sickle cell anemia and abnormal results on transcranial Doppler ultrasonography. New England Journal of Medicine 1998;339:5—11.
[13] Adams RJ, McKie VC, Carl EM, Nichols FT, Perry R, Brock K, et al. Long-term stroke risk in children with sickle cell disease screened with transcranial Doppler. Annals of Neurology 1997;42(5):699—704.
[15] Nichols FT, Jones AM, Adams RJ. Stroke prevention in sickle cell disease (STOP) study guidelines for transcranial Doppler testing. Journal of Neuroimaging 2001;11: 354—63.
[16] Brazilian guidelines for transcranial Doppler in children and adolescents with sickle cell disease. Revista Brasileira de Hematologia e Hemoterapia 2011;33(1).
[17] Adams RJ, Brambilla DJ, Granger S, Gallagher D, Vichinsky E, Abboud MR, et al. Stroke and conversion to high risk in children screened with transcranial Doppler ultrasound during the STOP study. Blood 2004;103(10):3689—94.
[18] Adams RJ, Brambilla D. Discontinuing prophylactic transfusions used to prevent stroke in sickle cell disease. New England Journal of Medicine 2005;353:2769—78.
[19] Kwiatkowski JL, Granger S, Brambilla DJ, Brown RC, Miller ST, Adams RJ. British Journal of Haematology 2006;134: 333—9.
[20] Aliyu ZY, Tumblin AR, Kato GJ. Current therapy of sickle cell disease. Haematologica 2006;91(1):7—10.
[21] Arkuszewski M, Melhem ER, Krejza J. Neuroimaging in assessment of risk of stroke in children with sickle cell disease. Advances in Medical Sciences 2010;55(2):115—29.

Transcranial Doppler sonography in children with sickle cell disease and silent ischemic lesions

Filippo Maria Farina [a,*], Patrizia Rampazzo [a], Laura Sainati [b], Renzo Manara [c], Angelo Onofri [a], Raffaella Colombatti [b], Claudio Baracchini [a], Giorgio Meneghetti [a]

[a] Department of Neuroscience, University of Padua, Padua, Italy
[b] Department of Pediatrics, University of Padua, Padua, Italy
[c] Institute of Neuroradiology, University of Padua, Padua, Italy

KEYWORDS
Sickle cell disease;
Transcranial Doppler sonography;
Silent strokes

Summary

Background: Sickle cell disease (SCD) is considered the most frequent cause of stroke in childhood. According to the STOP (stroke prevention trial in sickle cell anemia study) criteria, patients with abnormal values (>200 cm/s) of time-averaged mean velocities of maximum blood flow (TAMM), detected by transcranial Doppler sonography (TCD), should undergo blood transfusion in order to reduce the risk of ischemic stroke. However, patients with normal TAMM might harbor silent strokes on magnetic resonance imaging (MRI) scan. Our aim was to verify whether SCD patients with normal velocities but with a significant side-to-side asymmetry of TAMM are more prone to develop silent strokes.

Subjects and methods: Thirty-one consecutive SCD patients, (15 females; mean age: 9.23 ± 3.66 years), categorized as "normal" according to the STOP protocol (<170 cm/s) and without a history of blood transfusions and TIA/stroke, underwent a cerebral MRI scan and complete TCD evaluation in order to detect significant asymmetries in the main intracranial arteries. Then, we subdivided this cohort into two groups according to the detection of TAMM asymmetry: "normal and symmetric" (NS), "normal and asymmetric" (NA).

Results: We found 13/31 patients (41.9%) harboring a significant TAMM asymmetry (NA group), while brain MRI detected silent ischemic lesions in 13/31 (41.9%) patients. No significant differences were found between NA and NS regarding silent strokes frequencies (Chi-square test with continuity correction, $\chi^2 = 0.598$), lesion number (*t*-student test, $p = 0.09$) and lesion burden (*t*-student test, $p = 0.227$).

Conclusion: According to our study, TAMM asymmetry is not a significant predictor of silent cerebral ischemia.
© 2012 Elsevier GmbH. All rights reserved.

Introduction

Sickle cell disease (SCD), is a hematologic disorder caused by an autosomic recessive inherited mutation in the hemoglobin genes (HbS), is considered the most frequent hemoglobinopathy in the world, with a peak incidence in

* Corresponding author at: Via N.Giustiniani 5, 35128 Padua (PD), Italy, Department of Neuroscience, University of Padua School of Medicine. Tel.: +39 0498213600; fax: +39 0498214366.
  E-mail address: farippo@gmail.com (F.M. Farina).

Table 1 Baseline characteristics and MRI findings of SCD patients.

	NA (13)	NS (18)	Total (31)	p values[a]
Age (mean ± SD)	8.80 ± 2.59	10.62 ± 4.15	9.23 ± 3.66	ns
Sex (males/females)	6/7	10/8	16/15	ns
Patients with ischemic lesions (%)	6 (46.2%)	7 (38.9%)	13 (41.9%)	ns
Number of lesions (mean ± SD)	3 ± 1.55	7.85 ± 6.41	5.61 ± 4.28	ns
Range of number of lesions	1—20	2—10	2—20	—
Dimension of lesions (mean ± SD)	8.62 ± 6.16	6.33 ± 4.71	7.56 ± 5.44	ns
Lesion burden (mean ± SD)	631 ± 275	289 ± 118	473 ± 344	ns

MRI = magnetic resonance imaging, SCD = sickle cell disease, NA = SCD patients with "normal and asymmetric" TAMM values, NS = SCD patients with "normal and symmetric" TAMM values, SD = standard deviation, NS = Not Significant.
[a] Tests the probability of a difference between NA and NS using the t-student test for continuous variable and chi-square test for frequencies.

the African population. SCD is reported as the first cause of stroke in childhood; children with homozygous HbS genes have a yearly first stroke risk of approximately 0.5% [1].

According to the STOP study (stroke prevention trial in sickle cell anemia) [2], the stroke risk in these patients could be predicted by TAMM (time-averaged mean of maximum blood flow) velocities detected by transcranial Doppler sonography (TCD) in the major intracranial arteries. Patients are categorized as "normal" if TAMM is <170 cm/s, "conditional" if TAMM is between 170 and 200 cm/s, "abnormal" if TAMM is >200 cm/s. Children with "abnormal" values are at the highest risk of stroke and are advised to undergo blood transfusion, in order to reduce that risk.

However, there are many reports of SCD patients with "normal" TAMM velocities harboring silent strokes at MRI; the prevalence of these lesions is higher than in the normal population [3,4]. For this reason, we conducted a study to investigate whether the detection of a significant side-to-side asymmetry in patients with normal TAMM values could identify those subjects, which are more prone to develop silent strokes.

Subjects and methods

We enrolled in this study thirty-one SCD patients (15 females; mean age: 9.23 ± 3.66 years; age range: 4—14 years), previously categorized as "normal" according to the STOP protocol, which never received blood transfusions, and did not have a clinical history of TIA/stroke.

A complete TCD examination was performed by an experienced neurosonographer, in a quiet atmosphere and without pharmacological sedation, using a 2 MHz pulsed-wave Doppler probe (Viasys Healthcare, Model Sonara) to explore the major intracranial arteries through the temporal bone-window: TAMM velocity was recorded bilaterally in the middle cerebral artery, anterior cerebral artery and posterior cerebral artery and stored on a database. Offline side-to-side comparison of TAMM values allowed detecting a significant asymmetry, as defined by Zanette et al. [5].

All patients also underwent brain magnetic resonance imaging (MRI) by means of a 1.5 T MR scanner (Achieva, Philips, Best, the Netherlands). The study protocol included axial fluid attenuated inversion recovery (FLAIR) sequence (repetition time 11,000 ms; echo time 140 ms; inversion time: 2800; echo train length 53; flip angle 90°; field of view 230 mm; matrix 256 × 256; slice thickness 5 mm; interslice gap 0.5 mm; number of averages 2) to disclose ischemic lesions. Lesion area was manually traced on all images by a neuroradiogist with experience in pediatric neuroradiology on a dedicated console and software (Medstation). Lesion burden was calculated according to the following formula: total lesion area × (slice thickness + interslice gap).

We categorized our cohort of patients into two groups according to the detection of TAMM asymmetry: "normal and symmetric" (NS), "normal and asymmetric" (NA).

Results

A significant TAMM asymmetry (NA Group) was observed in 13/31 patients (41.9%). Silent ischemic lesions were detected in 6/13 (46.2%) NA and 7/18 (38.9%) NS patients. No significant difference was found in silent stroke rate (Chi square test with continuity correction, $\chi^2 = 0.598$), lesion number (t-student test, $p = 0.09$) and lesion burden (t-student test, $p = 0.22$) between the two groups (Table 1).

Discussion

According to this study, TAMM asymmetry does not seem to be a significant predictor of silent cerebral ischemia as evaluated by brain MRI; in particular, it does not have a prognostic value in terms of silent stroke rate, lesion number and lesion burden.

Furthermore, this study confirms the high prevalence of brain ischemic lesions (>40%) in so-called "normals" and underlines the importance of stroke prevention even when TCD findings are within a normal range.

The lack of association between TAMM asymmetry detected by TCD and MRI findings might be related to the pathogenesis of ischemic stroke in sickle cell disease. Even though an increase in TAMM velocities has been proven to be a predictor of ischemic stroke, the site of brain ischemia does not correlate with the vessel in which blood flow velocity was found to be increased. This finding suggests that factors other than major cerebral artery stenosis concur to determine brain ischemia [6]. In fact, rheological or hemodynamic impairment might undermine parenchymal lesions. A recent study pointed out that SCD patients have an impaired cerebral blood flow autoregulation compared with age-matched healthy subjects, independently from their hemolysis rate [7]. Furthermore, small vessels disease might play a role in the stroke pathogenesis of these children.

Side-to-side asymmetry of blood flow velocity is a common finding during TCD examination of the major arteries, both in adult than in children, but it is considered pathological whenever velocity values lie outside a standard range [8]. Nevertheless, a recent study indicated that SCD patients have a slightly wider physiological range of blood flow velocity values than normal children [9]. Furthermore, since SCD patients harbor a widespread tortuosity of intracranial vessels [3,4], a significant TAMM asymmetry might just represent this anatomical variation and not necessarily a pathological finding.

Finally, we have also to consider some of the limits related to the TCD equipment: different location of the sample volume and/or angle of insonation when recording from each side; in fact, in children the temporal acoustic window is larger than in adults, allowing the operator to insonate the artery from different angles with potential measurement errors [9].

In conclusion, TAMM asymmetry does not seem to be useful in predicting silent cerebral ischemia in patients with SCD. Moreover, the presence of silent strokes in over 40% of ''TCD normal'' children suggests the urgent need to find a reliable predictor to detect those among them who are at risk for silent stroke.

References

[1] Ohene-Frempong K, Weiner SJ, Sleeper LA, Miller ST, Embury S, Moohr JW, et al. Cerebrovascular accidents in sickle cell disease: rates and risk factors. Blood 1998;91(1):288–94.

[2] Adams RJ, McKie VC, Hsu L, Files B, Vichinsky E, Pegelow C, et al. Prevention of a first stroke by transfusions in children with sickle cell anemia and abnormal results on transcranial Doppler ultrasonography. N Engl J Med 1998;339:5–11.

[3] Moser FG, Miller ST, Bello JA, Pegelow CH, Zimmerman RA, Wang WC, et al. The spectrum of brain MR abnormalities in sickle cell disease: a report from the Co-operative study of sickle cell disease. AJNR Am J Neuroradiol 1996;17:965–72.

[4] Steen RG, Emudianughe T, Hankins GM, Wynn LW, Wang WC, Xiong X, et al. Brain imaging findings in pediatric patients with sickle cell disease. Radiology 2003 Jul;228(1):216–25.

[5] Zanette EM, Fieschi C, Bozzao L, Roberti C, Toni D, Argentino C, et al. Comparison of cerebral angiography and transcranial Doppler sonography in acute stroke. Stroke 1989;20:899–903.

[6] Adams RJ. Big strokes in small persons. Arch Neurol 2007 Nov;64(11):1567–74.

[7] Kim YS, Nur E, van Beers EJ, Truijen J, Davis SC, Biemond BJ, et al. Dynamic cerebral autoregulation in homozygous sickle cell disease. Stroke 2009;40:808–14.

[8] Sorteberg W, Langmoen JT, Lindegaard IA, Nornes KF. Side-to-side differences and day-to-day variations of transcranial Doppler parameters in normal subjects. J Ultrasound Med 1990;9(July):403–9.

[9] Arkuszewski M, Krejza J, Chen R, Kwiatkowski JL, Ichord R, Zimmerman R, et al. Sickle cell disease: reference values and interhemispheric differences of nonimaging transcranial Doppler blood flow parameters. AJNR Am J Neuroradiol 2011;32(September):1444–50.

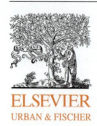
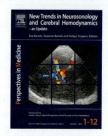

Bartels E, Bartels S, Poppert H (Editors):
New Trends in Neurosonology and Cerebral Hemodynamics — an Update.
Perspectives in Medicine (2012) 1, 272—274

journal homepage: www.elsevier.com/locate/permed

Intellectual impairment and TCD evaluation in children with sickle cell disease and silent stroke

Angelo Onofri [a,*], Maria Montanaro [b], Patrizia Rampazzo [a], Raffaella Colombatti [b], Filippo Maria Farina [a], Renzo Manara [c], Laura Sainati [b], Mario Ermani [a], Claudio Baracchini [a], Giorgio Meneghetti [a]

[a] Department of Neuroscience, University of Padua, Italy
[b] Department of Pediatrics, University of Padua, Italy
[c] Institute of Neuroradiology, University of Padua, Italy

KEYWORDS
Sickle cell disease;
Transcranial Doppler;
Silent strokes;
Cognitive impairment

Abstract

Background: Sickle cell disease (SCD) may impair intellectual activity; 25% of SCD patients have a significant cognitive deficit. Our aim was to verify in a cohort of children with HbSS if the presence of silent strokes or altered Time Averaged Mean velocities of Maximum blood flow (TAMM) detected by Transcranial Color Doppler (TCD) Sonography are indicators of impaired intellectual ability.

Methods: Thirty-five consecutive SCD patients (17 males; mean age: 8.6 ± 3.22) were subdivided into two groups according to neuro-psycological deficits. Cognitive function was assessed by WISC III (for the children aged 6—16 years) and WPPSI (for the children aged 4—6 years). All patients underwent a TCD scan of the main intracranial arteries, in order to detect any increase of TAMM velocities (normal <170 cm/s; altered >170 cm/s) and a cerebral MRI to reveal any silent stokes.

Results: According to the neuro-psycological evaluation, 29/35 (82.8%) patients (Group 1) had a ''normal'' Total Intelligence Quotient (TIQ $\geq$70), while 6/35 (17.2%) patients (Group 2) were defined intellectually impaired (TIQ <69).

TCD detected altered velocities in 8/35 (22.8%) patients. No significant differences were found in the percentage of altered TAMM velocities between the two groups (Fisher's exact test: $p = 0.42$).

MRI detected silent ischemic lesions in 14/35 patients (40.0%). No significant differences were found in silent stroke frequencies (Fisher's exact test: $p = 0.25$) between Group 1 and Group 2.

Conclusion: With the limitations of the study sample, according to our results, altered TAMM values and silent strokes do not seem to be indicators of impaired intellectual ability in SCD patients.

© 2012 Elsevier GmbH. All rights reserved.

* Corresponding author at: Department of Neuroscience, University of Padua School of Medicine, Via N. Giustiniani 5, 35128 Padua, Italy. Tel.: +39 0498213600; fax: +39 0498214366.
   E-mail address: angelo.onofri84@gmail.com (A. Onofri).

2211-968X/$ — see front matter © 2012 Elsevier GmbH. All rights reserved.
doi:10.1016/j.permed.2012.02.006

Introduction

Sickle cell disease (SCD), a hematological disorder caused by an autosomic recessive inherited mutation in the hemoglobin genes (HbS), is considered the most frequent hemoglobinopathy in the world, with a peak incidence in the African population. SCD also represents the first cause of stroke in childhood, with a yearly first stroke risk of approximately 0.5%. [1]

Several studies [2—4] reported neuropsychological deficits in children with SCD; in fact, Schatz et al. observed that 25% of SCD patients had a significant cognitive deficit [5—7]. Are these deficits correlated to ischemic strokes? Adams and colleagues [8—13] demonstrated the importance of Transcranial Doppler (TCD) to prevent ischemic stroke in children with SCD. In the STOP study (Stroke Prevention Trial in Sickle Cell Anemia) they found that the stroke risk in these patients could be predicted by measuring Time Averaged Mean velocities of Maximum blood flow velocities (TAMM) of the major intracranial arteries. In particular, patients were categorized as "normal" if TAMM was <170 cm/s, "conditional" if TAMM was between 170 and 200 cm/s, "abnormal" if TAMM was $\geq$200 cm/s. Children with "abnormal" values are at the highest risk of stroke and are advised to undergo blood transfusion, in order to reduce their stroke risk and their cognitive impairment. However, Watkins et al. [14] and Schatz et al. [15,16] reported intellectual impairment in patients with SCD but without silent strokes compared to healthy controls. Consequently, these authors suggested that besides ischemic silent strokes (ISS), also a persistent low level of hemoglobin saturation could impair the intellectual function. In fact the reduced capacity of transporting O_2 is correlated with an insufficient cerebral perfusion that might cause regions of hypoperfusion and contiguous cerebral areas of compensatory hyperperfusion. TCD could identify this area by detecting increased flow velocity values.

The aim of our study was to verify in a cohort of children with SCD if the presence of silent strokes or altered TAMM detected by TCD are indicators of impaired intellectual ability.

Materials and methods

Thirty-five consecutive SCD patients (17 males, 18 females; mean age: 8.6 ± 3.22) were subdivided into two groups according to the detection of neuropsychological deficits by means of a neuropsychological evaluation: Wechsler Intelligence Scale for Children (WISC III) for the children aged 6—16 years and Wechsler Preschool and Primary Scale of Intelligence (WPPSI III) test for children aged 4—6 years. The subtests were organized into Verbal and Performance scales, and provided scores for Verbal Intelligence Quotients (VIQ) and Performance Intelligence Quotient (PIQ) in order to assess the Total Intelligence Quotient (TIQ). TIQ score $\geq$70 was defined "normal". Moreover we calculated the difference between Verbal and Performance Intelligence Quotient (VIQ-PIQ). A VIP-PIQ score $\geq$ than 8 represents an abnormal development of Verbal ability in comparison to Performance ability and a score $\leq$ than −8 represent an abnormal development of Performance ability in comparison to Verbal ability.

All patients underwent a TCD evaluation of the main intracranial arteries in order to detect any increase of TAMM velocities (normal <170 cm/s, altered $\geq$170 cm/s according to the STOP protocol); TCD was performed by an experienced neurosonographer, in a quiet atmosphere and without pharmacological sedation, using a 2 MHz probe (Viasys Healthcare Sonara).

All patients underwent brain magnetic resonance imaging (MRI) by means of a 1.5 T MR scanner (Achieva, Philips, Best, The Netherlands). The study protocol included axial Fluid Attenuated Inversion Recovery (FLAIR) sequence (repetition time 11,000 ms; echo time 140 ms; inversion time: 2800; echo train length 53; flip angle 90°; field of view 230 mm; matrix 256 × 256; slice thickness 5 mm; interslice gap 0.5 mm; number of averages 2) to disclose ischemic lesions.

Results

Regarding the neuropsychological evaluation, 29/35 (82.8%) patients (Group 1) had a normal ($\geq$70) TIQ, while 6/35 (17.2%) patients (Group 2) were defined intellectually impaired (TIQ <69).

TCD detected altered velocities in 8/35 (22.8%) patients: 6 in Group 1 and 2 in Group 2. No significant differences were found in the percentage of altered TAMM velocities between the two groups (Fisher's exact test: $p = 0.42$).

MRI detected silent ischemic lesions in 14/35 patients (40.0%): 12 in Group 1 and 2 in Group 2. No significant differences were found in silent stroke frequencies (Fisher's exact test: $p = 0.25$) between Group 1 and Group 2.

VIQ-PIQ was normal in 16/35 (45.7%) patients and altered in 19/35 (54.2%) patients. TCD detected altered TAMM in 5 patients with normal VIQ-PIQ and in 3 patients with altered VIQ-PIQ. No significant differences were found in the percentage of altered TAMM velocities between these two groups (Fisher's exact test: $p = 0.28$).

MRI detected silent ischemic lesions in 6 patients with normal VIQ-PIQ and in 8 patients with altered VIQ-PIQ. No significant differences were found in silent stroke frequencies (Fisher's exact test: $p = 0.52$) between these two groups.

Discussion

According to our results, altered TAMM values and silent strokes do not seem to predict cognitive impairment in SCD patients. Our results do not seem to confirm the data found in literature, particularly the association between cognitive impairment and silent strokes [5,6].

The relationship between brain tissue injury and cognitive impairment in SCD is not well understood. In fact the increase of TAMM velocities have been proven to be a strong predictor of ischemic stroke but it can also be considered as a compensatory reaction to chronic hypoxia consequent to the diffuse vasculopathy induced by the low level of hemoglobin saturation. ISS could be seen as a cumulative and additional lesion to a cerebrovascular system already impaired by chronic hypoxia. Moreover a recent study [17] pointed out that children with SCD have an impaired cerebral blood flow autoregulation compared with age-matched healthy subjects, independently from their hemolysis rate. It suggests that children with SCD could have an impaired compensatory reaction to chronic hypoxia (that we consider a possible cause of cognitive impairment) without an increased intracranial blood flow velocities. So also a normal TAMM could be the expression of a pathological situation.

Furthermore we have to consider the particular anatomy of the vessels in these patients [18], with an increase of tortuous course not necessarily related to stroke development. This situation could cause an increase in TAMM velocities without a consequent cognitive impairment.

The higher brain plasticity of children compared to adult could explain why ISS detect by MRI do not correlate significantly with cognitive impairment. As altered TAMM are predictors of a high risk to develop ischemic stroke, it could express an initial damage that could induce a cognitive impairment after years. Only after a long-term follow-up of children with SCD and altered intracranial blood flow velocities a cognitive impairment could become clinically relevant.

This study has several intrinsic limits: the small sample size of the study population and the limits of TCD in children (large temporal acoustic windows with consequent errors in the measurements of intracranial blood flow velocities).

It is necessary to continue the study with a greater number of SCD children and to follow them up in order to assess the positive predictive value to develop cognitive impairment with a non invasive method (TCD) that already demonstrated a high potentiality in children with SCD.

References

[1] Ohene-Frempong K, Weiner SJ, Sleeper LA, Miller ST, Embury S, Moohr JW, et al. Cerebrovascular accidents in sickle cell disease: rates and risk factors. Blood 1998;91(1):288—94.

[2] Wasserman AL, Wilimas JA, Fairclough DL, Mulhern RK, Wang W. Subtle neuropsychological deficits in children with sickle cell disease. Am J Pediatr Hematol Oncol 1991;13:14—20.

[3] Knight S, Singhal A, Thomas P, Serjeant G. Factors associated with lowered intelligence in homozygous sickle cell disease. Arch Dis Child 1995;73:316—20.

[4] Armstrong FD, Thompson Jr RJ, Wang W, Miller S, Zimmerman R, Pegelow CH, et al. Cognitive functioning and brain MRI in children with SCD. Pediatrics 1996;97:864—70.

[5] Schatz J, Brown RT, Pascual JM, Hsu L, DeBaun MR. Poor school and cognitive functioning with silent cerebral infarcts and sickle cell disease. Neurology 2001;56(April (8)):1109—11.

[6] Schatz J, McClellan CB. Sickle cell disease as a neurodevelopmental disorder. Ment Retard Dev Disabil Res Rev 2006;12(3):200—7 [Review].

[7] Schatz J, McClellan CB, Puffer ES, Johnson K, Roberts CW. Neurodevelopmental screening in toddlers and early preschoolers with sickle cell disease. J Child Neurol 2008;23(January (1)):44—50.

[8] Adams RJ, Nichols FT, Figueroa R, McKie V, Lott T. Transcranial Doppler correlation with cerebral angiography in sickle cell disease. Stroke 1992;23:1073—7.

[9] Adams R, McKie V, Nichols F, Carl E, Zhang DI, McKie K, et al. The use of transcranial ultrasonography to predict stroke in sickle cell disease. N Engl J Med 1992;326:605—10.

[10] Adams RJ, McKie VC, Carl EM, Nichols FT, Perry R, Brock K, et al. Long term stroke risk in children with sickle cell disease screened with transcranial Doppler. Ann Neurol 1997;42:699—704.

[11] Adams RJ, Brambilla D, Optimizing Primary Stroke Prevention in Sickle Cell Anemia (STOP 2) Trial Investigators. Discontinuing prophylactic transfusions used to prevent stroke in sickle cell disease. N Engl J Med 2005;353(December (26)):2769—78.

[12] Adams RJ, McKie VC, Hsu L, Files B, Vichinsky E, Pegelow C, et al. Prevention of a first stroke by transfusions in children with sickle cell anemia and abnormal results on transcranial Doppler ultrasonography. N Engl J Med 1998;339:5—11.

[13] Nichols FT, Jones AM, Adams RJ. stroke prevention in sickle cell disease (STOP) study guidelines for transcranial doppler testing. J Neuroimaging 2001;11:354—62.

[14] Watkins KE, Hewes DK, Connelly A, Kendall BE, Kingsley DP, Evans JE, et al. Cognitive deficits associated with frontal-lobe infarction in children with sickle cell disease. Dev Med Child Neurol 1998;40(August (8)):536—43.

[15] Schatz J, Finke RL, Kellett JM, Kramer JH. Cognitive functioning in children with sickle cell disease: a meta-analysis. J Pediatr Psychol 2002;27(December (8)):739—48 [Review].

[16] Schatz J, White DA, Moinuddin A, Armstrong M, DeBaun MR. Lesion burden and cognitive morbidity in children with sickle cell disease. J Child Neurol 2002;17(December (12)):891—5.

[17] Kim Y-S, E Nur E, van Beers EJ, Truijen J, Davis SCAT, Biemond BJ, et al. Dynamic cerebral autoregulation in homozygous Sickle cell disease. Stroke 2009;40:808—14.

[18] Arkuszewski M, Krejza J, Chen R, Kwiatkowski JL, Ichord R, Zimmerman R, et al. Sickle cell disease: reference values and interhemispheric differences of nonimaging transcranial Doppler blood flow parameters. AJNR Am J Neuroradiol 2011;32(September (8)):1444—50.

8. Cerebral Autoregulation and Functional Testing

3. Cerebral Autoregulation and Functional Testing

Cerebral blood flow velocity in sleep

Jürgen Klingelhöfer

Department of Neurology, Medical Center Chemnitz, Dresdner Straße 178, 09131 Chemnitz, Germany

KEYWORDS
Transcranial doppler sonography;
Cerebral electrical activity;
CBF velocity during normal sleep and sleep disorders;
Sleep apnea syndrome

Summary   Sleep is the most conspicuous alteration of cerebral function during the circadian rhythm. It is composed of a cyclic sequence of stages defined on the basis of electrophysiological parameters. The underlying functional activity of the human brain is reflected by sleep correlated changes of cerebral blood flow (CBF), CBF velocity and cerebral metabolism (CM). Transcranial Doppler sonography (TCD) allows to analyze the rapid adaptation processes of cerebral hemodynamics due to TCD capabilities for high temporal resolution and continuous recording during sleep using modern ultrasonic probes with special fixation devices. After the onset of sleep there is a significant progressive reduction of CBF velocity from the waking state to slow wave sleep. The beginning of REM sleep is accompanied by a marked increase in CBF velocity. Furthermore, TCD enables the assessment of perfusion changes in pathological sleep conditions. In sleep apnea syndrome an apnea-associated increase in CBF velocity occurs, which is attributed to apnea-related hypercapnia, whereas a rapid normalization of flow velocity occurs at the end of each apneic episode. TCD is a useful method for long-term and on-line monitoring of dynamic changes in cerebral perfusion during normal sleep and in sleep disorders.
© 2012 Elsevier GmbH. All rights reserved.

Cerebral electrical activity, CBF and CM during normal sleep

The two basic types of sleep are non-rapid eye movement (NREM) and rapid eye movement (REM) sleep. In humans NREM sleep is further subdivided into four stages, each associated with distinct states of altered consciousness [1,2]. When compared with baseline levels during wakefulness, cerebral blood flow (CBF) and cerebral metabolism (CM) decrease with the onset of sleep and during sleep stages I–II and reach minimum values in all brain regions during slow-wave sleep (SWS; sleep stages III and IV) [3–10]. These changes are not uniformly distributed. Against this global fall in CBF are important regional variations with some brain regions (frontal cortex, basal ganglia, thalamus, pons, cerebellum) affected to a greater degree while others (temporal cortex) are relatively affected to a minor degree [7,11]. CBF and CM rise to or even exceed waking levels during rapid eye movement (REM) sleep [3,4,6,11–14]. In a study of regional CBF during REM sleep, Madsen et al. [15] showed that during REM sleep CBF increases in the associative visual area while it decreases in the inferior frontal cortex.

Electroencephalography studies show that there is a hyperfrontal distribution of the electrical activity of the brain during wakefulness [16]. The electroencephalogram (EEG) pattern is closely coupled with the state of conscious awareness. With increasing depth of sleep [17], this regional differentiation is lost and the EEG shows a generalized decrease of frequency. During REM sleep, high mixed frequencies occur [2,18]. A close correlation between the EEG frequency, CBF and CM during human sleep has been reported [7,16,19,20], corroborating the notion of a tight coupling between cerebral electrical activity, CBF and CM [21–25]. The changes in EEG frequency, CBF and CM have been attributed to variations of brain activity during sleep.

E-mail address: juergen_klingelhoefer@gmx.de

Transcranial Doppler sonography (TCD) allows continuous measurement of CBF velocity in the major cerebral arteries and with TCD the rapid adaptation processes of cerebral hemodynamics that occur during sleep may be analyzed with a high temporal resolution [26—29].

Ever since the beginning of clinical sleep research, the results of electroencephalographic recordings of the course of sleep have contradicted the findings of radioisotope tracer studies, which were obtained during a short sampling period for each sleep phase. The radioisotope studies revealed only a static picture of CBF and CM and were unable to demonstrate sleep as a dynamic state of changing cerebral function [3,30—32]. Because of TCD's capabilities for high temporal resolution and continuous recording using modern ultrasonic probes with special fixation devices, the relationship between EEG and cerebral perfusion changes over the course of the entire sleep period can now be recorded.

CBF velocity during normal sleep

In a study by Fischer et al. [33], the flow velocity (FV) in the right middle cerebral artery (MCA) was assessed during evening wakefulness, sleep stages II or IV of non-rapid eye movement (NREM) sleep and the morning waking stage in 5 healthy children (age: 5—13 years) and 6 adults (age: 24—42 years). Polysomnography was performed in all subjects. The MFV decreased during NREM sleep by an average of 21% in the adults and 32% in the children. An MFV increase was observed during awakening but, in both children and adults, the MFV was an average 19% less than during evening wakefulness. No significant change in pCO_2 was observed during sleep. From these findings, the authors concluded that the degree of wakefulness should be taken into account when assessing TCD study findings.

In another study by this group [34], the intracranial hemodynamics of sleep apnea syndrome (SAS) was assessed in 11 healthy adults (age: 37.1 ± 3.2 years), who served as the control group. The study design was the same as in the former study, except that, in this study, MFV measurements were also obtained during REM sleep. In this study, the MFV decreased by an average 17.5% during NREM sleep and a further slight decrease occurred in REM sleep. The MFV measured after awakening the next morning was an average 8.4% lower than the wakefulness value measured on the preceding evening. Changes in the pCO_2 during sleep were also detected in this test group; there was a 10.5% decrease during NREM sleep and a 3.2% decrease during REM sleep. The pCO_2 measured the next morning was 4.8% lower than the pCO_2 of the previous evening. After CO_2 correction of the MFV values [35], these researchers detected a significant MFV decrease during REM sleep and a slight MFV increase during NREM sleep compared with the values observed during evening wakefulness and after awakening the next morning. This group's findings on the MFV dynamics during sleep differ from those of other research groups [36—39].

Droste et al. [36], for example, obtained different results in their study of the MFV development in the MCA during nocturnal sleep in 10 healthy volunteers (age: 25—31 years). The MFV was significantly higher during REM sleep than in the

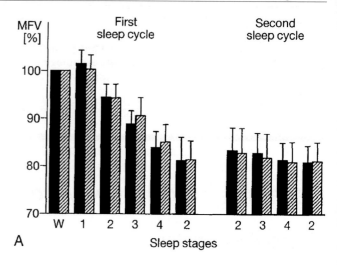

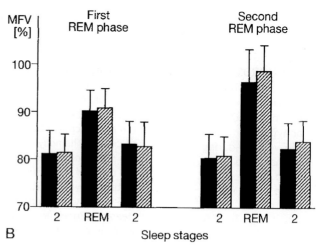

Figure 1 Relative mean flow velocities (related to the evening wakefulness values, W) detected in the middle cerebral artery (MCA). Black bars = left MCA, $n = 16$. Hatched bars = right MCA, $n = 18$. (A) During different NREM sleep stages (1st and 2nd sleep cycle) and (B) during REM sleep, together with sleep stage II prior to and after REM sleep (1st and 2nd sleep cycle). MFV: mean flow velocity (according to [39]).

NREM sleep stages and nocturnal wakeful states. After analyzing the results of their nocturnal TCD recordings using a fast Fourier transformation algorithm, they detected rhythmic fluctuations in the TCD curves, particularly during REM sleep, with wavelengths ranging from 20 to 75 s. Droste's group saw a causal relationship between the rhythmic oscillations and the B-waves of nocturnal intracranial pressure (ICP) fluctuations.

Klingelhöfer et al. [39] measured the MFV in the right ($n = 18$) and left MCA ($n = 16$) as well as heart rate, peripheral arterial blood pressure and pCO_2 in 18 healthy male volunteers (age: 24—34 years) during two nights. Polysomnography, performed in all volunteers, included an EEG, bilateral electrooculogram, electromyogram (submental and anterior tibial muscle), ECG, measurement of nasal and oral airflow during chest and abdominal wall respiratory movements, blood pressure, pulsoximetry and capnometry. The MFV changes and pCO_2 changes during the manually determined sleep stages of the first, second and last sleep cycles were determined with reference to the evening wakefulness values (Fig. 1). For assessment of sleep events (EEG), all sleep spindles, K-complexes with and without sleep spindles, EEG arousals and movement arousals (EEG arousals with an increase in EMG activity) during the last sleep cycle were manually determined from polysomnograms obtained during 12 nights and time-correlated to the corresponding MFV values and vegetative parameters. After a total of 980 EEG events, the reactions of the MFV and autonomic nervous system were assessed.

Long-term analysis in healthy subjects (whole night period)

After the onset of sleep, there> was a significant ($p < 0.001$) progressive reduction of the MFV from the waking state to stage IVa of the first sleep cycle (Figs. 1 and 2). In spite of the subsequent decrease in the depth of sleep, MFV decreased further from stages IVa to IIc preceding the REM period. MFVs in stage IIa of the second and last sleep cycles were significantly ($p < 0.01$) lower than those in stage IIa during the first NREM cycle. A special pattern in the MFV profile was seen during passage through the second and subsequent NREM sleep cycles. MFV values were low during sleep stages IIa and IVa following REM sleep, increased moderately during intermediate sleep stage IIb and decreased again gradually with consecutive sleep stages IIIb, IVb and IIc. The decrease in MFV values was less during the second and last NREM sleep stages than during the first sleep cycle. MFV values in all sleep stages did not differ significantly during the NREM sleep stages in the second and last NREM sleep cycles studied.

The beginning of REM sleep was accompanied by a marked increase in MFV. MFV values markedly exceeded values of the preceding sleep stages II and IV but did not reach waking values in the first, second and last sleep cycle. The MFV during alpha-frequency wakefulness that follows NREM

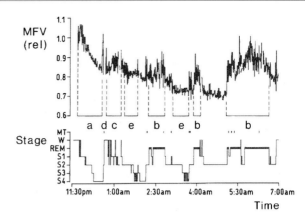

Figure 3 Course of the MFV (relative values) of the right MCA and the corresponding sleep profile in a 26-year-old healthy subject. Lower-case letters characterize (a) progressive MFV reduction; (b) increased MFV during REM sleep; (c) reduced MFV while awakening; (d) movement artifact; and (e) unaltered MFV during changes from stage II to slow-wave sleep (according to [66]).

sleep was lower than waking values preceding sleep onset (Fig. 3). After morning awakening, patients lying awake often required more than half an hour to reach MFV values corresponding to the waking state of the previous evening. MFV profiles were occasionally interrupted by movement artifacts in all healthy subjects (Fig. 3).

Short-term analysis in healthy subjects (dynamics of rapid FV fluctuations)

Rapid fluctuations in FV lasting seconds occurred during SWS as well as stage II and REM sleep. Fig. 4 shows the FV curve with corresponding sleep stages in a typical healthy subject [39]. There were no major fluctuations of FV during stage IV. Moderate fluctuations appeared during sleep stage II. During REM sleep, the amplitude and the duration of fluctuations were markedly increased. Large fluctuations in FV lasting seconds were accompanied by fluctuations

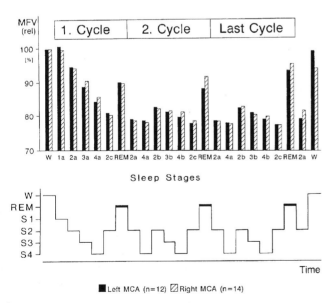

Figure 2 Relative MFV in the right ($n = 14$) and left ($n = 12$) MCA during different sleep stages in healthy male volunteers (according to [38]).

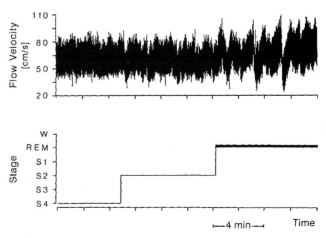

Figure 4 Dynamics of rapid FV fluctuations in the left MCA during the transition from sleep stage IV to REM sleep via stage II in the first sleep cycle in a 25-year-old healthy subject (according to [39]).

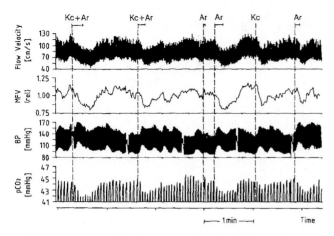

Figure 5 Relationship between FV (right MCA), MFV, blood pressure, end-expiratory CO_2 concentration, and sleep events (Kc, K-complex; Ar, arousal) in sleep stage II in a healthy 27-year-old subject (according to [39]).

in blood pressure. However, the changes in peripheral blood pressure and pulse were not always accompanied by corresponding changes in FV. Fluctuations in FV also occurred following sleep events such as K-complexes and arousal. Immediately after the sleep event there was a moderate increase followed by a pronounced decrease in MFV. During REM sleep, increases in velocity that appeared during phases of rapid eye movements (phasic REM) often persisted for several minutes.

Fig. 5, showing a typical recording of about 6 min duration during sleep stage II, illustrates FV fluctuations that correlated with cardiovascular and respiratory parameters. K-complexes and arousal initiated the observed alterations in FV, MFV, blood pressure and CO_2. Blood pressure increased in the subsequent cardiac cycles, reaching a maximum after about 5 s, then returned to normal during the next 5–15 s. Increases in MFV did not always occur despite rising blood pressure in stage II but were usually found with greater rises of blood pressure in REM sleep. Blood pressure and MFV curves did not follow a parallel course. Hyperventilation with 2–3 mmHg decrease in CO_2 often persisted for more than 30 s during sleep (Fig. 5). A close correlation was found between decreases in MFV and reduction of CO_2.

In their interpretation of these findings, the authors concluded that the reduction in MFV during NREM sleep is a reflection of reduced cerebral activity and that the later increase during REM sleep corresponds to the active brain processes associated with frequent dream phases. The findings in the first sleep cycle are in agreement with the results of CBF measurements and they confirm the close relationship between cerebral perfusion and brain electrical activity, even during human sleep. Continuous measurement over the entire sleep period, as permitted by TCD, demonstrated that, in the later sleep cycles, the course of MFV development is independent of the NREM sleep stages. This finding, together with the finding of delayed MFV increase after morning awakening, may indicate an uncoupling of brain electrical activity from cerebral perfusion in sleep. This suggests that other mechanisms besides locally active mechanisms may also be involved in the regulation of cerebral perfusion during sleep. The MFV changes after EEG events can be interpreted as a result of cardiovascular and respiratory reactions that occur during the waking reaction. Primary constriction of the cerebral arteries mediated by the activated sympathetic nervous system may also be hypothesized. Quantitative differences in the MFV fluctuations after K-complexes, EEG arousal and movement arousal correspond to the increasing intensity of the associated awakening reactions. The absence of MFV responses and autonomic nervous system responses during the occurrence of sleep spindles support the theory that sleep spindles are sleep-protective events.

Droste et al. [40] studied intracranial pressure B-waves and their association with rhythmic changes in CBF velocity (B-wave equivalents) by TCD monitoring. In overnight TCD recordings in 10 normal young adults, these rhythmic changes in CBF velocity were higher and more frequent during REM sleep and sleep stage I than during other sleep stages. B-wave equivalents also had a longer wavelength during REM sleep. These results support the hypothesis that ICP B-waves are caused by vasodilation.

The MFV dynamics in the right and left MCAs of 12 healthy volunteers (age: 25–34 years) was also studied by Hajak et al. [38] using the same test design. The MFV values measured during NREM sleep were lower than those detected during wakefulness and the values measured during the second and last sleep cycle were significantly lower than in the first sleep cycle. The MFVs in sleep stage II at the end of an NREM sleep period were lower than in the preceding slow-wave sleep. At the onset of REM sleep, the MFV increased rapidly and reached a level significantly higher than in the preceding NREM sleep period. MFV fluctuations occurred in all sleep stages; the most significant fluctuations occurred during REM sleep and the least pronounced fluctuations were observed in slow-wave sleep. In the later sleep cycles, the MFV changes from one sleep stage to another were less pronounced than in the first sleep cycle. During the transition from NREM sleep to wakefulness, the MFV remained lower than in the evening pre-sleep stage. Even after the patients awoke the next morning, it took several minutes for the MFV to reach the value measured during the pre-sleep phase of the previous evening. There were no significant side-to-side differences between the left and right MCA. When changes in the sleep stages were provoked using brief tone pulses or clicks, the EEG frequency rose, but the MFV remained low or even decreased for a few seconds before rising to the earlier level.

CO_2 reactivity during normal sleep

CO_2 retention by holding one's breath or CO_2 stimulation will lead to a vessel dilatation of the cerebral resistance vessels and to a decrease of vascular resistance. Therefore, the relative CO_2 reactivity can be defined as the percentage of FV change per percentage of mmHg CO_2 change. Although the CO_2 test is used as a matter of routine [41,42] and although approximately more than 30% of all cerebral ischemias occur at night time, so far little is known about CO_2 reactivity during normal sleep. We, therefore, tried to perform a CO_2 stimulation during sleep in healthy subjects. During 19 nights the authors [Klingelhöfer J et al., unpublished data] were able to evaluate on 106 CO_2 stimulation periods. In order to be admitted into evaluation, the healthy subjects had

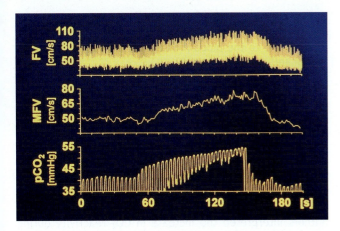

Figure 6 Original recording of the left MCA of a 23-year-old sleeping healthy subject during CO_2 stimulation: original envelope curve, course of MFV, end-expiratory CO_2 concentration. The increase of velocity during CO_2 stimulation is clearly visible (according to [Kingelhöfer J et al., unpublished data]).

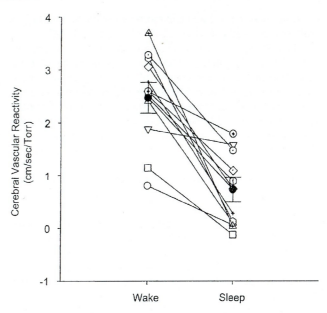

Figure 7 Changes in cerebral vascular reactivity from wake to sleep. The cerebral vascular reactivity to CO_2 from wake to NREM sleep is reduced in each individual. Open symbols: individual values; solid symbols: group mean values (according to [45]).

to reach at least an end-expiratory CO_2 concentration of more than 50 mmHg. They also had to be able to tolerate a CO_2 accumulation period for a minimum of 90 s. Fig. 6 shows an original recording of the left MCA of a 23-year-old subject during sleep. The topmost recording demonstrates the original envelope curve, the middlemost the course of MFV and the lowermost the CO_2 concentration during CO_2 stimulation. The increase of velocity is clearly visible. From these data the authors calculated the relative CO_2 reactivity during different sleep stages for the whole healthy collective. The results show that CO_2 stimulation presented no significant differences in light, slow wave and REM sleep as compared to the waking state in healthy subjects. The authors concluded that cerebrovascular CO_2 reactivity is maintained during normal sleep. In healthy subjects no significant differences as compared to the waking state have been revealed. During CO_2 stimulation in healthy sleepers an increase of mean EEG frequencies in slow wave sleep has been explained as a sign of growing activity within an arousal reaction.

A second study examining CO_2 reactivity in normal sleep was accomplished by Meadows et al. [43,44]. The authors investigated the effects of stable stage III/IV NREM sleep on the CBF response to CO_2 using TCD to determine MCA velocity as an index of CBF [43,45]. Meadows et al. determined that, in normal human subjects, hypercapnic cerebral vascular reactivity is reduced by 70% compared to wakefulness (Fig. 7). The authors concluded that this marked reduction in cerebral vascular reactivity during sleep indicates that the regulation of CBF is significantly altered compared with wakefulness. The functional advantage of such a reduction in the sleep-related cerebral vascular reactivity could not be explained by the authors.

Spontaneous hemodynamic behavior during normal sleep and sleep transitions characterized with near-infrared spectroscopy

In a current study Näsi et al. [46] carried out 30 all-night sleep measurements with combined near-infrared spectroscopy (NIRS) and polysomnography to investigate spontaneous hemodynamic behavior in slow wave sleep compared to light sleep and REM sleep. Their results indicated that slow spontaneous cortical and systemic hemodynamic activity was reduced in slow wave sleep compared to light sleep, REM sleep and wakefulness. This behavior was explained by neuronal synchronization observed in electrophysiological studies of slow wave sleep and a reduction in autonomic nervous system activity. Also, sleep stage transitions were asymmetric, so that the slow wave sleep-to-light sleep and light sleep-to-REM sleep transitions, which are associated with an increase in the complexity of cortical electrophysiological activity, were characterized by more dramatic hemodynamic changes than the opposite transitions. Thus, it appeared to the authors that while the onset of slow wave sleep and termination of REM sleep occurred only as gradual processes over time, the termination of slow wave sleep and onset of REM sleep may be triggered more abruptly by a particular physiological event or condition.

Pathophysiology, cerebral hemodynamics and CBF in sleep apnea syndrome

All sleep apnea syndromes — whether of the central, the obstructive, or the mixed type — are characterized by a disorder of breathing during sleep. For diagnostic purposes, apnea is defined as a cessation of airflow at the nose and mouth lasting at least 10 s [47]. The diagnosis of SAS is made when at least 30 apneic episodes are observed during REM and NREM stages over 7 h of nocturnal sleep. Some of the apneic episodes must appear in a repetitive sequence during NREM sleep [48]. Sleep apnea syndromes have been associated with medical complications such as pulmonary and arterial hypertension, cardiovascular disease, excessive daytime sleeping, fatigue and morning headache [48,49], as well as increased risk of cerebral infarction [50—54].

The etiology of SAS remains equivocal, but several mechanisms (e.g., instability of central respiratory regulation, reduction in the responsiveness of medullary chemoreceptors and relaxation of the upper airway musculature during sleep) have been proposed as factors in the genesis of nocturnal apnea phases [55—60]. Longobardo et al. [56] believe that an increase in circulation time between receptors in the brainstem respiratory centers and controlled alveolar ventilation is the cause of periodic cessation of breathing. Because apnea is accompanied by hypoxia and hypercapnia and pCO_2 and perivascular pH are major regulatory determinants of CBF and flow velocity, changes in cerebral hemodynamics are to be expected in patients with SAS [35,41,42,61]. These theoretic considerations have been confirmed by a limited number of studies. Meyer et al. [62] performed CBF measurements during daytime sleeping and waking states in 13 patients with narcolepsy and 7 with SAS. In the waking state, brainstem, cerebellar and bihemispheric flow were below normal in both patient groups. After sleep onset, CBF decreased further; maximum changes of regional flow values were seen in brainstem regions, indicating a critically reduced brainstem functional activity during sleep in SAS. Alterations of flow velocities during apnea-associated changes of CO_2 were also reported in obstructive SAS [63].

CBF velocity during sleep apnea syndrome

Now that several studies have shown that transcranial Doppler sonography is a useful method for long-term and on-line monitoring of dynamic changes in cerebral perfusion during sleep, researchers have begun using TCD for the assessment of perfusion changes in pathological sleep conditions. Various studies have been performed to assess cerebral flow velocity changes during nocturnal apneic episodes in patients with SAS. Siebler et al. [64] were the first to observe a cerebral flow velocity increase during nocturnal apneic phases in a patient with obstructive SAS and their findings have since been confirmed by various independent work groups in larger numbers of patients [65—67]. Fischer et al. [34], who compared the MFV changes in SAS patients with those of a comparable control group, observed lower MFV values in SAS patients during wakefulness, NREM sleep and REM sleep than in normals. They therefore concluded that altered cerebral perfusion occurs in SAS patients.

However, a sleep stage-correlated CBF velocity assessment in SAS patients and normal control subjects determined that the course of CBF velocity changes in apneic patients during night sleep were comparable to those observed in healthy control subjects. These findings indicate that the general pattern of cerebral perfusion changes associated with sleep remains preserved in SAS and they contradict the hypothesis of the existence of cerebral hypoperfusion in SAS [65,66]. Klingelhöfer et al. [66] observed MFV increases of 19—219%, reaching a maximum in REM sleep, during apneic episodes in 6 patients with SAS (age: 34—55 years, mean age: 49 years) (Fig. 8). There was also a significant increase in blood pressure (12.5—83.1%) during apneic episodes. A multiple linear regression analysis revealed that the flow velocity increase was not only attributable to the blood pressure increase alone, but was significantly linked to apnea.

Siebler and Nachtmann [67] compared the flow velocity responses during apneic episodes in SAS patients with those observed during arbitrary apnea in healthy control subjects. They detected comparable MFV increases in both groups and concluded that cerebral CO_2 reactivity is preserved in SAS. Klingelhöfer et al. [66] also observed normal CO_2 reactivity ($4.4 \pm 1.2\%$) in SAS patients during wakefulness, but the reactivity values increased significantly during sleep stages I and II and reached a maximum during REM sleep with rises of CO_2 reactivity up to three times the waking values. The authors interpreted the increase in CO_2 reactivity during sleep as hypersensitivity of intracranial CO_2 or pH receptors in SAS patients and attributed this to a possible disorder of the central catecholaminergic and cholinergic systems in SAS. They presume that the marked flow velocity fluctuations during apneic episodes and the associated changes in vessel wall tension place a chronic strain on the cerebral blood vessels, thereby promoting the development of micro- and macroangiopathy. This, among other factors, could be a reason for the increased incidence of cerebral ischemia in patients with SAS.

In addition to the apnea-associated increase in CBF velocity, which most authors attribute to apnea-related hypercapnia [64—67], it is also notable that a rapid normalization of flow velocity occurs at the end of each apneic episode. Hajak et al. [65] demonstrated in 10 patients (mean age: 37 years) that, in addition to its connection with the restoration of breathing and the associated occurrence of normocapnia, this flow velocity reduction is also regularly associated with the occurrence of EEG arousal or movement arousal. Because arousals represent a type of neuronal activation, the authors concluded that this indicates a direct neuronal influence on flow velocity during apneic episodes.

Franklin [68] compared cerebral hemodynamics in obstructive sleep apneas and central sleep apneas. Cerebral and cardiovascular changes display a different pattern during central and obstructive sleep apneas. By means of their study they revealed that the CBF velocity according to TCD increases during an obstructive apnea and decreases after apnea termination concomitant with changes in arterial pressure. Their interpretation of the results was: the changes in cerebral circulation during obstructive apneas could be an immediate effect of rapid changes in blood pressure because cerebral autoregulation is overridden. The opposite pattern was seen during a central apnea, with a decrease in CBF velocity during apnea and an increase after apnea termination (Fig. 9). Changes during obstructive apneas are probably hazardous, with adverse cardiovascular effects including stroke. This may not be the case during central apneas, as Cheyne—Stokes respiration with central apneas is a result of an underlying disorder such as heart failure and stroke and is not a disease entity in itself.

Contrary to every study using TCD during obstructive sleep apnea [65—67,69,70], Netzer et al. reported in 1998 [71] that the CBF velocity declined during 80% of obstructive sleep apneas. They also recorded a decline in CBF velocity during central apnea but only in 14% of central apneas, which contradicts the studies by Franklin et al. [68,72],

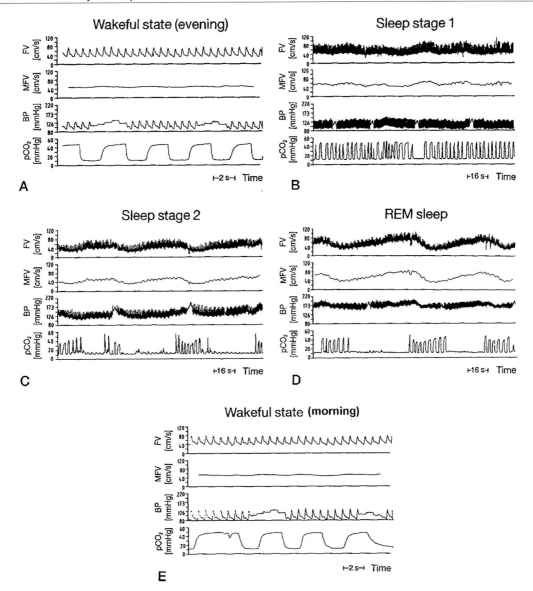

Figure 8 Changes in flow velocity (FV) and mean flow velocity (MVF) of the right middle cerebral artery (MCA), and changes in blood pressure (BP) and end-tidal CO_2 concentration (pCO_2) in a 35-year-old man with severe sleep apnea syndrome (A, E) during the wakeful state and (B—D) during different sleep stages. Due to methodological reasons, the measured rise in pCO_2 is too low after some apneic episodes. In these cases, expiration of air did not take place exclusively through the nose, where the sensor for the end-tidal pCO_2 determination was located. These apneic episodes were excluded from the CO_2 reactivity calculations. FV: flow velocity; BP: blood pressure; MFV: mean flow velocity (according to [66]).

which reports a consistently low CBF velocity during central apnea. The reason for these contradictory results is unclear and the authors do not discuss their findings in comparison with others.

The cerebral vascular reactivity to hypercapnia in patients with obstructive sleep apnea syndrome (OSAS) was investigated by Diomedi et al., 1998 [73] and Placidi et al., 1998 [74] to evaluate the influence of hemodynamic changes caused by OSAS. They studied cerebral vascular reactivity to hypercapnia calculated by means of the breath holding index. The investigation was performed in the early morning, soon after awakening and in the late afternoon. OSAS patients showed significantly lower breath holding index values with respect to controls both in the morning (0.57 vs. 1.40; $p < 0.0001$) and in the afternoon (1.0 vs. 1.51; $p < 0.0001$). In patients, breath holding index values in the afternoon were significantly higher than in the morning. The authors concluded that the data demonstrate a diminished vasodilator reserve in obstructive OSAS patients, particularly evident in the morning. This reduction of the possibility of cerebral vessels to adapt functionally in response to stimulation could be linked to hyposensitivity of cerebrovascular chemoreceptors after the continuous stress caused by nocturnal hypercapnia.

Droste et al. [75] studied the potential effect of continuous positive airway pressure (CPAP) on cerebral perfusion. They investigated 23 patients with OSAS and 16 healthy young adults in the waking state. As compared with

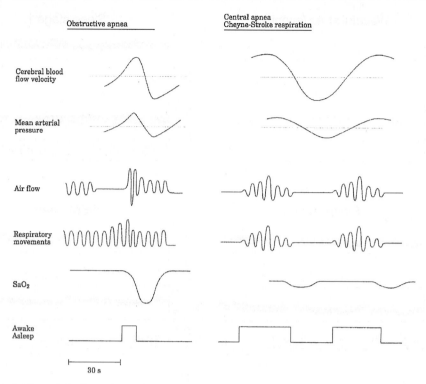

Figure 9 Outline of the hemodynamic pattern during obstructive and central apnea (according to [68]).

normal breathing CBF velocity of MCA and pCO_2 remained unchanged during CPAP. Systolic and diastolic blood pressure increased slightly by 1.2 mmHg and 1.1 mmHg, respectively. Cerebrovascular reactivity did not differ in the two groups. From their findings the authors concluded that nasal CPAP of 9 cmH$_2$O is a safe treatment with respect to the maintenance of CBF. The study gives further evidence for the autoregulation's capacity to maintain CBF velocity constant during different levels of intrathoracic pressure and different cerebral perfusion pressures.

Another group of scientists [76] analyzed whether increasing levels of CPAP may affect cerebral hemodynamics, assessed by TCD in normal humans. They found that even low levels of CPAP delivered through a mouthpiece in awake, young volunteers led to a decrease in CBF velocity, measured by TCD. This fall in CBF velocity was associated with hypocapnia and with an increase in both cerebrovascular resistance and anxiety due to breathing against positive pressure.

In a recent study Furtner et al. [63] investigated CBF velocity changes and vascular compliance in patients with OSAS using TCD and cerebral pulse transit time. Cerebrovascular reactivity was assessed by calculation of apnea and hypopnea-related CBF velocity changes. Arterial compliance was characterized by cerebral pulse transit time derived from phase difference analysis between ECG and TCD signals. Sleep time was dichotomized into periods with high density of consecutive respiratory events vs. periods with low density of consecutive respiratory events. TCD measurements of CBF velocity showed a regular, undulating pattern with flow minima immediately before apneas or hypopneas and maxima closely after their termination, reciprocally to peripheral O$_2$ saturation. CBF velocity reactivity was significantly diminished in consecutive respiratory events compared to non-consecutive respiratory event periods. The authors discussed severe disturbances of cerebrovascular reactivity in OSAS patients and interpreted their data as a sign of loss of vasoreactivity and increase of arterial stiffness.

Conclusion

The combined long-term recordings of intracranial flow patterns and polysomnography constitute an important method for evaluating dynamic aspects of brain function and cerebral perfusion during sleep. Numerous studies concerning this scientific field using this technique have contributed to a better understanding of the physiology of the normal sleep and the pathophysiology of sleep disorders as well as that of nocturnal stroke.

References

[1] Krueger JM, Rector DM, Roy S, Van Dongen HPA, Belenky G, Panksepp J. Sleep as a fundamental property of neuronal assemblies. Nat Rev Neurosci 2008;9:910—9.

[2] Rechtschaffen A, Kales A. A manual for standardized terminology, techniques and scoring system for sleep stages of human subjects. In: US public health service. Washington, DC: US Government Printing Office; 1968.

[3] Sakai F, Meyer JS, Karacan I, Derman S, Yamamoto M. Normal human sleep: regional cerebral hemodynamics. Ann Neurol 1980;17:471—8l.

[4] Gozukirmizi E, Meyer JS, Okabe T, Amano T, Mortel K, Karacan I. Cerebral blood flow during paroxysmal EEG activation induced by sleep in patients with complex partial seizures. Sleep 1982;5:329—42.

[5] Kennedy C, Gillin JC, Mendelson W, Suda S, Miyaoka M, Ito M, et al. Local cerebral glucose utilization in nonrapid eye movement sleep. Nature 1982;297:325—7.

[6] Heiss WD, Pawlik G, Herholz K, Wagner R, Wienhard K. Regional cerebral glucose metabolism in man during wakefulness, sleep, and dreaming. Brain Res 1985;327:362—6.

[7] Meyer JS, Ishikawa Y, Hata T, Karacan I. Cerebral blood flow in normal and abnormal sleep and dreaming. Brain Cogn 1987;6:266—94.

[8] Meyer JS, Amano T, Karacan I, Derman S, Hartse K, Nakajima S. Changes in LCBF measured by CT scan during REM and non-REM human sleep. J Cereb Blood Flow Metab I 1981;(Suppl. 1):465—6.

[9] Madsen PL, Schmidt JF, Wildschiødtz G, Friberg L, Holm S, Vorstrup S, et al. Cerebral oxygen metabolism and cerebral blood flow in humans during deep and rapid-eye-movement sleep. J Appl Physiol 1991;70:2597—601.

[10] Zoccoli G, Walker AM, Lenzi P, Franzini C. The cerebral circulation during sleep: regulation mechanisms and functional implications. Sleep Med Rev 2002;6(6):443—55.

[11] Buchsbaum MS, Gillin JC, Wu J, Hazlett E, Sicotte N, Dupont RM, et al. Regional cerebral glucose metabolic rate in human sleep assessed by positron emission tomography. Life Sci 1989;45:1349—56.

[12] Maquet P, Dive D, Salmon E, Sadzot B, Franco G, Poirrier R, et al. Cerebral glucose utilization during sleep-wake cycle in man determined by positron emission tomography and [18F]2-fluoro-2-deoxy-D-glucose method. Brain Res 1990;513:136—43.

[13] Reivich M, Isaacs G, Evarts E, Kety S. The effect of slow wave sleep and REM sleep on regional cerebral blood flow in cats. J Neurochem 1968;15:301—6.

[14] Lenzi P, Cianci T, Guidalotti PL, Leonardi GS, Franzini C. Brain circulation during sleep and its relation to extracerebral hemodynamics. Brain Res 1987;415:14—20.

[15] Madsen PL, Holm S, Vorstrup S, Friberg L, Wildschiødtz G. Human regional cerebral blood flow during rapid-eye-movement sleep. J Cereb Blood Flow Metab 1991;11:502—7.

[16] Ingvar DH, Rosen I, Johannesson G. EEG related to cerebral metabolism and blood flow. Pharmakopsychiatry 1979;12:200—9.

[17] Massimini M, Tononi G, Huber R. Slow waves, synaptic plasticity and information processing: insights from transcranial magnetic stimulation and high density EEG experiments. Eur J Neurosci 2009;29(9):1761—70.

[18] Kubota Y, Takasu NN, Horita S, Kondo M, Shimizu M, Okada T, et al. Dorsolateral prefrontal cortical oxygenation during REM sleep in humans. Brain Res 2011;1389:83—92.

[19] Meyer JS. Regulation of cerebral hemodynamics in health and disease. Eur Neurol 1983;22(Suppl. 1):47—60.

[20] Uchida-Ota M, Tanaka N, Sato H, Makia. A intrinsic correlations of electroencephalography rhythms with cerebral hemodynamics during sleep transitions. NeuroImage 2008;42:357—68.

[21] Raichle ME, Grubb Jr RL, Gado MH, Eichling JO, Ter-Pogossian MM. Correlation between regional cerebral blood flow and oxidative metabolism. In vivo studies in man. Arch Neurol 1976;33:523—6.

[22] Mazzilotta JC, Phelps ME, Miller J, Kuhl DE. Tomographic mapping of human cerebral metabolism: normal unstimulated state. Neurology 1981;31:503—16.

[23] Phelps ME, Kuhl DE, Mazziotta JC. Metabolic mapping of the brain's response to visual stimulation: studies in humans. Science 1981;211:1445—8.

[24] Kuschinsky W, Wahl M. Local chemical and neurogenic regulation of cerebral vascular resistance. Physiol Rev 1978;58:656—89.

[25] Sokoloff L. Relationships among local functional activity, energy metabolism, and blood flow in the central nervous system. Fed Proc 1981;40:2311—6.

[26] Aaslid R. Visually evoked dynamic blood flow response on the human cerebral circulation. Stroke 1987;18(4):771—5.

[27] Conrad B, Klingelhöfer J. Dynamics of regional blood flow for various visual stimuli. Exp Brain Res 1989;77:437—41.

[28] Aaslid R, Lindegaard KF, Sorteberg W, Nomes H. Cerebral autoregulation dynamics in humans. Stroke 1989;20:45—52.

[29] Klingelhöfer J, Matzander G, Sander D, Schwarze JJ, Boecker H, Bischoff C. Assessment of functional hemispheric asymmetry by bilateral simultaneous cerebral blood flow velocity monitoring. J Cereb Blood Flow Metab 1997;17:577—85.

[30] Lassen NA. Measurement of regional cerebral blood flow in humans with single photonemitting radioisotopes. In: Sokoloff L, editor. Brain imaging and brain function. New York: Raven Press; 1985. p. 9—20.

[31] Madsen PL, Schmidt JF, Holm S, Vorstrup S, Lassen NA, Wildschiodtz G. Cerebral oxygen metabolism and cerebral blood flow in man during light sleep (stage 2). Brain Res 1991;557:217—20.

[32] Phelps ME, Mazziotta JC, Huang SC. Review: study of cerebral function with positron computed tomography. J Cereb Blood Flow Metab 1982;2:113—62.

[33] Fischer AQ, Taonruna MA, Akhtar B, Chaudhary BA. The effect of sleep on intracranial hemodynamics: a transcranial Doppler study. J Child Neurol 1991;6:155—8.

[34] Fischer AQ, Chaudhary BA, Taormina MA, Akhtar B. Intracranial hemodynamics in sleep apnea. Chest 1992;102:1402—6.

[35] Markwalder TM, Grolimund P, Seiler RW, Roth F, Aaslid R. Dependency of blood flow velocity in the middle cerebral artery on end-tidal carbon dioxide partial pressure — a transcranial ultrasound Doppler study. J Cereb Blood Flow Metab 1984;4:368—72.

[36] Droste DW, Berger W, Schuler E, Krauss JK. Middle cerebral artery blood flow velocity in healthy persons during wakefulness and sleep: a transcranial Doppler study. Sleep 1993;16:603—9.

[37] Hajak G, Klingelhöfer J, Schulz-Varszegi M, Matzander G, Conrad B, Ruther E. New views into the dynamic changes of cerebral blood flow during sleep. In: Home J, editor. Sleep'90. Bochum: Pontenagel Press; 1990. p. 78—81.

[38] Hajak G, Klingelhöfer J, Schulz-Varszegi M, Matzander G, Sander D, Conrad B, et al. Relationship between cerebral blood flow velocities and cerebral electrical activity in sleep. Sleep 1994;17:11—9.

[39] Klingelhöfer J, Hajak G, Matzander G, Schulz-Varszegi M, Sander D, Rüther E, et al. Dynamics of cerebral blood flow velocities during normal human sleep. Clin Neurol Neurosurg 1995;97:142—8.

[40] Droste DW, Krauss JK, Berger W, Schuler E, Brown MM. Rhytmic oscillations with a wavelength of 0.5—2 min in transcranial Doppler recordings. Acta Neurol Scand 1994;90(2):99—104.

[41] Ringelstein EB, Sievers C, Ecker S, Schneider PA, Otis SM. Noninvasive assessment of CO_2-induced cerebral vasomotor response in normal individuals and patients with internal carotid artery occlusions. Stroke 1988;19:963—9.

[42] Widder B, Paulat K, Hackspacher J, Mayr E. Transcranial Doppler CO_2-test for the detection of hemodynamically critical carotid artery stenoses and occlusions. Eur Arch Psychiatry Neurol Sci 1986;236:162—8.

[43] Meadows GE, Dunroy HM, Morell MJ, Corfield DR. Hypercapnic cerebral vascular reactivity is decreased, in human, during sleep compared with wakefulness. J Appl Physiol 2003;94:2197—202.

[44] Meadows GE, O'Driscoll DM, Simonds AK, Morell MJ, Corfield DR. Cerebral blood flow response to isocapnic hypoxia during slow-wave sleep and wakefulness. J Appl Physiol 2004;97:1343—8.

[45] Corfield DR, Meadows GE. Control of cerebral blood flow during sleep and the effects of hypoxia. Adv Exp Med Biol 2006;588:65—73.

[46] Näsi T, Virtanen J, Noponen T, Toppila J, Salmi T, Ilmoniemi RJ. Spontaneous hemodynamic oscillations during human sleep and sleep stage transitions characterized with near-infrared spectroscopy. PLoS ONE 2011;10:e25415.

[47] Guilleminault C, Eldridge FL, Simmon FB, Dement WC. Sleep apnea syndrome: can it induce hemodynamic changes? West J Med 1975;123:7—16.

[48] Guilleminault C, Tilkian A, Dement WC. The sleep apnea syndromes. Annu Rev Med 1976;27:465—84.

[49] Guilleminault C. Clinical features and evaluation of obstructive sleep apnea. In: Kryger MH, Roth T, Dement WC, editors. Principles and practice of sleep medicine. Philadelphia: WB Saunders; 1989.

[50] Partinen M, Palomaki H. Snoring and cerebral infarction. Lancet 1985;2(8468):1325—6.

[51] Bassetti C, Aldrich MS, Chervin RD, Quint D. Sleep apnea in patients with transient ischemic attack and stroke: a prospective study of 59 patients. Neurology 1996;47(5):1167—73.

[52] Silvestrini M, Rizzaro B, Placidi F, BarutTaldi R, Bianconi A, Diomedi M. Carotid artery wall thickness in patients with obstructive sleep apnea syndrome. Stroke 2002;33(7):1782—5.

[53] Nachtmann A, Stang A, Wang YM, Wondzinski E, Thilmann AF. Association of obstructive sleep apnea and stenotic artery disease in ischemic stroke patients. Atherosclerosis 2003;169(2):301—7.

[54] Hsieh SW, Lai CL, Liu CF, Hsu CY. Obstructive sleep apnea linked to wake-up strokes. J Neurol 2012;4.

[55] Onal E, Lopata M. Periodic breathing and the pathogenesis of occlusive sleep apneas. Am Rev Respir Dis 1982;126:667—80.

[56] Longobardo GS, Gothe B, Goldman MD, Cherniack MS. Sleep apnea considered as a control system instability. Respir Physiol 1982;50:311—33.

[57] Patrick GB, Strohl KP, Rubin SB, Altose MD. Upper airway and diaphragm muscle responses to chemical stimulation and loading. J Appl Physiol 1982;53:1133—7.

[58] Strohl KP, Saunders NA, Sullivan CE. Sleep apnea syndromes. In: Saunders NS, Sullivan CE, editors. Sleep breathing. New York/Basel: Marcel Decker; 1984.

[59] Ayalon L, Peterson S. Functional central nervous system imaging in the investigation of obstructive sleep apnea. Curr Opin Pulm Med 2007;13(6):479—83.

[60] Desseilles M, Dang-Vu T, Schabus M, Sterpenich V, Maquet P, Schwartz S. Neuroimaging insights into the pathophysiology of sleep disorders. Sleep 2008;31(6):777—94.

[61] Kirkham FJ, Padayachee TS, Parsons S, Seargeant LS, House FR, Gosling RG. Transcranial measurement of blood velocities in the basal cerebral arteries using pulsed Dopple ultrasound: velocity as an index of flow. Ultrasound Med Biol 1986;12:15—21.

[62] Meyer JS, Sakai F, Karacan I, Derman S, Yamamoto M. Sleep apnea, narcolepsy, and dreaming: regional cerebral hemodynamics. Ann Neurol 1980;7:479—85.

[63] Furtner M, Staudacher M, Frauscher B, Brandauer E, Esnaola y Rojas MM, Gschliesser V, et al. Cerebral vasoreactivity decreases overnight in severe obstructive sleep apnea syndome: a study of cerebral hemodynamics. Sleep 2009;10:875—81.

[64] Siebler M, Daffertshofer M, Hennerici M, Freund HJ. Cerebral blood flow velocity alterations during obstructive sleep apnea syndrome. Neurology 1990;40:1461—2.

[65] Hajak G, Klingelhöfer J, Schulz-Varszegi M, Sander D, Rüther E. Sleep apnea syndrome and cerebral hemodynamics. Chest 1996;110:670—9.

[66] Klingelhöfer J, Hajak G, Sander D, Schulz-Varszegi MC, Ruther E, Conrad C. Assessment of intracranial hemodynamics in sleep apnea syndrome. Stroke 1992;23:1427—33.

[67] Siebler M, Nachtmann A. Cerebral hemodynamics in obstructive sleep apnea. Chest 1993;103:1118—9.

[68] Franklin KA. Cerebral haemodynamics in obstructive sleep apnoea and Cheyne—Strokes respiration. Sleep Med Rev 2002;6(6):429—41.

[69] Rieke K, Poceta JA, Mitler MM, Ley LR, Torruella AK, Adams HP, et al. Continuous blood flow velocity measurements in obstructive sleep apnoea syndrome. J Neuroimaging 1992;2:202—7.

[70] Bålfors EM, Franklin KA. Impairment of cerebral perfusion during obstructive sleep apnoeas. Am J Respir Crit Care Med 1994;150:1587—91.

[71] Netzer N, Werner P, Jochums I, Lehmann M, Strohl KP. Blood flow of the middle cerebral artery with sleep-disordered breathing: correlation with obstructive hypopneas. Stroke 1998;29:87—93.

[72] Franklin KA, Sandström E, Johansson G, Bålfors EM. Hemodynamics, cerebral circulation and oxygen saturation in Cheyne—Strokes respiration. J Appl Physiol 1997;83:1184—91.

[73] Diomedi M, Placidi F, Cupini LM, Bernardi G, Silvestrini. Cerebral hemodynamic changes in sleep apnea syndrome and effect of continuous positive airway pressure treatment. Neurology 1998;51:1051—6.

[74] Placidi F, Diomedi M, Cupini LM, Bernadi G, Silvestrini M. Impairment of daytime cerebrovascular reactivity in patients with obstructive sleep apnoea syndrome. J Sleep Res 1998;7:288—92.

[75] Droste DW, Lüdemann P, Anders F, Kemény V, Thomas M, Krauss JK, et al. Middle cerebral artery blood flow velocity, end-tidal pCO_2 and blood pressure in patients with obstructive sleep apnea and in healthy subjects during continuous positive airway pressure breathing. Neurol Res 1999;21:737—41.

[76] Scala R, Turkington PM, Wanklyn P, Bamford J, Elliot MW. Effects of incremental levels of continuous positive airway pressure on cerebral blood flow velocity in healthy adult humans. Clin Sci 2003;104:633—9.

Asymmetry of cerebral autoregulation does not correspond to asymmetry of cerebrovascular pressure reactivity

Bernhard Schmidt[a],*, Marek Czosnyka[b], Jürgen Klingelhöfer[a]

[a] Department of Neurology, Chemnitz Medical Center, Germany
[b] Academic Neurosurgical Unit, Addenbrooke's Hospital, Cambridge, UK

KEYWORDS
Cerebral autoregulation;
Cerebrovascular reactivity;
Cerebral perfusion pressure;
Cerebral blood flow;
Transcranial Doppler ultrasonography

Summary

Background: Small cerebral vessels respond to variations of cerebral perfusion pressure (CPP) by changes of vessel diameter inducing changes of blood flow resistance and keeping cerebral blood flow constant. This mechanism is called cerebral autoregulation (CA). Recently stronger reactions of CA during pressure increase than during decrease were reported. Aim of this study was to assess the symmetry behavior of CA during spontaneous CPP changes and compare it to cerebrovascular pressure reactivity (CVR).

Methods: In 238 patients with traumatic brain injury or stroke, correlation indices between CPP and cerebral blood flow velocity (CBFV) were calculated during periods of increasing (upMx) and decreasing CPP (downMx). The indices range from −1 to +1, values ≤0 indicating intact, values >0 indicating impaired autoregulation. Similar correlation between arterial blood pressure (ABP) and ICP was calculated during increasing (upPRx) and decreasing ABP (downPRx), negative values indicating intact, positive values indicating impaired CVR. Only recordings with strong pressure changes (CPP/ABP > 10 mmHg) were evaluated.

Results: CA was assessed in 62 patients. On average (mean ± SD) upMx was 0.06 ± 0.52, downMx was 0.15 ± 0.55 ($P < 0.005$). CVR was assessed in 47 patients. On average upPRx was 0.45 ± 0.43, downPRx was 0.38 ± 0.48 ($P < 0.05$). In 40 patients both Mx and PRx were calculated. On average upMx was 0.21 ± 0.55 and downMx was 0.27 ± 0.56 ($P = 0.05$), upPRx was 0.35 ± 0.43 and downPRx was 0.27 ± 0.47 ($P < 0.05$).

Conclusions: During pressure increase the autoregulatory response was significantly stronger than during decrease, while in contrast the cerebrovascular reactivity was significantly weaker. The reason for this opposed behavior remains unclear and needs further exploration.
© 2012 Elsevier GmbH. All rights reserved.

Introduction

The mechanism of cerebral autoregulation (CA) minimizes fluctuations of cerebral blood flow (CBF) during changes of cerebral perfusion pressure (CPP). Pressure triggered dilatation or constriction of small artery vessels may

* Corresponding author at: Dresdner Str. 178, 09131 Chemnitz, Germany. Tel.: +49 371 33312358; fax: +49 371 33310530.
E-mail address: B.Schmidt@skc.de (B. Schmidt).

control cerebral blood flow resistance and prevent the brain from ischemia during decrease as well as from hyperemia during increase of CPP. This so-called cerebrovascular pressure reactivity (CVR) is a pre-condition of a working CA. While cerebral autoregulation is characterized by its regulating effect on cerebral blood flow, CVR describes the state of its underlying mechanism. Since CA may be affected in patients with severe brain injuries [1,2] its monitoring provides important information for clinical treatment. Various monitoring methods are based on the concept of dynamic CA [3] which not only describes a steady-state relationship between CPP and CBF [1] but also assesses the flow dynamics during rapid pressure changes. During monitoring these pressure changes may either be induced under controlled conditions [4,5] or due to spontaneous oscillations of ABP or CPP [6,7].

In recent publications the question whether CA was symmetric, i.e. whether CA response was equally effective during increase and decrease of pressure challenge, was subject to investigation and partly contradictive results. For the first time Aaslid reported a stronger response of dynamic autoregulation during increasing ABP compared to decreasing ABP [8]. This effect was demonstrated in 14 patients with traumatic brain injuries (TBI) during cyclic changes of ABP which have been induced by sequentially repeated leg cuff tests. The asymmetric behavior of autoregulation was explained by a non-linearity of the dynamic autoregulation mechanism [9]. No asymmetry was observed in 10 healthy persons. The authors analyzed CA during spontaneous CPP oscillations in 53 patients with severe TBI [10]. They observed a slightly but significantly stronger autoregulatory response during increase of CPP compared to decrease of CPP. The degree of asymmetry observed in the current study was weaker than formerly reported by Aaslid which may be explained by different methods of CA assessment as well as the usage of different CA stimuli (induced ABP versus spontaneous CPP changes). Asymmetry of CA was also confirmed by Tzeng et al. [11] during pharmacologically induced ABP changes. The population, however, consisted of 10 healthy persons which contradicted the former results [8].

The reasons for the asymmetry of CA are still not clear. The purpose of the current study was to investigate whether a stronger CA response during pressure increase was accompanied by a stronger reaction of small cerebral vessels, in other words whether asymmetry of CA corresponded to an asymmetry (in same direction) of CVR.

Materials and methods

Patient population

238 patients (mean age 37 ± 18 years, 191 male/47 female) were studied. They suffered either from traumatic brain injury (TBI) ($N=210$) or stroke ($N=28$). At the time of data recording all the patients were sedated, paralyzed and mechanically ventilated. Their arterial partial pressure of CO_2 ranged from 30 to 40 mmHg. The patients were treated either in Addenbrooke's Hospital, Cambridge, UK ($N=171$; TBI only) or in Chemnitz Medical Center (39 TBI and 28 strokes).

Monitoring

TCD measurements were taken by different MHz pulsed Doppler devices (TC 2-64B, EME, Überlingen, Germany or Multidop-P, DWL, Sipplingen, Germany – in Chemnitz; Scimed, Bristol, UK or Neuroguard, Medasonics, CA – in Cambridge). The envelope curve of FV in MCA was continuously recorded in the hemisphere ipsilateral to brain lesion. Blood pressure was measured with a standard manometer line inserted into the radial artery.

ICP was measured using either implanted intraparenchymal or intraventricular microsensors (Camino Laboratories, San Diego, CA, USA; Codman Group Inc., Andover, MA, USA; Raumedic GmbH, Rehau, Germany), a sensor with air pouch probes (Spiegelberg Plc/Ltd./Co., Hamburg, Germany), or an external ventricular drainage.

The signals were recorded for the duration of 20–120 min, the sampling frequencies ranged from 25 Hz to 50 Hz. In total 808 recordings were created between 1992 and 2005.

Monitoring was a routine clinical practice used for daily patients' management and did not require individual consents. Local Ethical Committees approved these procedures.

Assessment of cerebral autoregulation and cerebrovascular pressure reactivity

In a retrospective analysis the recorded signal data of ICP, ABP, CPP (CPP = ABP – ICP), and FV was initially filtered by a 0.1 Hz low-pass filter. Cerebral autoregulation was assessed in terms of Pearson's correlation of CPP and FV during 5-min intervals. The correlation indices were averaged over the whole recording time and resulted in the autoregulation index Mx [6]. Predominant positive correlation between CPP and FV (i.e. Mx > 0) indicated passive dependence of blood flow on CPP. Zero or negative value of Mx indicated active regulation of blood flow.

In order to assess the autoregulation during increasing CPP, the index upMx was introduced. Only CPP values and their time-corresponding FV values during sequences of pressure increase of at least 10 mmHg were taken for a correlation analysis (Fig. 1). The required high CPP signal dynamic was important for the comparability with the before-mentioned study of Aaslid [8] where asymmetry of dynamic but not of static cerebral autoregulation [1,4] has been reported. The index downMx for assessment of CA during decrease in CPP was computed completely analogous to upMx by evaluating periods of strongly (at least 10 mm Hg) decreasing CPP. Being correlation coefficients, the indices, Mx, upMx and downMx are normalized in values (+1 to −1).

In a similar way the pressure reactivity index PRx [12] was used for assessment of CVR. PRx is based on Pearson's correlation of CPP and FV and calculated completely analogous to Mx. Moreover, the indices upPRx and downPRx for assessment of CVR during increase and decrease of ABP were introduced corresponding to upMx and downMx. In this case pressure changes of at least 10 mm Hg of ABP instead of CPP were required for calculation.

A signal recording was included for CA analysis if both upMx and downMx could be calculated and included for CVR analysis if both upPRx and downPRx could be calculated.

The difference upMx − downMx of each included recording was considered a measure of the asymmetry between the autoregulatory response to increasing and to decreasing CPP. The difference upPRx − downPRx was considered a measure for the asymmetry of cerebrovascular reaction to increasing and to decreasing ABP.

Results

Strong CPP fluctuations with pressure changes of more than 10 mmHg were found in 95 recordings of 62 patients. From this data 95 pairs of upMx and downMx were calculated. On average (±SD) upMx was 0.06 ± 0.52 and downMx was 0.15 ± 0.55 (difference was significant at $P < 0.005$). The lower value of upMx indicated stronger autoregulatory responses to increasing CPP than to decreasing CPP.

Strong fluctuations of ABP were found in 67 recordings of 47 patients. On average (±SD) in these recordings upPRx was 0.45 ± 0.43 and downPRx was 0.38 ± 0.48 (difference was significant at $P < 0.05$). The higher value of upPRx indicated a weaker cerebrovascular reaction to increasing ABP than to decreasing ABP. Therefore, the asymmetry was opposite to the asymmetry of CA. In 51 recordings of 40 patients both Mx and PRx could be calculated. Mx and PRx correlated moderately ($R = 0.52$; $P < 0.001$) (Fig. 1). On average upMx was 0.21 ± 0.55 and downMx was 0.27 ± 0.56 ($P = 0.05$), upPRx was 0.35 ± 0.43 and downPRx was 0.27 ± 0.47 ($P < 0.05$). Again Mx and PRx showed asymmetries in different directions (Fig. 2). The difference upPRx − downPRx was significantly higher in recordings in which decrease of ABP was accompanied by increase of ICP ($N = 15$; mean ± SD: 0.30 ± 0.31) compared to the other recordings ($N = 36$; 0.00 ± 0.21) ($P < 0.001$) (Fig. 3a). The difference upMx − downMx did not significantly vary between both groups ($N = 15$; -0.08 ± 0.38 | $N = 36$; -0.05 ± 0.22 | $P = 0.5$, n.s.). The difference upPRx − downPRx did not significantly vary between recordings in which increase of ABP was accompanied by decrease of ICP ($N = 12$; -0.03 ± 0.29) and the other recordings ($N = 39$; 0.12 ± 0.28) ($P = 0.2$, n.s.) (Fig. 3b). The differences upMx − downMx and

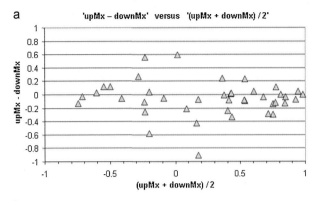

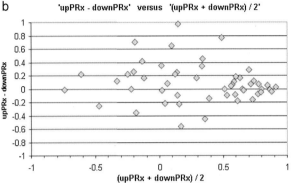

Figure 2 (a) Bland—Altman plot for comparison of upMx and downMx. Fifty-one values of indices upMx and downMx (x-axis) are plotted against their differences (y-axis). In spite of a high variation of the upMx − downMx differences a slight shift toward values below the $y = 0$ line confirms the calculated result that on average upMx was significantly lower than downMx, i.e. that CA was regulating more effective during CPP increase than during decrease. (b) Bland—Altman plot for comparison of upPRx and downPRx. Fifty-one values of indices upPRx and downPRx (x-axis) are plotted against their differences (y-axis). In contrast to (a) the upPRx − downPRx differences showed a slight prevalence above the $y = 0$ line. The diagram confirms the calculated result that on average upPRx was significantly higher than downPRx, i.e. that CVR was stronger during ABP decrease than during increase.

upPRx − downPRx did not correlate significantly with ICP or CPP.

Discussion

The observed stronger autoregulatory response during increase of CPP compared to decrease was in accordance to former results [8,10]. However, the converse behavior of cerebrovascular reactivity was surprising (Fig. 2). While Mx and PRx showed moderate correlation (Fig. 1), CVR was found stronger during ABP decrease than during increase. In view of CVR being the underlying mechanism of CA parallel asymmetries of CVR and CA would have been expected in addition (to correlation of related indices). PRx indirectly assesses small vessel motion (constriction or dilatation) by its impact on ICP. Even though being influenced by various other parameters as well, e.g. the cerebral compliance [13—15], PRx has been shown to provide information about vessel activities [12]. One possible explanation

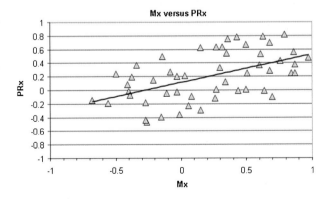

Figure 1 Scatter plot of Mx versus PRx. Fifty-two pairs of CA related indices Mx and CVR related PRx together with a regression line are plotted. The indices correlated moderately, the regression coefficient being 0.52 ($P < 0.001$). The correlation of both indices is consistent with the close relationship between CA and CVR (CA, cerebral autoregulation; CVR, cerebrovascular pressure reactivity).

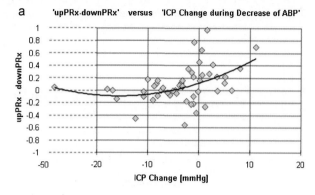

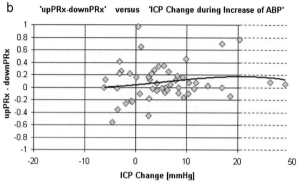

Figure 3 (a) Scatter plot of 'upPRx-downPRx' and 'ICP change during decrease of ABP'. A curve fitting of a 3-degree polynomial illustrates significant higher upPRx − downPRx values in case of increasing ICP (ICP change > 0). This might be interpreted as a stronger imbalance toward vasoreactivity during decrease of ABP. (b) Scatter plot of 'upPRx − downPRx' and 'ICP change during increase of ABP'. The curve fitting of 3-degree polynomial emphasizes the optical impression that upPRx − downPRx values are independent from the direction of ICP change during increase of ABP, i.e. the asymmetry of vasoreactivity remains the same whether ICP decreases or not.

might be that regulation of decreasing pressure is generally less effective and needs stronger vascular compensation to sustain cerebral blood flow than regulation during pressure increase. First point is that a decrease of cerebral flow resistance due to dilatations of small cerebral arteries do not influence flow resistance caused by other parts of the cerebrovascular system. This might delimit the effectiveness of regulation during decrease of pressure but not during increase. Furthermore, compensatory vasodilatation during ABP decrease may increase ICP which aggravates ABP decrease and reduces the benefit of lowered blood flow resistance. This effect may be called 'false impairment of autoregulation' in analogy to the more familiar occurrence of 'false autoregulation' [16]. A hazardous variation of this effect is assumed to be the reason for the formation of ICP plateau waves in patients with exhausted cerebral compliance [13–15,17]. 'False autoregulation' occurs during ABP increase in case of non-reacting small cerebral vessels. Cerebral blood volume increases leading to increase of ICP and dampening rise of CPP. This effect may facilitate the vascular regulation task during event of increasing pressure. These hypotheses are supported by the result that asymmetry of PRx was significantly higher (i.e. the predomination of CVR during pressure decrease was more pronounced)

in those recordings with combined decrease of ABP and increase of ICP ('false impairment of CA') (Fig. 3a) while the asymmetry of CA remained constant. It seems that vessels have to react stronger during pressure decrease to provide a constant effectiveness of CA. It is unlikely that the raised asymmetry of PRx can be simply explained by the special selection of just those recordings with downPRx < 0 (decrease of ABP and increase of ICP). In this case one might have expected the inverse effect as well, i.e. a significantly lower asymmetry of PRx in those recordings with upPRx < 0 (increase of ABP accompanied by decrease of ICP). But in these recordings upPRx − downPRx did not deviate from the remaining data (Fig. 3b).

The results to the subject of CA asymmetry published so far [8,10,11] and our current results concordantly show a stronger effectiveness of CA during increase of driving pressure which was considered either ABP or CPP. However, there have been contradictive results as well. No asymmetry was found by Aaslid et al. in healthy persons while Tseng et al. solely studied healthy subjects. The asymmetry was much weaker in our investigations then reported by Aaslid. It remains unclear whether these differing results might be caused by the use of differing methods of CA assessment. In this study CA was compared to CVR for a deeper understanding of the mechanisms of CA and possible reasons of the observed asymmetry. However, the made considerations about CA and CVR still are just hypotheses. Further studies with bigger population to analyze the CA−CVR interaction appear warranted.

Conclusion

During pressure increase the autoregulatory response was significantly stronger than during decrease, while in contrast the cerebrovascular reactivity was significantly weaker. The reason for this opposed behavior remains unclear and needs further exploration.

Sources of support

M. Czosnyka was supported by National Institute of Health Research, Biomedical Research Center Cambridge (Neuroscience Theme).

Acknowledgment

M. Czosnyka is on leave from Warsaw University of Technology, Poland.

References

[1] Lassen NA. Control of cerebral circulation in health and disease. Circ Res 1974;34(June (6)):749–60.
[2] Enevoldsen EM, Jensen FT. Autoregulation and CO_2 responses of cerebral blood flow in patients with severe head injury. J Neurosurg 1978;48:689–703.
[3] Tiecks FP, Lam AM, Aaslid R, Newell DW. Comparison of static and dynamic cerebral autoregulation measurements. Stroke 1995;26:1014–9.
[4] Aaslid R, Lindegaard KF, Sorteberg W, Nornes H. Cerebral autoregulation dynamics in humans. Stroke 1989;20:45–52.

[5] Diehl RR, Linden D, Lücke D, Berlit P. Phase relationship between cerebral blood flow velocity and blood pressure: a clinical test of autoregulation. Stroke 1989;20:1—3.

[6] Czosnyka M, Smielewski P, Kirkpatrick P, Menon DK, Pickard JD. Monitoring of cerebral autoregulation in head-injured patients. Stroke 1996;27:1829—34.

[7] Panerai RB, White RP, Markus HS, Evans DH. Grading of cerebral dynamic autoregulation from spontaneous fluctuations in arterial blood pressure. Stroke 1998;29(November (11)):2341—6.

[8] Aaslid R, Blaha M, Sviri G, Douville CM, Newell DW. Asymmetric dynamic cerebral autoregulatory response to cyclic stimuli. Stroke 2007;38:1465—9.

[9] Giller CA, Mueller M. Linearity and non-linearity in cerebral hemodynamics in humans. Med Eng Phys 2003;25:633—46.

[10] Schmidt B, Klingelhöfer J, Perkes I, Czosnyka M. Cerebral autoregulatory response depends on the direction of change in perfusion pressure. J Neurotrauma 2009;26:1—6.

[11] Tzeng YC, Willie CK, Atkinson G, Lucas SJE, Wong A, Ainslie PN. Cerebrovascular regulation during transient hypotension and *hypertension* in humans. Hypertension 2010;56:268—73.

[12] Czosnyka M, Smielewski P, Kirkpatrick P, Laing RJ, Menon D, Pickard JD. Continuous assessment of the cerebral vasomotor reactivity in head injury. Neurosurgery 1997;41:11—9.

[13] Lundberg N. Continuous recording and control of ventricular fluid pressure in neurosurgical practice. Acta Psych Neurol Scand (Suppl) 1960;149:1—93.

[14] Lundberg N, Cronqvist S, Kjallqvist A. Clinical investigations on interrelations between intracranial pressure and intracranial hemodynamics. Prog Brain Res 1968;30:70—5.

[15] Rosner MJ, Becker DP. Origin and evolution of plateau waves: experimental observations and a theoretical model. J Neurosurg 1984;60:312—24.

[16] Enevoldsen EM, Jensen FT. ''False'' autoregulation of cerebral blood flow in patients with acute severe head injury. Acta Neurol Scand Suppl 1977;64:514—5.

[17] Schmidt B, Czosnyka M, Schwarze JJ, Sander D, Gerstner W, Lumenta CB, et al. Cerebral vasodilatation causing acute intracranial hypertension — a method for non-invasive assessment. J Cereb Blood Flow Metab 1999;19:990—6.

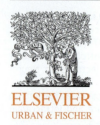
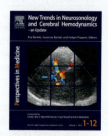

Adaptation of cerebral pressure-velocity hemodynamic changes of neurovascular coupling to orthostatic challenge

Pedro Castro [a,*], Rosa Santos [a], João Freitas [b], Bernhard Rosengarten [c], Ronney Panerai [d], Elsa Azevedo [a]

[a] Dept. Neurology, Hospital São João, Faculty of Medicine of University of Porto, Portugal
[b] Autonomic Unit, Hospital São João, Faculty of Medicine of University of Porto, Portugal
[c] Dept. Neurology, University of Giessen, Germany
[d] Dept. Cardiovascular Sciences, University of Leicester, United Kingdom

KEYWORDS
Transcranial Doppler;
Brain activation studies;
Cerebral hemodynamics;
Neurovascular coupling;
Cerebral autoregulation;
Critical closing pressure

Summary Neurovascular coupling (NVC), analysed by a control system approach, was shown to be unaffected by orthostatic challenge, but data is lacking regarding the mechanism of this interplay and the behaviour of other cerebrovascular reactivity parameters. We investigated the changes in different pressure–velocity models during functional transcranial Doppler (TCD), under different orthostatic conditions.

Thirteen healthy volunteers performed a reading test stimulation task in sitting, supine and head-up tilt (HUT) positions. CBF velocity was monitored with TCD in the posterior cerebral artery, and blood pressure was monitored with Finapres. Cerebrovascular resistance index (CVRi) was compared to a two-parameter model including resistance-area product (RAP) and critical closing pressure (CrCP), in the maximal and in the stable phases of flow response to visual stimulation.

All cerebrovascular resistance parameters decreased with visual stimulation but the magnitude of their variation in each orthostatic condition was not similar. From supine to HUT, CrCP variation decreased (both maximal and stable phase $p = 0.001$). CVRi variation increased from sitting to HUT positions (maximal $p = 0.039$; stable phase $p = 0.033$). RAP variation to visual stimulation did not change between the three positions (maximal $p = 0.077$; stable phase $p = 0.188$).

Abbreviations: NVC, neurovascular coupling; ABP, arterial blood pressure; TCD, transcranial Doppler; CBF, cerebral blood flow; BFV, blood flow velocity; MCA, middle cerebral artery; PCA, posterior cerebral artery; HR., heart rate; CVRi, cerebrovascular resistance index; CrCP, critical closing pressure; RAP, resistance-area product.
* Corresponding author at: Dept. Neurology, Hospital São João, Faculty of Medicine of University of Porto, Alameda Professor Hernani Monteiro, 4200-319 Porto, Portugal. Tel.: +351 931725181; fax: +351 220919086.
E-mail addresses: pedromacc@gmail.com (P. Castro), rosampsantos2@gmail.com (R. Santos), jppafreitas@sapo.pt (J. Freitas), Bernhard.Rosengarten@neuro.med.uni-giessen.de (B. Rosengarten), rp9@leicester.ac.uk (R. Panerai), elsaazevedo@netcabo.pt (E. Azevedo).

2211-968X/$ — see front matter © 2012 Elsevier GmbH. All rights reserved.
doi:10.1016/j.permed.2012.02.052

A 2-parameter model of vascular resistance provided better discrimination for the effects of posture on NVC as shown by the adaptive changes in CrCP with orthostatic challenge, in comparison with the classical use of CVRi. These findings suggest that although NVC seemed unaffected by orthostatic challenge, more complex vasoregulative mechanisms are activated in different orthostatic conditions that could potentially be of diagnostic or prognostic value.
© 2012 Elsevier GmbH. All rights reserved.

Introduction

The brain has the capability of maintaining continuous vascular supply of oxygen and glucose to support active neuronal populations [1–3]. Neurovascular coupling (NVC) matches cerebral blood flow (CBF) to different cortical areas metabolic demand [1,2]. Another physiological mechanism, cerebral autoregulation, maintains CBF stable against changes in cerebral perfusion pressure and thus changes in arterial blood pressure (ABP) [4,5].

The NVC is studied with different techniques such as MRI, PET, SPECT and transcranial Doppler (TCD). Due to technical reasons the postural condition of the patients varies with these approaches. A recent focus on a disturbed NVC has been outlined in stroke [6], Alzheimer [7], and autonomic failure [8] diseases. For these reasons, a better understanding of NVC mechanism in different orthostatic conditions can have an impact both in scientific and clinical grounds.

There have been remarkable developments in the two last decades about our understanding of the underlying neurogenic, myogenic and metabolic components driving NVC [9,10]. Neurons, as well as astrocytes, seem to play an important role in focal CBF activation leading to upstream vasodilation from the microvasculature through pial arteries supplying focal activated area [11–13]. Probably, the same resistance vessels play an important role in the cerebral autoregulation [14], so that the vascular tonus of the cortical arterioles might be adjusted in accordance to the needs of both the cerebral autoregulation as well as the NVC. A previous study [15] has shown that activity-induced flow velocity responses under different orthostatic conditions can be compared with each other, but the mechanisms that keep NVC unaffected under orthostatic stress remained obscure. To further investigate this issue, we studied the behaviour of systemic and cerebral pressure–velocity parameters during functional TCD (fTCD) monitoring, under different orthostatic conditions, by extending the classical representation of cerebrovascular resistance to a more realistic 2-parameter model [21–23].

Materials and methods

Subjects

This study was performed in Hospital São João, a 1200-bed university hospital in Oporto. The local institutional ethical committee approved the study. After information and instruction each volunteer gave informed consent to participate in the study.

Thirteen young adult volunteers (8 male) with mean ± SD age 26.4 ± 8.7 years (range 18–48 years), were included. These subjects lacked classical cardiovascular risk factors and did not take any medication, except for birth control pills. They abstained from caffeine more than 12 h before the tests. Previously to the study, the volunteers performed a cervical and transcranial duplex scan, with a HDI 5000 device (Philips, USA). Normal findings and a good temporal acoustic bone window to ensure a good acquisition of velocity curves during the whole test were required as an inclusion criterion.

Measurements

The study was carried out in a quiet room with a constant temperature of approximately 22 °C. Systolic, mean and diastolic blood pressure and heart rate were monitored with a non-invasive finger cuff Finapres device (model 2300; Ohmeda, Englewood, CO, USA) holding the finger at heart level. A hand support was used to allow a constant position throughout the tests in the three different postural conditions [15,16].

For insonation through the temporal transcranial ultrasonic bone window, 2 MHz pulsed wave Doppler monitoring probes of a Multidop T2 Doppler device (DWL, Singen, Germany) were mounted on an individually fitted headband, to record flow velocity in the P2 segment of the left posterior cerebral artery (PCA), and the M1 segment of the right middle cerebral artery (MCA), as described elsewhere [15,17,18]. Beat-to-beat peak systolic, mean and end diastolic blood flow velocities (BFV), ABP, calculated heart rate (HR) and stimulus marker were digitally recorded in the Doppler device. Recordings were considered acceptable when the blood flow velocities could be detected bilaterally, with a clear envelope of the velocity spectrum during the entire cardiac cycle.

Visual-evoked paradigm

The visual-evoked paradigm consisted of 10 cycles, each with a resting phase of 20 s with closed eyes and a stimulating phase of 40 s of silent reading text columns. The text that the study subjects read was the same for all participants and free of strong emotional content. Changes between phases were signalled acoustically using a tone. The complete test cycle had a total duration of 10 min, and was repeated in each position — supine, sitting and 70° head-up tilt (HUT). The reading test and its reliability have been already validated against a checkerboard stimulation paradigm [19].

Data analysis

All signals were visually inspected to identify artifacts or noise, and narrow spikes were removed by linear interpolation. The heart–MCA distance was used to obtain estimates of ABP in the MCA (ABP-MCA). Cerebrovascular resistance index (CVRi) was estimated by the ratio of mean ABP to mean BFV for each heartbeat. For both PCA and MCA, the instantaneous relationship between ABP and BFV was also used to estimate the critical closing pressure (CrCP) of the cerebral circulation, by extrapolation of the linear regression $BFV = a \times ABP + b$, as previously described [20–22]. The inverse of the linear regression slope was also obtained for each cardiac cycle, and it is referred to as "resistance area product" ($RAP = 1/a$) to differentiate it from CVRi [22,23]. The CrCP can be obtained from the value of ABP where BFV = 0, that is, $CrCP = -b/a$.

All beat-to-beat estimates were interpolated with a third-order polynomial and resampled at 0.2-s intervals to generate a time series with a uniform time base.

To become independent from the insonation angle, all parameters were normalized by the averaged value of the 5 s period prior to activation [8,15,17,19]. Ten cycles of 20 s rest (closed eyes) and 40 s stimulation (silent reading) were averaged for each volunteer at each position.

For each parameter, two different variables were calculated from the evoked CBF in response to visual task: (1) the maximal velocity variation during the 40 s of stimulation and (2) the averaged last 20 s corresponding to a stable phase of flow evoked response. The first one corresponds to the classical overshoot phase used in other fTCD investigations [24–29]; the second was included since it seems to be the most stable phase during activation, after the initial overshooting, and allows some comparison with the gain parameter of a second order analysis [14,15,19].

Statistics

Data were expressed as mean ± standard deviation (SD). Normal distribution of all variables was confirmed by Shapiro–Wilk test and homogeneity of the variances was assured by Levene's test.

Repeated-measures ANOVA with lower-bound adjustments for degrees of freedom were applied to compare absolute and relative data in the three positions — supine, sitting and HUT. Simple contrasts were applied to compare each two different positions in case of statistical significance, which was assumed for $p < 0.05$.

Results

Table 1 shows absolute resting values and relative maximal and stable phase (last 20 s) variations to visual stimulation of HR, mean ABP, mean BFV, CVRi, CrCP, and RAP, for PCA and MCA, in supine, sitting and HUT conditions.

Regarding only resting values, repeated-measures ANOVA showed a step increase in HR from supine to HUT positions ($p = 0.0001$), and of mean ABP from supine to sitting ($p = 0.0004$), then stabilizing. There was a step decrease in mean BFV of MCA from supine to HUT conditions ($p = 0.0004$) but for the PCA it seemed to remain constant ($p = 0.054$) in all positions. Concerning resting data of cerebrovascular resistance models, RAP did not change between different positions, while CVRi and CrCP resting values progressively increased from supine to HUT conditions, in both MCA ($p = 0.00001$ and $p = 0.0002$, respectively) and PCA ($p = 0.0002$ and $p = 0.00005$, respectively), although not reaching statistical significance between sitting and HUT in the case of CVRi of PCA ($p = 0.053$).

The variation of the parameters with visual stimulation can be visualized in Fig. 1A–F. Mean BFV in the PCA, had similar responses to visual stimulation in all positions (Fig. 1A, maximal $p = 0.076$; stable phase $p = 0.176$). All cerebrovascular resistance parameters decreased with visual stimulation in the three positions, but showed different patterns in response to orthostatic challenge: variation of CrCP diminished progressively between supine and HUT (maximal and stable phase $p = 0.001$); CVRi decreased slightly but significantly more from sitting to HUT positions (maximal $p = 0.036$; stable phase $p = 0.033$). RAP seemed to have decreased more in HUT conditions but there was no statistical significance (maximal $p = 0.077$; stable phase $p = 0.188$).

Although the MCA territory was used as a control, being theoretically a non-stimulated territory, it registered, similarly across all conditions, a small amplitude increment in mean BFV (5–10%), as well as a decrement of CVRi (6–9%), RAP (9–11%) and CrCP (11–17%) at maximal evoked flow phase, which then tended to decrease in the stable phase. For the MCA significant changes were only observed for BFV in maximal ($p = 0.035$) and CVRi in maximal ($p = 0.029$) and stable phases ($p = 0.043$).

Regarding systemic hemodynamic data, the changes of ABP and HR with stimulation ranged no more than 4%, with no significant differences between positions, except for maximal increment of ABP which was inferior during HUT compared to supine condition ($p = 0.045$).

Discussion

Main findings

We confirmed previous findings showing that the BFV response to a reading paradigm was not altered by different orthostatic challenges [15], but have also demonstrated that the sensitivity of NVC to orthostasis is in fact manifested by regulatory mechanisms influencing the instantaneous pressure–velocity relationship.

Specifically, variation of CrCP following visual stimulation was progressively reduced, more than a half, during orthostatic challenge. Opposed to this pattern, RAP and CVRi seemed to decrease slightly more during HUT. From the changes in CVRi, one would assume that despite rising baseline resting values with seating and HUT, the correspondingly larger decreases with orthostasis during NVC activation (Table 1) would simply reflect arteriolar vasodilation to match the increased demand for O_2. The problems with the single-parameter model of CVR are two-fold. First, it has been demonstrated that instantaneous pressure–velocity relationships of the cerebral circulation do not tend to intercept the pressure axis at the origin [20,22]. Second, CVRi cannot explain the complexities of the interplay between NVC and dynamic cerebral autoregulation [32]. This complexity can be appreciated by the changes in CrCP and RAP. Although the temporal response of RAP (Fig. 1) was not significantly different for the three body positions considered, overall it tends to reflect the myogenic response of dynamic

Table 1 Absolute resting values and relative maximal and stable phase (last 20 s) variations to visual stimulation of HR, mean ABP, mean BFV, CVRi, CrCP, and RAP, for PCA and MCA, in supine, sitting and HUT conditions.

	Supine	Sitting	Tilt	ANOVA p¶
HR				
Resting (bpm)	68.7 ± 9.4	76.3 ± 11.9*	86.3 ± 9.0*,†	0.0001
Maximal vel. phase (%)	4.4 ± 3.3	2.9 ± 3.2	2.8 ± 2.0	0.279
Stable phase (%)	0.7 ± 2.6	0.2 ± 3.6	−1.4 ± 2.6	0.067
Mean ABP				
Resting (mmHg)	73.2 ± 11.7	89.8 ± 9.3*	93.8 ± 9.7*	0.0004
Maximal vel. phase (%)	3.2 ± 2.0	2.1 ± 1.2	1.4 ± 1.2*	0.045
Stable phase (%)	−0.2 ± 1.6	−0.5 ± 1.6	−1.1 ± 2.0	0.223
MCA				
Mean BFV				
Resting (mmHg cm^{-1} s^{-2})	60.4 ± 12.4	56.0 ± 10.6*	52.1 ± 10.1*,†	0.0004
Maximal vel. phase (%)	5.5 ± 1.7	7.0 ± 2.5	9.5 ± 4.2*	0.035
Stable phase (%)	1.2 ± 3.1	2.1 ± 2.7	4.7 ± 3.8	0.011
CVRi				
Resting (mmHg cm^{-1} s^{-2})	1.3 ± 0.4	1.6 ± 0.2*	1.9 ± 0.3*,†	0.00002
Maximal vel. phase (%)	−6.2 ± 2.7	−6.0 ± 1.7	−9.3 ± 3.7*,†	0.029
Stable phase (%)	−1.9 ± 4.4	−3.0 ± 1.8	−6.0 ± 3.8*,†	0.043
RAP				
Resting (mmHg cm^{-1} s^{-2})	0.8 ± 0.2	0.9 ± 0.2	0.8 ± 0.1	0.338
Maximal vel. phase (%)	−11.2 ± 8.0	−8.8 ± 5.4	−11.0 ± 4.2	0.567
Stable phase (%)	−2.5 ± 5.4	−1.5 ± 3.5	−1.5 ± 3.3	0.773
CrCP				
Resting (mmHg)	26.5 ± 13.9	42.4 ± 9.0*	51.5 ± 9.1*,†	0.0004
Maximal vel. phase (%)	−17.3 ± 12.3	−11.2 ± 6.6	−11.0 ± 5.6	0.061
Stable phase (%)	0.5 ± 6.5	−1.7 ± 4.9	−4.7 ± 3.6	0.070
PCA				
Mean BFV				
Resting (mmHg cm^{-1} s^{-2})	36.7 ± 6.8	33.6 ± 6.7	33.0 ± 5.8	0.054
Maximal vel. phase (%)	−32.0 ± 6.4	−33.9 ± 9.5	−37.7 ± 8.1	0.076
Stable phase (%)	−23.4 ± 5.6	−24.2 ± 7.6	−26.4 ± 6.8	0.176
CVRi				
Resting (mmHg cm^{-1} s^{-2})	2.1 ± 0.6	2.8 ± 0.6*	2.9 ± 0.6*	0.00006
Maximal vel. phase (%)	−25.0 ± 4.5	−25.2 ± 4.9	−27.6 ± 3.7*,†	0.039
Stable phase (%)	−21.5 ± 5.1	−22.4 ± 4.8	−24.9 ± 4.4*,†	0.033
RAP				
Resting (mmHg cm^{-1} s^{-2})	1.2 ± 0.3	1.3 ± 0.3	1.2 ± 0.2	0.077
Maximal vel. phase (%)	−15.6 ± 5.6	−14.7 ± 4.9	−19.9 ± 6.1	0.077
Stable phase (%)	−9.4 ± 5.4	−6.4 ± 6.1	−11.4 ± 8.3	0.188
CrCP				
Resting (mmHg)	29.3 ± 9.9	46.6 ± 7.0*	56.5 ± 9.4*,†	0.00002
Maximal vel. phase (%)	−44.1 ± 19.9	−27.2 ± 12.8*	−18.9 ± 6.3*,†	0.001
Stable phase (%)	−27.2 ± 12.2	−17.9 ± 10.0*	−11.7 ± 5.1*,†	0.001

Heart rate (HR), arterial blood pressure (ABP), middle cerebral artery (MCA), posterior cerebral artery (PCA), cerebral blood flow velocity (BFV), cerebrovascular resistance index (CVRi), resistance area product (RAP), critical closing pressure (CrCP). Resting and activation values are presented in mean ± SD and normalized percentual variation, respectively.
¶ Repeated-measures ANOVA p test comparing three positions.
* Repeated-measures ANOVA $p < 0.05$ for contrast to supine position.
† Repeated-measures ANOVA $p < 0.05$ for contrast between sitting and head-up tilt position.

autoregulation, mainly as a compensation for the drop in ABP following neural stimulation (Fig. 1E). It is likely that some of its change also contributed to the rise in CBV during the response (Fig. 1A). On the other hand, it can be speculated that the changes in CrCP are mainly reflecting the action of metabolic mechanisms [22,33]. If this is the case, then it is not possible to say that the NVC response to reading is entirely indifferent to orthostasis, since reading and HUT seem to require less metabolic-coupled changes than responses in the supine position.

Some studies have shown significant [30,35—37] or no statistically significant [38] increases in ABP and HR during mental activation. Moody et al. [30] analysed the hemodynamic changes of cerebral and systemic responses, putting

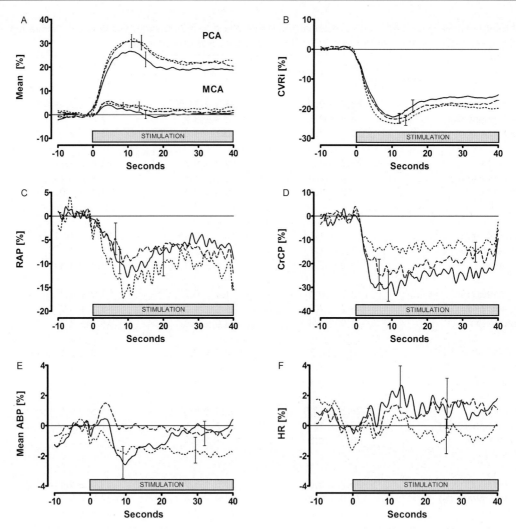

Figure 1 Group averaged normalized mean BFV (A), CVRi (B), RAP(C) and CrCP (D) of PCA [and mean BFV of MCA as a control (A)] and mean ABP (E) and HR (F) changes before and during 40 s of reading task (gray bar at bottom) in supine (*continuous line*), sitting (*dashed line*) and tilt (*dotted line*) positions. For clarity, only the largest ±SE is represented at the point of occurrence. (First 10 s of resting phase not shown only for graphical proposal.)

into evidence an initial ABP peak, ~5 s after MCA cortical activation, that would drive an early-phase cerebral vasoconstriction reflected in increased CVRi and RAP, followed by metabolic vasodilatation. Our results showed non-significant changes in HR and ABP responses. A watchful eye through the curves of ABP in Fig. 1E might identify an initial ABP peak at ~5 s only at sitting condition. Also, the previously described possible initial 'vasoconstriction response' [30] could not be demonstrated. With the same as ours activation paradigm, Rosengarten et al. [37] found no relevance of HR effects in regulative features of the activity—flow coupling during reading task. A possible explanation to discrepant findings between the studies can be a less demanding visual paradigm related to the PCA territory as compared to MCA-activation paradigm, rendering a less pronounced systemic/sympathetic response. On the other hand, even in a PCA evoked flow paradigm a small activation can sometimes be measured in the MCA territory, as in our study, which might reflect some activation of cortical areas, probably related to visual processing.

Limitations of the study

CO_2, a major determinant of cerebrovascular tone [31,33,34], was not evaluated, and could have influenced our results. However, we can speculate that relative hypocapnia in orthostasis [34], namely during HUT, and an assumed inverse relationship between CO_2 and CrCP [22], would cause absolute CrCP to increase from supine to HUT conditions and also would prevent a substantial decrease with cortical activation in HUT. Also, it is known that induced hypocapnia impairs NVC with a similar experimental protocol [29]. Given that these changes were not observed in our study, it is more likely that $PaCO_2$ remained relatively constant during the orthostatic challenges. The importance of CO_2 changes during mental activation was studied previously in a MCA-based protocol which analysed also CrCP—RAP variations [30] and found significant changes of CO_2 interacting with cerebral and systemic hemodynamic parameters. Nevertheless, the study by Moody et al. [35] adopted cognitive paradigms that can be much more stressful than plain reading and hence might have caused significantly greater hyperventilation.

Conclusions

Taken together, we conclude that NVC has different pressure-autoregulatory adaptation mechanisms with orthostatic challenge, in spite of preserved cerebral evoked flow responses.

Analysis of the NVC response to reading based solely on the inspection of the BFV amplitude response gives the false impression of a lack of effect of orthostatic challenges. In reality, by looking separately at changes in RAP and CrCP, it is possible to appreciate the complex interplay of these responses at different levels of orthostatic challenge. Further work is needed to assess the response of these mechanisms in different cerebrovascular conditions and their potential diagnostic and prognostic value.

References

[1] Iadecola C. Neurovascular regulation in the normal brain and in Alzheimer's disease. Nat Rev 2004;5(5):347—60.
[2] Iadecola C. Regulation of the cerebral microcirculation during neural activity: is nitric oxide the missing link? Trends Neurosci 1993;16(6):206—14.
[3] Hossmann KA. Viability thresholds and the penumbra of focal ischemia. Ann Neurol 1994;36(4):557—65.
[4] Aaslid R, Lindegaard KF, Sorteberg W, Nornes H. Cerebral autoregulation dynamics in humans. Stroke: J Cereb Circ 1989;20(1):45—52.
[5] Paulson OB, Strandgaard S, Edvinsson L. Cerebral autoregulation. Cerebrovasc Brain Metab Rev 1990;2(2):161—92.
[6] Lin WH, Hao Q, Rosengarten B, Leung WH, Wong KS. Impaired neurovascular coupling in ischaemic stroke patients with large or small vessel disease. Eur J Neurol 2010;18(5):731—6.
[7] Rosengarten B, Paulsen S, Burr O, Kaps M. Neurovascular coupling in Alzheimer patients: effect of acetylcholine-esterase inhibitors. Neurobiol Aging 2009;30(12):1918—23.
[8] Azevedo E, Castro P, Santos R, Freitas J, Coelho T, Rosengarten B, et al. Autonomic dysfunction affects cerebral neurovascular coupling. Clin Auton Res 2011.
[9] Hamel E. Perivascular nerves and the regulation of cerebrovascular tone. J Appl Physiol 2006;100(3):1059—64.
[10] Iadecola C, Nedergaard M. Glial regulation of the cerebral microvasculature. Nat Neurosci 2007;10(11):1369—76.
[11] Cox SB, Woolsey TA, Rovainen CM. Localized dynamic changes in cortical blood flow with whisker stimulation corresponds to matched vascular and neuronal architecture of rat barrels. J Cereb Blood Flow Metab 1993;13(6):899—913.
[12] Ngai AC, Ko KR, Morii S, Winn HR. Effect of sciatic nerve stimulation on pial arterioles in rats. Am J Physiol 1988;254(1 (Pt 2)):H133—9.
[13] Silva AC, Lee SP, Iadecola C, Kim SG. Early temporal characteristics of cerebral blood flow and deoxyhemoglobin changes during somatosensory stimulation. J Cereb Blood Flow Metab 2000;20(1):201—6.
[14] Rosengarten B, Huwendiek O, Kaps M. Neurovascular coupling and cerebral autoregulation can be described in terms of a control system. Ultrasound Med Biol 2001;27(2):189—93.
[15] Azevedo E, Rosengarten B, Santos R, Freitas J, Kaps M. Interplay of cerebral autoregulation and neurovascular coupling evaluated by functional TCD in different orthostatic conditions. J Neurol 2007;254(2):236—41.
[16] Omboni S, Parati G, Frattola A, Mutti E, Di Rienzo M, Castiglioni P, et al. Spectral and sequence analysis of finger blood pressure variability. Comparison with analysis of intra-arterial recordings. Hypertension 1993;22(1):26—33.
[17] Azevedo E, Santos R, Freitas J, Rosas MJ, Gago M, Garrett C, et al. Deep brain stimulation does not change neurovascular coupling in non-motor visual cortex: an autonomic and visual evoked blood flow velocity response study. Parkinsonism Relat Disord 2010;16(9):600—3.
[18] Aaslid R, Markwalder TM, Nornes H. Noninvasive transcranial Doppler ultrasound recording of flow velocity in basal cerebral arteries. J Neurosurg 1982;57(6):769—74.
[19] Rosengarten B, Huwendiek O, Kaps M. Neurovascular coupling in terms of a control system: validation of a second-order linear system model. Ultrasound Med Biol 2001;27(5): 631—5.
[20] Aaslid R, Lash SR, Bardy GH, Gild WH, Newell DW. Dynamic pressure—flow velocity relationships in the human cerebral circulation. Stroke: J Cereb Circ 2003;34(7): 1645—9.
[21] Dawson SL, Panerai RB, Potter JF. Critical closing pressure explains cerebral hemodynamics during the Valsalva maneuver. J Appl Physiol 1999;86(2):675—80.
[22] Panerai RB. The critical closing pressure of the cerebral circulation. Med Eng Phys 2003;25(8):621—32.
[23] Evans DH, Levene MI, Shortland DB, Archer LN. Resistance index, blood flow velocity, and resistance-area product in the cerebral arteries of very low birth weight infants during the first week of life. Ultrasound Med Biol 1988;14(2):103—10.
[24] Aaslid R. Cerebral hemodynamics. New York: Raven Press; 1992.
[25] Conrad B, Klingelhofer J. Dynamics of regional cerebral blood flow for various visual stimuli. Exp Brain Res 1989;77(2):437—41.
[26] Gomez SM, Gomez CR, Hall IS. Transcranial Doppler ultrasonographic assessment of intermittent light stimulation at different frequencies. Stroke: J Cereb Circ 1990;21(12): 1746—8.
[27] Wittich I, Klingelhöfer J, Sander D, Schwarze JJ. Visual evoked perfusion changes in the posterior cerebral artery during activity of various visual field sections. In: Klingelhöfer J, Bartels E, Ringelstein EB, Ebner TJ, editors. New trends in cerebral hemodynamics and neurosonology. Doetinchen: Elsevier; 1997. p. 548—56.
[28] Sturzenegger M, Newell DW, Aaslid R. Visually evoked blood flow response assessed by simultaneous two-channel transcranial Doppler using flow velocity averaging. Stroke: J Cereb Circ 1996;27(12):2256—61.
[29] Szabo K, Lako E, Juhasz T, Rosengarten B, Csiba L, Olah L. Hypocapnia induced vasoconstriction significantly inhibits the neurovascular coupling in humans. J Neurol Sci 2011;309(1—2):58—62.
[30] Moody M, Panerai RB, Eames PJ, Potter JF. Cerebral and systemic hemodynamic changes during cognitive and motor activation paradigms. Am J Physiol Regul Integr Comp Physiol 2005;288(6):R1581—8.
[31] Carey BJ, Eames PJ, Panerai RB, Potter JF. Carbon dioxide, critical closing pressure and cerebral haemodynamics prior to vasovagal syncope in humans. Clin Sci (Lond) 2001;101(4):351—8.
[32] Panerai RB, Moody M, Eames PJ, Potter JF. Cerebral blood flow velocity during mental activation: interpretation with different models of the passive pressure—velocity relationship. J Appl Physiol 2005;99(6):2352—62.
[33] Ainslie PN, Duffin J. Integration of cerebrovascular CO_2 reactivity and chemoreflex control of breathing: mechanisms of regulation, measurement, and interpretation. Am J Physiol Regul Integr Comp Physiol 2009;296(5):R1473—95.

[34] Serrador JM, Hughson RL, Kowalchuk JM, Bondar RL, Gelb AW. Cerebral blood flow during orthostasis: role of arterial CO_2. Am J Physiol Regul Integr Comp Physiol 2006;290(4): R1087—93.

[35] Sitzer M, Knorr U, Seitz RJ. Cerebral hemodynamics during sensorimotor activation in humans. J Appl Physiol 1994;77(6):2804—11.

[36] Tiecks FP, Haberl RL, Newell DW. Temporal patterns of evoked cerebral blood flow during reading. J Cereb Blood Flow Metab 1998;18(7):735—41.

[37] Rosengarten B, Budden C, Osthaus S, Kaps M. Effect of heart rate on regulative features of the cortical activity—flow coupling. Cerebrovasc Dis 2003;16(1): 47—52.

[38] Klingelhofer J, Matzander G, Sander D, Schwarze J, Boecker H, Bischoff C. Assessment of functional hemispheric asymmetry by bilateral simultaneous cerebral blood flow velocity monitoring. J Cereb Blood Flow Metab 1997;17(5): 577—85.

Are impaired endothelial function in the posterior cerebral circulation and intact endothelial function in the anterior cerebral and systemic circulation associated with migraine: A post hoc study

Denis Perko*, Janja Pretnar-Oblak, Bojana Žvan, Marjan Zaletel

University Medical Centre Ljubljana, Department of Neurology, Zaloška Cesta 2, 1000 Ljubljana, Slovenia

KEYWORDS
Transcranial Doppler;
Flow mediated dilatation;
Endothelium;
Dysfunction;
Migraine;
Association

Summary It seems that migraine patients might suffer from localized and not systemic endothelial dysfunction. However, the probability whether impaired endothelial function in the posterior cerebral circulation, and intact endothelial function elsewhere is associated with migraine is not known. This is a post hoc study based on two of our previous published studies that evaluated cerebral and systemic endothelial function in 40 migraine patients (20 with (MwA) and 20 without aura (MwoA)) without comorbidities, and 20 healthy subjects. Cerebrovascular reactivity (CVR) to L-arginine in the middle (MCA) and posterior (PCA) cerebral artery as well as flow mediated vasodilatation (FMD) were used for this purpose. The logistic regression analysis was used to evaluate the association between CVR to L-arginine, FMD and migraine. We found a significant association between CVR to L-arginine in the PCA and migraine (OR: 0.38; CI 95%: 0.19–0.79; $p=0.01$), but not between CVR to L-arginine in the MCA and migraine (OR: 0.74; CI 95%: 0.34–1.59; $p=0.44$). Similar results were obtained in MwA and MwoA. We did not find any significant association between FMD and migraine (OR: 0.99; CI 95%: 0.83–1.19; $p=0.96$). The same conclusion was reached in both migraine groups (MwA OR: 1.0; CI 95%: 0.83–1.19; $p=0.99$, MwoA OR: 0.99; CI 95%: 0.81–1.21; $p=0.99$). We could conclude that impaired endothelial function in the posterior cerebral circulation is associated with migraine, both MwA and MwoA, while intact endothelial function in the anterior cerebral and systemic circulation is not associated only with migraine.
© 2012 Elsevier GmbH. All rights reserved.

Introduction

There is some evidence that migraine patients might have endothelial dysfunction [1]. In this context, it is proposed that migraine could lead to endothelial dysfunction or endothelial dysfunction could lead to migraine [1]. Nevertheless, endothelial dysfunction could be important in the pathophysiology of vascular diseases in migraine patients. Namely, several studies have shown that migraine is associated with disorders of the cerebrovascular, coronary, retinal and peripheral vasculatures [1]. However, it must be emphasized that in many studies the authors did not exclude vascular risk factors, or perhaps, besides excluding

* Corresponding author. Tel.: +386 1 522 37 38; fax: +386 1 522 22 08.
E-mail address: perkodenis@yahoo.com (D. Perko).

many vascular risk factors, they did not evaluate carotid intima—media thickness (IMT), a morphological marker of the early atherosclerotic process [2—7]. Therefore, all the already mentioned vascular disorders in migraine patients might be a consequence of vascular risk factors, or of an unrecognized atherosclerotic process.

Despite this fact, it was still unclear whether endothelial dysfunction in migraine patients could be isolated or systemic. In accordance with that, we have conducted two studies to assess whether migraine patients have systemic or just isolated cerebral endothelial dysfunction [8,9]. The methods of cerebrovascular reactivity (CVR) to L-arginine and flow-mediated vasodilatation (FMD) were used to assess the anterior and posterior cerebral and systemic endothelial function [10—17]. We also measured carotid IMT, gathered medical history, performed physical and neurological examinations, as well as ran clinical laboratory tests. Only migraine patients without comorbidities and with normal IMT were included.

In our first study we have shown that migraine patients without comorbidities, both with or without aura, might have intact systemic endothelial function [8].

In our second study we have found reduced vasodilatatory capacity in the territory of the posterior cerebral artery (PCA), and intact in the territory of the middle cerebral artery (MCA) which could indicate impaired cerebral endothelial function in the posterior cerebral circulation in migraine patients without comorbidities [9].

The aim of this post hoc study was to evaluate whether impaired endothelial function of the posterior cerebral circulation and intact endothelial function of the anterior cerebral and systemic circulation are associated with migraine. These comparisons have not yet been performed.

Materials and methods

This post hoc study was performed using data obtained from our two previous studies, which were approved by the National Medical Ethics Committee of the Republic of Slovenia. Forty migraine patients and twenty healthy subjects participated. All subjects gave written informed consent before being included in the study. Migraine patients were diagnosed according to the International Headache Society criteria (2nd edition) [18]. Healthy subjects were randomly selected from hospital staff and acquaintances after completing a questionnaire. Migraine patients were randomly selected from a headache clinic. All subjects had a normal somatic and neurological examination. Migraine patients were divided into two groups, 20 patients with migraine with aura (MwA), and 20 patients without aura (MwoA). The three groups were matched for gender and age. None of the subjects in the control group were suffering from headache when the study was conducted, and none had migraine or other headache. Migraine patients had the last migraine episode more than 24 h before the investigations were conducted.

The major exclusion criteria were: history of cardiovascular disease, arterial hypertension (systolic blood pressure (SBP) > 140 mmHg or diastolic blood pressure (DBP) > 90 mmHg), body mass index (BMI) < 18 and $\geq 25\,kg/m^2$, hypercholesterolemia (total cholesterol > 5.5 mmol/L), diabetes, IMT > 1.0 mm, pregnancy or lactation and regular use of vasoactive drugs (except triptane, or other transient vasoactive antimigraine drugs). Therefore, all subjects had normal values of SBP, DBP, BMI, total cholesterol, HDL, LDL, triglycerides, IMT, and glucose [8,9].

Color-coded duplex sonography of the carotid and vertebral arteries was performed with all patients. IMT was measured according to the Mannheim Intima—Media Thickness Consensus on both sides 2 cm below the bifurcation on the far wall of the common carotid artery [19]. The distance between the characteristic echoes from the lumen—intima and media—adventitia interfaces was measured. The final IMT value was based on the mean value of three maximal IMT measurements. Subjects with plaques (focal structures that encroached into the arterial lumen of at least 0.5 mm or 50% of the surrounding IMT value or demonstrated a thickness > 1.5 mm) were excluded from the study.

FMD of the right brachial artery was performed according to the recommendations of Corretti et al. in a quiet room under constant conditions between 7.30 and 10.30 am after a fasting period of at least 10 h [20]. A high-resolution ultrasound system with a 10-MHz linear array transducer located 2—10 cm above the antecubital fossa was used. The brachial artery was scanned in the longitudinal section, and the end-diastolic mean arterial diameter was measured at the end of the diastole period, incident with the R-wave on the simultaneously recorded electrocardiogram. A hyperemic flow increase was then induced by inflation of a blood pressure cuff to a pressure of 50 mm Hg higher than the measured systolic blood pressure for 4 min. The hyperemic diameter was recorded within 1 min after cuff deflation, and the final scan was performed 4 min later. FMD was expressed as the percentage change in the artery diameter after reactive hyperemia relative to the baseline scan.

CVR to L-arginine was simultaneously measured in the anterior and posterior cerebral circulation. For this purpose, the middle (MCA) and the posterior cerebral artery (PCA) were chosen. The experiment consisted of a 10-min baseline period, a 30-min intravenous infusion of 100 mL 30% L-arginine, and a 10-min period after L-arginine application. The mean arterial velocity (v_m) in the MCA was recorded through the left temporal acoustic window at a depth of 50—60 mm, and in the PCA through the right temporal acoustic window at a depth of 50—60 mm, with a mechanical probe holder maintaining a constant probe position. TCD Multi-Dop X4 software was used to determine v_m during the 5-min baseline period and the 5-min period after L-arginine infusion. CVR to L-arginine in the PCA and the MCA was expressed as the percentage change in the v_m after stimulation with L-arginine.

The variables FMD, CVR, migraine and healthy subjects were statistically analyzed by the statistic software SPSS 18.0. For this purpose, binary logistic regression analysis was used to analyze a possible association between FMD, CVR and migraine. The dependent variable was the presence of migraine (yes = 1, no = 0). In a further analysis, the dependent variable was the presence of migraine type (MwA = 1, MwoA = 0). Independent variables CVR to L-arginine in the MCA, CVR to L-arginine in the PCA and FMD were transformed into attributive variables.

Table 1 The association of cerebrovascular reactivity (CVR) to L-arginine in the posterior cerebral artery (PCA) and in the middle cerebral artery (MCA) with migraine.

	B	P	Exp (B) or OR	CI 95%
CVR PCA	−0.95	0.01	0.38	0.19—0.79
CVR MCA	−0.29	0.44	0.74	0.34—1.59

Table 2 The association of CVR to L-arginine in the PCA and the MCA with migraine with (MwA) and without aura (MwoA).

	B	P	Exp (B) or OR	CI 95%
CVR PCA MwA	−0.93	0.01	0.39	0.19—0.80
CVR PCA MwoA	−1.01	0.02	0.36	0.15—0.86
CVR MCA MwA	−0.33	0.39	0.71	0.33—1.54
CVR MCA MwoA	−0.34	0.47	0.71	0.27—1.83

Table 3 The association of flow mediated dilatation (FMD) with migraine, and separately with migraine with (MwA) and without aura (MwoA).

	B	P	Exp (B) or OR	CI 95%
FMD	−0.00	0.96	0.99	0.83—1.19
FMD MwA	0.00	0.99	1.00	0.83—1.19
FMD MwoA	−0.01	0.99	0.99	0.81—1.21

Results

In step one, we evaluated a possible association of CVR to L-arginine in the MCA and the PCA with migraine, and also of CVR to L-arginine in the MCA and the PCA with MwA and MwoA.

We found a significant negative association between CVR to L-arginine in the PCA and migraine ($p = 0.01$), but not between CVR to L-arginine in the MCA and migraine ($p = 0.44$). The results are summarized in Table 1.

Similarly, we found a significant negative association between CVR to L-arginine in the PCA on MwA ($p = 0.01$) and between CVR to L-arginine in the PCA and MwoA ($p = 0.02$). Again we did not find any association between CVR to L-arginine in the MCA and MwA ($p = 0.39$) and also between CVR to L-arginine and MwoA ($p = 0.47$). The results are summarized in Table 2.

In step two, we evaluated a possible association of FMD with migraine, and repeated the procedure separately with MwA and MwoA. The results are represented in Table 3. The binary logistic regression did not show any association between FMD and migraine ($p = 0.96$) and also between FMD and MwA ($p = 0.99$) and MwoA ($p = 0.99$).

Discussion

The main original finding of our post hoc study is that we have found a significant negative association between CVR to L-arginine in the posterior cerebral circulation and migraine, and no association between CVR to L-arginine in the anterior cerebral circulation and migraine.

In recent years it has been proposed that migraine affects not only systemic but also cerebral circulation [1]. Namely, ischemic stroke can occur between or during migraine attacks, particularly in MwA and young women [21—24]. The territory of the posterior cerebral artery is preferentially affected [25]. In addition to clinical strokes, focal ischemic and hyperintensive, ischemic-like lesions have been found in the territory of the posterior cerebral circulation [22,26,27]. In our previous study we showed a lower CVR to L-arginine in the PCA and normal CVR to L-arginine in the MCA in migraine patients without comorbidities compared to healthy subjects [9]. In such circumstances this could be applied to cerebral endothelial dysfunction localized only in the territory of the posterior cerebral circulation. However, a confirmation from another point of view was still missing. For this purpose we analyzed the association between migraine and parameters of systemic, as well as cerebral endothelial function. The findings of this study have shown that impaired posterior cerebral endothelial function could be associated with migraine, while intact anterior cerebral endothelial function could not be only associated with migraine but it could be also attributed to physiological conditions.

The other main finding of our study is that we did not find any association between CVR to L-arginine in the MCA, FMD and migraine. In other words, our study showed that intact endothelial function in the anterior cerebral and systemic circulation could not be only associated with migraine but again this could be also attributed to physiological conditions. This again is in accordance with one of our previous findings that migraine patients without comorbidities and early atherosclerotic process probably have intact systemic endothelial function [8]. This has also been suggested by Vanmolkot and de Hoon [28]. In recent years it has been proposed that migraine is associated with disorders of the coronary, retinal and peripheral vasculature [1]. However, in many studies the authors did not exclude vascular risk factors, or perhaps they excluded many vascular risk factors, but did not evaluate IMT, a morphological marker of the early atherosclerotic process and associated endothelial dysfunction, which consequently might have biased their findings [2—7]. Therefore, according to the previous sentence, the findings of our current and previous studies might suggest that behind vascular disorders could not be systemic endothelial dysfunction but perhaps localized endothelial dysfunction or other pathological vascular conditions.

Conclusion

Taking into account all the presented findings of this and previous studies, the following can be concluded in migraine patients without comorbidities: (I) impaired endothelial function in the posterior cerebral circulation is associated with migraine; (II) intact endothelial function in the anterior cerebral and systemic circulation is not associated only with migraine.

Acknowledgments

The authors express their gratitude to Valentin Beznik and Marjeta Švigelj for technical assistance, and especially to all the volunteers.

References

[1] Tietjen GE. Migraine as a systemic vasculopathy. Cephalalgia 2009;29:989—96.
[2] Stang PE, Carson AP, Rose KM, Mo J, Ephross SA, Shahar E, et al. Headache, cerebrovascular symptoms, and stroke: the Atherosclerosis Risk in Communities Study. Neurology 2005;64:1573—7.
[3] Rose KM, Wong TY, Carson AP, Couper DJ, Klein R, Sharrett AR. Migraine and retinal microvascular abnormalities: the Atherosclerosis Risk in Communities Study. Neurology 2007;68:1694—700.
[4] Tietjen GE, Al Qasmi MM, Shukairy MS. Livedo reticularis and migraine: a marker for stroke risk? Headache 2002;42:352—5.
[5] O'Keeffe ST, Tsapatsaris NP, Beetham Jr WP. Association between Raynaud's phenomenon and migraine in a random population of hospital employees. J Rheumatol 1993;20:1187—8.
[6] Yetkin E, Ozisik H, Ozcan C, Aksoy Y, Turhan H. Increased dilator response to nitrate and decreased flow-mediated dilatation in migraineurs. Headache 2007;47:104—10.
[7] Silva FA, Rueda-Clausen CF, Silva SY, Zarruk JG, Guzmían JC, Morillo CA, et al. Endothelial function in patients with migraine during the interictal period. Headache 2007;47:45—51.
[8] Perko D, Pretnar-Oblak J, Sabovic M, Zvan B, Zaletel M. Endothelium-dependent vasodilatation in migraine patients. Cephalalgia 2011;31(6):654—60.
[9] Perko D, Pretnar-Oblak J, Sabovič M, Zvan B, Zaletel M. Cerebrovascular reactivity to L-arginine in the anterior and posterior cerebral circulation in migraine patients. Acta Neurol Scand 2011;124:269—74.
[10] Micieli G, Bosone D, Zappoli F, Marcheselli S, Argenteri A, Nappi G. Vasomotor response to CO_2 and L-arginine in patients with severe internal carotid artery stenosis; pre- and postsurgical evaluation with transcranial Doppler. J Neurol Sci 1999;163:153—8.
[11] Okamoto M, Etani H, Yagita Y, Kinoshita N, Nukada T. Diminished reserve for cerebral vasomotor response to L-arginine in the elderly: evaluation by transcranial Doppler sonography. Gerontology 2001;47:131—5.
[12] Zvan B, Zaletel M, Pogačnik T, Kiauta T. Testing of cerebral endothelium function with L-arginine after stroke. Int Angiol 2002;21:256—9.
[13] Zimmermann C, Wimmer M, Haberl RL. L-Arginine-mediated vasoreactivity in patients with risk of stroke. Cerebrovasc Dis 2004;17:128—33.
[14] Rosenblum WI, Nishimura H, Nelson GH. Endothelial dependent L-arginin and L-NMMA-sensitive mechanisms regulate tone of brain microvessels. Am J Physiol 1990;259:H1395—401.
[15] Reutens DC, McHugh MD, Toussaint PJ, Evans AC, Gjedde A, Meyer E, et al. L-Arginine infusion increases basal but not activated cerebral blood flow in humans. J Cereb Blood Flow Metab 1997;17:309—15.
[16] Raitakari OT, Celermajer DS. Flow-mediated dilatation. Br J Clin Pharmacol 2000;50:397—404.
[17] Celermajer DS, Sorensen KE, Gooch VM, Spiegelhalter DJ, Miller OI, Sullivan ID, et al. Non-invasive detection of endothelial dysfunction in children and adults at risk of atherosclerosis. Lancet 1992;340:1111—5.
[18] Olesen J. The international classification of headache disorders. 2nd ed. (ICHD-II). Rev Neurol (Paris) 2005;161:689—91.
[19] Touboul PJ, Hennerici MG, Meairs S, Adams H, Amarenco P, Desvarieux M, et al. Advisory board of the 3rd watching the risk symposium. 13th European stroke conference. Mannheim intima—media thickness consensus. Cerebrovasc Dis 2004;18:346—9.
[20] Corretti MC, Anderson TJ, Benjamin EJ, Celermajer D, Charbonneau F, Creager MA, et al. Guidelines for the ultrasound assessment of endothelial-dependent flow-mediated vasodilation of the brachial artery. A report of the international brachial artery reactivity task force. J Am Coll Cardiol 2002;39:257—65.
[21] Bousser MG, Welch KM. Relation between migraine and stroke. Lancet Neurol 2005;4:533—42.
[22] Kruit MC, Launer LJ, Ferrari MD, van Buchem MA. Infarcts in the posterior circulation territory in migraine. The population-based MRI CAMERA study. Brain 2005;128:2068—77.
[23] Tzourio C, Tehindrazanarivelo A, Iglesias S, Alperovitch A, Chedru F, D'Anglejan-Chatillon J, et al. Case—control study of migraine and risk of ischemic stroke in young women. BMJ 1995;310:830—3.
[24] Kurth T, Gaziano JM, Cook NR, Logroscino G, Diener HC, Buring JE. Migraine and risk of cardiovascular disease in women. JAMA 2006;296:283—91.
[25] Broderick JP, Swanson JW. Migraine-related strokes. Clinical profile and prognosis in 20 patients. Arch Neurol 1987;44(8):868—71.
[26] Kruit MC, Launer LJ, Ferrari MD, van Buchem MA. Brain stem and cerebellar hyperintense lesions in migraine. Stroke 2006;37:1109—12.
[27] Milhaud D, Bogousslavsky YJ, Melle G, Liot P. Ischemic stroke and active migraine. Neurology 2001;57:1805—11.
[28] Vanmolkot FH, de Hoon JN. Endothelial function in migraine: a cross-sectional study. BMC Neurol 2010;10:119.

Effect of helium on cerebral blood flow: A n = 1 trial in a healthy young person

Sanne M. Zinkstok[a], Daniela Bertens[b], Jelle R. de Kruijk[c], Selma C. Tromp[d,*]

[a] Department of Neurology, Academic Medical Center, University of Amsterdam, PO Box 22660, 1100 DD Amsterdam, The Netherlands
[b] Department of Neurology, VU University Medical Center, De Boelelaan 1117, 1081 HV Amsterdam, The Netherlands
[c] Department of Neurology, Tergooiziekenhuizen, Rijksstraatweg 1, 1261 AN Blaricum, The Netherlands
[d] Department of Clinical Neurophysiology, St. Antonius Hospital, PO Box 2500, 3430 EM Nieuwegein, The Netherlands

KEYWORDS
Transcranial Doppler;
Helium;
Heliox

Summary Several experimental studies have shown that noble gases can have neuroprotective effects in cerebral ischemia. The exact mechanism is unknown; increased cerebral blood flow may play a role. In order to investigate this concept we performed a n = 1 trial measuring cerebral blood flow velocity by means of transcranial Doppler (TCD) in a healthy young woman inhaling air or heliox. Peak systolic velocity, mean flow velocity and pulsatility index were measured in the right middle cerebral artery, and oxygen saturation and heart rate were measured with pulse oximetry. After a baseline of 3 min breathing normal air, heliox (79% helium, 21% oxygen) was inhaled though an oral nasal mask for 5 min, followed by a washout period of 5 min breathing normal air. This protocol was repeated four times. No significant changes were observed in hemodynamic parameters, except for a small increase in pulsatility index during heliox inhalation (from 0.91 to 0.95; $p = 0.01$).

In conclusion, inhalation of heliox does not influence cerebral blood flow in a healthy young person. Any beneficial effects of helium in stroke patients are more likely due to other neuroprotective effects than to hemodynamic changes.
© 2012 Elsevier GmbH. All rights reserved.

Introduction

Given the narrow therapeutic time window for reperfusion in acute ischemic stroke, there is a strong need for neuroprotective strategies aiming at preservation of tissue at risk for infarction to increase the number of patients eligible for reperfusion. Former clinical trials in neuroprotection led to disappointing results due to poor interpretation and translation from an experimental to a clinical setting.

When selecting agents for neuroprotection not only proof of efficacy but also easy implementation in acute stroke care is of great importance. Gas therapy and especially the noble gas helium might be a promising neuroprotective strategy that meets criteria for every day practical use [1–3]. Helium is directly available in the hyperacute prehospital phase, is well-tolerated and lacks toxicity or interactions [4,5]. The exact neuroprotective mechanism of helium is not well known but egression of nitrogen from neural mitochondria is suggested. This might facilitate oxygen reuptake during

* Corresponding author. Tel.: +31 30 609 2452;
fax: +31 30 609 2327.
E-mail addresses: s.m.zinkstok@amc.uva.nl (S.M. Zinkstok),
d.bertens@vumc.nl (D. Bertens), jdekruijk@tergooiziekenhuizen.nl
(J.R. de Kruijk), s.tromp1@antoniusziekenhuis.nl (S.C. Tromp).

2211-968X/$ — see front matter © 2012 Elsevier GmbH. All rights reserved.
doi:10.1016/j.permed.2012.02.009

Table 1 Results of the measurements in the two conditions.

	Heliox	Room air (washout)	P-Value
MFV (cm/s)	48.5 ± 3.4	47.8 ± 2.8	0.21
PSV (cm/s)	77.0 ± 5.7	75.2 ± 4.7	0.09
PI	0.95 ± 0.07	0.91 ± 0.06	0.01
Oxygen saturation (%)	98.96 ± 0.35	98.94 ± 0.24	0.40
Heart rate (beats/min)	77.6 ± 5.8	76.5 ± 4.6	0.20

MFV = mean flow velocity; PSV = peak systolic velocity; PI = pulsality index. Means and standard deviations are given.

reperfusion [6]. Another supposed mechanism of neuroprotection by gas therapy is an increase of cerebral blood flow. Rats with distal middle cerebral artery occlusion breathing 100% oxygen had an increase in cerebral blood flow (CBF), while infarct size was decreased compared to rats breathing 30% oxygen. Since the concentration of oxyhemoglobin in the infarct core was increased in the 100% oxygen group, a better tissue delivery of oxygen due to a higher CBF might explain the results [7]. On the other hand, increased blood flow might cause reperfusion damage or hypertensive hemorrhage in the infarction area during reperfusion.

Before studying any neuroprotective effect of helium in acute ischemic stroke in humans, it is necessary to know if helium influences cerebral blood flow in healthy people. In order to investigate this, we performed a $n = 1$ trial measuring cerebral blood flow parameters by means of transcranial Doppler (TCD) in a healthy young women alternatingly inhaling air or helium.

Methods

To measure cerebral blood flow TCD was performed with a pulsed Doppler transducer (Pioneer TC4040, EME Überlingen, Germany), gated at a focal depth of 50 mm. Our female 29-year-old healthy volunteer was positioned laying on the back and the transducer (2 MHz) was placed at the right temporal bone. When the main stem of the right middle cerebral artery was found, the transducer was fixed with a head strap. The mean flow velocity (MFV), peak systolic velocity (PSV), and pulsatility index (PI) were measured continuously and recorded every minute. Furthermore, heart rate frequency and blood oxygen saturation were measured with a fingertip monitor (pulse oximetry) in order to exclude possible confounding factors.

At baseline all parameters were measured during 3 min while breathing normal room air. After baseline measurement, Heliox (helium 79%, oxygen 21%) was administered for 5 min using an oral nasal mask. This intervention was followed by a washout of 5 min breathing room air. This block of 5 min Heliox intervention and 5 min washout was repeated four times. At the end, all measurements were performed during another period of 5 min breathing room air.

The null hypothesis was that there would not be any difference in the hemodynamic parameters during helium inhalation or room air inhalation. For analysis we used a one tailed Student's t-test. We considered a P-value of less than 0.05 as statistically significant.

Results

No adverse events occurred during helium administration except for temporary changes in voice pitch. Median baseline values were: MFV 50 cm/s, PSV 79 cm/s, PI 0.92, heart rate 77 min^{-1} and oxygen saturation 99%. Heart rate frequency and blood oxygen saturation were stable and did not differ significantly between the periods of breathing helium and room air. MFV in the right middle cerebral artery as well as the PSV did also not differ significantly in the two test conditions (Table 1).

The PI had a mean of 0.95 in Heliox compared to 0.91 in room air inhalation; this difference was significant with a P-value of 0.01.

Discussion

The present study investigated the effect of helium inhalation on cerebral blood flow in a healthy young person. We found that inhalation of helium did not influence cerebral blood flow as compared to inhalation of room air. The mean flow velocity and peak systolic velocity in the right middle cerebral artery as well as heart rate frequency and blood oxygen saturation did not differ during helium or room air (washout) inhalation.

Although the pulsatility index (PI) was significantly higher during helium inhalation, this effect was only small (0.95 versus 0.91), and the values stayed well within the normal range (0.6—1.1). A rise in PI can have different causes, such as a rise in intracranial pressure with reduced vessel compliance, bradycardia or hyperventilation. In our study the latter two did not contribute to the changes in PI, since heart rate frequency, blood oxygen saturation and cerebral blood flow did not change. Increased intracranial pressure has not been described after inhalation of a mixture of helium and oxygen before, although it has been widely used in pulmonary diseases. In addition, another noble gas xenon has been shown not to have any effect on intracranial pressure [8]. Therefore, increased intracranial pressure is not likely to be the cause of the minimal increase in PI.

In accordance to our findings, Pan et al. [3] did not find any significant differences in hemodynamic parameters in animals breathing helium as compared to animals breathing normal air. The present study confirms these findings in a healthy human being.

Conclusions

Inhalation of helium does not influence cerebral blood flow in a healthy young person. If proven in future, beneficial effects of helium in stroke patients will be more likely due to other neuroprotective effects than to hemodynamic changes.

References

[1] Coburn M, Maze M, Franks NP. The neuroprotective effects of xenon and helium in an in vitro model of traumatic brain injury. Crit Care Med 2008;36:588—95.
[2] David HN, Haelewyn B, Chazalviel L, Lecocq M, Degoulet M, Risso JJ, et al. Post-ischemic helium provides neuroprotection in rats subjected to middle cerebral artery occlusion-induced ischemia by producing hypothermia. J Cereb Blood Flow Metab 2009;29:1159—65.
[3] Pan Y, Zhang H, VanDeripe DR, Cruz-Flores S, Panneton WM. Heliox and oxygen reduce infarct volume in a rat model of focal ischemia. Exp Neurol 2007;205:587—90.
[4] Hess DR, Fink JB, Venkataraman ST, Kim IK, Myers TR, Tano BD. The history and physics of heliox. Respir Care 2006;51:608—12.
[5] Hurford WE, Cheifetz IM. Respiratory controversies in the critical care setting. Should heliox be used for mechanically ventilated patients? Respir Care 2007;52:582—91.
[6] VanDeripe DR. The swelling of mitochondria from nitrogen gas; a possible cause of reperfusion damage. Med Hypotheses 2004;62:294—6.
[7] Shin HK, Dunn AK, Jones PB, Boas DA, Lo EH, Moskowitz MA, et al. Normobaric hyperoxia improves cerebral blood flow and oxygenation, and inhibits peri-infarct depolarizations in experimental focal ischemia. Brain 2007;130:1631—42.
[8] Marion DW, Crosby K. The effect of stable Xenon on ICP. J Cereb Blood Flow Metab 1991;11:347—50.

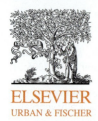
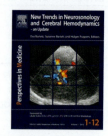

Bartels E, Bartels S, Poppert H (Editors):
New Trends in Neurosonology and Cerebral Hemodynamics — an Update.
Perspectives in Medicine (2012) 1, 304—308

journal homepage: www.elsevier.com/locate/permed

Cerebral blood flow in the chronic heart failure patients

Toplica Lepic [a,*], Goran Loncar [b], Biljana Bozic [c], Dragana Veljancic [a], Boban Labovic [a], Zeljko Krsmanovic [a], Milan Lepic [a], Ranko Raicevic [a]

[a] Department of neurology, Military Medical Academy, Belgrade, Serbia
[b] Department of cardiology, Clinical Center Zvezdara, Belgrade, Serbia
[c] Institute for Physiology and Biochemistry, University of Belgrade, Serbia

KEYWORDS
Cerebral blood flow;
Carotid Doppler;
Chronic heart failure;
Left ventricle ejection fraction

Abstract

Background: Global cerebral blood flow (CBF), as a measure of cerebral perfusion, can be noninvasively studied using Doppler sonography. Chronic heart failure (CHF) increases the risk of stroke and dementia. One of the possible causes may be cerebral hypoperfusion in CHF patients. Therefore, we aimed to investigate the relationship between CBF and CHF severity.

Methods: The study was performed in 76 ischemic or idiopathic dilatative cardiomyopathy patients, left ventricular ejection fraction (LVEF) < 40%, with no clinical evidence of decompensation and 20 healthy volunteers. Each CHF patient was categorized according to the New NYHA criteria. All patients underwent Doppler echocardiography examination (GE Vivid 7). The LVEF was quantified using the Simpson method. CBF was estimated by a 7.0-MHz linear transducer of a computed sonography system (Toshiba Power vision 6000). CBF volume was determined as the sum of the flow volumes of the ICA and the VA of both sides.

Results: Atrial fibrillation was noted in 30%, left bundle branch block in 26%, while pacemaker was implanted in 9% of patients with CHF. History of myocardial infarction was presented in 64% of patients. No differences in age, waist/hip ratio, body mass index and lipid profile were found between CHF patients and healthy subjects. CBF was calculated in 71 of 76 patients. Three patients had occlusion of ICA, while VA was occluded in another two patients. Others did not have a hemodynamically significant ICA and VA stenosis. CBF volume was decreased in CHF patients, (677 ± 170) according to control (783 ± 128).

Conclusion: Our results of noninvasive sonographic measurement of CBF according to LVEF and NYHA criteria, suggest on significantly reduced CBF in CHF patients.
© 2012 Elsevier GmbH. All rights reserved.

* Corresponding author. Tel.: +381 112477164; fax: +381 113609458.
  E-mail address: lepict@gmail.com (T. Lepic).

2211-968X/$ — see front matter © 2012 Elsevier GmbH. All rights reserved.
doi:10.1016/j.permed.2012.02.057

Introduction

Brain dysfunction associated with structural brain changes, are the important but under-recognised complication of chronic heart failure (CHF) [1—3]. In addition, CHF increases the risk of dementia and Alzheimer disease in later life [4]. One of the possible causes may be cerebral hypoperfusion secondary to low cardiac output in patients with CHF apart from biohumoral, clinical, socio-demographic and other potentially relevant factors [5,6]. Cerebral blood flow (CBF), as a measure of cerebral perfusion, can be noninvasively studied by flow volume measurements in extracranial cerebral arteries using Doppler and duplex methods [7]. Relationship of CBF to different markers of heart failure severity was only modestly presented in previous papers. Therefore, we aimed to investigate the relationship between CBF and CHF severity as well as to evaluate its determinants among different parameters of cardiac dysfunction.

Methods

Study design

Based on reviewed medical history archives on the baseline visit we screened 152 males aged 55 years and above with CHF due to ischemic or idiopathic dilated cardiomyopathy. Following the baseline visit 76 patients were selected all of whom met the study inclusion criteria. Inclusion criteria were as follows: duration of CHF for longer than 1 year; echocardiographically assessed left ventricular ejection fraction (LVEF) < 40%; etiology of CHF: ischemic or idiopathic dilated cardiomyopathy; NYHA functional class II and III; unchanged medication regimen within the previous 6 weeks; clinically stable condition with no clinical evidence of decompensate heart failure, such as raised jugular venous pressure, ascites, hepatomegaly. Exclusion criteria were as follows: diabetes mellitus determined by either self reported histories or evidence within the hospital case notes; primary lung disease including chronic obstructive pulmonary disease; musculoskeletal diseases; uncontrolled hypertension of more than 170/110 mmHg; myocardial infarction or unstable angina within previous 3 months; acute or chronic infection, inflammatory diseases such as sepsis, arthritis or systemic connective tissue disease; symptomatic peripheral vascular disease; alcohol abuse; serum creatinine 200 mmol/l; valvular cardiomyopathy or artificial heart valve; malignant disease, significant liver, thyroid, suprarenal gland or pituitary disease; cardiac cachexia defined as unintentional weight loss of 7.5% body weight over 6 months [8]. Finally, we included 71 patients because 3 patients were characterised by occlusion of internal carotid artery, while vertebral artery was not visualised in 2 patients.

The control group consisted of 20 healthy male volunteers aged 55 years and above, who did not take medications. No previous medical illness was reported (including diabetes or any other cardiovascular disease).

Clinical, cardiovascular and carotid color duplex sonography assessment

After the patient gave his written consent, the medical history was reviewed, including the cause of heart failure, comorbidities and medical history. Each patient with CHF was categorised according to the New York Heart Association (NYHA) criteria [9]. A physical exam was performed to assess CHF stability. The 6-min walk test was performed according to the standard protocol [10].

All patients underwent a two-dimensional Doppler echocardiography examination (GE Vivid 7). Systolic function was quantified by measurement of LVEF using the Simpson method. We also measured left ventricular end-diastolic diameter (LVEDD), right ventricular systolic pressure (RVSP) and left atrial volume (LAV) according to the ASE recommendation [11].

During an initial 20 min of rest with the subjects in a supine position, the extracranial arteries, i.e., the common carotid arteries, internal carotid arteries (ICA) and the vertebral arteries (VA) of both sides were explored with a 7.0 MHz linear transducer of a computed sonography system (Toshiba PowerVision 6000). The examination followed a previously described protocol [7]. CBF volume was determined as the sum of the flow volumes of the ICA and the VA of both sides. Resistance index, as a measure of cerebrovascular resistance, was calculated as follows: (peak systolic velocity end diastolic velocity)/peak systolic velocity [12]. Included subjects did not have hemodynamically significant stenosis of the common carotid artery, ICA and VA. The peak systolic velocity value averaged from both ICA and VA was used, as well. Intima-media thickness was measured on the far wall of the right and left common carotid artery, the carotid bulb, and the ICA [13]. The carotid intima-media thickness was defined as the mean of intima-media thickness measurements at these six sites.

Quality of life was estimated from The 'Minnesota — Living with Heart Failure Questionnaire' [14]. The Tei index is defined as the sum of isovolumic contraction and relaxation time divided by the ejection time. This index is a sensitive indicator of overall cardiac dysfunction in patients with mild-to-moderate CHF [15].

Statistical analysis

Descriptive statistics were presented as mean values with standard deviation or median with interquartile range for numeric variables, or as absolute numbers with percentages for categorical variables. Evaluation of normality was performed with Kolmogorov—Smirnov test. Student t-test was used to calculate differences between mean values. Mann—Whitney U-test was used to determine differences between median values. The Pearson coefficient was used for measuring linear correlation between variables. Partial correlation analysis was performed to adjust for age and body mass index. Finally, since variables are inter-related, multivariate regression analysis, backward method, was performed to assess the independent variables that may explain CBF. A p value 50.05 was considered to indicate statistical significance. Statistical analysis was performed using the

Table 1 Demographic, clinical characteristics, color duplex sonography of neck arteries, assessment of endothelial function and echocardiogaphic measurements of CHF patients and healthy subjects.

Variable	CHF patients (n=71)	Healthy subjects (n=20)	p value
Age (years)	68±7	67±7	0.909
Waist/hip ratio	1.03±0.04	1.01±0.06	0.086
BMI (kg/m^2)	28±5	28±3	0.496
Duration of disease (years)	5±4	—	
Smoking former/active, n (%)	16(22)/10(14)	3(15)/5(25)	0.454
Ischemic/idiopathic dilatated CMP, n (%)	56(79)/15(21)	—	
NYHA class II/III, n (%)	54(76)/17(24)	—	
MLHFQ	30±14	—	
Six-minute walking distance (m)	406±84	578±64	<0.0001
Mean blood pressure (mmHg)	101±12	103±7	0.387
ICA flow (ml/min)	505±144	593±118	0.014
VA flow (ml/min)	172±68	190±72	0.298
CBF (ml/min)	677±170	783±128	0.011
PSV (cm/s)	50±10	55±8	0.041
RI	0.65±0.08	0.67±0.06	0.244
CIMT (mm)	1.00±0.12	0.92±0.12	0.009
LAV (ml)	95±42	46±14	<0.0001
LVEDD (mm)	66±9	49±4	<0.0001
LVMi (g/m^2)	159±44	81±12	<0.0001
LVWT (mm)	20±4	19±1	0.018
LVEF (%)	29±8	65±5	<0.0001
RVSP (mmHg)	46±16	29±3	<0.0001
Tei index	0.61±0.22	0.28±0.12	<0.0001

Data are expressed as mean ± standard deviation (Mean ± SD) or median ± interquartile range (Me ± IQR) or as absolute number (%).
BMI = body mass index; CMP = cardiomyopathy; hs CRP = high sensitive C reactive protein; MLHFQ = Minnesota Living with Heart Failure Questionnaire; NYHA = New York Heart Association; CBF = cerebral blood flow; CIMT = carotid intima-media thickness; FMD = flow mediated dilatation; ICA = internal carotid artery; LAV = left atrial volume; LVEF = left ventricular ejection fraction; LVMi = left ventricular mass index; LVWT = left ventricular wall thickness; PSV = peak systolic velocity; RI = resistance index; RVSP = = right ventricular systolic pressure (n = 65/10, CHF patients/healthy controls); VA = vertebral artery.

SPSS software for Windows, version 15 (SPSS, Inc., Chicago, IL).

Results

Basic characteristics of CHF patients and healthy subjects

The basic clinical and biohumoral parameters of studied subjects are shown in Table 1. Atrial fibrillation was noted in 31%, left bundle branch block in 25%, while pacemaker was implanted in 9% of patients with CHF. History of myocardial infarction was presented in 63% of patients. Angiotensinconverting enzyme inhibitors were presented in 80% of patients, 75% were on b-blockers, 80% of patients were on loop diuretics, 55% were on spironolactone, 65% were on aspirin and 27% on statins. No differences in age, waist/hip ratio, body mass index and lipid profile were found between patients with CHF and healthy subjects.

Color duplex sonography of neck arteries and echocardiogaphic measurements

Color duplex sonography of neck arteries and echocardiogaphic measurements in studied subjects are presented in Table 1. CBF was decreased in patients with CHF, while there was no difference in resistance index between studied groups. CBF decreased according to NYHA class ($p < 0.0001$), with those in NYHA class III having level of CBF 542 ± 104 ml/min that was 25% lower than CBF in NYHA class II patients (719 ± 166 ml/min). Carotid intima-media thickness was significantly greater in patients with CHF compared to healthy controls. Echocardiographic variables of systolic and diastolic function were impaired in patients with CHF. CBF in patients with CHF was positively correlated with decreased LVEF (Fig. 1).

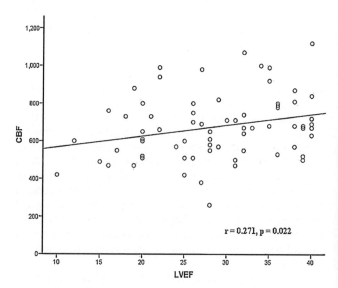

Fig. 1 Scatter plots of the association between CBF and LVEF in elderly patients with CHF. CBF = cerebral blood flow; LVEF = left ventricular ejection fraction.

Table 2 Multivariate regression analysis (backward model) with cerebral blood flow as dependent variable in elderly CHF males.

Variable	B	p value	F (p)
CBF (Constant)	0.454	5.121	
MLHFQ	−0.003	0.049	(0.001)
LVEF	0.006	0.031	
FMD	0.184	0.099	
Tei index	0.220	0.021	
$r^2 = 0.289$			

B = parameter estimate; F = Fisher test. CBF = cerebral blood flow; FMD = low mediated dilatation; LVEF = left ventricular ejection fraction; MLHFQ = Minnesota Living with Heart Failure Questionnaire.

Multivariate regression analysis

Multivariate regression analysis with backward model was used to asses the independent variables that may affect CBF (Table 2). The independent variables entered in the model were: age, body mass index, mean blood pressure, quality of life score, 6-min walk distance, LVEF and Tei index. LVEF was independently associated with reduced CBF in patients with CHF.

Discussion

The objective of this study was to investigate the association of CBF with different parameters of heart failure severity in elderly males. The major observations in this study are that: (1) elderly men with CHF demonstrated reduced CBF compared to healthy controls; (2) reduced CBF was also associated with deteriorated physical performance capacity (6-min walk distance), impaired quality of life, and pulmonary hypertension; (4) clinically more advanced CHF, expressed as NYHA class, was related to greater reduction of CBF. In this study, CBF was significantly reduced by 14% in elderly patients with CHF compared to healthy controls. Similarly, Choi et al. [16] have shown that global CBF (measured by radionuclide angiography) was decreased by approximately 19% in patients with CHF compared with normal controls. Patients with heart failure showed damage to multiple brain regions that play significant roles in autonomic nervous system control and cognitive function including mood regulation, memory processing, pain and language [3]. One of the major factors that may lead to cognitive impairment is cerebral hypoperfusion demonstrated in our as well as in previous studies [17]. CBF is regulated by perfusion pressure and vascular resistance. The autoregulation of blood flow over a wide range of perfusion pressures is one of the characteristics of brain circulation. Compensatory mechanisms maintain perfusion to vital organs, such as brain in response to the progressive reduction of cardiac output. One of the chronic adaptations of the circulatory system is peripheral vasoconstriction which may be provoked by the heart failure-induced activation of neurohormonal systems [18]. In agreement with our results, cerebral vascular resistance, expressed by resistance index, was not elevated in patients with mild-to-moderate CHF compared to healthy controls [19]. Therefore, decreased perfusion pressure as a consequence of reduced systolic left ventricular function in patients with CHF may be marked as principal factor of reduced CBF. Low LVEF was the independent determinant of impaired CBF in our patients with CHF. Thus, it can be speculated that cerebral hypoperfusion due to left ventricular systolic dysfunction may contribute to brain injury secondary to low cardiac output. A correlation between cardiac index and intracranial hemodynamics has been reported [20]. However, Eicke et al. [21] showed no correlation between LVEF and CBF supporting the concept that CBF is independent of cardiac output. In addition, Choi et al. [16] showed that CBF was not correlated to LVEF in patients with CHF, suggesting that the LVEF was not a factor determining the degree of breakdown of the autoregulation of CBF. This discrepancy may be explained that in the patients with more severe CHF such as those in the study of Choi et al., factors other than LVEF contributed more to CBF, such as NYHA functional class and neurohormonal activation. Our recent published data presents relation between CBF reduction and neurohormonal activation in CHF patients [22].

The same study reported an inverse association between CBF with RVSP which is in agreement with our finding. Finally, reduced CBF in our study was significantly associated with impaired physical performance; measured by 6-min walk test contrary to previous data [19]. The 6-min walk test is a safe and simple clinical tool that strongly and independently predicts morbidity and mortality in patients with CHF [23].

Color duplex volumetric test of the brain-feeding arteries can only yield information about the relative contributions of the anterior and posterior cerebral circulation to global CBF volume. We found a contribution of the VA to global CBF volume of 25% which remained almost constant with increasing age. Previously, it was estimated that the VA contribute 24% of the global CBF volume in healthy subjects [24]. To date, there are no reports on the relative contributions of the anterior and posterior circulation to global CBF volume in patients with CHF. Carotid intima-media thickness was greater in our patients with CHF compared to healthy controls. High carotid intima-media thickness was marked as an independent risk factor for incidence of heart failure requiring hospitalisation [25]. Increased carotid intima-media thickness was shown to be a powerful predictor of coronary and cerebrovascular events, as well [26]. Although both parameters were impaired in our patients, the lack of a link between them suggests that they may represent independent surrogates that measure different pathophysiological aspect of heart failure progression.

The limitation of our study is a relatively small number of studied patients. Our cohort comprised a highly selected CHF sample and is thus less representative of the overall CHF population. The relations between CBF and different variables were examined in a cross-sectional study, which cannot prove a causal relation between these variables. color duplex volumetric examination of the brain feeding extracranial arteries is a highly reproducible and noninvasive technique. The reliability of the method should be confirmed in comparative studies with established radionuclide procedures which is difficult for ethical reasons. However, reduction of CBF in our patients with CHF compared to healthy controls was similar to the value obtained by radionuclide technique. In this study, we did not perform evaluation of mental status or brain imaging. Therefore, we cannot say that reduced CBF was associated with neuropsychiatric or brain morphologic disorders among patients with CHF. Finally, it would be of interest to evaluate the impact of diminished CBF on major clinical outcomes in future studies.

In conclusion, we have shown that CBF was reduced in elderly males with mild to moderate CHF, and was independently associated with factors that represent the severity of CHF. Reduced CBF was associated with impaired physical performance, and deteriorated quality of life, as well. Future studies are now needed to tease out possible association of CBF with cerebral disorders known to be more potentiated in the population with heart failure as well as to investigate the possible underlying mechanisms.

References

[1] Zuccalà G, Cattel C, Manes-Gravina E, Di Niro MD, Coecchi A, Bernabei R. Left ventricular dysfunction: a clue to cognitive impairment in older patients with heart failure. J Neurol Neurosurg Psychiatry 1997;63:509—12.

[2] Woo MA, Kumar R, Macey PM, Fonarow GC, Harper RM. Brain injury in autonomic, emotional, and cognitive regulatory areas in patients with heart failure. J Card Fail 2009;15:214—23.

[3] Beer C, Ebenezer E, Fenner S, Lautenschlager NT, Arnolda L, Flicker L, et al. Contributors to cognitive impairment in congestive heart failure: a pilot case-control study. Intern Med J 2009;39:600—5.

[4] Qiu C, Winblad B, Marengoni A, Klarin I, Fastbom J, Fratiglioni L. Heart failure and risk of dementia and Alzheimer disease: a population-based cohort study. Arch Intern Med 2006;166:1003—8.

[5] Pullicino PM, Hart J. Cognitive impairment in congestive heart failure? Embolism vs hypoperfusion. Neurology 2001;57:1945—6.

[6] Staniforth AD, Kinnear WJM, Cowley AJ. Cognitive impairment in heart failure with Cheyne-Stokes respiration. Heart 2001;85:18—22.

[7] Scheel P, Ruge C, Petruch UR, Schöning M. Color duplex measurement of cerebral blood flow volume in healthy adults. Stroke 2000;31:147—50.

[8] Anker SD, Ponikowski P, Varney S, Chua TP, Clark AL, Webb-Peploe KM, et al. Wasting as independent risk factor for mortality in chronic heart failure. Lancet 1997;349:1050—3.

[9] The Criteria Committee of the New York Heart Association Nomenclature and Criteria for Diagnosis of Diseases of the Heart and Great Vessels. 9th ed. Boston, Mass: Little, Brown & Co; 1994:253—256.

[10] ATS statement: guidelines for the six-minute walk test. ATS Committee on Proficiency Standards for Clinical Pulmonary Function Laboratories. Am J Respir Crit Care Med 2002;166:111—117.

[11] Silvestry FE, Kerber RE, Brook MM, Carroll JD, Eberman KM, Goldstein SA, et al. Echocardiography-guided interventions. J Am Soc Echocardiogr 2009;22:213—31.

[12] Pourcelot L. Applications cliniques de l'examen Doppler transcutane. Coloques de l'Inst Natl Santeï Rech Med 1974;12:1376—80.

[13] Chambless LE, Heiss G, Folsom AR, Rosamond W, Szklo M, Sharrett AR, et al. Association of coronary heart disease incidence with carotid arterial wall thickness and major risk factors: the Atherosclerosis Risk in Communities (ARIC) Study, 1987—1993. Am J Epidemiol 1997;146:483494.

[14] Rector TS, Cohn JN. Assessment of patient outcome with the Minnesota Living with Heart Failure questionnaire: reliability and validity during a randomized, double-blind, placebocontrolled trial of pimobendan. Pimobendan Multicenter Research Group. Am Heart J 1992;124:1017—25.

[15] Bruch C, Schmermund A, Marin D, Katz M, Bartel T, Schaar J, et al. Tei-index in patients with mild-to-moderate congestive heart failure. Eur Heart J 2000;21:1888—95.

[16] Choi BR, Kim JS, Yang YJ, Park KM, Lee CW, Kim YH, et al. Factors associated with decreased cerebral blood flow in congestive heart failure secondary to idiopathic dilated cardiomyopathy. Am J Cardiol 2006;97:1365—9.

[17] Romaïn GC. Brain hypoperfusion: a critical factor in vascular dementia. Neurol Res 2004;26:454—8.

[18] Macrae IM, Robinson MJ, Graham DI, Reid JL, McCulloch J. Endothelin-1-induced reductions in cerebral blood flow: dose dependency, time course, and neuropathological consequences. J Cereb Blood Flow Metab 1993;13: 276—84.

[19] van Langen H, van Driel VJ, Skotnicki SH, Verheugt FW. Alterations in the peripheral circulation in patients with mild heart failure. Eur J Ultrasound 2001;13:7—15.

[20] Saha M, Muppala MR, Castaldo JE, Gee W, Reed III JF, Morris DL. The impact of cardiac index on cerebral hemodynamics. Stroke 1993;24:1686—90.

[21] Eicke BM, von Schlichting J, Mohr-Ahaly S, Schlosser A, von Bardeleben RS, Krummenauer F, et al. Lack of association between carotid artery volume blood flow and cardiac output. J Ultrasound Med 2001;20:1293—8.

[22] Loncar G, Bozic B, Lepic T, Dimkovic S, Prodanovic N, Radojicic Z, et al. Relationship of reduced cerebral blood flow and heart failure severity in elderly males. Aging Male 2011;14(March (1)):59—65. Epub 2010 Sep 27.

[23] Bittner V, Weiner DH, Yusuf S, Rogers WJ, McIntyre KM, Bangdiwala SI, et al. Prediction of mortality and morbidity with a 6-minute walk test in patients with left ventricular dysfunction. SOLVD Investigators. JAMA 1993;270: 1702—7.

[24] Kashimada A, Machida K, Honda N, Mamiya T, Takahashi T, Kamano T, et al. Measurement of cerebral blood flow with two-dimensional cine phase-contrast mR imaging: evaluation of normal subjects and patients with vertigo. Radiat Med 1995;13:95—102.

[25] Engström G, Melander O, Hedblad B. Carotid intima-media thickness, systemic inflammation, and incidence of heart failure hospitalizations. Arterioscler Thromb Vasc Biol 2009;29:1691—5.

[26] O'Leary DH, Polak JF, Kronmal RA, Manolio TA, Burke GL, Wolfson SK. Carotid-artery intima and media thickness as a risk factor for myocardial infarction and stroke in older adults. N Engl J Med 1999;340:14—22.

Withdraw of statin improves cerebrovascular reserve in radiation vasculopathy

John J. Volpi [a,b,*], Rasadul Kabir [a], Zsolt Garami [b,c], Pamela New [a,b]

[a] The Methodist Hospital Neurological Institute, 6560 Fannin, Suite 802, Houston, TX 77030, USA
[b] The Methodist Hospital Research Institute, 6565 Fannin, Houston, TX 77030, USA
[c] Methodist DeBakey Heart and Vascular Center, Houston, 6550 Fannin, Suite 1401, TX 77030, USA

KEYWORDS
Functional TCD;
Vasomotor reactivity;
Statin;
Radiation vasculopathy

Summary Cerebrovascular reserve is impaired in radiation vasculopathy from radiation injury to small arteries and arterioles. Few interventions or medications have been shown to be effective in this disease. We report a unique finding in which a statin contributed to worsening of the cerebrovascular reserve.
© 2012 Elsevier GmbH. All rights reserved.

Introduction

Radiation vasculopathy affects patients with primary brain tumor and causes significant morbidity from ischemia related to hemodynamic insufficiency [1,2]. In these patients, medical management for secondary stroke prevention commonly includes HMG-CoA reductase inhibitors, or statins. Previous studies have shown that statin use improves cerebrovascular reactivity [3]. We report a contradictory finding in a unique patient with radiation vasculopathy and suggest broader implications for patients with hemodynamic insufficiency.

Abbreviations: ACA, anterior cerebral artery; MCA, middle cerebral artery; TCD, transcranial Doppler; BHI, breath holding index; GTP, guanosine triphosphate; NO, nitric oxide; eNOS, endothelial nitric oxide synthase.
* Corresponding author at: 6560 Fannin, Suite 802, Houston, TX 77030, USA. Tel.: +1 713 441 3951; fax: +1 713 793 7019.
E-mail address: jjvolpi@tmhs.org (J.J. Volpi).

Methods

A 66 year old man who underwent surgery and radiation for glioblastoma multiforme presented 6 months post surgery with new onset left sided weakness. He was found with a right middle cerebral artery infarct and placed on simvastatin along with aspirin. He underwent a baseline transcranial Doppler (TCD) and then had his statin withdrawn. He was then brought back to the clinic 6 weeks later for follow-up study.

Results

Initial TCD showed no significant stenoses by velocity criteria in the proximal vessels of the circle of Willis. Interestingly, however, there was flow diversion on the right with ACA > MCA velocity, suggesting distal stenosis. The breath holding index was 0.42. 6 weeks later, after statin withdraw, TCD showed persistent flow diversion, but significant improvement in the BHI to 0.78.

Discussion

The data from this patient suggests small arteriolar disease from radiation vasculopathy causing poor hemodynamic flow to the right hemisphere. Although the precise means by which statins worsen the hemodynamic flow to the affected hemisphere is unknown, the mechanism we propose below for this finding is based on previous studies in which statins have been shown to improve cerebrovascular flow [3]. While these findings seem to be contradictory, the finding in radiation vasculopathy is actually a logical extension of the larger theory regarding statin effects on cerebral blood flow and in fact corroborates the other findings of flow augmentation.

Statins have the effect of decreasing cholesterol synthesis, and do so by inhibiting the upstream enzyme HMG CoA reductase. The downstream effect of this inhibition is the decreased production of not only cholesterol, but also geranyl pyrophosphate, a constituent of the family of small GTPases known as Rho. In the absence of geranyl pyrophosphate, less of the Rho GTPases are active [4].

The role of the Rho GTPases is key to the statin effect in the endothelium. Through a series of downstream effects, the Rho GTPases inhibit NO production in the endothelium by decreasing eNOS expression and activity [4]. Less eNOS activity results in a paucity of the vasodilatory effects of NO. In essence, the Rho GTPases causes arteriolar vasoconstriction. By inhibiting their production, statins ''turn off the off switch'' and thus promote eNOS activity and vasodilation.

Based on this theory, the expected result of statin administration would be increased cerebral blood flow with statins, which has been shown in healthy subjects [3]. In radiation vasculopathy, however, the situation is quite different from healthy controls in that the affected hemisphere has diffuse arteriolar vasculopathy, while the contralateral hemisphere is spared this pathology. We suggest that the contradictory finding we observed is a special result of the rule of vasodilation and an example of cerebral steal. At baseline, we hypothesize that there is maximal vasodilation in the pathological hemisphere. The addition of the statin could not improve the already maximally dilated vessels on the pathological hemisphere. Statins and the addition of eNOS activity would, however, increase vessel dilation to the healthy hemisphere, shifting it from a neutral amount of vessel tone to a dilated state. This shift to a more dilated stated on the healthy hemisphere seems to exacerbate the underlying hemodynamic inequity and causes a steal syndrome. By withdraw of statin, the healthy hemisphere tone returns to normal, and the pathological hemisphere was able to shunt more flow and improve.

Conclusion

In healthy subjects or those with diffuse bihemispheric cerebrovascular disease, the addition of statins will likely improve vasomotor tone and augment cerebral blood flow. In the special circumstance of a patient with isolated high-grade cerebrovascular disease in a single vascular bed, the addition of a statin may lead to a cerebral steal phenomenon.

References

[1] Acker JC, Marks LB, Spencer DP, Yang W, Avery MA, Dodge RK, et al. Serial in vivo observations of cerebral vasculature after treatment with a large single fraction of radiation. Radiat Res 1998;149(April (4)):350—9.
[2] Chu CN, Chen SW, Bai LY, Mou CH, Hsu CY, Sung FC. Increase in stroke risk in patients with head and neck cancer: a retrospective cohort study. Br J Cancer 2011;105(October (9)):1419—23.
[3] Sander K, Hof U, Poppert H, Conrad B, Sander D. Improved cerebral vasoreactivity after statin administration in healthy adults. J Neuroimaging 2005;15(3):266—70.
[4] Srivastava K, Bath PM, Bayraktutan U. Current therapeutic strategies to mitigate the eNOS dysfunction in ischaemic stroke. Cell Mol Neurobiol 2011;(December).

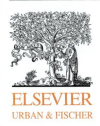
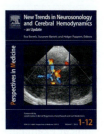

Bartels E, Bartels S, Poppert H (Editors):
New Trends in Neurosonology and Cerebral Hemodynamics — an Update.
Perspectives in Medicine (2012) 1, 311—315

journal homepage: www.elsevier.com/locate/permed

Informativity of pulsatility index and cerebral autoregulation in hydrocephalus

Vladimir Semenyutin[a,*], Vugar Aliev[a], Valery Bersnev[a], Andreas Patzak[b], Larisa Rozhchenko[a], Alexandr Kozlov[a], Shakhob Ramazanov[a]

[a] Russian Polenov Neurosurgical Institute, St. Petersburg, Russian Federation
[b] University Hospital Charite, Humboldt-University of Berlin, Johannes-Mueller Institute of Physiology, Berlin, Germany

KEYWORDS
Cerebrospinal fluid;
Hydrocephalus;
Intracranial pressure;
Cerebral autoregulation;
Transcranial Doppler

Summary
Background: A high correlation between transcranial Doppler pulsatility index (PI) increase and intracranial hypertension has been recently demonstrated in most neurosurgical patients. But in patients with hydrocephalus PI is sometimes controversial. This may be due to a different degree of cerebral autoregulation (CA) under condition of cerebral perfusion pressure decrease.
Purpose: To compare the results of PI and CA assessment in patients with hydrocephalus.
Material and methods: Twenty-six patients (aged 16—52; male — 9, female — 17) with various types of hydrocephalus were studied. We monitored blood flow velocity in middle cerebral arteries with Multi Dop X and systemic blood pressure with Finapres-2300. CA was assessed with cuff test (evaluation of ARI) and cross-spectral analysis of spontaneous oscillations of cerebral and systemic hemodynamics within the range of Mayer's waves (evaluation of phase shift in radians — PS).
Results: Depending on presence of intracranial hypertension (ICH), all patients have been divided in two groups. Mean values of PI did not differ significantly in both groups. At the same time ARI and PS were considerably ($p < 0.01$) higher in patients without signs of ICH. In group of patients with ICH postoperative clinical improvement was accompanied with considerable ($p < 0.05$) increase of PS. In group of patients without ICH we did not observe any positive changes in neurological state postoperatively.
Conclusion: Preoperative CA assessment being more informative than PI evaluation can increase transcranial Doppler valuability in noninvasive diagnostics of cerebral spinal fluid dynamics and may be helpful in clarifying indications for operation in patients with hydrocephalus.
© 2012 Elsevier GmbH. All rights reserved.

* Corresponding author.
E-mail address: lbcp@mail.ru (V. Semenyutin).

Introduction

The disturbance of cerebrospinal fluid (CSF) circulation in system of CSF pathways owing to the various reasons (impairment of CSF production and absorption, the mechanical block) can cause development of hydrocephalus. Depending on compensating capabilities of brain this pathology may not have clinical symptoms or, being accompanied by increase of intracranial pressure (ICP), can give a clinical picture of intracranial hypertension (ICH) syndrome. In the latter case carrying out surgical treatment — correction of the disturbed CSF circulation by means of shunting or endoscopic intervention — is required. Nevertheless in some cases, when ICH is doubtful or has temporal character, the data of clinical examination, computed tomography/magnetic resonance scanning of the brain appear insufficient for defining indications for operations.

For today long-term monitoring of ICP with infusion tests (IT) in various modifications (external lumbar drainage test [11], Marmarou's bolus method [15], Katzman—Hussey's method with constant-rate infusion of physiologic saline [2,12]) is used as "the gold standard" and can help to make the correct solution. They allow to define not only ICP or pressure of CSF, but also to estimate other parameters, such as rate of CSF production, resistance of outflow, elasticity, pressure—volume index, compliance, which characterize system of CSF pathways as a whole. Besides, monitoring of ICP, at least within 30 min, and according to some authors up to 24 h, plays an essential role for an estimation of occurrence and amplitude of slow intracranial B-waves and plateau-waves [4,23].

The received data can be very important for the choice of tactics of treatment, particularly, in patients with idiopathic normal pressure hydrocephalus (INPH). But at the same time, it is necessary to recognize, that IT are invasive and potentially bear the risk of development of inflammatory complications that limits their wide application as the tool of preoperative diagnostics in many neurosurgical clinics.

Thus search of adequate noninvasive methods for estimation of functional state of CSF pathways system seems to be an actual task from clinical and fundamental point of view. Occurrence of various symptoms of hydrocephalus are supposed to be connected with different morphological changes in white matter among which brain tissue distortion, diffusion of CSF containing vasoactive metabolites into periventricular areas [17] are most evident. Decrease of cerebral perfusion pressure (CPP) in case of impaired cerebral autoregulation (CA) can lead to decrease of cerebral blood flow and an ischemia. Surgical treatment of hydrocephalus, as a rule, restores CPP up to normal values, improves CA which is accompanied with regression of neurologic deterioration. At present time there are various noninvasive methods which are used for an estimation of cerebral blood flow (SPECT, pwMRI, PET-Xe^{133}) [14,19,21,22] but they are cumbersome and expensive. As an accessible and adequate method for its evaluation can be used transcranial Doppler (TCD), allowing the bedside registration of blood flow velocity (BFV) in the basal cerebral arteries. It was established that this parameter is an equivalent of cerebral blood flow if the diameter of insonated vessel during registration remains constant [18]. Possibility of noninvasive diagnostics of ICH by means of pulsatility index (PI) on the base of TCD was shown in different pathologies [8,9,16]. However in patients with hydrocephalus PI is not always informative. It could be explained with various degree of CA impairment under conditions of decreased CPP. The results of CA estimation by means of TCD in patients with hydrocephalus are limited or inconsistent [3].

Purpose

To compare the results of PI and CA assessment in patients with hydrocephalus.

Materials and methods

Twenty-six patients (aged 16—52; male — 9, female — 17) with various types of hydrocephalus were studied: INPH — 15, hypertensive hydrocephalus — 11 (communicating — 3, occlusive — 8). The obstruction of CSF pathways was diagnosed at the level of cerebral aqueduct or foramen of Monro. It was caused by inflammatory process or tumor located in the region of the third or fourth ventricle.

The primary diagnosis of hydrocephalus was based on the results of computed tomography (CT) and magnetic resonance (MR) imaging. The main complaints on admission were different types of headache, dizziness, and in some cases Hakim triad (gait disturbance, incontinence, memory and behaviour disfunctions).

An examination was carried out according to standard neurosurgical protocol, which contained basic clinical, neurologic, ophthalmologic inspection of the patient. The size of ventricles according to CT/MR imaging was assessed with the help Evans's craniocerebral index [7,20]. The degree of psychopathologic disorders was estimated with Frontal assessment battery (FAB) score [6].

All patients on admission underwent non-invasive monitoring of systemic blood pressure (BP) with Finapres-2300 (Ohmeda) and BFV in both middle cerebral arteries (MCA) with Multi Dop X (DWL). In operated patients postoperative investigation was carried out 10 days after surgery. During monitoring a patient was in supine position with his head tilted up to 30°. Continuous recording was carried out during 10 min. It was done at rest and spontaneous breathing, corresponding to normal ventilation [13]. CA was assessed by cuff test [1] and cross-spectral analysis of slow spontaneous oscillations of BP and BFV in MCA within the range of Mayer's waves (80—120 mHz) [5]. An index of autoregulation (ARI) and phase shift (PS) between Mayer's waves (M-waves) of BP and BFV were defined, correspondently.

The software "Statistica 7.0 for Windows" (Time Series and Prognostication module) was used for cross-spectral analysis of spontaneous oscillations of BP and BVF in accordance with standard algorithm. PS between BP and BFV was calculated in radians (rad) at frequency with maximum amplitude of M-waves in BP spectra. While calculating PS, we used a high coherence criterion at that frequency, where a coherence index between M-waves of BP and BFV was more than 0.6.

In some cases we measured the CSF pressure and performed IT in lumbar cistern with use of lumbar needle (21 gauge Whitacre) and external transducer (Becton Dickinson, USA); in subdural space with use of latex ballon or optosensor probe (Codman, a Johnson & Johnson Company, Raynham, MA); intraventricularly with use of ventricular catheter and external transducer (Becton Dickinson). Signals of CSF pressure through an analog input submitted to Multi Dop X (DWL) where multichannel monitoring of all parameters, including BP, BFV in MCA was carried out.

Resistance of CSF outflow (R_{out}) was assessed by Katzman—Hussey's method [12] with constant-rate (1.5 ml/min) infusion of physiologic saline. In case of communicating hydrocephalus we used lumbar access with two needles on adjacent levels. In cases of occlusive hydrocephalus we used intraventricular access with ventricular catheter and 3-way stopcock. The measurement of CSF pressure in the lateral ventricles was carried out on the next day after ventricular catheterization and then catheter was removed. A strict aseptic technique was used to keep all the prefilled tubing and the probes sterile. There were not any inflammatory complications after procedure.

Indications to surgery ($n = 16$) were based mainly on the data of clinical examination and the results of CT/MR imaging. If the blockage of CSF pathways was caused by big size tumor, their restoration was achieved by removing the tumor ($n = 5$). In other cases of occlusive hydrocephalus and in cases of INPH ventricular-peritoneal shunting ($n = 8$) or endoscopic intervention — perforation of the bottom of the third ventricle ($n = 3$) — were performed. Valves with middle-pressure range and antisiphon device (Codman, a Johnson & Johnson Company, Raynham, MA) were chosen for shunting.

Data were processed with applying conventional statistical programs (Statistica 7.0 for Windows, Excel). Parametric (Student) and non-parametric (Kolmogorov—Smirnov) criteria were used. Difference was considered to be reliable in $p < 0.05$.

The protocol of the study was approved by the Ethical Committee of the Polenov Research Neurosurgical Institute. Participation in the study was possible only after receiving a patient's written consent.

Results

Depending on presence of ICH symptoms, all patients have been divided in two groups. The first group included 11 patients with hydrocephalus and signs of ICH on admission to the hospital, the second group included 15 patients with hydrocephalus and without signs of ICH.

Mean values of PI did not differ significantly in the 1st (0.81 ± 0.14 — on the left, 0.82 ± 0.13 — on the right) and 2nd groups (0.86 ± 0.16 — on the left, 0.82 ± 0.13 — on the right).

At the same time preoperative ARI (6.5 ± 1.5 — on the left, 6.1 ± 1.7 — on the right) and PS (0.9 ± 0.2 rad — on the left, 1.0 ± 0.3 rad — on the right) were considerably ($p < 0.01$) higher in patients without signs of ICH than preoperative ARI (3.7 ± 0.5 — on the left, 3.6 ± 0.6 — on the right) and PS (0.5 ± 0.2 rad — on the left, 0.5 ± 0.1 rad — on the right) in patients with signs of ICH.

The surgery was performed in all 11 patients with clinical signs of ICH and in 5 out of 15 patients without signs of ICH.

In the first group of patients postoperative clinical improvement was accompanied with considerable ($p < 0.05$) increase of PS on both sides (right — 0.9 ± 0.2, left — 0.9 ± 0.1 rad). In the second group of operated patients without signs of ICH we did not observe any positive changes in neurological state postoperatively. Mean values of ARI (right — 6.3 ± 1.5, left — 6.0 ± 1.0) and PS (right — 1.0 ± 0.2, left — 1.0 ± 0.3 rad) prior to operation in the second group were considerably higher than the same values in operated

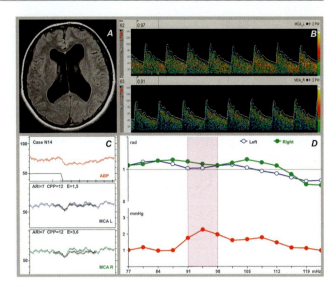

Figure 1 Results of examination of the 35 years old female patient with INPH. (A) MR image; (B) BFV spectra in both MCA; (C) dynamics of BP and BFV and ARI during cuff test; (D) PS between BP and BFV and amplitude spectra of BP within the range of M-waves.

patients of the first group. After surgery in patients of the second group PS had a tendency to insignificant decrease of PS (right — 0.9 ± 0.2, left — 0.9 ± 0.1 rad).

Fig. 1 illustrates the results of examination of the female patient with INPH. She suffered of headache, but without dizziness and nausea. Evans's index was 0.26, the level of mental abilities according to FAB score was high — 15 points. Baseline CSF pressure in lumbar cistern was normal (12 mmHg), R_{out} corresponded to the upper level of the normal range (15 mmHg/ml/min).

BFV in both MCA were also within the normal range, but PI was high and indicated the presence of ICH.

At the same time PS and ARI corresponded to normal values and testified an absence of CA disturbance despite enlarged ventricles according to the brain scan imaging. Taking into account minimal clinical symptoms and positive results of CSF monitoring it has been decided to refuse from surgery and to conduct dynamic observation. Further improvement was noted and the patient was discharged from the hospital on 10th day.

Fig. 2 illustrates the results of examination of the male patient with communicating hydrocephalus and clinical signs of ICH.

He suffered of headache, gait disturbance, incontinence. Evans's index was 0.28, the level of mental disorders according to FAB score — 9 points. Baseline CSF pressure in lumbar cistern was 18 mmHg, R_{out} 17 mmHg/ml/min. BFV in both MCA were within the normal range, but PI was low and indicated an absence of ICH. However, significant decrease of ARI and PS testified marked CA disturbance.

The patient underwent ventriculo-peritoneal shunting which led to a significant regression of neurological symptoms. Evans's index was decreased to 0.12, and the level of mental abilities according to FAB score increased up to 15 points.

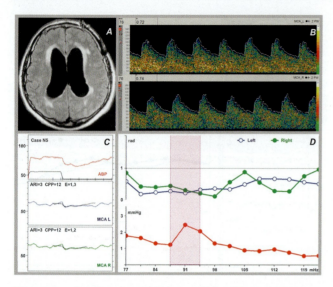

Figure 2 Results of examination of the 42 years old male patient with communicating hydrocephalus and signs of moderate ICH prior to ventriculo-peritoneal shunting. Notations are as in Fig. 1.

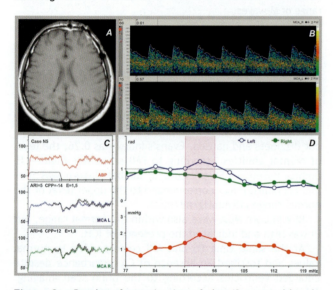

Figure 3 Results of examination of the 42 years old male patient with communicating hydro-cephalus and signs of moderate ICH after ventriculo-peritoneal shunting. Notations are as in Fig. 1.

Fig. 3 illustrates the results of examination of the same male patient with communicating hydrocephalus and clinical signs of ICH on the 10th day after operation.

After shunting we observed significant increase of both PS and ARI which testified improvement of CA. There has been a further decline in the PI, but without marked changes of BFV. The patient was discharged in fair condition on 12th day after operation.

Discussion

The problem of surgical treatment of patients with hydrocephalus has not been completely solved yet. Considering the high rate of ineffective surgical interventions in hydrocephalus, reliable diagnostic and prognostic indication criteria for surgical operations are required [10]. Monitoring of CSF dynamics, including IT, together with methods of neuroimaging and evaluation of neurological and psychological status, is still necessary and included in recommendations for management of patients with hydrocephalus. However, the use of ICP monitoring and IT is limited in clinical practice. The leading cause of their limited usage despite their high informativity and sensitivity seems to be invasiveness of these methods and long duration of investigation that may increase the risk of inflammatory complications.

Thus, search of noninvasive methods of evaluation of CSF dynamics as well as cerebral hemodynamics in these patients seems to be an actual purpose. TCD due to its noninvasiveness, informativity and possibility of bedside monitoring may be used as a method of choice. According to data of cerebral hemodynamics assessment received by TCD in patients with hydrocephalus, PI does not always indicate ICH. However, there is a reliable difference in CA in patients with ICH and without it.

Positive correlation in all patients was revealed by correlation analysis between ARI and PS ($r = 0.82$, $p < 0.05$), which indicate possibility of replacement of cuff test by cross-spectral analysis. The latter seems more physiological especially in patients with intellectual disfunction making the cuff test more problematic.

It should be mentioned that some patients may have discrepancies between PS and ARI. In cuff test the decrease of BP may get below the lower limit of CA while cross-spectral analysis of slow oscillations is usually performed within the limits of CA. Technical reasons may also cause discrepancies between PS and ARI. Cross-spectral analysis requires precise calibration and reliable fixation of transducers measuring BFV, BP and ICP, high signal/noise ratio during all time of registration and high sampling rate of registering devices.

Postoperative registration of CA allows evaluation of surgical operation efficacy. In this study the group of patients with normotensive hydrocephalus was presented with patients who either did not meet indications for surgery or operation was not effective and did not significantly improve quality of their lives. Confirmation of informativity of CA parameters in choosing management strategy requires further studies of patients with normotensive hydrocephalus compromising cerebral hemodynamics. It seems important to compare CA parameters with MR and CT imaging not only in the short-term follow-up, but also in the long-term one — after six and twelve months after operation.

Conclusion

Preoperative CA assessment being more informative than PI evaluation can increase TCD valuability in noninvasive diagnostics of CSF dynamics' state and may be helpful in clarifying indications for operation in patients with hydrocephalus.

Appendix A. Supplementary data

Supplementary data associated with this article can be found, in the online version, at http://dx.doi.org/10.1016/j.permed.2012.03.006.

References

[1] Aaslid R, Lindegaard K, Sorteberg W, Nornes H. Cerebral autoregulation dynamics in humans. Stroke 1989;20: 45–52.

[2] Czosnyka Z, Czosnyka M, Lavinio A, Keong N, Pickard JD. Clinical testing of CSF circulation. European Journal of Anaesthesiology 2008;25(S42):142–5.

[3] Czosnyka Z, Czosnyka M, Whitfield PC, Donovan T, Pickard JD. Cerebral autoregulation among patients with symptoms of hydrocephalus. Neurosurgery 2002;50(3):526–33.

[4] Czosnyka M, Czosnyka Z, Keong N, Lavinio A, Smielewski P, Momjian S, et al. Pulse pressure waveform in hydrocephalus: what it is and what it isn't? Neurosurgical Focus 2007;22: 1–7.

[5] Diehl R, Linden D, Lucke D, Berlit P. Phase relationship between cerebral blood flow velocity and blood pressure. A clinical test of autoregulation. Stroke 1995;26:1801–4.

[6] Dubois B, Slachevsky A, Litvan I, Pillon B. The FAB: a Frontal Assessment Battery at bedside. Neurology 2000;55(11):1621–6.

[7] Evans WA. An encephalographic ratio for estimating ventricular enlargement and cerebral atrophy. Archives of Neurology and Psychiatry 1942;47(6):931–7.

[8] Georgia A. Pulsatility index may predict poor outcome after intracerebral hemorrhage. Covering Neurology 2003;61:1051–6.

[9] Hanlo PW, Gooskens R, Nijhuis I, Faber J, Peters R, Huffelen A, et al. Value of transcranial Doppler indices in predicting raised ICP in infantile hydrocephalus. Child's Nervous System 1995;11:595–603.

[10] INPH Guidelines Study Group. Guidelines for the diagnosis and management of idiopathic normal-pressure hydrocephalus. Neurosurgery 2005;57(3):1–39.

[11] Kahlon B, Sundbärg G, Rehncrona S. Lumbar infusion test in normal pressure hydrocephalus. Acta Neurologica Scandinavica 2005;111:379–84.

[12] Katzman R, Hussey F. A simple constant infusion manometric test for measurement of CSF absorption. Neurology 1970;20:534–44.

[13] Lavinio A, Schmidt EA, Haubrich C, Smielewski P, Pickard JD, Czosnyka M. Noninvasive evaluation of dynamic cerebrovascular autoregulation using Finapres plethysmograph and transcranial Doppler. Stroke 2007;38(2):402–4.

[14] Mamo HL, Meric PC, Ponsin JC, Rey AC, Luft AG, Seylaz JA. Cerebral blood flow in normal pressure hydrocephalus. Stroke 1987;18(6):1074–80.

[15] Marmarou A, Shulman K, Rosende RM. A nonlinear analysis of the cerebrospinal fluid system and intracranial pressure dynamics. Journal of Neurosurgery 1978;48:332–44.

[16] Martí-Fàbregas J, Belvís R, Guardia E, Cocho D, Muñoz J, Marruecos L, et al. Prognostic value of Pulsatility Index in acute intracerebral hemorrhage. Neurology 2003;61(8):1051–6.

[17] Momjian S, Owler BK, Czosnyka Z, Czosnyka M, Pena A, Pickard JD. Pattern of white matter regional cerebral blood flow and autoregulation in normal pressure hydrocephalus. Brain 2004;127:965–72.

[18] Newell D, Weber J, Watson R. Effect of transient moderate hyperventilation on dynamic cerebral autoregulation after severe head injury. Neurosurgery 1996;39:35–43.

[19] Owler BK, Pickard JD. Cerebral blood flow and normal pressure hydrocephalus. A review. Acta Neurologica Scandinavica 2001;104:325–42.

[20] Synek V, Reuben JR, Du Boulay GH. Comparing Evans' index and computerized axial tomography in assessing relationship of ventricular size to brain size. Neurology 1976;26(3):231–3.

[21] Vorstrup S, Christensen J, Gjerris F, Sorensen PS, Thomsen AM, Paulson OB. Cerebral blood flow in patients with normal-pressure hydrocephalus before and after CSF shunting. Journal of Neurosurgery 1987;66:379–87.

[22] Waldemar G, Schmidt JF, Delecluse F, Andersen AR, Gjerris F, Paulson OB. High resolution SPECT with [99mTc]-d,l-HMPAO in normal pressure hydrocephalus before and after shunt operation. Journal of Neurology, Neurosurgery, and Psychiatry 1993;56:655–64.

[23] Weerakkody RA, Czosnyka M, Schuhmann MU, Schmidt E, Keong N, Santarius T, et al. Clinical assessment of cerebrospinal fluid dynamics in hydrocephalus. Guide to interpretation based on observational study. Acta Neurologica Scandinavica 2011;124(2):85–98.

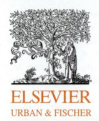
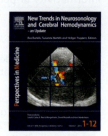

Bartels E, Bartels S, Poppert H (Editors):
New Trends in Neurosonology and Cerebral Hemodynamics — an Update.
Perspectives in Medicine (2012) 1, 316—320

journal homepage: www.elsevier.com/locate/permed

The long-term effects of hypobaric and hyperbaric conditions on brain hemodynamic: A transcranial Doppler ultrasonography of blood flow velocity of middle cerebral and basilar arteries in pilots and divers

Seyed-Mohammad Fereshtehnejad [a,b,*], Masoud Mehrpour [c], Seyed Mohammad Hossein Mahmoodi [d], Poorang Bassir [d], Banafsheh Dormanesh [e], Mohammad Reza Motamed [c]

[a] Firoozgar Clinical Research Development Center (FCRDC), Tehran University of Medical Sciences, Tehran, Iran
[b] Department of Neurobiology, Care Sciences and Society (NVS), Karolinska Institutet, Stockholm, Sweden
[c] Firoozgar Clinical Research Development Center (FCRDC), Neurology Department, Tehran University of Medical Sciences, Tehran, Iran
[d] Student Scientific Research Committee (SSRC), Tehran University of Medical Sciences, Tehran, Iran
[e] AJA University of Medical Sciences, Tehran, Iran

KEYWORDS
Hypobaric condition;
Hyperbaric condition;
Brain hemodynamic;
Transcranial Doppler ultrasonography;
Blood flow velocity

Summary
Background: Nowadays, more attention is paid to the potential risk factors of cerebrovascular events including some environmental conditions. We aimed to compare the long-term effects of hypobaric condition of pilots versus hyperbaric condition of divers as two possible occupational risk factors on blood flow velocity of middle cerebral and basilar arteries.
Methods: This cross-sectional study was performed in Firoozgar Hospital, Tehran, Iran between March 2009 and June 2010. A final number of 15 pilots and 16 divers were referred to the Neurology Laboratory of Firoozgar Hospital. Afterward, Transcranial Doppler ultrasonography was performed to evaluate blood flow velocity of middle cerebral (MCA) and basilar arteries.
Results: Comparison of the TCD findings between these two groups showed that resistance index was significantly higher in divers [0.57 (SD = 0.03) vs. 0.52 (SD = 0.06), $P = 0.008$]. A significant inverse correlation was also found between total working index of the pilots and the mean velocities ($r = -0.58$, $P = 0.027$) of right MCA even after eliminating the confounding effect of age.

* Corresponding author at: Firoozgar Hospital, Beh-Afarin St., Valiasr Ave., Tehran, Iran. Tel.: +98 21 82141367/9125207595; fax: +98 21 82141321.
E-mail addresses: sm.fereshtehnejad@ki.se (S.-M. Fereshtehnejad), m-mehrpour@tums.ac.ir (M. Mehrpour), homahmoodi@gmail.com (S.M.H. Mahmoodi), pbassir@yahoo.com (P. Bassir), smf681@yahoo.com (B. Dormanesh), mrmotamed2005@yahoo.com (M.R. Motamed).

2211-968X/$ — see front matter © 2012 Elsevier GmbH. All rights reserved.
doi:10.1016/j.permed.2012.01.002

Conclusion: In our report, some considerable associations were found especially with regard to the long-term effects of hyperbaric condition of divers on blood flow velocity of middle cerebral and basilar arteries using Transcranial Doppler ultrasonography. Chronic exposure to the hyperbaric condition of diving seems to have some probable effects on brain hemodynamics in the long-term which are in favor of decreasing blood flow and increasing of RI and PI.
© 2012 Elsevier GmbH. All rights reserved.

Introduction

With an annual incidence of about 795,000 in the United States [1], and a various incidence rate of 8–43.2 per 100,000 in Iran [2,3], stroke is a highly burdened disease [4] which is estimated to cause 5.7 million deaths in the year 2004 worldwide [5]. As a global considerable problem, much attention is currently paid to the potential risk factors of stroke. Although the previous well-known risk factors (e.g. hypertension, current smoking, diabetes mellitus, alcohol intake, depression, psychosocial, and lack of regular physical activity) were recently confirmed in a multicenter case—control study [6], more attempts are made to find out other probable risk factors.

Some evidence proposed hypobaric environment as a potential risk factor for cerebrovascular events. In a review by Clarke it was concluded that stroke and transient ischemic attack (TIA) occur more frequently than one might expect at high altitudes [7]. Another review by Wilson also revealed a considerable incidence of brain edema and headache following cerebral blood flow disturbance and cellular hypoxia induced by ascent to high altitudes [8]. Moreover, the experiences of TIA are reported in some cases of pilots [9,10].

On the other hand, hyperbaric condition of divers is also thought to be associated with a higher incidence of cerebral ischemic events [11–14]. Even though patent foramen ovale (PFO) is mostly introduced to be accompanied with these attacks, a recent study confirms the association between hyperbaric condition and cerebral ischemic events regardless of PFO [13].

Being exposed to long-term hypobaric and hyperbaric environments, pilotage and diving might be considered as occupational risk factors for brain ischemic events and consequent stroke. According to the literature review, most of the previous studies either have indirectly evaluated this relationship in artificial situation of high altitudes or reported only a limited number of cases of pilots. Furthermore, none of them have addressed the comparison between hypobaric and hyperbaric effects on brain hemodynamic. Thus, our study was designed to perform this comparison between pilots and divers. We aimed to evaluate the long-term effects of hypo/hyperbaric conditions on flow velocity of middle cerebral and basilar arteries by means of Transcranial Doppler (TCD) ultrasonography.

Methods and subjects

Individual enrollment

This cross-sectional study was performed in Firoozgar Hospital affiliated to Tehran University of Medical Sciences (TUMS), Tehran, Iran between March 2009 and June 2010.

The study protocol was approved by research committee of both Tehran University of Medical Sciences (TUMS) and AJA University of Medical Sciences. Moreover, a verbal consent form was taken from all the recruited cases. All the eligible persons had at least 2 years of working history without any previous history of cerebrovascular or cardiovascular events. Finally, a total number of 15 pilots and 16 divers were selected by snowball sampling method and referred to the Neurology Laboratory of Firoozgar Hospital.

Blood flow velocity measurements

After recruitment, Transcranial Doppler (TCD) ultrasonography was performed to evaluate blood flow velocity of middle cerebral (MCA) and basilar arteries for all of the cases. All the TCD measurements were performed by the same two experienced neurologists. Cerebral blood flow was estimated by a 2 MHz Transcranial Doppler ultrasound probe (Transcranial Doppler, Esaote, Genoa, Italy) fixed over temporal window to insonate the proximal segment of middle cerebral artery (MCA). Also in order to assess basilar artery, foramen magnum window was used. Once the optimal signal-to-noise ratio was obtained, the probe was covered with an adhesive ultrasonic gel and secured with a headband device (Multigon) to maintain optimal insonation position and angle throughout the protocol. Optimization of the Doppler signals from the MCA and basilar artery was performed by varying the sample volume depth in incremental steps and at each depth, varying the angle of insonance to obtain the best-quality signals from the Doppler frequency. In addition to basilar artery, both right and left MCAs' velocities were monitored reporting the main indexes including peak systolic velocity, end diastolic velocity and mean flow velocities. Consequently, other indexes such as systolic/diastolic velocity ratio, pulsatility index (PI) and resistance index (RI) were calculated using following formulas [15]:

$$PI = \frac{V_{peak\,systolic} - V_{end\,diastolic}}{V_{mean}}$$

$$RI = \frac{V_{peak\,systolic} - V_{end\,diastolic}}{V_{peak\,systolic}}$$

In addition to flow velocity indexes, baseline characteristics (e.g. smoking history, family history of cerebrovascular diseases, diabetes mellitus, and hypertension), laboratory variables (e.g. liver function test, lipid profile, blood sugar) and occupational indexes (duration of working, height or depth of working, working hours per week) were also recorded for each person.

Statistical analysis

Qualitative and quantitative variables were described by frequency percentages, mean and standard deviation (SD), respectively. Univariate comparisons were performed using independent sample t-test and Mann—Whitney U-test. Afterwards, analysis of covariance (ANCOVA) and partial correlation methods were used to adjust the comparisons by controlling for confounders in multivariate procedures. All the analytical processes were performed by SPSS v.16 software (Chicago, IL, USA). A P-value less than 0.05 was considered to be statistically significant.

Results

A total of 15 pilots and 16 divers aged 21—60 years participated in this study. All participants were male with a mean work history of 21 (SD = 12.53) years. None of demographic, baseline and laboratory characteristics were significantly different in two groups except for age ($P < 0.001$) and work history ($P = 0.004$).

TCD findings of right and left MCA and basilar artery were compared between two groups of this study, pilots and divers. Resistance index, pulsatility index and systolic to diastolic velocity ratio of right MCA were all significantly lower in pilots in comparison with divers ($P = 0.008$ and 0.045 and 0.021, respectively). However, speed values including mean flow velocities and end diastolic velocities were not statistically different in bivariate analysis (Tables 1—3).

Considering the age as a confounder of comparisons, a set of statistical methods employed for eliminating its effect. Analysis of covariance (ANCOVA) for controlling the variable age, revealed a significantly higher mean flow velocity of right MCA in pilots with estimated mean of 44.09 ($\pm$2.48) cm/s versus 35.74 ($\pm$2.48) cm/s of divers ($P = 0.040$). A similar difference was found between end diastolic velocity of this artery in these two groups; pilots with adjusted mean of 32.30 ($\pm$1.85) cm/s were significantly different from divers with adjusted mean of 25.02 ($\pm$1.85) cm/s ($P = 0.018$). By controlling the effect of age with partial correlation analysis, a significant reverse correlation was also detected between index of total working and mean flow velocity of right MCA in pilots ($r = -0.58$, $P = 0.027$).

Discussion

Little is known about the effect of hypobaric and hyperbaric condition on brain hemodynamic in pilots and divers according to literature review. Our study was performed to assess and compare blood flow velocity indexes between pilots and divers as representatives of hypobaric and hyperbaric conditions. While trying to explore these new features of cerebrovascular investigations, some novel findings were expected to be revealed.

In this study, with controlling the effect of age, divers appeared to have lower flow velocities including peak systolic and end diastolic as well as mean flow velocity. On the other hand, divers have also a significantly higher resistance index (RI) and pulsatility index (PI) which is in favor of low stage atherosclerotic changes of brain arteries. Although the divers were significantly younger than the pilots, these hemodynamic findings remained or even strengthened after adjusting the age effect between two study groups. These results were more significant in the right MCA which is mostly considered artery for brain hemodynamic studies in previous researches where they have shown no systematic differences in MCA flow velocities measured from the right or left sides by use of similar methodology [16,17].

Considering the normal range of PI between 0.6 and 1.1 [18], most of the cases have values within the normal range. However, a PI of lower than 0.6 (stenosis) was detected in the basilar artery of four individuals which all belonged to divers' group (25% vs. none, $P < 0.05$). Furthermore, another 2 divers had a PI of higher than 1.1 which is in favor of attenuated blood flow in basilar artery. In pilots' group, the entire measured PI's were found to be within the normal range despite the significantly higher mean age in this group.

Table 1   Comparison of TCD findings of right MCA between pilots and divers.

Velocity index	Unadjusted values		P-value	Adjusted values		P-value
	Groups of study			Groups of study		
	Pilots (n = 15)	Divers (n = 16)		Pilots (n = 15)	Divers (n = 16)	
Peak systolic velocity (cm/s)	63.67 ± 16.12	61.20 ± 13.07	0.775	67.68	57.18	0.105
Range	(41—90)	(41—92)		(59—75)	(48—65)	
End diastolic velocity (cm/s)	30.53 ± 7.72	26.80 ± 5.57	0.148	32.30	25.02	0.018*
Range	(20—45)	(21—41)		(28—36)	(21—28)	
Mean flow velocity (cm/s)	41.58 ± 10.13	38.27 ± 7.89	0.412	44.09	35.74	0.040*
Range	(27.00—58.67)	(29.67—58.00)		(30—49)	(30—40)	
Systolic/diastolic velocity ratio	2.11 ± 0.25	2.32 ± 0.23	0.021*	2.11	2.31	0.074
Range	(1.56—2.55)	(1.71—2.71)		(1.96—2.25)	(2.17—2.45)	
Resistance index	0.52 ± 0.06	0.57 ± 0.03	0.008*	0.52	0.57	0.029*
Range	(0.36—0.61)	(0.53—0.63)		(0.49—0.55)	(0.54—0.60)	
Pulsatility index	0.80 ± 0.14	0.90 ± 0.12	0.045*	0.79	0.89	0.111
Range	(0.47—1.02)	(0.57—1.07)		(0.72—0.87)	(0.81—0.97)	

* Statistical significant difference ($P < 0.05$).

Table 2 Comparison of TCD findings of left MCA between pilots and divers.

Velocity index	Unadjusted values		P-value	Adjusted values		P-value
	Groups of study			Groups of study		
	Pilots (n = 15)	Divers (n = 16)		Pilots (n = 15)	Divers (n = 16)	
Peak systolic velocity (cm/s)	67.08 ± 15.36	68.29 ± 15.97	0.830	73.69	62.14	0.094
Range	(47—95)	(45—105)		(64—82)	(53—70)	
End diastolic velocity (cm/s)	31.38 ± 8.24	30.71 ± 8.44	1	33.88	28.39	0.169
Range	(21—48)	(18—50)		(28—39)	(23—33)	
Mean flow velocity (cm/s)	43.28 ± 10.40	43.24 ± 10.50	0.981	47.15	39.64	0.117
Range	(31.00—63.67)	(29.33—68.33)		(40.96—53.34)	(33.73—45.55)	
Systolic/diastolic velocity ratio	2.18 ± 0.28	2.29 ± 0.41	0.519	2.21	2.26	0.751
Range	(1.89—2.86)	(1.74—3.17)		(1.97—2.44)	(2.04—2.49)	
Resistance index	0.54 ± 0.05	0.55 ± 0.07	0.616	0.54	0.54	0.969
Range	(0.47—0.65)	(0.43—0.68)		(0.50—0.58)	(0.50—0.58)	
Pulsatility index	0.83 ± 0.14	0.88 ± 0.19	0.488	0.85	0.86	0.891
Range	(0.67—1.15)	(0.58—1.26)		(0.74—0.96)	(0.75—0.96)	

These findings could probably emphasize the potential harmful role of hyperbaric working situation of divers compared with hypobaric environment of pilots.

A previous study by Boussuges et al. [19] showed numerous hemodynamic changes after an open-sea scuba dive. Although they have investigated hemodynamic changes after 1 h post-diving, an increase in heart rate and decrease in systolic flow velocity were demonstrated. Afterwards, they proposed two possible factors to explain these hemodynamic alterations including low volemia secondary to immersion, and venous gas embolism induced by nitrogen desaturation occurred in divers [19]. Another recent study by Moen et al. [20] that was performed on Norwegian professional divers shows widespread diffusion and perfusion abnormalities in different parts of brain hemodynamic of divers compared with controls. They concluded that several mechanisms could be contributing differently in various regions, depending for instance on the brain vessel size [20]. Compared to these previous studies, our samples of professional divers were younger in age and it is very important to show these brain hemodynamic changes in an age-group where it is not expected to have senile atherosclerotic changes yet.

Not only have they been evaluated in brain hemodynamics, but also there are some previous evidence which show that some other brain damages are more prevalent in divers including abnormalities of the electroencephalogram (EEG) [21,22] and even impaired function in some cognitive domains [23,24].

By contrast to the divers, no brain hemodynamic abnormality was detected within pilots' group. Even though the pilots were significantly more aged than the divers, measured flow velocities were higher and the mean RI and PI were lower which are in favor of a better brain hemodynamic. It must be noted that the other well-known risk factors for cerebrovascular events such as lipid profile, family history of stroke, myocardial infarction, diabetes mellitus. hypertension, and smoking history were not significantly different between two groups of study. However,

Table 3 Comparison of TCD findings of basilar artery between pilots and divers.

Velocity index	Unadjusted values		P-value	Adjusted values		P-value
	Groups of study			Groups of study		
	Pilots (n = 15)	Divers (n = 16)		Pilots (n = 15)	Divers (n = 16)	
Peak systolic velocity (cm/s)	43.43 ± 17.53	46.38 ± 14.44	0.402	45.28	44.38	0.913
Range	(25—92)	(26—83)		(34—55)	(33—55)	
End diastolic velocity (cm/s)	19.71 ± 4.58	21.77 ± 7.68	0.583	21.05	20.33	0.817
Range	(12—28)	(14—43)		(17—24)	(16—24)	
Mean flow velocity (cm/s)	27.62 ± 8.42	29.97 ± 9.77	0.550	29.12	28.35	0.865
Range	(16.33—48.67)	(18.67—56.33)		(23.37—34.88)	(22.31—34.38)	
Systolic/diastolic velocity ratio	2.16 ± 0.50	2.18 ± 0.34	0.550	2.09	2.25	0.458
Range	(1.69—3.42)	(1.77—2.92)		(1.82—2.36)	(1.97—2.54)	
Resistance index	0.52 ± 0.08	0.53 ± 0.07	0.583	0.50	0.54	0.297
Range	(0.41—0.71)	(0.43—0.66)		(0.45—0.55)	(0.49—0.59)	
Pulsatility index	0.82 ± 0.22	0.83 ± 0.17	0.616	0.77	0.86	0.367
Range	(0.55—1.34)	(0.59—1.12)		(0.65—0.90)	(0.73—0.99)	

after controlling for age, still a significant reverse correlation was also detected between index of total working and mean flow velocity of right MCA in pilots demonstrating that the higher the working duration and height of pilotage are, the lower flow velocities are expected which could be explained by hopoxic hypobaric effects of their working condition. Although not as strong as the divers, this association may be implied as the effect of pilots' chronic hypobaric condition.

Although our study has some limitations including cross-sectional design and small sample size, it must be taken into account that our TCD findings could explain some of the long-term clinical symptoms commonly reported among professional divers. In conclusion, chronic exposure to the hyperbaric condition of diving seems to have some probable effects on brain hemodynamics in the long-term which are in favor of decreasing blood flow and increasing of RI and PI. It is strongly recommended to evaluate the changes of brain hemodynamics in this working group (diving) by performing some longitudinal studies assessing the alteration of TCD indexes over the time in divers.

Acknowledgments

The authors would like to thank Dr Elham Rahmani and Dr Somayyeh Barati for their help and support in the study performance. The authors would also like to appreciate Research Deputy of AJA University of Medical Sciences for the financial support.

References

[1] Lloyd-Jones D, Adams R, Carnethon M, De Simone G, Ferguson TB, Flegal K, et al. Heart disease and stroke statistics 2009 update: a report from the American Heart Association Statistics Committee and Stroke Statistics Subcommittee. Circulation 2009;119:480—6.

[2] Ghandehari K, Izadi-M ood Z, Moud ZI. Khorasan stroke registry: analysis of 1392 stroke patients. Arch Iran Med 2007;10(3):327—34.

[3] Ghandehari K, Moud ZI. Incidence and etiology of ischemic stroke in Persian young adults. Acta Neurol Scand 2006;113(2):121—4.

[4] Akala FA, El-Saharty S. Public-health challenges in the Middle East and North Africa. Lancet 2006;367(9515):961—4.

[5] WHO. Burden of disease statistics. Geneva, Switzerland: World Health Organization; 2009. Visited on 12 May 2009 http://www.who.int/healthinfo/bod/en/index.html.

[6] O'Donnell MJ, Xavier D, Liu L, Zhang H, Chin SL, Rao-Melacini P, et al. Risk factors for ischaemic and intracerebral haemorrhagic stroke in 22 countries (the INTERSTROKE study): a case—control study. Lancet 2010;376(9735):112—23.

[7] Clarke C. Acute mountain sickness: medical problems associated with acute and subacute exposure to hypobaric hypoxia. Postgrad Med J 2006;82(973):748—53.

[8] Wilson MH, Newman S, Imray CH. The cerebral effects of ascent to high altitudes. Lancet Neurol 2009;8(2):175—91.

[9] Radimer MC. Cases from the aerospace medicine residents' teaching file. Transient ischemic attack in an aviator with patent foramen ovale and Factor V Leiden. Aviat Space Environ Med 2003;74(12):1303—5.

[10] Zhou CD, Han DX, Liu YH, Zhai YJ, Li YS. Dominant frequency uncertainty analysis of EEG alpha activity in pilots with transient ischemic attacks. Space Med Med Eng (Beijing) 1999;12(2):84—7.

[11] Knauth M, Ries S, Pohimann S, Kerby T, Forsting M, Daffertshofer M, et al. Cohort study of multiple brain lesions in sport divers: role of a patent foramen ovale. BMJ 1997;314(7082):701—5.

[12] Lier H, Schroeder S, Hering R. Patent foramen ovale: an underrated risk for divers? Dtsch Med Wochenschr 2004;129(1—2):27—30.

[13] Schwerzmann M, Seiler C, Lipp E, Guzman R, Lövblad KO, Kraus M, et al. Relation between directly detected patent foramen ovale and ischemic brain lesions in sport divers. Ann Intern Med 2001;134(1):21—4.

[14] Honek T, Veselka J, Tomek A, Srámek M, Janugka J, Sefc L, et al. Paradoxical embolization and patent foramen ovale in scuba divers: screening possibilities. Vnitr Lek 2007;53(2):143—6.

[15] Gosling RG, Dunbar G, King DH, Newman DL, Side CD, Woodcock JP, et al. The quantitative analysis of occlusive peripheral arterial disease by a nonintrusive ultrasonic technique. Angiology 1971;22:52—5.

[16] Klingelhofer J, Hajak G, Sander D, Schulz-Varszegi M, Ruther E, Conrad B. Assessment of intracranial hemodynamics in sleep apnea syndrome. Stroke 1992;23:1427—33.

[17] Netzer N, Werner P, Jochums I, Lehmann M, Strohl KP. Blood flow of the middle cerebral artery with sleep-disordered breathing: correlation with obstructive hypopneas. Stroke 1998;29:87—93.

[18] Dikanovic M, Hozo I, Kokic S, Titlic M, Jandric M, Balen I, et al. Transcranial Doppler ultrasound assessment of intracranial hemodynamics in patients with type 2 diabetes mellitus. Ann Saudi Med 2005;25(6):486—8.

[19] Boussuges A, Blanc F, Carturan D. Hemodynamic changes induced by recreational scuba diving. Chest 2006;129:1337—43.

[20] Moen G, Specht K, Taxt T, Sundal E, Grøning M, Thorsen E, et al. Cerebral diffusion and perfusion deficits in North Sea divers. Acta Radiol 2010;51(9):1050—8.

[21] Todnem K, Nyland H, Kambestad BK, Aarli JA. Influence of occupational diving upon the nervous system: an epidemiological study. Br J Ind Med 1990;47:708—14.

[22] Todnem K, Skeidsvoll H, Svihus R, Rinck P, Riise T, Kambestad BK, et al. Electroencephalography, evoked potentials and MRI brain scans in saturation divers. An epidemiological study. Electroencephalogr Clin Neurophysiol 1991;79:322—9.

[23] Vaernes RJ, Kl ø ve H, Ellertsen B. Neuropsychologic effects of saturation diving. Undersea Biomed Res 1989;16:233—51.

[24] Tetzlaff K, Friege L, Hutzelmann A, Reuter M, Holl D, Leplow B. Magnetic resonance signal abnormalities and neuropsychological deficits in elderly compressed-air divers. Eur Neurol 1999;42:194—9.

Oscillating transcranial Doppler patterns of brain death associated with therapeutic maneuvers

Pedro Cardona [a,*], Helena Quesada [a], Luis Cano [a], Jaume Campelacreu [a], Anna Escrig [b], Paloma Mora [c], Francisco Rubio [a]

[a] *Department of Neurology, Bellvitge University Hospital, Spain*
[b] *Department of Neurology, Sant Boi Hospital, Spain*
[c] *Department of Neuroradiology, Bellvitge University Hospital, Barcelona, Spain*

KEYWORDS
Brain death;
Transcranial Doppler (TCD);
Intracranial pressure (ICP);
Patterns;
Oscillating flow;
Spikes

Summary

Background: Transcranial Doppler (TCD) is a specific test for brain death diagnosis. Several Doppler patterns could change slightly during an increase of intracranial pressure related to mass effect.

Methods: We present two patients with a clinical diagnosis of brain death after massive brain hemorrhage. A Doppler pattern of reverse flow with small diastolic positive flow in both middle cerebral arteries and basilar arteries was observed in both cases.

Results: TCD was repeated 6 h later, showing an increase of systolic and diastolic flow associated with high intracranial pressure (ICP) in the first patient and a decrease of ICP in the second patient associated with polyuria. Transient improvements of blood cerebral flow could be related to the use of adrenergic drugs or the use of osmotic drugs to decrease ICP. Finally the patients showed a pattern of low spikes that led to the diagnosis of cerebrovascular arrest and brain death.

Conclusions: Therapeutics drugs to decrease ICP and several physiological processes can change several patterns of TCD associated with progression of brain death.
© 2012 Elsevier GmbH. All rights reserved.

Background

Transcranial Doppler (TCD) is a sensitive and specific test for brain death diagnosis [1].

Cerebral circulatory arrest is initially associated with Doppler evidence of oscillatory movement of blood in the large arteries at the base of the brain, but net flow is zero. This is mainly due to the elasticity of the arterial wall and the compliance of the vasculature distal to the recording site. This first pattern, diagnostic of brain death, has been validated with angiographic vascular arrest in the literature [2,3]. These oscillations eventually become low amplitude spectral spikes and finally no pulsations are detectable. In vivo experiments show that around 10—15 min of total cerebral ischemia lead to irreversible total loss of cerebral function. Therefore, a short time of cerebral circulatory arrest demonstrated by ultrasounds is sufficient to confirm irreversibility and hence cerebral death [4,5].

Several Doppler patterns could change slightly during an increase of intracranial pressure related to mass effect. We

* Corresponding author. Tel.: +34 932607919; fax: +34 932607882.
E-mail address: pcardonap@bellvitgehospital.cat (P. Cardona).

2211-968X/$ — see front matter © 2012 Elsevier GmbH. All rights reserved.
doi:10.1016/j.permed.2012.02.059

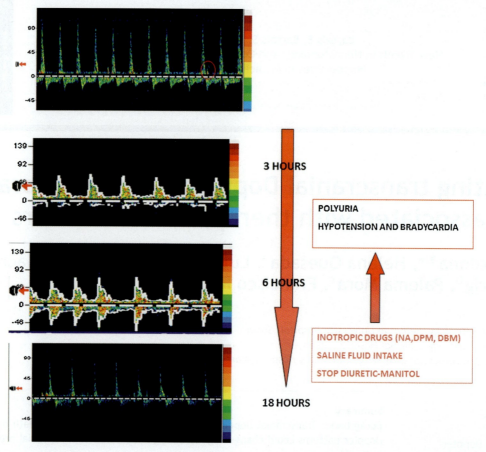

Figure 1 TCD showing reverberating flow (top image), but with brief diastolic positive spikes, that was incompatible with brain death. After a few hours TCD showed improvement of diastolic flow with a high and positive pattern possibly related to the polyuric phase and use of inotropic drugs. The last Doppler image shows isolated brief systolic flow with spikes. At that moment the patient was diagnosed of brain death.

present two patients with severe changes in Doppler patterns during evaluation of brain death.

Methods and Results

We present two patients with a clinical diagnosis of brain death but with positive blood benzodiazepine levels.

Both suffered a hemorrhagic stroke consisting of lobar hematoma and massive subarachnoid hemorrhage, with an initial exam of coma in the emergency room (GCS 3—5), and they underwent oral intubation. TCD (DWL-Multidop 2 MHz probe) was performed 24 h after hospital admission.

A Doppler pattern of reverse flow with small diastolic positive flow in both middle cerebral arteries and basilar arteries was observed in both cases. The patients were maintained with respiratory support in an intensive care unit. TCD was repeated 6 h later, showing an increase of systolic and diastolic flow associated with high intracranial pressure (ICP) in the first patient and a decrease of ICP in the second patient associated with polyuria. A new TCD examination 6 h later finally showed a pattern of low spikes that led to the diagnosis of cerebrovascular arrest and brain death.

Discussion

Extensive death of hemispheric tissue, intracranial bleeding or brain swelling can cause severe increase of ICP. If the ICP equals the diastolic arterial pressure, the brain is perfused only in systole and if ICP rises over the systolic arterial pressure, cerebral perfusion will cease [2]. Oscillating flow or systolic spikes are typical Doppler-sonographic flow signals found in the presence of cerebral circulatory arrest, which if irreversible, results in brain death. This first diagnostic pattern of brain death has been validated with angiography in the literature.

Transient improvements of blood cerebral flow could be related to the use of adrenergic drugs or the use of osmotic drugs to decrease ICP.

The use of adrenergic drugs is very common to treat hypotension associated with brain herniation and failure of the autonomic nervous system. The use of osmotic drugs is mandatory to improve intracranial pressure but is not

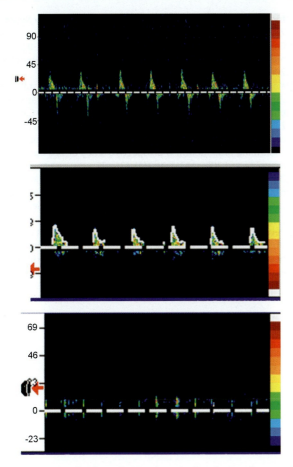

Figure 2 Cerebral and intraventricular hemorrhage with oscillation of high intracranial pressure (ICP catheter Camino).

the follow-up process of brain vascular arrest. Besides, physiological disturbances previous to death and associated with herniation, such as the polyuric phase and the inhibition of vasopressin, can decrease ICP and improve agonic blood flow. Different physiological responses after brain death lead to hemodynamic instability that could be associated with an oscillation of TCD patterns, like catecholamine output, syndrome of inappropriate antidiuretic hormone secretion, polyuria, hypothermia, decrease of thyroid hormones, decrease of cortisol or soft tissue edema [6,7].

In 1998 the Task Force Group on cerebral death of the Neurosonology Research Group of the World Federation of Neurology described that, theoretically, vital flow may reappear after a longer period of cessation of flow due to remittance of brain swelling resulting in a false negative result. However, such a case had not been observed [1].

Our cases support this hypothesis, and therefore a prolonged monitoring of cerebral flow by TCD (30 min) is recommendable when the patient has been recently treated with manitol/hiperosmotic fluids, adrenergic drugs or dosage of these treatments has been changed due to an increase of ICP or decrease of blood pressure [8,9] (Figs. 1—3).

justified in patients with irreversible and progressive neurological deterioration.

These therapeutic maneuvers can improve systemic organ perfusion and delay progression of TCD patterns associated with brain death, but may lead to mistakes in

Conclusions

The use of therapeutic drugs to decrease ICP and several physiological processes in patients with large cerebral mass effect can change several patterns of TCD associated with progression of brain death. In case of doubt, additional tests like EEG may be applied in order to confirm brain death, but an exhaustive evaluation of new treatments or dosage previously administered and repeated TCD can increase the sensitivity and specificity of ultrasound test when certain adrenergic or osmotic treatments are used.

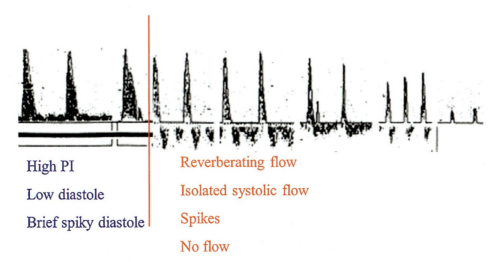

Figure 3 TCD patterns associated with progressive increase of intracranial pressure (blue) and patterns of brain death (red). (For interpretation of the references to color in this figure legend, the reader is referred to the web version of the article.)

References

[1] Ducrocq X, Hassler W, Moritake K, Newell DW, von Reutern GM, Shiogai T, et al. Consensus opinion on diagnosis of cerebral circulatory arrest using Doppler-sonography: Task Force Group on cerebral death of the Neurosonology Research Group of the World Federation of Neurology. J Neurol Sci 1998;159(August (2)):145—50.

[2] Sorrentino E, Budohoski KP, Kasprowicz M, Smielewski P, Matta B, Pickard JD, et al. Critical thresholds for transcranial Doppler indices of cerebral autoregulation in traumatic brain injury. Neurocrit Care 2011;14(April (2)):188—93.

[3] Karakitsos D, Poularas J, Karabinis A, Dimitriou V, Cardozo A, Labropoulos N. Considerations for the utilization of transcranial Doppler sonography in the study of progression towards cerebral circulatory arrest. Intensive Care Med 2010;36(December (12)):2163—4.

[4] Segura T, Calleja S, Irimia P, Tembl JI. Recommendations for the use of transcranial Doppler ultrasonography to determine the existence of cerebral circulatory arrest as diagnostic support for brain death. Spanish Society of Neurosonology. Rev Neurosci 2009;20(3—4):251—9.

[5] Calderón CV, Portela PC. Recommendations of the transcranial Doppler in the diagnosis of brain death]. Neurologia 2008;23(July—August (6)):397—8.

[6] Monteiro LM, Bollen CW, van Huffelen AC, Ackerstaff RG, Jansen NJ, van Vught AJ. Transcranial Doppler ultrasonography to confirm brain death: a meta-analysis. Intensive Care Med 2006;32(December (12)):1937—44.

[7] de Freitas GR, André C. Sensitivity of transcranial Doppler for confirming brain death: a prospective study of 270 cases. Acta Neurol Scand 2006;113(June (6)):426—32.

[8] Ducrocq X, Braun M, Debouverie M, Junges C, Hummer M, Vespignani H. Brain death and transcranial Doppler: experience in 130 cases of brain dead patients. J Neurol Sci 1998;160(September (1)):41—6.

[9] Petty GW, Mohr JP, Pedley TA, Tatemichi TK, Lennihan L, Duterte DI, et al. The role of transcranial Doppler in confirming brain death: sensitivity, specificity, and suggestions for performance and interpretation. Neurology 1990;40(February (2)):300—3.

9. Transcranial Duplex Ultrasonography

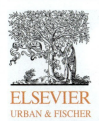

Bartels E, Bartels S, Poppert H (Editors):
New Trends in Neurosonology and Cerebral Hemodynamics — an Update.
Perspectives in Medicine (2012) 1, 325—330

journal homepage: www.elsevier.com/locate/permed

Transcranial color-coded duplex ultrasonography in routine cerebrovascular diagnostics

Eva Bartels

Center for Neurological Vascular Diagnostics, Munich, Germany

KEYWORDS
Transcranial color-coded duplex ultrasonography;
Middle cerebral artery;
Stenosis;
Occlusion;
Stroke;
Arteriovenous malformation

Summary Transcranial color-coded duplex ultrasonography (TCCS) enables the visualization of basal cerebral arteries through the intact skull by color-coding of blood flow velocity. The arteries of the circle of Willis can be identified by their anatomic location with respect to the brain stem structures and by the determination of the flow direction. TCCS is an important neuroimaging method due to its excellent time resolution. In addition to the diagnostics of intracranial vascular disease, this technique is valuable in intensive care and stroke units, e.g. for follow-up examinations in vasospasm after subarachnoid hemorrhage, and for intraoperative monitoring as well. In difficult anatomical conditions, the application of echo contrast agents can improve the diagnostic reliability of the examination. This paper reviews the examination technique and the clinical application of this method in routine cerebrovascular diagnostics.
© 2012 Elsevier GmbH. All rights reserved.

Introduction

Seventy years ago, as early as 1942, the Austrian neurologist Karl Theodor Dussik published the first paper on medical ultrasonics. Inspired by a report on the application of ultrasound in radar underwater technology, together with his brother Fritz Dussik, he introduced in Vienna a device that was able to produce sonographic images of the head and brain [1,2]. This method, named hyperphonography, however, was not accepted as a possible diagnostic tool at that time, because ultrasonic waves were attenuated by the skull in a high extend.

In the early 1950s, echoencephalography was introduced. This technique made it possible to image the position of midline echoes of the brain [3—5]. Further development of ultrasonographic techniques enabled the two-dimensional B-mode imaging of cerebral parenchyma at the end of the 1970s. However, this was only possible through the fontanel in young children [6,7].

Parallel to this development, Aaslid presented transcranial Doppler (TCD) sonography for the examination of cerebral hemodynamics in 1982 [8]. Using a pulsed Doppler system with low transmitter frequency, this method allows blood flow velocities to be recorded from basal cerebral arteries through the intact skull. With this method, intracranial arteries are examined by using transtemporal, suboccipital and transorbital approaches. The Doppler signal obtained is assigned to a specific artery based on indirect parameters: the depth of the sample volume, the position of the transducer, and the flow direction [9]. Exact differentiation between individual vessels can be in some cases difficult using the TCD method. Mistakes can occur because of the lack of anatomical structures for orientation, especially in distinguishing between arteries of the same direction of flow, or in the presence of anatomical variations. To perform compression tests of the common carotid artery in this case, however, is not recommended because during the compression thromboembolic complications cannot be

E-mail address: bartels.eva@t-online.de

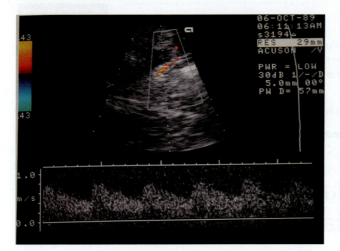
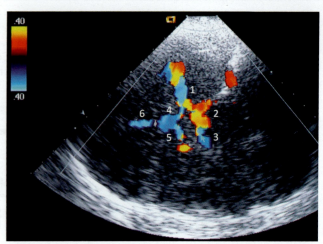

Figure 1 View of a color-coded image of the middle cerebral artery with a corresponding Doppler spectral analysis, performed under visual control using a transtemporal insonation in a healthy adult (the sample volume is placed in 57 mm depth). Documentation of this probably oldest printed image of a transcranial color-coded examination was performed on October 6, 1989 during the "Dreiländertreffen 1989" Congress in Hamburg.

Figure 2 View of the basal cerebral arteries in the axial plane with transtemporal insonation. Color-coded duplex sonography of the ipsilateral middle cerebral artery (MCA) = 1, ipsilateral posterior cerebral artery (PCA) = 2, contralateral PCA = 3, A1 segment of the ipsilateral anterior cerebral artery (ACA) = 4, A1 segment of the contralateral ACA = 5, and A2 segment of the ipsilateral and/or contralateral ACA = 6. Due to insufficient resolution, a side differentiation of the A2 segments (of both sides) is not possible.

ruled out in patients with atherosclerotic vascular disease [10].

Transcranial color-coded duplex ultrasonography (TCCS), on the other hand, enables the visualization of the basal cerebral arteries through the intact skull by color-coding of blood flow velocity. TCCS was first applied in studies of children [11]. The development of high-resolution ultrasonic systems and high performance sector transducers has opened up new perspectives for transcranial examination in adults as well [12—14]. Fig. 1 demonstrates our very first recording of the blood flow in the middle cerebral artery in October 1989 using a high resolution Acuson XP equipment (Acuson, Montain View, CA).

Examination technique

A sector transducer with an operating frequency of 2.0—3.5 MHz with a small aperture size is used for imaging intracranial vessels. As in conventional TCD, three different approaches are used to insonate intracranial arteries: transtemporal, transnuchal (suboccipital), and transorbital.

Using the transtemporal approach the basal cerebral arteries can best be displayed in the axial scanning plane. An imaging depth of 140—160 mm is most convenient. At the 1998 meeting of the European Transcranial Color-Coded Duplex Sonography Study Group (TCCS Study Group) the following standard transtemporal axial scanning planes were recommended:

1. An axial scanning plane through the *mesencephalic* brain stem — achieved by scanning in the orbitomeatal axial plane
2. An axial scanning plane through the *diencephalon* — achieved by slightly angling the transducer 10 degrees apically
3. An axial scanning plane through the *cella media* — achieved by angling the transducer 30 degrees apically.

For easier anatomical orientation on the screen, firstly, the cerebral structures in the midline — the hypoechogenic butterfly-shaped mesencephalic brain stem, surrounded by the hyperechogenic basal cistern — are displayed with B-mode ultrasonography. Subsequently, the color mode can be added to render the basal cerebral arteries visible (Fig. 2). The arteries of the circle of Willis can be identified by their anatomical location to the brain stem structures and by the determination of their flow direction based on specific color coding of the blood flow velocity. The middle cerebral artery (MCA), along with the P1 and proximal P2 segments of the posterior cerebral artery (PCA), is coded red due to their flow direction toward the transducer. In contrast, the A1 and A2 segments of the ipsilateral anterior cerebral artery (ACA), and the distal P2 segment of the PCA are coded blue, because the flow in these vessels is directed away from the transducer. Accordingly, the contralateral A1 segment of the ACA is coded red and the contralateral MCA is coded blue.

The limitations of the transtemporal insonation are mainly related to an unfavorable acoustic "bone window", in particular with elderly people. In middle-aged patients, similar to the conventional TCD, the TCCS examination is technically not possible in 10—20% [15]. The inability to image intracranial vessels in these cases can be overcome with echo contrast agents [14].

The transnuchal (suboccipital) insonation is used for the examination of the proximal portion of the basilar artery and the intracranial segment of the vertebral arteries. To make the orientation on the screen easier, first the hypoechoic structure of the foramen magnum is visualized on the B-mode image. In the next step, switching to the color mode,

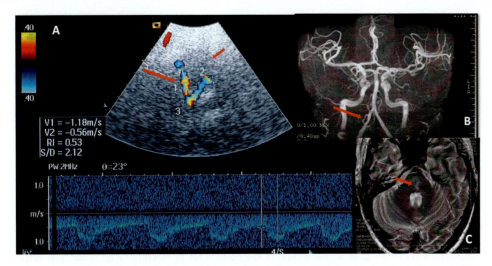

Figure 3 Imaging of the basal cerebral arteries by transnuchal (suboccipital) insonation in a 52-year-old woman with a left paramedian pons ischemia and a minor stenosis of the right vertebral artery. (A) Visualization of the right vertebral artery (VA) = 1, of the left VA = 2 and the basilar artery (BA) = 3 by insonating through the great foramen (short arrow). The spectral waveform of the right VA shows slightly increased blood flow velocities in the V4 segment (long arrow). V1 = maximum systolic velocity (118 cm/s). (B) Magnetic resonance angiogram (MRA) shows a moderate stenosis of the right VA in V4 segment (arrow). (C) Magnetic resonance image (MRI) of a left paramedian pons ischemia (arrow). (MRI, MRA images: Courtesy - Radiologie Dr. Sollfrank, München, with permission.)

the two vertebral arteries appear on both sides within the foramen magnum. Since their direction of flow is away from the transducer, these arteries are coded blue (Fig. 3).

In the transorbital color-coded ultrasonography the acoustic power should be reduced to 10—15% of the power usually used in the transtemporal approach. The duration of the insonation should be kept to a minimum in order not to damage the eye lens. The examination enables visualization of the ophthalmic artery and the carotid siphon.

As compared to the conventional TCD, the advantages of TCCS are related especially to its imaging component. A complete circle of Willis is found only in 20% of the population [16]. Most often variations are observed in which one or several vascular segments may be hypoplastic or aplastic. Especially in the axial plane, these anatomical variations can be displayed easily using TCCS (Fig. 5b and c).

In addition, by using TCD, the angle between the insonated vessel and the ultrasonic beam is not known. Because the position of the pulsed sample volume and the insonation angle cannot be visually controlled, the flow velocity within the artery can be underestimated. With TCD, a small angle of insonation (0°—30°) is assumed [8]. Accordingly, if the angle of insonation ranges from 0° to 30°, the cosine varies between 1.00 and 0.86, yielding a maximum error of less than 15% [17]. Our data show that the angle of insonation is more variable than currently assumed [18,19]. Using TCCS the sample volume is placed under visual control in the vessel segment of interest, and the insonation angle can be measured by positioning the cursor parallel to the vessel course. The mean angle of insonation was less than 30° only in the basilar artery. Although values of angle corrected blood flow velocity are not absolute values, they are more precise than those obtained by conventional TCD examination. Nevertheless, in tortuous vessels the blood flow velocity increases in proportion to the increase in the angle of insonation. This is of considerable importance in assessment of blood flow velocities in pathological conditions, especially in quantification of the stenosis of an intracranial artery.

Clinical aspects

During the last two decades TCCS found its important role in the routine diagnostics of cerebrovascular diseases, despite the technical difficulties at the beginning of the transcranial duplex ultrasonography period.

In the second part of this article a short overview of the possible indications for TCCS in the clinical routine in the examination of the intracranial arteries will be presented. The imaging of the cerebral parenchyma disorders and the examination of the cerebral veins are described in other chapters of this book [20,21].

Findings in cerebral occlusive disease

Data concerning the sensitivity and specificity of TCCS in *intracranial stenosis* and normal values of flow velocities have been established by several investigators [22—25]. The classification is based on conventional TCD studies.

The degree of stenosis is estimated on the basis of the changes of the Doppler spectrum (increased flow velocities in the area of the stenosis, and flow disturbances upstream and downstream from the lesion). TCCS provides information on the localization of the stenosis. Using the frequency dependent color-coding, the site of the stenosis can be more easily recognized due to the aliasing phenomenon (Figs. 3 and 4).

An increase in flow velocity is also measured in the case of *vasospasm*. In a stenosis the aliasing phenomenon is usually visible in a circumscribed, short section of the vessel, corresponding to the extension of the stenotic segment, whereas

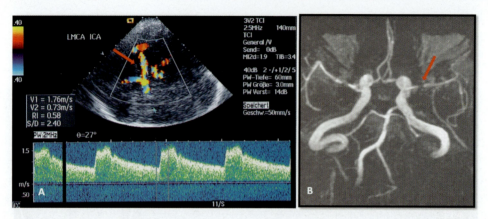

Figure 4 Bilateral MCA stenosis in the case of a 62-year-old-man with vasculitis. (A) Imaging of a moderate stenosis of the left MCA. The sample volume is placed in 60 mm depth (arrow), V1 = maximum systolic velocity (178 cm/s). An aliasing phenomenon can be seen in all visualized arteries because of the setting of the color scale by 40 cm/s mean blood flow velocity. (B) MRA of the bilateral MCA stenosis (the arrow indicates the sonographically examined artery). (MRA image: Courtesy - Radiologie Dr. Sollfrank, München, with permission.)

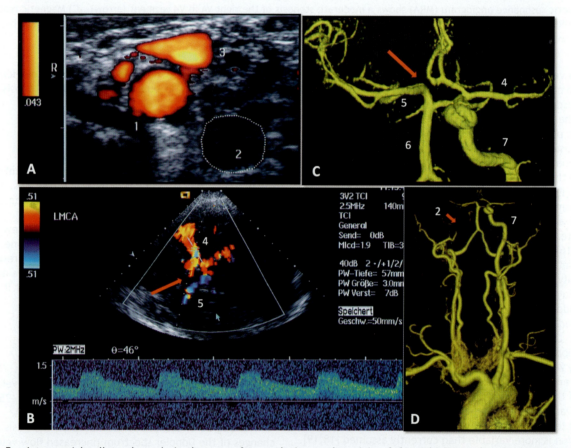

Figure 5 Intracranial collateral supply in the case of an occlusion at the origin of the right internal carotid artery (ICA) in a 67-year-old man without neurological symptoms. (A) Power mode image of the occlusion of the right ICA at the origin in transverse plane. The nonperfused lumen of the ICA [2] beside the perfused lumens of the external carotid artery (ECA) [1] and the jugular vein (JV) [3] can readily be delineated. (B) With transtemporal insonation of the left side a good collateral supply of the right hemisphere via the vertebrobasilar system can be visualized. The circle of Willis is incomplete in this patient — with an aplastic right anterior cerebral artery (arrow). (C) Intracranial MRA showing the aplastic right anterior cerebral artery (arrow), and a good collateral supply. (D) Extracranial MRA image of the occlusion of the right ACI at the origin (the arrow points at the ICA area without flow signal). 1: right ECA, 2: right ICA, 3: right JV, 4: left MCA, 5: right MCA, 6: BA, and 7: left ICA. (MRA images: Courtesy - Diagnoseklinik München, with permission.)

with a vasospasm several vessels are often affected simultaneously. This can be impressively demonstrated due to the aliasing phenomenon in all imaged vessels facilitating the differentiation between a stenosis and vasospasm [14].

Ultrasonographic diagnosis of an *occlusion* of a cerebral artery can be made when a color-coded signal cannot be obtained at depths of insonation corresponding to that artery, although neighboring arteries can be imaged well.

Criteria for the diagnosis of MCA occlusion include lack of detectable flow in the MCA, a sufficient visibility of the other arteries (of the ipsilateral PCA, or ACA), or veins (deep middle cerebral vein), and the detection of a collateral flow.

TCCS has become a standard diagnostic technique to assess the intracranial status in acute stroke. It is increasingly used for the evaluation of prognosis and the success of revascularization in clinical trials. Recommendations on the methodology how examinations should be performed in the time limited situation of acute stroke, for monitoring of recanalization, and on documentation are summarized in the "*Consensus Recommendations for Transcranial Color-Coded Duplex Sonography for the assessment of Intracranial Arteries in Clinical Trials on Acute Stroke*" which were approved during a meeting of the consensus group in October 2008 in Giessen, Germany [26].

In an *extracranial* occlusion of the internal carotid artery the *presence of collateral pathways* imaged by transcranial sonography allow a prognosis to be made in the case of an acute vessel obstruction. To assess the effects of an extracranial occlusion of the internal carotid artery on cerebral hemodynamics, indirect extra- and intracranial findings must be considered (Fig. 5) [14,27].

Findings in cerebral vascular malformations

An *arteriovenous malformation* (*AVM, angioma*) is a massive collection of abnormal vessels in which the arterial circulation flows directly into the venous circulation, bypassing the capillary network. With TCCS, the pathological vascular convolutions of an AVM can be displayed directly on the screen. Furthermore, the typical Doppler spectrum of the angiomatous vessels can be recorded under visual control. Visualization of an AVM depends on its localization, rather than its size. The detection of AVMs located in the temporal and deep basal brain regions, in particular, is usually highly successful. AVMs located near the parietal, frontal, occipital or cerebellar cortex, on the other hand, are difficult to image, even if their diameters are larger [28].

If an AVM cannot be visualized directly, detection of feeding arteries in the circle of Willis makes the diagnosis very probable. Hereby, especially the low pulsatility of the Doppler spectrum is typical.

An *aneurysm* is imaged as a color-coded appendix next to a normal vessel. The most typical color coded feature is the presence of two areas with inversely directed flow: Half of the aneurysm is coded blue, and the other half is coded red, with the colors corresponding to the direction of in- and outflowing blood. Between these two areas, a black separation zone without color coding and with undetectable blood flow can be recognized.

Visualization of an aneurysm depends on its localization and size (>5 mm). Aneurysms located in the proximal segment of the arteries of the circle of Willis can be recognized more easily than those situated in the periphery. Special software, such as three-dimensional reconstruction tools, can make these lesions assessable in a high number of patients [29]. In addition, power Doppler imaging can be useful in detecting low flow velocities within aneurysms. The reliability of the investigation can also be improved by using echo contrast agents [30].

TCCS should not be used for screening of AVM. On the other hand, as a noninvasive method this technique is suitable for postoperative follow-up examination and for *embolization monitoring* in patients with intracranial angioma or fistulae. After embolization, a decrease of vascular convolutions, a reduction in flow velocities, and an increase of the reduced pulsatility indices can be observed [14].

Conclusion

Transcranial color-coded duplex ultrasonography is an important neuroimaging method due to its excellent time resolution. In addition to the diagnostics of intracranial vascular disease, this technique is valuable in intensive care and stroke units for follow-up examinations in vasospasm after subarachnoid hemorrhage and for intraoperative monitoring. In difficult anatomical conditions, the application of echo contrast agents can improve the diagnostic reliability of the examination. Based on advances in computer and transducer technology TCCS as a noninvasive method has a great potential in further innovative imaging and therapeutic solutions such as cerebral perfusion imaging, sonothrombolysis, and site targeted ultrasound contrast agents for drug delivery to the brain.

References

[1] Dussik KT. Über die Möglichkeit, hochfrequente mechanische Schwingungen als diagnostisches Hilfsmittel zu verwerten. Z Ges Neurol Psychiat 1942;174:153—68.

[2] Dussik KT, Dussik F, Wyt L. Auf dem Weg zur Hyperphonographie des Gehirns. Wiener Medizinische Wochenschrift 1947;97:425—9.

[3] French LA, Wild JJ, Neal D. The experimental application of ultrasonic to the localization of brain tumors. Journal of Neurosurgery 1951;8:198—203.

[4] Leksell L. Kirurgisk behandling av skallskador. In: Vortrag: Meeting of Svenska Läkasaällskapet. 1954.

[5] Bartels E. Transcranial color-coded ultrasonography. In: Babikian V, Wechsler L, editors. Transcranial doppler ultrasonography. Boston: Butterworth-Heinemann; 1999. p. 271—84.

[6] Cook RWI. Ultrasound examination of neonatal heads. Lancet 1979;1:38.

[7] Babcock DS, Han BK, LeQuesne GW. B-mode gray scale ultrasound of the head in newborn and young infant. American Journal of Neuroradiology 1980;1:181—92.

[8] Aaslid R, Markwalder T-M, Nornes H. Noninvasive transcranial Doppler ultrasound recording of velocity in basal cerebral arteries. Journal of Neurosurgery 1982;57:769—74.

[9] Arnolds BJ, von Reutern G-M. Transcranial Doppler sonography, examination technique and normal reference values. Ultrasound in Medicine and Biology 1986;12:115—23.

[10] Khaffaf N, Karnik R, Winkler W-B, Valentin A. Embolic stroke by compression maneuver during transcranial Doppler sonography. Stroke 1994;25:1056–7.

[11] Schöning M, Grunert D, Stier B. Transkranielle Duplexsonographie durch den intakten Knochen: Ein neues diagnostisches Verfahren. Ultraschall in der Medizin 1989;10:66–71.

[12] Furuhata H. New evolution of transcranial tomography (TCT) and transcranial color Doppler tomography (TCDT). Neurosonology 1989;2:8–15.

[13] Bogdahn U, Becker G, Winkler J, Greiner K, Perez J, Meurers B. The transcranial colour coded real-time sonography in adults. Stroke 1990;21:1680–8.

[14] Bartels E. Transcranial Color-Coded Ultrasonography (TCCS) — Cerebral arteries and Parenchyma. In: Bartels E, editor. Color-Coded Duplex Ultrasonography of the Cerebral Vessels/Atlas and Manual [Farbduplexsonographie der hirnversorgenden Gefäße/Atlas und Handbuch]. Stuttgart: Schattauer; 1999. p. 187–220.

[15] Grolimund P, Seiler RW. Age dependence of the flow velocity in the basal cerebral arteries: a transcranial Doppler ultrasound study. Ultrasound in Medicine and Biology 1988;14:191–8.

[16] Riggs HE, Rupp C. Variation in form of circle of Willis. Archives of Neurology 1963;8:24–30.

[17] Ringelstein EB, Kahlscheurer B, Niggermeyer E, et al. Transcranial Doppler sonography: anatomical landmarks and normal velocity values. Ultrasound in Medicine and Biology 1990;16:745–61.

[18] Bartels E. Transkranielle farbkodierte Duplexsonographie: Möglichkeiten und Grenzen der Methode im Vergleich zu der konventionellen transkraniellen Dopplersonographie. Ultraschall in der Medizin 1993;14:272–8.

[19] Bartels E, Flügel KA. Quantitative measurements of blood flow velocity in basal cerebral arteries with transcranial color Doppler imaging. Journal of Neuroimaging 1994;4:77–81.

[20] Walter U. Transcranial sonography of the cerebral parenchyma: update on clinically relevant applications. In: Bartels E, Bartels S, Poppert H, editors. New trends in neurosonology and cerebral hemodynamics — an update. Elsevier, Perspectives in Medicine, in press.

[21] Stolz E. Ultrasound examination techniques of extra- and intracranial veins. In: Bartels E, Bartels S, Poppert H, editors. New trends in neurosonology and cerebral hemodynamics — an update. Elsevier, Perspectives in Medicine, in press.

[22] Martin P, Evans D, Naylor A. Transcranial colour-coded sonography of the basal cerebral circulation. Reference data from 115 volunteers. Stroke 1994;25:390–6.

[23] Baumgartner RW. Transcranial color-coded duplex sonography. Journal of Neurology 1999;246:637–47.

[24] Baumgartner RW. Transcranial color duplex sonography in cerebrovascular disease: a systematic review. Cerebrovascular Diseases 2003;16:4–13.

[25] Krejza J, Baumgartner RW. Clinical applications of transcranial color-coded duplex sonography. Journal of Neuroimaging 2004;14:215–25.

[26] Nedelmann M, Stolz E, Gerriets T, Baumgartner RW, Malferrari G, Seidel G, et al. Consensus recommendations for transcranial color-coded duplex sonography for the assessment of intracranial arteries in clinical trials in acute stroke. Stroke 2009;40:3238–44.

[27] Baumgartner RW, Baumgartner I, Mattle HP, Schroth G. Transcranial color-coded duplex sonography in the evaluation of collateral flow through the circle of Willis. American Journal of Neuroradiology 1997;18:127–33.

[28] Bartels E. Evaluation of arteriovenous malformations with transcranial color-coded duplex ultrasonography. Does the location of an AVM influence its ultrasonic detection? Journal of Ultrasound in Medicine 2005;24:1511–7.

[29] Klötzsch C, Bozzato A, Lammers G, Mull M, Noth J. Three-dimensonal transcranial color-coded sonography of cerebral aneurysms. Stroke 1999;30:2285–90.

[30] Droste DW, Boehm T, Ritter MA, Dittrich R, Ringelstein EB. Benefit of echocontrast-enhanced transcranial arterial color-coded duplex ultrasound. Cerebrovascular Diseases 2005;20: 332–6.

Evaluation of very early recanalization after tPA administration monitoring by transcranial color-coded sonography

Hidetaka Mitsumura [a,*], Makiko Yogo [a], Renpei Sengoku [a], Hiroshi Furuhata [b], Soichiro Mochio [a]

[a] *The Jikei University School of Medicine, Department of Neurology, 3-25-8, Nishi Shimbashi, Minato-ku, Tokyo 1058461, Japan*
[b] *The Jikei University School of Medicine, ME Laboratory, Japan*

KEYWORDS
Transcranial ultrasound;
Acute ischemic stroke;
Recanalization;
Tissue plasminogen activator;
Magnetic resonance angiography

Summary

Background/aims: Cerebrovascular ultrasonography was useful clinically for evaluating cerebral hemodynamics rapidly and in real-time for patients with acute ischemic stroke. We analyzed if the patients had early recanalization or not using transcranial color-coded sonography (TCCS) in order to evaluate the usefulness of real-time monitoring in systemic thrombolysis.

Methods: Subjects were patients who had acute ischemic stroke with intravenous tissue plasminogen activator (tPA) within 3 h from onset. We evaluated occlusion of intracranial arteries from transtemporal or suboccipital window by TC-CFI with Thrombolysis in Brain Ischemia (TIBI) flow-grading system and monitored residual flow in real-time every 15 min until 120 min after the t-PA bolus.

Results: We could monitor residual flow in 5 patients who had good echo windows (4 male, mean age; 60.8 ± 6.4 years). Two patients had proximal occlusion of the middle cerebral artery (MCA), one patient had distal occlusion of MCA, one patient had M2 occlusion and one patient had distal occlusion of unilateral vertebral artery. Four patients had early complete recanalization within 60 min after the t-PA bolus (two patients within 60 min and other two patients within 30 min), however, occlusion persisted during 120 min monitoring in one patient with proximal occlusion of MCA. NIH Stroke Scale of two patients with very early recanalization was 0 at the end of the treatment. There was no symptomatic and asymptomatic intracranial hemorrhage in 4 patients except for the patients without recanalization.

Conclusions: It is anticipated that real-time ultrasound monitoring is useful for evaluating a very early thrombolytic effect of tPA connected with early clinical recovery.
© 2012 Elsevier GmbH. All rights reserved.

Introduction

The National Institute of Neurological Disorders and Stroke trial of recombinant tissue plasminogen activator (tPA) showed that intravenous thrombolysis with acute ischemic stroke within 3 h from onset had favorable clinical recovery compared with placebo-treated patients [1]. However, a thrombolytic effect was not evaluated with monitoring of occlusion artery in this study. Cerebrovascular ultrasonography was useful clinically for evaluating cerebral hemodynamics rapidly and in real-time for the patients with acute ischemic stroke compared with magnetic resonance

* Corresponding author.
  E-mail address: hmitsumura@mac.com (H. Mitsumura).

angiography (MRA). The timing and speed of recanalization after (tPA) therapy monitoring by transcranial Doppler (TCD) correlates with clinical recovery [2,3]. These real-time flow informations are useful in developing next therapies and in selection for interventional treatment.

The aim of this study was to analyze if the patients had early recanalization or not using transcranial color-coded sonography (TCCS) in order to evaluate the usefulness of real-time monitoring in systemic thrombolysis.

Material and methods

Consecutive patients who had acute ischemic stroke with intravenous tPA within 3 h from onset between April 2010 and January 2011 were included in this study. tPA was administered in a dose of 0.6 mg/kg (10% bolus, 90% continuous infusion during 1 h) according to Japanese standard protocol [4]. The patients with insufficient acoustic window were excluded.

An experienced neuro-sonographer performed all TCCS studies using a EUB-7500 or 8500 with a 2 MHz sector transducer (S50A, HITACHI Medical Corporation, Japan). We evaluated occlusion of intracranial arteries from transtemporal or suboccipital window by TCCS with Thrombolysis in Brain Ischemia (TIBI) flow-grading system [5] and monitored residual flow in real-time every 15 min until 120 min after the t-PA bolus. An insonation time with TCCS was not longer than 5 min in each examination. No head frame was used during insonation. Complete recanalization was defined as TIBI 0—3 to 5, and partial recanalization was defined as TIBI 0—2 to 3.

National Institutes of Health Stroke Scale (NIHSS) scores were obtained before tPA treatment, every 15 min until 1 h and every 30 min after 1 h by a neurologist. Dramatic clinical recovery was defined as a decrease in the total NIHSS score to <3 at the end of tPA infusion.

All patients had magnetic resonance imaging (MRI) including diffusion-weighted imaging (DWI) and MRA before tPA administration. Follow-up MRA was performed immediately after the end of tPA infusion, if possible.

Results

We could monitor residual flow in 5 patients who had good echo windows (4 male, mean age; 60.8 ± 6.4 years). Two patients had proximal occlusion of the middle cerebral artery (MCA), one patient had distal occlusion of the MCA, one patient had a M2 occlusion and one patient had a distal occlusion of the unilateral vertebral artery. One patient with proximal MCA occlusion had an insufficient acoustic window, but we could monitor residual flow at M2.

Four patients had early complete recanalization within 60 min after the t-PA bolus - two patients at 60 min and other two patients at 30 min. In the patient who could be monitored at M2, one of M2 (M2a) was partial at 30 min, another M2 (M2b) was complete at 30 min. On the other hand, the occlusion persisted during 120 min monitoring in one patient with proximal occlusion of MCA.

NIH Stroke Scale of two patients with very early recanalization (within 30 min) was 0 at the end of the treatment (dramatic clinical recovery).

In three patients a follow-up MRA could be performed after the end of tPA infusion. Follow-up MRA showed early recanalization in two patients and no recanalization in one patient. These findings of MRA were consistent with diagnosis of TCCS. There was no symptomatic and asymptomatic intracranial hemorrhage in 4 patients except for the patients without recanalization. Table 1 shows clinical detail data of 5 patients, and Fig. 1 shows the information of TCCS und MRA in patients with very early recanalization (within 30 min).

Discussion

The present study showed that patients with early recanalization had a favorable outcome after tPA therapy. In these

Table 1 Clinical data of subjects.

Case	Age	Sex	TIBI	MRA	Early recanalization	NIHSS before treatment	NIHSS after treatment[c]	Symptomatic ICH
1	68	M	TIBI 3 at Rt M1	Rt M1 distal occlusion	Complete[a]	10	6	—
2	58	M	TIBI 3 at Rt VA	Rt VA distal occlusion	Complete[a]	4	2	—
3[d]	52	M	TIBI 3 at Lt M1	Lt M2 occlusion	Complete[b]	2	0	—
4[d]	60	F	TIBI 0 at Rt M2	Rt M1 proximal occlusion	M2a; partial M2b; complete[b]	10	0	—
5	66	M	TIBI 0 at Lt M1	Lt M1 proximal occlusion	No recanalization	18	19	+

M, male; F, female; Rt, right; Lt, left; VA, vertebral artery; ICH, intracerebral hemorrhage.
Case 4; one branch of M2 had complete recanalization < 30 min, the other branch had partial recanalization at 30 min and complete recanalization at 120 min.
[a] Recanalization < 60 min.
[b] Recanalization < 30 min.
[c] NIHSS at 120.
[d] Two patients with gray shaded values had very early recanalization (within 30 min). Details are shown in Fig. 1.

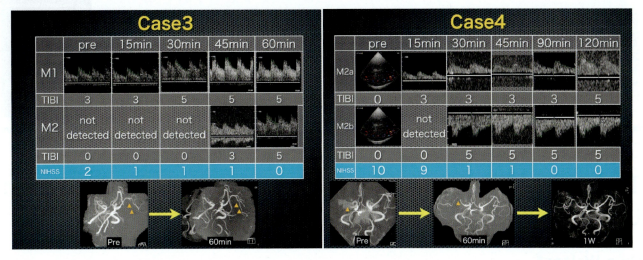

Figure 1 Angiographic information of patients with very early recanalization (see also case 3 and case 4 on table). Upper table is sonogram of residual flow and NIHSS at each examination point. Lower pictures are MRA before and after tPA therapy. Case 3 was M2 occlusion and case 4 with proximal MCA occlusion had insufficient acoustic window, but we could monitor residual flow at M2. Case 3 had very early complete recanalization within 30 min after the t-PA bolus. In case 4, one of M2 (M2a) was partial at 30 min, and another M2 (M2b) was complete at 30 min. MRA findings of these cases were consistent with diagnosis of TCCS.

studies, recanalization after tPA was evaluated by MRA [6,7] or TCD [2,3]. There are different benefits and limitations between MRA and TCD/TCCS in their diagnostic ability and characteristics as a diagnostic device. MRI is the standard device for the detection of vessel occlusion or stenosis, however, it cannot be monitored during tPA infusion because patients who get a MRI have to be transferred to the MRI laboratory. On the other hand, TCD/TCCS is useful for real-time evaluation of intracranial hemodynamics at patient's bedside. Several cases, however, had an insufficient acoustic window especially in Asian elderly female.

In TCD study (2), 25% patients recanalized within the first 30 min, 50% recanalized within 30—60 min, 11% recanalized 61—120 min, and 14% recanalized after first 2 h after tPA bolus administration. The timing of arterial recanalization after stroke onset detected with TCD correlated with early improvement in the NIHSS scores within the next hour after recanalization (S-shaped curve demonstrates correlation between timing of recanalization on TCD and early recovery from ischemic stroke).

Our data showed patients with complete early recovery after tPA treatment recanalized within the first 30 min on TCCS monitoring. It is anticipated that early arterial recanalization correlated with early clinical improvement like present studies.

In other TCD study (3), the speed of intracranial arterial recanalization on TCD correlates with short-term improvement after tPA therapy. Short duration (sudden < 1 min and stepwise 1—29 min) of arterial recanalization is associated with better short-term improvement because of faster and more complete clot breakup with low resistance of the distal circulatory bed. Slow (>30 min) flow improvement and dampened flow signal that indicate partial recanalization are less favorable prognostic signs.

However, our study did not use continuous TCCS monitoring, the speed of clot lysis as well as timing of arterial recanalization is useful information for evaluating effect of thrombolytic therapy. This real-time and noninvasive information using TCD/TCCS are the advantage over MRA.

Conclusions

Very early recanalization within 30 min after tPA administration correlated with complete early on TCCS monitoring. It is anticipated that real-time ultrasound monitoring is useful for evaluating very early thrombolytic effect of tPA connected with early clinical recovery.

References

[1] The National Institutes of Neurological Disorders and Stroke rt-PA Stroke Study Group. Tissue plasminogen activator for acute ischemic stroke. N Engl J Med 1995;333:1581—7.
[2] Christou I, Alexandrov AV, Burgin WS, Mojner AW, Felberg RA, Malkoff M, et al. Timing of recanalization after tissue plasminogen activator therapy determined by transcranial Doppler correlates with clinical recovery from ischemic stroke. Stroke 2000;31:1812—6.
[3] Alexandrov AV, Burgin WS, Demchuck AM, El-Mitwalli A, Grotta JC. Speed of intracranial clot lysis with intravenous tissue plasminogen activator therapy. Sonographic classification and short-term improvement. Circulation 2001;103:2897—902.
[4] Yamaguchi T, Mori E, Minematsu K, Nakagawara J, Hashi K, Saito I, et al. Alteplase at 0.6 mg/kg for acute ischemic stroke within 3 h of onset: Japan Alteplase Clinical Trial (J-ACT). Stroke 2006;37:1810—5.
[5] Demchuk AM, Burgin WS, Christou I, Felberg RA, Barber PA, Hill MD, et al. Thrombolysis in brain ischemia (TIBI) transcranial Doppler flow grades predict clinical severity, early recovery, and mortality in patients treated with intravenous tissue plasminogen activator. Stroke 2001;32:89—93.
[6] Mori E, Minematsu K, Nakagawara J, Yamaguchi T, Sasaki M, Hirano T, et al. Effects of 0.6 mg/kg Intravenous alteplase on vascular and clinical outcome in middle cerebral artery occlusion. Japan Alteplase Clinical Trial II (J-ACT II). Stroke 2010;41:461—5.
[7] Kimura K, Iguchi Y, Shibasaki K, Aoki J, Watanabe M, Kobayashi K, et al. Recanalization within one hour after intravenous tissue plasminogen activator is associated with favorable outcome in acute stroke patients. Eur Neurol 2010;63:331—6.

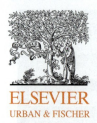
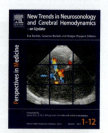

Bartels E, Bartels S, Poppert H (Editors):
New Trends in Neurosonology and Cerebral Hemodynamics — an Update.
Perspectives in Medicine (2012) 1, 334—343

journal homepage: www.elsevier.com/locate/permed

Transcranial sonography of the cerebral parenchyma: Update on clinically relevant applications

Uwe Walter*

Department of Neurology, University of Rostock, Gehlsheimer Str. 20, D-18147, Rostock, Germany

KEYWORDS
Transcranial ultrasound;
Stroke;
Parkinsonism;
Substantia nigra;
Basal ganglia;
Electrode position control

Summary Transcranial B-mode sonography (TCS) is a neuroimaging technique that displays the brain parenchyma and the intracranial ventricular system through the intact skull. Sophisticated TCS systems can currently achieve a higher image resolution of echogenic deep brain structures than MRI under clinical conditions. The different imaging principle of TCS allows visualization of characteristic changes in several neurodegenerative diseases that can hardly be visualized with other imaging methods, such as substantia nigra hyperechogenicity in Parkinson's disease (PD), and lenticular nucleus hyperechogenicity in atypical Parkinsonian syndromes. The intracranial ventricular system and a midline shift due to space-occupying brain lesions (e.g., intracerebral hematomas) are reliably assessed with TCS. The present paper reviews recent studies on diagnostic TCS applications that, as a result, can be recommended for routine use in clinical practice. These applications include the bedside monitoring of space-occupying lesions in acute stroke patients, the early and differential diagnosis of PD, and the postoperative position control of deep brain stimulation electrodes. Novel technologies such as in-time fusion of TCS with MRI scans, automated detection of intracranial target structures, and improved 3D-image analysis promise an even wider application of TCS in the coming years.
© 2012 Elsevier GmbH. All rights reserved.

Introduction

Transcranial B-mode sonography (TCS) is a neuroimaging technique that displays the brain parenchyma and the intracranial ventricular system through the intact skull. Its different imaging principle allows visualization of characteristic changes in several neurodegenerative diseases that can hardly be visualized with other imaging methods, such as substantia nigra (SN) hyperechogenicity in Parkinson's disease (PD) [1,2]. While TCS has been performed in children already in the 1980s and 1990s of the last century [3,4], the clinical application of TCS in adults has developed only subsequently since the TCS imaging conditions are much more difficult in adults because of the thickening of temporal bones with increasing age [5]. In the 1990s first studies showed that TCS allows the visualization of major parenchymal structures, as well as lesions (mainly tumors and bleeding) from the lower brainstem up to the parietal lobe [6—10], and well reproducible measurements of the whole ventricular system [11]. Due to the technological advances of the past decade a high-resolution imaging of deep brain structures is meanwhile possible in the majority of adults [2,12,13]. Present-day TCS systems can achieve a higher image resolution in comparison not only to former-generation systems, but currently also to MRI under clinical conditions (Fig. 1) [13]. A sophisticated clinical high-end TCS system was shown to gain an in-plane image

* Tel.: +49 381 4949696; fax: +49 381 4944794.
E-mail address: uwe.walter@med.uni-rostock.de

2211-968X/$ — see front matter © 2012 Elsevier GmbH. All rights reserved.
doi:10.1016/j.permed.2012.02.014

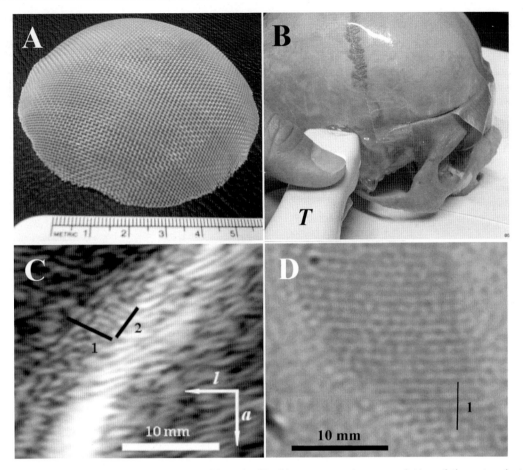

Figure 1 Comparison of transcranial sonography (TCS) and MRI with respect to image resolution of the network structure of a kitchen strainer placed within a human skull phantom filled with ultrasound gel. (A) Photograph of the kitchen strainer consisting of polyamide threads forming a 1.1 mm × 0.8 mm network. (B) The transducer (T) was placed at preauricular position for TCS. (C) Using a contemporary TCS system, the network structure of the intracranially located strainer could be clearly visualized (a = axial direction, l = lateral direction, 1 = bar indicating five threads with 1.1 mm distance, 2 = bar indicating five threads with 0.8 mm distance). (D) With MRI, simulating clinical conditions, the network structure was not visualized (1 = bar indicating five threads with 1.1 mm distance) [13].

resolution of intracranial structures in the focal zone of about 0.7 mm × 1.1 mm [13]. Beside high image resolution, contemporary TCS systems also offer high mobility, and TCS images of good quality are meanwhile obtained with distinct hand-held TCS systems [14]. Further advantages of TCS are its non-invasiveness, low costs, high acceptance by the patients, and relative independence from movement artefacts. This has promoted the development of a number of clinical TCS applications especially in patients with movement disorders, and in patients who need bedside assessment. An important milestone was the establishment of consensus guidelines on TCS in movement disorders [1], which was triggered by an activity of the European Society of Neurosonology and Cerebral Hemodynamics (ESNCH) in 2004. The use of ultrasound contrast agents offers an improved assessment on TCS of patients with acute stroke [15—17], with brain tumors [18], and inflammatory brain disorders [19], but is still on an experimental level and will be reviewed in another chapter of this serial.

The present paper reviews TCS studies without contrast agent application published in the past decade that assessed novel TCS applications, which can be, as a result, recommended for clinical use. These applications include the monitoring of space-occupying lesions in acute stroke patients, the early and differential diagnosis of PD, and the postoperative position control of deep brain stimulation (DBS) electrodes.

TCS system settings and scanning procedures

For TCS, a contemporary high-end ultrasound system, as applied also for transcranial color-coded cerebrovascular ultrasound, equipped with a 2.0- to 3.5- (1.0- to 5.0-) MHz transducer can well be used. It has to be considered that certain measurements, e.g., of the size of a hyperechogenic area are dependent on the applied ultrasound system and the individual system settings. System parameters, such as the width of ultrasonic beam, the line density, and even the age of the probe influence the image resolution. Therefore, reference values need to be obtained (and ideally updated for the same probe every 2—3 years) separately for each ultrasound system. The following system settings are recommended: penetration depth 14—16 cm,

Table 1 Ultrasound system settings for transcranial sonography.

Parameter	Settings
Ultrasound system	
Penetration depth	Start with 14—16 cm, reduce if needed
Dynamic range	45—55 dB
Postprocessing function	Moderate suppression of low echo signals
Time gain compensation	Adjust manually as needed, or use the 'tissue optimization' function if available
Image brightness	Adjust manually, not too high, or use the 'tissue optimization' function if available
Ultrasound transducer	
Crystal/channel	As high as possible, ideally: 'matrix' probe
Insonation frequency (center frequency)	2.0—3.5 MHz, preferably 2.5 MHz

dynamic range 45—55 dB, and if selectable a post-processing preset with moderate suppression of low echogenic signals (Table 1). Image brightness and time gain compensation are adapted visually and/or with using automated image optimization (available with high-end ultrasound systems). For the examination, the patient is posed in a supine position, and the examiner usually sits at the head of the examination table. The investigation is usually performed through the transtemporal bone window consecutively from each side with preauricular position of the ultrasound probe (Fig. 2). Other transcranial approaches used for specific questions are the foramen magnum, the transfrontal, and the transoccipital bone window. The latter two, however are more frequently insufficient to insonate in adults. The structures assessed at different planes and windows are detailed below. There are two standard transtemporal axial scanning planes, defined by cerebral landmark structures (midbrain, thalamus), that are recommended to be applied especially at any diagnostic examination in patients with movement disorders [1,2], although the course of the examination may be individually adapted according to the diagnostic question [12,20].

To display the plane at midbrain level, the examination starts with the identification of the hypo- to anechogenic butterfly-shaped structure of mesencephalic brainstem surrounded by the highly echogenic basal cisterns in the axial scanning plane. The mesencephalic brainstem surrounded by the highly echogenic basal cisterns can easily be delineated in 90—95% of individuals, even in those with only partially sufficient acoustic bone windows. Within the brainstem, several structures of increased echogenicity, including SN, red nucleus, the midline raphe, and the aqueduct can be visualized. For the clinical applications described in this article, the assessment of SN echogenicity is most important. To date, the best-validated method to grade SN echogenicity is the planimetric measurement of SNs echogenic signals in axial plane [1,2,20]. Semiquantitative visual grading was less reliable [20,21]. Efforts to quantify SN echogenicity in

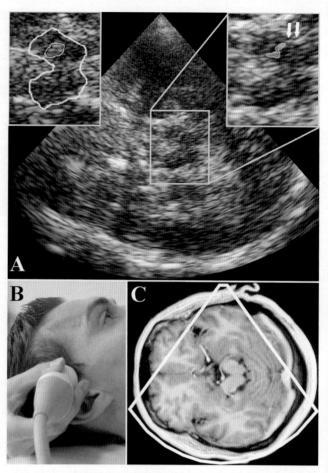

Figure 2 Illustration of transcranial sonography (TCS) of substantia nigra (SN). (A) TCS axial image of the brain at midbrain level obtained in a patient with normal appearance of SN. In the center of the image, the butterfly-shaped, weakly echogenic midbrain is displayed which is surrounded by the highly echogenic basal cisterns. The rectangle corresponds to the zoomed image of the midbrain shown in the insert panel in the right upper corner; in this panel, the echosignals of the SN are surrounded (here: normal echogenic area). Note the typical imaging artifact from the basal cistern (arrows) that should not be mistaken for SN echosignals. For comparison, an exemplary image obtained in another patient with markedly hyperechogenic SN is shown in the insert panel in the left upper corner. (B) Transducer position for TCS. (C) MR image corresponding to the TCS plane shown in (A).

a less rater-dependent way, e.g., by measuring echointensity of SN relative to surrounding parenchyma, volumetry, semi-automatic SN detection, or complex mathematical echo-signal analysis have either failed, or are not ripe for clinical application [20]. According to consensus guidelines [1], a marked SN hyperechogenicity is considered, if the measured echogenic area exceeds a cut-off value defined by the 90% percentile of measures in normal population, and moderate hyperechogenicity, if the measured area ranges in-between the 75% and 90% percentile of measures in normal population. Most authors use the larger of bilaterally measured sizes for rating SN echogenicity.

Table 2 Reported cut-off values for the discrimination between normoechogenic and hyperechogenic substantia nigra with different ultrasound systems.

Manufacturer/ultrasound system	Probe/frequency (MHz)	Cut-off value (cm^2) SN-h	References
Esaote/AU4	Phased-array/2.5	≥0.20	[23]
Esaote/MyLab25 Gold	PA240/2.5	≥0.20	[14]
Esaote/MyLab Twice	PA240/2.5	≥0.24	(Own data)
Esaote/Technos MP	Sector/2.5	≥0.19	[26]
General Electric/Logiq 7	3S/2.5	≥0.24	[24]
General Electric/Logiq 9	3S/2.5	≥0.20	[28]
Philips/HP Sonos 4500	S3/2.25	≥0.20	[25]
Philips/HP Sonos 5500	Adult cardiac/1.8—3.6	≥0.20	[27]
Siemens/Acuson Antares	PX4-1/2.5	≥0.24	[21]
Siemens/Sonoline Elegra	2.5PL20/2.6	≥0.20	[22]

Abbreviations: SN-h, substantia nigra hyperechogenicity.

Hitherto, standard reference values on echogenic sizes of the SN have been published for a number of ultrasound systems as listed in Table 2 [14,21—28].

To display the plane at thalamus level the ultrasound probe is tilted 10—20° in upward direction. An important landmark of the thalamus level is the usually calcified, and therefore highly echogenic pineal gland (Fig. 3). At this plane, the third ventricle, anterior horns of the lateral ventricles, the thalami and the anatomic site of the basal ganglia are depicted. The thalami are typically displayed as hypoechogenic oval structures; the thalami and the frontal horns help to discern the anatomical site of caudate nucleus and lenticular nucleus. At this level, the transverse diameters of the third ventricle, and of the frontal horn of the contralateral lateral ventricle can be measured [1,11]. Hydrocephalus can be easily diagnosed on TCS. In addition, early brain atrophy and associated risk of cognitive impairment can be detected with TCS by measurement of third-ventricle width [29]. Furthermore, the echogenicity of contralateral thalamus, contralateral lenticular nucleus and contralateral caudate nucleus should be evaluated semi-quantitatively. Normally, these structures are invisible, i.e., isoechogenic to the surrounding brain parenchyma. Sometimes, the borders of the ipsilateral internal capsule can be detected, allowing a separation of the thalamus from the lenticular nucleus. An increased echogenicity ('hyperechogenicity') of thalamus, lenticular nucleus or caudate nucleus compared with surrounding white matter is considered to be abnormal. Hyperechogenicity of deep brain structures is often caused by trace metal accumulation or by calcification [2]. In the latter case, the echosignals are very bright, similar to that of pineal gland [30].

TCS for monitoring of acute stroke patients

Two of the earliest published TCS applications in adults were the detection of intracranial hematomas in acute stroke or trauma patients [8,10,31], and the assessment of the ventricular system [11]. While computed tomography (CT) and MRI today represent the gold standard in the diagnosis of intracranial hemorrhage [32,33], TCS can well be used for the bedside monitoring for the size and resorption of hematomas, and, especially for the monitoring of

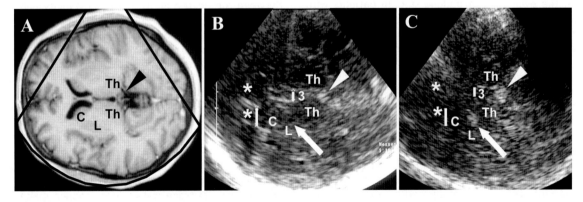

Figure 3 Transcranial sonography (TCS) axial brain scan at thalamus level. C = caudate nucleus, L = lenticular nucleus, Th = thalamus; 3 = third ventricle (width indicated by bar); *frontal horn of lateral ventricle (width of contralateral frontal horn indicated by bar); triangle indicates pineal gland. (A) MRI scan corresponding to the TCS images shown in (B and C). (B) TCS axial scan through the brain at thalamus level of an individual with normal TCS findings. The increased echogenicity of pineal gland (triangle) is normal since this structure usually contains chalk. The lenticular nucleus is displayed with low (normal) echogenicity (arrow). (C) TCS axial scan through the brain at thalamus level of a subject with an atypical Parkinsonian syndrome (multiple-system atrophy). The increased echogenicity ('hyperechogenicity') of the lenticular nucleus (arrow) is a characteristic finding.

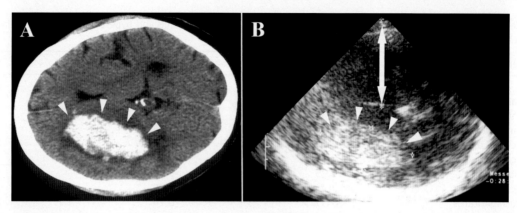

Figure 4 Transcranial sonography (TCS) axial brain scan at thalamus level showing a large intracerebral hematoma. (A) Computed tomography (CT) image corresponding to the TCS image shown in (B). The triangles indicate the hematoma. (B) TCS image showing the highly echogenic hematoma in the acute phase. The midline shift at level of third ventricle can be calculated after measuring the distance d of the temporally placed transducer face to the third ventricle (indicated by double arrow) from both sides: midline shift = $(d1 - d2)/2$.

midline shift. In the acute phase, intracerebral hemorrhage (ICH) appears homogenous, sharply demarcated and hyperechogenic (Fig. 4) [31]. In 1993, Seidel et al. [8] were the first to describe an alteration of the sonographic appearance of ICH over time with a decrease in echo intensity beginning at the center of the lesion. They were able to detect the ICH with ultrasound in 18 of 23 patients (78%). Insufficient insonation conditions were found in 13% of patients. In a prospective TCS study of 151 patients with acute hemiparesis of whom 60 had an ICH on CT, TCS differentiated correctly between ischemia and hemorrhage in 95% of the assessable patients [34]. Insufficient insonation conditions were found in 12% of patients. In a more recent study of 25 patients with confirmed subdural hematoma, TCS detected the hematoma in 22 (88%) patients while the temporal bone window was insufficient in 3 (12%) patients [35]. Large hemorrhagic transformations of ischemic infarctions have also been reliably detected with TCS [36,37]. A recent study found a good agreement between TCS and CT measures of hematoma volumes [38].

The first TCS studies that specifically addressed the value of TCS in the evaluation of midline shift in patients with space-occupying brain infarctions were published by the group of Kaps and co-workers [39—41]. In these studies a high correlation between TCS and CT measures of midline shift at the level of third ventricle was found. All patients with an MLS < 4 mm at 32 h survived, whereas patients with an MLS > 4 mm died, as a result of cerebral herniation with an exception of one patient who underwent decompressive hemicraniectomy [40,41]. Subsequent studies performed by independent groups confirmed the reliability of TCS in the assessment of midline shift in patients with space-occupying stroke, ICH and traumatic brain injury [42—45]. In a recent study, the widths of lateral ventricles (frontal horns) were monitored with TCS in 37 patients with intraventricular hemorrhage [46]. The authors reported a cut-off value for increase of lateral ventricular width of 5.5 mm that yielded high sensitivity (100%) and specificity (83%) in combination with a 100% negative predictive value for reopening of the external ventricular or lumbar drainage.

In conclusion, TCS can be regarded as a reliable tool for monitoring the midline shift, as well as the ventricular width in patients with acute supratentorial brain lesions who have adequate acoustic bone windows (>80% of patients). In many neurological and neurosurgical departments with appropriate expertise in neurosonology, TCS is already today routinely used for this purpose.

TCS for the early and differential diagnosis of Parkinson's disease

Substantia nigra hyperechogenicity in Parkinson's disease

Becker et al. [47] were the first to describe the TCS finding of SN hyperechogenicity in PD patients (Fig. 2). In the past decade, this finding has been confirmed by a number of independent groups [23—25,27,28,48—54]. This TCS finding, present in about 90% of PD patients at cross-section is independent from PD duration and severity [55,56], and was found to be stable in a 5-year follow-up study of PD patients [57]. Also there was no correlation found between the degree of SN hyperechogenicity and the striatal uptake of N-omega-fluoropropyl-2beta-carbomethoxy-3beta-4-[(123)I]iodophenyl-nortropane (FP-CIT) on SPECT, which is thought to represent a correlate for the degeneration of presynaptic dopaminergic neurons in PD [58]. These findings indicate that SN hyperechogenicity is not a correlate of the progressive degeneration of SN neurons.

However, a close correlation between SN echogenicity and tissue iron content has been shown in post-mortem studies of human brains [59], suggesting that SN hyperechogenicity in PD is at least in part, caused by an elevated iron content of the SN. Also in a number of other neurodegenerative disorders TCS was demonstrated to detect accumulation of trace metals (iron, copper, manganese) in the basal ganglia with higher sensitivity than MRI supporting the idea that TCS can display trace metal accumulation in deep brain structures [59—62]. On the other hand, increased iron content alone cannot be the only explanation for SN hyperechogenicity since iron accumulates over time in the SN of PD patients, and other iron-rich brain structures, such as red nucleus or globus pallidus internus normally show no increased echogenicity on TCS [2]. Therefore, additional factors, such as abnormal iron—protein bindings were proposed to contribute to SN hyperechogenicity [59]. The close correlation of the TCS finding of SN hyperechogenicity with increased iron content in the SN [59], together with an apparently autosomal dominant inheritance of this echofeature in relatives of patients with idiopathic PD [63], supports the idea of a primary role of disturbed iron metabolism in PD. Subsequent mutation analyses of genes encoding for iron-transport and iron-regulatory proteins known to be associated with Parkinsonism led to the discovery of specific mutations in the *ferritin-H*, the *iron-regulatory protein 2*, and the *hemochromatosis* gene, respectively, in single PD patients with SN hyperechogenicity [64—66]. The most striking association was found in the *ceruloplasmin* gene: of five exonic missense mutations, the I63T mutation was only found in one PD patient, the D544E and R793H mutations in far more PD patients than in ethnically matched controls [67]. The *ceruloplasmin* gene mutations were clearly associated to the TCS finding of SN hyperechogenicity in PD patients and healthy control subjects [67].

Early diagnosis of Parkinson's disease

The question of whether the TCS finding of SN hyperechogenicity, present in 90% of PD patients but also in 9% of healthy adults, really indicates an increased risk of later developing PD is currently being studied in large longitudinal studies. First clues were reported by Becker et al. [47] who observed that one of the healthy subjects in whom marked SN hyperechogenicity was detected in an early TCS study, two years later developed PD [22]. Meanwhile, there is growing evidence supporting the idea that SN hyperechogenicity indeed is an indicator for an increased risk of PD. FDOPA-PET studies in young healthy adults as well as in young asymptomatic *parkin* mutation carriers revealed that SN hyperechogenicity is associated with a subclinical malfunction of the nigrostriatal dopaminergic system [22,68]. In psychiatric patients the degree of SN hyperechogenicity was clearly correlated with the severity of Parkinsonian symptoms induced by neuroleptic therapy [69]. SN hyperechogenicity was related to subtle motor asymmetry in non-depressive and, even more frequently, in depressive subjects [70,71]. TCS studies in populations known to have an increased risk of PD showed 2- to 4-fold increased frequencies of SN hyperechogenicity in first-degree relatives of PD patients [63], in individuals with idiopathic hyposmia [72], in patients with unipolar depressive disorders [73], individuals with essential tremor [24], and individuals with idiopathic REM sleep behavior disorder [74,75]. In these groups, the subjects with SN hyperechogenicity were more liable to show subtle Parkinsonian motor signs and reduced striatal radiotracer uptake on FP-CIT SPECT or F-DOPA PET studies than subjects with normal SN echogenicity [63,71—75]. Recently, the first follow-up data came out of an ongoing longitudinal study since 2004, conducted at the Universities of Tübingen (Germany), Innsbruck (Austria) and Homburg (Germany) [76,77]. This study included more than 1800 healthy individuals older than 50 years who were examined with respect to SN echogenicity and epidemiologic risk factors, as well as premotor symptoms of PD like depression, autonomic and smelling dysfunction, neuropsychological deficits and slight motor signs. The 37-months prospective follow-up data obtained in this cohort suggest a 17-fold increased risk of subsequently developing PD in individuals with SN hyperechogenicity. A prospective follow-up study of individuals with idiopathic REM sleep behavior disorder showed an 100% sensitivity and a 55% specificity of combined ^{123}I-FP-CIT SPECT and TCS to predict the conversion to a synucleinopathy (mainly PD) after 2.5 years [78].

It appears reasonable to combine TCS with other, ideally non-invasive, methods to enhance the predictive value in the early diagnosis of PD. In a prospective study we have assessed more than 500 patients with early parkinsonism (PD, vascular parkinsonism, atypical parkinsonian syndromes, essential tremor, major depressive disorder with motor slowing) on the Unified PD Rating Scale for motor asymmetry, on the 12-item Sniffin' Sticks test for hyposmia, and on TCS for SN hyperechogenicity. Results of this study showed that the combination of these measures markedly improves the prediction of PD, with a specificity of nearly 100% if all three key findings were present [79].

The combined assessment of motor asymmetry, hyposmia and SN hyperechogenicity could be used as a cost-effective tool for the screening of populations at risk of developing PD. This assessment battery is applicable in an ambulatory setting using the Sniffin' Sticks test or similar tests, and a portable TCS system [14]. Subjects assessed to have an increased liability of developing PD, as well as subjects with signs of mild Parkinsonism, but still an unclear diagnose, might be included in a follow-up program at specialized centers [80]. Such a program might offer further diagnostic steps, including elaborate motor and neuropsychological analysis, advanced structural and functional brain imaging, and genetic testing. Even though the ethical issues of such an approach need to be resolved, the early correct diagnosis of PD promises enhanced success of disease-modifying therapies.

Differential diagnosis of Parkinson's disease

The TCS feature of SN hyperechogenicity, which is a characteristic for PD is usually not found in patients with atypical or secondary Parkinsonian disorders such as multiple-system atrophy (MSA) and progressive supranuclear palsy (PSP) [50,81—84], posttraumatic Parkinsonism [85], vascular Parkinsonism [86], and welding-related, supposedly manganese-induced Parkinsonism [62]. According to a meta-analysis of five independent TCS studies [50,81—84], the finding of SN hyperechogenicity discriminates PD from atypical Parkinsonian syndromes (MSA and PSP) with a sensitivity of 92% and a specificity of 80% [2]. On the other hand, hyperechogenic lesions of the lenticular nucleus can be typically seen on TCS in primary degenerative atypical Parkinsonian disorders but rarely in PD [62,81—83] (Fig. 3). While TCS of SN alone is helpful for discriminating a number of atypical Parkinsonian syndromes from PD already at early disease stages [81,84], the specificity for the diagnosis of MSA and PSP can be increased to 98—100% at the cost of sensitivity (65—84%) by combining TCS of SN, lenticular nucleus and third ventricle [82,83], or by combining SN TCS with testing for hyposmia and motor asymmetry [79]. Since clinical

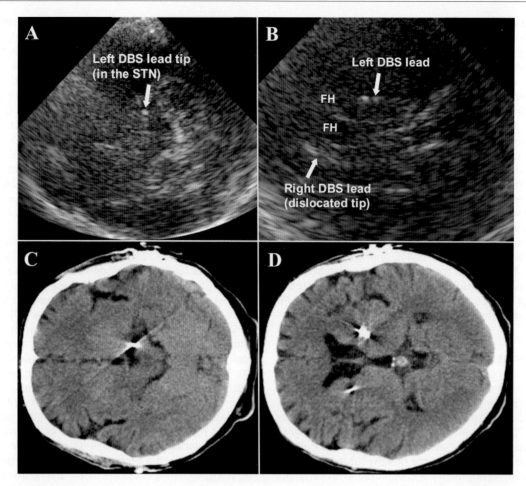

Figure 5 Post-operative transcranial sonography (TCS) of a patient with deep brain stimulation (DBS) in whom unilateral DBS lead displacement was diagnosed. The lead dislocation on the right side was first detected on TCS and subsequently confirmed on CT. (A) TCS image showing the left-sided DBS lead tip (arrow) correctly located within the subthalamic nucleus while the right-sided DBS electrode is not displayed due to dislocation. (B) TCS image showing the more cranial parts of the left-sided DBS lead (arrow) and the tip of the dislocated right-sided lead (arrow) lateral from the caudate nucleus. (C) CT image corresponding to the TCS image in (A). (D) CT image corresponding to the TCS image in (B).

and other neuroimaging methods often do not allow a clear differentiation of atypical Parkinsonian syndromes versus PD in the early disease stages, TCS is a valuable tool for early diagnosis, and may promote a sooner initiation of disease specific therapies.

TCS for post-operative localization of brain implants

In patients with DBS, there are discrepancies of up to 4 mm (average 2 mm) between the initial selected target and the final DBS lead location caused mainly by caudal brain shift that occurs once the cranium is open [87]. Moreover, the DBS lead may get displaced postoperatively, e.g., by delayed brain shift or head injury. Provided sufficient imaging conditions (sufficient bone window, contemporary high-end ultrasound system), TCS is a valuable tool for the post-operative monitoring of the DBS electrode location [88,89]. Gross DBS lead dislocation is easily detected with TCS (Fig. 5). A detailed overview and recommendations on the application of TCS for the post-operative localization of DBS electrodes are given in chapter XX3 of this serial.

Conclusions and outlook

In the past decade, the technological advances realized in the commercially available ultrasound systems went along with an enormous progress in the application of TCS in patients with brain disorders. The present article focused on the clinically most relevant applications of TCS that are supported each by the results of prospective studies. Novel technologies, such as the in-time fusion of TCS with MRI images [90], automated detection of intracranial target structures [91], and improved 3D-image analysis [92] promise an even wider application of TCS in the coming years.

References

[1] Walter U, Behnke S, Eyding J, Niehaus L, Postert T, Seidel G, et al. Transcranial brain parenchyma sonography in

[1] movement disorders: state of the art. Ultrasound Med Biol 2007;33:15—25.
[2] Berg D, Godau J, Walter U. Transcranial sonography in movement disorders. Lancet Neurol 2008;7:1044—55.
[3] Machado HR, Martelli N, Assirati Júnior JA, Colli BO. Infantile hydrocephalus: brain sonography as an effective tool for diagnosis and follow-up. Childs Nerv Syst 1991;7:205—10.
[4] Babcock DS. Sonography of the brain in infants: role in evaluating neurologic abnormalities. AJR Am J Roentgenol 1995;165:417—23.
[5] Wijnhoud AD, Franckena M, van der Lugt A, Koudstaal PJ, Dippel ED. Inadequate acoustical temporal bone window in patients with a transient ischemic attack or minor stroke: role of skull thickness and bone density. Ultrasound Med Biol 2008;34:923—9.
[6] Becker G, Perez J, Krone A, Demuth K, Lindner A, Hofmann E, et al. Transcranial color-coded real-time sonography in the evaluation of intracranial neoplasms and arteriovenous malformations. Neurosurgery 1992;31:420—8.
[7] Becker G, Krone A, Koulis D, Lindner A, Hofmann E, Roggendorf W, et al. Reliability of transcranial colour-coded real-time sonography in assessment of brain tumours: correlation of ultrasound, computed tomography and biopsy findings. Neuroradiology 1994;36:585—90.
[8] Seidel G, Kaps M, Dorndorf W. Transcranial color-coded duplex sonography of intracerebral hematomas in adults. Stroke 1993;24:1519—27.
[9] Mäurer M, Becker G, Wagner R, Woydt M, Hofmann E, Puls I, et al. Early postoperative transcranial sonography (TCS), CT, and MRI after resection of high grade glioma: evaluation of residual tumour and its influence on prognosis. Acta Neurochir (Wien) 2000;142:1089—97.
[10] Woydt M, Greiner K, Perez J, Becker G, Krone A, Roosen K. Transcranial duplex-sonography in intracranial hemorrhage. Evaluation of transcranial duplex-sonography in the diagnosis of spontaneous and traumatic intracranial hemorrhage. Zentralbl Neurochir 1996;57:129—35.
[11] Seidel G, Kaps M, Gerriets T, Hutzelmann A. Evaluation of the ventricular system in adults by transcranial duplex sonography. J Neuroimaging 1995;5:105—8.
[12] Kern R, Perren F, Kreisel S, Szabo K, Hennerici M, Meairs S. Multiplanar transcranial ultrasound imaging: standards, landmarks and correlation with magnetic resonance imaging. Ultrasound Med Biol 2005;31:311—5.
[13] Walter U, Kanowski M, Kaufmann J, Grossmann A, Benecke R, Niehaus L. Contemporary ultrasound systems allow high-resolution transcranial imaging of small echogenic deep intracranial structures similarly as MRI: a phantom study. Neuroimage 2008;40:551—8.
[14] Go CL, Frenzel A, Rosales RL, Lee LV, Benecke R, Dresser D, et al. Assessment of substantia nigra echogenicity in German and Filipino population using a portable ultrasound system. J Ultrasound Med 2012;31:191—6.
[15] Seidel G, Meairs S. Ultrasound contrast agents in ischemic stroke. Cerebrovasc Dis 2009;27(Suppl. 2):25—39.
[16] Kern R, Kablau M, Sallustio F, Fatar M, Stroick M, Hennerici MG, et al. Improved detection of intracerebral hemorrhage with transcranial ultrasound perfusion imaging. Cerebrovasc Dis 2008;26:277—83.
[17] Alonso A, Della Martina A, Stroick M, Fatar M, Griebe M, Pochon S, et al. Molecular imaging of human thrombus with novel abciximab immunobubbles and ultrasound. Stroke 2007;38:1508—14.
[18] van Leyen K, Klötzsch C, Harrer JU. Brain tumor imaging with transcranial sonography: state of the art and review of the literature. Ultraschall Med 2011;32:572—81.
[19] Reinhardt M, Hauff P, Linker RA, Briel A, Gold R, Rieckmann P, et al. Ultrasound derived imaging and quantification of cell adhesion molecules in experimental autoimmune encephalomyelitis (EAE) by Sensitive Particle Acoustic Quantification (SPAQ). Neuroimage 2005;27:267—78.
[20] Skoloudík D, Walter U. Method and validity of transcranial sonography in movement disorders. Int Rev Neurobiol 2010;90:7—34.
[21] van de Loo S, Walter U, Behnke S, Hagenah J, Lorenz M, Sitzer M, et al. Reproducibility and diagnostic accuracy of substantia nigra sonography for the diagnosis of Parkinson's disease. J Neurol Neurosurg Psychiatry 2010;81:1087—92.
[22] Berg D, Becker G, Zeiler B, Tucha O, Hofmann E, Preier M, et al. Vulnerability of the nigrostriatal system as detected by transcranial ultrasound. Neurology 1999;53:1026—31.
[23] Ressner P, Skoloudík D, Hlustík P, Kanovský P. Hyperechogenicity of the substantia nigra in Parkinson's disease. J Neuroimaging 2007;17:164—7.
[24] Stockner H, Sojer M, K KS, Mueller J, Wenning GK, Schmidauer C, et al. Midbrain sonography in patients with essential tremor. Mov Disord 2007;22:414—7.
[25] Huang YW, Jeng JS, Tsai CF, Chen LL, Wu RM. Transcranial imaging of substantia nigra hyperechogenicity in a Taiwanese cohort of Parkinson's disease. Mov Disord 2007;22:550—5.
[26] Mijajlović M, Dragasević N, Stefanova E, Petrović I, Svetel M, Kostić VS. Transcranial sonography in spinocerebellar ataxia type 2. J Neurol 2008;255:1164—7.
[27] Mehnert S, Reuter I, Schepp K, Maaser P, Stolz E, Kaps M. Transcranial sonography for diagnosis of Parkinson's disease. BMC Neurol 2010;10:9.
[28] Fedotova Elu, Chechetkin AO, Shadrina MI, Slominskiĭ PA, Ivanova-Smolenskaia IA, Illarioshkin SN. Transcranial sonography in Parkinson's disease. Zh Nevrol Psikhiatr Im S S Korsakova 2011;111:49—55.
[29] Wollenweber FA, Schomburg R, Probst M, Schneider V, Hiry T, Ochsenfeld A, et al. Width of the third ventricle assessed by transcranial sonography can monitor brain atrophy in a time- and cost-effective manner — results from a longitudinal study on 500 subjects. Psychiatry Res 2011;191:212—6.
[30] Brüggemann N, Schneider SA, Sander T, Klein C, Hagenah J. Distinct basal ganglia hyperechogenicity in idiopathic basal ganglia calcification. Mov Disord 2010;25:2661—4.
[31] Becker G, Winkler J, Hofmann E, Bogdahn U. Differentiation between ischemic and hemorrhagic stroke by transcranial color-coded real-time sonography. J Neuroimaging 1993;3:41—7.
[32] Azar-Kia B, Fine M. Evaluation of intracerebral hematoma by computed tomography. Comput Tomogr 1977;1:339—48.
[33] Fiebach JB, Schellinger PD, Gass A, Kucinski T, Siebler M, Villringer A, et al. Stroke magnetic resonance imaging is accurate in hyperacute intracerebral hemorrhage: a multicenter study on the validity of stroke imaging. Stroke 2004;35:502—6.
[34] Mäurer M, Shambal S, Berg D, Woydt M, Hofmann E, Georgiadis D, et al. Differentiation between intracerebral hemorrhage and ischemic stroke by transcranial color-coded duplex-sonography. Stroke 1998;29:2563—7.
[35] Niesen WD, Burkhardt D, Hoeltje J, Rosenkranz M, Weiller C, Sliwka U. Transcranial grey-scale sonography of subdural haematoma in adults. Ultraschall Med 2006;27:251—5.
[36] Seidel G, Cangür H, Albers T, Meyer-Wiethe K. Transcranial sonographic monitoring of hemorrhagic transformation in patients with acute middle cerebral artery infarction. J Neuroimaging 2005;15:326—30.
[37] Seidel G, Cangür H, Albers T, Burgemeister A, Meyer-Wiethe K. Sonographic evaluation of hemorrhagic transformation and arterial recanalization in acute hemispheric ischemic stroke. Stroke 2009;40:119—23.
[38] Matsumoto N, Kimura K, Iguchi Y, Aoki J. Evaluation of cerebral hemorrhage volume using transcranial color-coded duplex sonography. J Neuroimaging 2011;21:355—8.

[39] Stolz E, Gerriets T, Fiss I, Babacan SS, Seidel G, Kaps M. Comparison of transcranial color-coded duplex sonography and cranial CT measurements for determining third ventricle midline shift in space-occupying stroke. AJNR Am J Neuroradiol 1999;20:1567–71.

[40] Gerriets T, Stolz E, Modrau B, Fiss I, Seidel G, Kaps M. Sonographic monitoring of midline shift in hemispheric infarctions. Neurology 1999;52:45–9.

[41] Gerriets T, Stolz E, König S, Babacan S, Fiss I, Jauss M, et al. Sonographic monitoring of midline shift in space-occupying stroke: an early outcome predictor. Stroke 2001;32: 442–7.

[42] Llompart Pou JA, Abadal Centellas JM, Palmer Sans M, Pérez Bárcena J, Casares Vivas M, Homar Ramírez J, et al. Monitoring midline shift by transcranial color-coded sonography in traumatic brain injury. A comparison with cranial computerized tomography. Intensive Care Med 2004;30:1672–5.

[43] Tang SC, Huang SJ, Jeng JS, Yip PK. Third ventricle midline shift due to spontaneous supratentorial intracerebral hemorrhage evaluated by transcranial color-coded sonography. J Ultrasound Med 2006;25:203–9.

[44] Horstmann S, Koziol JA, Martinez-Torres F, Nagel S, Gardner H, Wagner S. Sonographic monitoring of mass effect in stroke patients treated with hypothermia. Correlation with intracranial pressure and matrix metalloproteinase 2 and 9 expression. J Neurol Sci 2009;276:75–8.

[45] Kukulska-Pawluczuk B, Książkiewicz B, Nowaczewska M. Imaging of spontaneous intracerebral hemorrhages by means of transcranial color-coded sonography. Eur J Radiol 2011; in press, doi:10.1016/j.ejrad.2011.02.066.

[46] Kiphuth IC, Huttner HB, Struffert T, Schwab S, Köhrmann M. Sonographic monitoring of ventricle enlargement in posthemorrhagic hydrocephalus. Neurology 2011;76:858–62.

[47] Becker G, Seufert J, Bogdahn U, Reichmann H, Reiners K. Degeneration of substantia nigra in chronic Parkinson's disease visualized by transcranial color-coded real-time sonography. Neurology 1995;45:182–4.

[48] Walter U, Wittstock M, Benecke R, Dressler D. Substantia nigra echogenicity is normal in non-extrapyramidal cerebral disorders but increased in Parkinson's disease. J Neural Transm 2002;109:191–6.

[49] Hagenah JM, König IR, Becker B, Hilker R, Kasten M, Hedrich K, et al. Substantia nigra hyperechogenicity correlates with clinical status and number of Parkin mutated alleles. J Neurol 2007;254:1407–13.

[50] Okawa M, Miwa H, Kajimoto Y, Hama K, Morita S, Nakanishi I, et al. Transcranial sonography of the substantia nigra in Japanese patients with Parkinson's disease or atypical parkinsonism: clinical potential and limitations. Intern Med 2007;46:1527–31.

[51] Kim JY, Kim ST, Jeon SH, Lee WY. Midbrain transcranial sonography in Korean patients with Parkinson's disease. Mov Disord 2007;22:1922–6.

[52] Kolevski G, Petrov I, Petrova V. Transcranial sonography in the evaluation of Parkinson disease. J Ultrasound Med 2007;26:509–12.

[53] Doepp F, Plotkin M, Siegel L, Kivi A, Gruber D, Lobsien E, et al. Brain parenchyma sonography and 123I-FP-CIT SPECT in Parkinson's disease and essential tremor. Mov Disord 2008;23: 405–10.

[54] Vlaar AM, de Nijs T, van Kroonenburgh MJ, Mess WH, Winogrodzka A, Tromp SC, et al. The predictive value of transcranial duplex sonography for the clinical diagnosis in undiagnosed parkinsonian syndromes: comparison with SPECT scans. BMC Neurol 2008;8:42.

[55] Berg D, Siefker C, Becker G. Echogenicity of the substantia nigra in Parkinson's disease and its relation to clinical findings. J Neurol 2001;248:684–9.

[56] Walter U, Dressler D, Wolters A, Wittstock M, Benecke R. Transcranial brain sonography findings in clinical subgroups of idiopathic Parkinson's disease. Mov Disord 2007;22: 48–54.

[57] Berg D, Merz B, Reiners K, Naumann M, Becker G. Five-year follow-up study of hyperechogenicity of the substantia nigra in Parkinson's disease. Mov Disord 2005;20:383–5.

[58] Spiegel J, Hellwig D, Möllers MO, Behnke S, Jost W, Fassbender K, et al. Transcranial sonography and [123I]FP-CIT SPECT disclose complementary aspects of Parkinson's disease. Brain 2006;129:1188–93.

[59] Berg D, Roggendorf W, Schröder U, Klein R, Tatschner T, Benz P, et al. Echogenicity of the substantia nigra: association with increased iron content and marker for susceptibility to nigrostriatal injury. Arch Neurol 2002;59:999–1005.

[60] Berg D, Weishaupt A, Francis MJ, Miura N, Yang XL, Goodyer ID, et al. Changes of copper-transporting proteins and ceruloplasmin in the lentiform nuclei in primary adult-onset dystonia. Ann Neurol 2000;47:827–30.

[61] Walter U, Krolikowski K, Tarnacka B, Benecke R, Czlonkowska A, Dressler D. Sonographic detection of basal ganglia lesions in asymptomatic and symptomatic Wilson disease. Neurology 2005;64:1726–32.

[62] Walter U, Dressler D, Lindemann C, Slachevsky A, Miranda M. Transcranial sonography findings in welding-related Parkinsonism in comparison to Parkinson's disease. Mov Disord 2008;23:141–5.

[63] Ruprecht-Dörfler P, Berg D, Tucha O, Benz P, Meier-Meitinger M, Alders GL, et al. Echogenicity of the substantia nigra in relatives of patients with sporadic Parkinson's disease. Neuroimage 2003;18:416–22.

[64] Felletschin B, Bauer P, Walter U, Behnke S, Spiegel J, Csoti I, et al. Screening for mutations of the ferritin light and heavy genes in Parkinson's disease patients with hyperechogenicity of the substantia nigra. Neurosci Lett 2003;352:53–6.

[65] Deplazes J, Schöbel K, Hochstrasser H, Bauer P, Walter U, Behnke S, et al. Screening for mutations of the IRP2 gene in Parkinson's disease patients with hyperechogenicity of the substantia nigra. J Neural Transm 2004;111:515–21.

[66] Akbas N, Hochstrasser H, Deplazes J, Tomiuk J, Bauer P, Walter U, et al. Screening for mutations of the HFE gene in Parkinson's disease patients with hyperechogenicity of the substantia nigra. Neurosci Lett 2006;407:16–9.

[67] Hochstrasser H, Bauer P, Walter U, Behnke S, Spiegel J, Csoti I, et al. Ceruloplasmin gene variations and substantia nigra hyperechogenicity in Parkinson disease. Neurology 2004;63:1912–7.

[68] Walter U, Klein C, Hilker R, Benecke R, Pramstaller PP, Dressler D. Brain parenchyma sonography detects preclinical parkinsonism. Mov Disord 2004;19:1445–9.

[69] Berg D, Jabs B, Merschdorf U, Beckmann H, Becker G. Echogenicity of substantia nigra determined by transcranial ultrasound correlates with severity of parkinsonian symptoms induced by neuroleptic therapy. Biol Psychiatry 2001;50:463–7.

[70] Ruprecht-Dörfler P, Klotz P, Becker G, Berg D. Substantia nigra hyperechogenicity correlates with subtle motor dysfunction in tap dancers. Parkinsonism Relat Disord 2007;13:362–4.

[71] Hoeppner J, Prudente-Morrissey L, Herpertz SC, Benecke R, Walter U. Substantia nigra hyperechogenicity in depressive subjects relates to motor asymmetry and impaired word fluency. Eur Arch Psychiatry Clin Neurosci 2009;259:92–7.

[72] Sommer U, Hummel T, Cormann K, Mueller A, Frasnelli J, Kropp J, et al. Detection of presymptomatic Parkinson's disease: combining smell tests, transcranial sonography, and SPECT. Mov Disord 2004;19:1196–202.

[73] Walter U, Hoeppner J, Prudente-Morrissey L, Horowski S, Herpertz SC, Benecke R. Parkinson's disease-like midbrain

sonography abnormalities are frequent in depressive disorders. Brain 2007;130:1799—807.
[74] Unger MM, Möller JC, Stiasny-Kolster K, Mankel K, Berg D, Walter U, et al. Assessment of idiopathic rapid-eye-movement sleep behavior disorder by transcranial sonography, olfactory function test, and FP-CIT-SPECT. Mov Disord 2008;23: 596—9.
[75] Stockner H, Iranzo A, Seppi K, Serradell M, Gschliesser V, Sojer M, et al. Midbrain hyperechogenicity in idiopathic REM sleep behavior disorder. Mov Disord 2009;24:1906—9.
[76] Berg D, Seppi K, Liepelt I, Schweitzer K, Wollenweber F, Wolf B, et al. Enlarged hyperechogenic substantia nigra is related to motor performance and olfaction in the elderly. Mov Disord 2010;25:1464—9.
[77] Berg D, Seppi K, Behnke S, Liepelt I, Schweitzer K, Stockner H, et al. Enlarged substantia nigra hyperechogenicity and risk for Parkinson disease: a 37-month 3-center study of 1847 older persons. Arch Neurol 2011;68:932—7.
[78] Iranzo A, Lomeña F, Stockner H, Valldeoriola F, Vilaseca I, Salamero M, et al. Decreased striatal dopamine transporter uptake and substantia nigra hyperechogenicity as risk markers of synucleinopathy in patients with idiopathic rapid-eye-movement sleep behaviour disorder: a prospective study. Lancet Neurol 2010;9:1070—7.
[79] Busse K, Heilmann R, Kleinschmidt S, Abu-Mugheisib M, Hoeppner J, Wunderlich C, et al. Value of combined midbrain sonography, olfactory and motor function assessment in the differential diagnosis of early Parkinson's disease. J Neurol Neurosurg Psychiatry 2012; doi:10.1136/jnnp-2011-301719, in press.
[80] Walter U. Transcranial brain sonography findings in Parkinson's disease: implications for pathogenesis, early diagnosis and therapy. Expert Rev Neurother 2009;9:835—46.
[81] Walter U, Niehaus L, Probst T, Benecke R, Meyer BU, Dressler D. Brain parenchyma sonography discriminates Parkinson's disease and atypical parkinsonian syndromes. Neurology 2003;60:74—7.
[82] Behnke S, Berg D, Naumann M, Becker G. Differentiation of Parkinson's disease and atypical parkinsonian syndromes by transcranial ultrasound. J Neurol Neurosurg Psychiatry 2005;76:423—5.
[83] Walter U, Dressler D, Probst T, Wolters A, Abu-Mugheisib M, Wittstock M, et al. Transcranial brain sonography findings in discriminating between parkinsonism and idiopathic Parkinson disease. Arch Neurol 2007;64:1635—40.
[84] Gaenslen A, Unmuth B, Godau J, Liepelt I, Di Santo A, Schweitzer KJ, et al. The specificity and sensitivity of transcranial ultrasound in the differential diagnosis of Parkinson's disease: a prospective blinded study. Lancet Neurol 2008;7(May (5)):417—24.
[85] Kivi A, Trottenberg T, Kupsch A, Plotkin M, Felix R, Niehaus L. Levodopa-responsive posttraumatic parkinsonism is not associated with changes of echogenicity of the substantia nigra. Mov Disord 2005;20:258—60.
[86] Tsai CF, Wu RM, Huang YW, Chen LL, Yip PK, Jeng JS. Transcranial color-coded sonography helps differentiation between idiopathic Parkinson's disease and vascular parkinsonism. J Neurol 2007;254:501—7.
[87] Khan MF, Mewes K, Gross RE, Skrinjar O. Assessment of brain shift related to deep brain stimulation surgery. Stereotact Funct Neurosurg 2008;86:44—53.
[88] Walter U, Wolters A, Wittstock M, Benecke R, Schroeder HW, Müller JU. Deep brain stimulation in dystonia: sonographic monitoring of electrode placement into the globus pallidus internus. Mov Disord 2009;24:1538—41.
[89] Walter U. Transcranial sonography-assisted stereotaxy and follow-up of deep brain implants in patients with movement disorders. Int Rev Neurobiol 2010;90:274—85.
[90] Ewertsen C. Image fusion between ultrasonography and CT, MRI or PET/CT for image guidance and intervention — a theoretical and clinical study. Dan Med Bull 2010;57:B4172.
[91] Schreiber J, Sojka E, Licev L, Sknourilova P, Gaura J, Skoloudik D. A new method for the detection of brain stem in transcranial ultrasound images. Proc Biosignals 2008;2:478—83.
[92] Ahmadi SA, Baust M, Karamalis A, Plate A, Boetzel K, Klein T, et al. Midbrain segmentation in transcranial 3D ultrasound for Parkinson diagnosis. Med Image Comput Comput Assist Interv 2011;14:362—9.

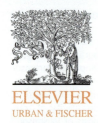
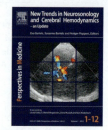

Bartels E, Bartels S, Poppert H (Editors):
New Trends in Neurosonology and Cerebral Hemodynamics — an Update.
Perspectives in Medicine (2012) 1, 344—348

journal homepage: www.elsevier.com/locate/permed

Intra- and post-operative monitoring of deep brain implants using transcranial ultrasound

Uwe Walter*

Department of Neurology, University of Rostock, Gehlsheimer Str. 20, D-18147 Rostock, Germany

KEYWORDS
Transcranial sonography;
Deep brain stimulation;
Ultrasound-guided procedure;
Post-operative monitoring;
Electrode position control

Summary   Transcranial sonography (TCS) of the brain parenchyma meanwhile allows a high-resolution imaging of deep brain structures in the majority of adults. A new application of TCS is the intra- and post-operative visualization with TCS and the TCS-assisted insertion of deep brain stimulation (DBS) electrodes. In pilot studies it has been shown that the TCS-assisted insertion of DBS electrodes into the subthalamic nucleus and the globus pallidus interna is feasible and safe provided the exact knowledge on the extent of electrode TCS imaging artifacts. Even more, TCS can be recommended for the post-operative monitoring of DBS electrode position. Dislocation of a DBS electrode can be easily detected. In a recent longitudinal study we could demonstrate that TCS measures of lead coordinates agreed with MRI measures in anterior—posterior and medial—lateral axis, and that the TCS-based grading of optimal vs suboptimal lead location predicts the clinical 12 months outcome of patients with movement disorders. Currently, an international multi-center study is being planned to further prove the value of TCS in the post-operative monitoring of DBS electrode position. This trial is intended to start in 2012, and is still open for joining. The obvious advantages of TCS will promote its increasing use for the intra- and post-operative monitoring of deep brain implants.
© 2012 Elsevier GmbH. All rights reserved.

Introduction

Transcranial B-mode sonography (TCS) of the brain parenchyma and the intracranial ventricular system has been performed in children already in the 80s and 90s of the last century [1,2]. Also, the guidance of programming a shunt valve system in the treatment of a fluctuating child hydrocephalus has been shown to be well possible with TCS [3].

In adults, the TCS imaging conditions are much more difficult than in children because of the thickening of temporal bones with increasing age [4]. Nevertheless, due to the technological advances of the past decades a high-resolution imaging of deep brain structures is meanwhile possible even in the majority of adults [5,6]. Present-day TCS systems can achieve a higher image resolution in comparison not only to former-generation systems, but currently also to MRI under clinical conditions [7]. A sophisticated clinical high-end TCS system was shown to gain an in-plane image resolution of intracranial structures in the focal zone of about $0.7\,mm \times 1.1\,mm$ [7]. With the type of phased-array probes usually applied for TCS in adults, using a center frequency of 2.0—3.5 MHz, the focal zone of maximum resolution is in a distance of 5—7 (4—8) cm from the contact plane of the probe. This means that the best quality images of intracranial structures are obtained in deep brain areas near the midline.

* Tel.: +49 381 4949696; fax: +49 381 4944794.
E-mail address: uwe.walter@med.uni-rostock.de

2211-968X/$ — see front matter © 2012 Elsevier GmbH. All rights reserved.
doi:10.1016/j.permed.2012.02.012

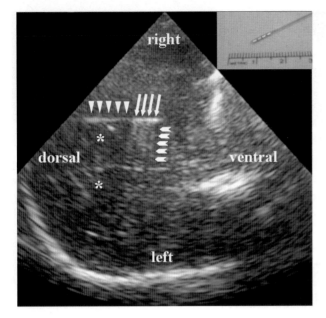

Figure 1 Longitudinal-section transcranial sonography (TCS) image of intracranial deep brain stimulation (DBS) lead (coronal image of a patients' head; * lateral ventricles). The DBS lead array with the four metal contacts (arrows) can be distinguished from the cable (triangles) by the reverberation artifacts originating from the metal contacts (arrow heads). The inserted panel in the right upper corner shows a photograph of the DBS lead.

This opens a new field of TCS application, the intra-operative assistance of deep brain implant placement and the post-operative monitoring of brain implant position. The present paper reviews the current literature and the experience of our lab in the application of TCS for the localization of deep brain stimulation (DBS) electrodes in patients with movement disorders.

TCS imaging artifacts and safety issues

Intracranial devices containing metal parts such as DBS electrodes cause several imaging artifacts on TCS due to their high echogenicity. First, due to poorer lateral image resolution compared to axial image resolution, the DBS electrode appears more extended in lateral direction than in axial direction. Second, reverberation artifacts are generated behind the DBS electrode (Fig. 1). We have performed human skull phantom studies, applying the TCS system Acuson Antares (Siemens; Erlangen, Germany) [8—10]. In lateral direction of insonation, usually applied to monitor DBS electrode depth intra- and post-operatively, the highly echogenic imaging artefact of the metal part of the DBS lead used for globus pallidus interna (GPI) stimulation in dystonia exceeded the 1 mm rubber tip by minimum 0.1 mm (range, 0.1—1.5 mm, depending on image brightness). In axial direction of insonation, the imaging artifact exceeding the real boundary of the DBS lead was smaller (range, 0.3—0.6 mm; resulting seeming DBS lead diameter, 1.9—2.5 mm, depending on image brightness; real diameter, 1.27 mm) [8,10]. It should be stressed that, before any application of TCS for intra-operative guiding the positioning of DBS lead in patients, the sizes of imaging artifacts need to be estimated separately for each different ultrasound system and each different DBS lead type to account for differences of imaging technologies and lead shape [9].

Using a skull phantom, it was also investigated whether the insonation of intracranially located DBS electrodes might be associated with a heating of the electrode. A constant temperature of the intracranial DBS lead was found when exposed to TCS or transcranial color-coded sonography (TCCS) for 30 min each with ultrasound frequencies of 2.0, 2.5, or 3.1 MHz (ultrasound intensity: mechanical index 1.4) [8]. Therefore it is unlikely that a heating of DBS electrodes occurs during TCS application, considering also the effective heat transfer within the brain due to the intense blood perfusion of the brain [9].

TCS for intra-operative implant monitoring

While a considerable number of studies have dealt with the intra-operative application of sonography in patients with open cranium [11—15], applications of intra-operative TCS have been rarely described. White et al. reported on preliminary findings using a novel intra-operative brain-shift monitor using shear-mode transcranial ultrasound [16]. Despite the advantages of ultrasound in an intra-operative setting compared to other imaging methods [9], such as high temporal resolution, portability, and non-ionizing mode of radiation, the application of commercially available TCS systems for intra-operative monitoring of DBS electrode placement has been reported only rarely so far.

One early study applied a former-generation TCS system (Sonoline Elegra, Siemens; Erlangen, Germany) during implantation of DBS electrodes into the targeted subthalamic nucleus (STN) in patients with Parkinson's disease [17]. The authors reported an easy visualization of the 0.8 mm thick electrode. The position of the imaging artefact of the tip of the DBS electrode appeared to be within in the anatomic region of substantia nigra that usually is of high echogenicity in patients with Parkinson's disease. Additionally, the segment of the laterally running posterior cerebral artery at the corresponding level could also be displayed. The authors found the appearing correct position of the DBS electrode tip on TCS at a place just touching the echo-signals of the substantia nigra. The results of this pilot study were limited by the poorer lateral image resolution of the TCS system applied compared to contemporary TCS systems [7], and the missing estimation of the exact size of the electrode imaging artifacts which caused some uncertainty with regard to the exact electrode tip position.

In a more recent study, a contemporary TCS system (Acuson Antares, Siemens; Erlangen, Germany) was applied intra-operatively to monitor the placement of DBS electrode into the GPI in patients with idiopathic dystonia [8]. In this study not only the visualization of the final DBS electrodes was possible but also the simultaneous visualization of 2—5 closely located microelectrodes used for detection of the optimal trajectory of the final electrode (Fig. 2A). Another advantage of the intra-operative TCS monitoring was that the distance of the DBS electrode tip to the artery at the anatomic target (penetrating branch of the posterior communicating artery) could be assessed (Fig. 2B).

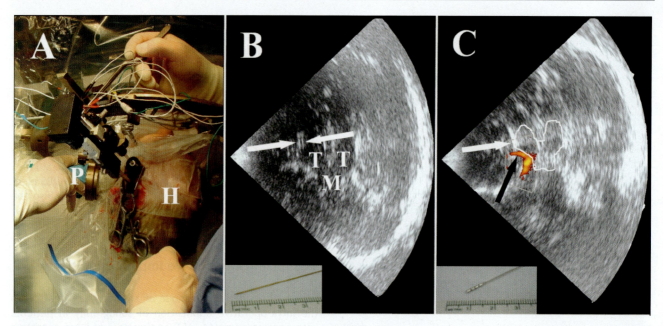

Figure 2 Transcranial sonography (TCS) images of deep brain stimulation (DBS) electrodes obtained during stereotactic implantation. (A) Position of the TCS probe (P) placed at the temporal plane of the patients head (H). (B) Coronal TCS image of the patients head. T indicates thalamus; M, midbrain. Two closely located microelectrodes (arrows) of 0.5 mm diameter are visualized in the target region. The inserted panel in the left lower corner shows a photograph of a microelectrode. (C) Coronal TCS image showing the tip of the final DBS lead (white arrow) and its distance to the perforating branch (black arrow) of the posterior communicating artery. The midbrain and thalami are surrounded for better recognition. The inserted panel in the left lower corner shows a photograph of the DBS lead.

This was possible since the extent of the imaging artefact of the electrode had been estimated in advance for the referring TCS system and implant [8]. This even enabled intra-operatively the decision to insert the final DBS electrode somewhat deeper than it would have been done using only the pre-operatively planned navigation data [8]. Simultaneous visualization of the artery at the anatomic target prevented hemorrhages at the target site.

The possibility to intra-operatively optimize the electrode position is of high interest since discrepancies of up to several millimeters between the initial target, selected on pre-operative MRI, and the final DBS lead location are caused mainly by caudal brain shift that occurs after opening the dura [16,18]. Intra-operative MRI may be an option to overcome this discrepancy but is expensive and not widely available [19]. The higher mobility and temporal resolution achieved with TCS may promote an increasing use for the intra-operative guidance of deep brain implant placement [9].

TCS for post-operative localization of implants

Despite advances in stereotactic pre-operative MRI techniques [20], there are discrepancies of up to 4 mm (average 2 mm) between the initial selected target and the final DBS lead location caused mainly by caudal brain shift that occurs once the cranium is open [18]. Moreover, the DBS lead may get displaced post-operatively, e.g. by delayed brain shift or head injury [21,22]. Therefore, poor post-operative outcome or unexpected change in neurological state requires brain imaging to check the lead location. Computed tomography (CT) is frequently used for this purpose but has the disadvantages of patient's exposure to radiation and considerable imaging artifacts caused by the metal tip of the electrodes. On the other hand, performing MRI in patients with neurostimulators may be associated with several risks such as heating of electrodes, magnetic field interactions, functional device disruption, and induced electrical current, which might lead to irreversible tissue damage [23]. Therefore, head MRI in DBS patients was recommended to be performed only if a number of technical restrictions and guidelines were followed. Provided sufficient imaging conditions (sufficient bone window, contemporary high-end ultrasound system), TCS may be a good alternative for the post-operative monitoring of the DBS electrode location. Compared to the intra-operative setting, it is even easier to localize DBS electrodes post-operatively on TCS since the patients and the investigator are in a much more comfortable setting. Especially, there is less constriction in finding the optimal temporal acoustic bone in order to achieve high-quality brain images. Measuring electrodes as well as DBS electrodes were easily identified at different targets [9,10,24,25]. Typical aspects of DBS electrodes targeting the pars ventralis intermedius (VIM) of the thalamus and the STN are shown in Fig. 3. It is recommendable to define some landmarks that can be used as reference points for estimating the exact position of the DBS electrode tip. Typical measures are the shortest distance of the electrode tip from the midline and/or the outer boundary of the third ventricle (VIM, GPI, STN), the distance of the electrode tip from the pineal gland (VIM, GPI), and the position of the electrode in relation to highly echogenic neighboring structures such as the internal capsule (VIM, GPI) and the substantia nigra (STN)

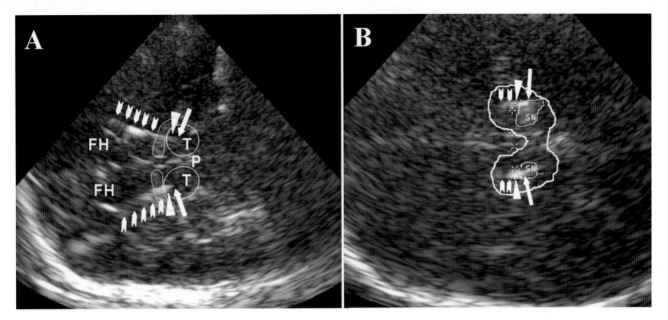

Figure 3 Transcranial sonography (TCS) images obtained for the post-operative control of deep brain stimulation (DBS) electrode position in two patients. (A) Semi-coronal TCS scan through the brain of a patient with severe essential tremor in whom DBS bilaterally of the nucleus ventralis intermedius (VIM) of the thalamus was performed. The thalami are surrounded for better recognition. The lead tips of the bilateral DBS electrodes are visualized in the right and the left thalamus (virtual tip position: arrows; true tip position: arrow heads). FH denotes frontal horn of lateral ventricle, P, pineal gland, T, thalamus. (B) Axial (transverse) TCS scan in a patient with Parkinson's disease in whom DBS bilaterally of the subthalamic nucleus (STN) was performed. The midbrain and the bilateral markedly echogenic ("hyperechogenic") substantia nigra are surrounded for better recognition. Considering the lower lateral than axial image resolution on TCS, the real position of the lead tips of the bilateral DBS electrodes is exactly within the STN (arrow heads), even though on the TCS image the virtual lead tip is within the substantia nigra (arrows).

[9,10,25]. We have recently proposed criteria for grading optimum vs suboptimum DBS electrode position for the DBS targets VIM, GPI and STN [10].

In our experience, the detection of slight differences of 2 mm and more between right- and left-sided electrode with respect to their distance to midline, but also in their rostro-caudal position, is possible with TCS [10]. Electrode dislocation can easily be diagnosed with TCS [9].

Conclusions and outlook

The results of the studies published so far [8–10,17,24,25] support the use of TCS for the monitoring of intracranial electrode position. It can be expected that the obvious advantages of TCS in comparison to other neuroimaging methods, such as high mobility, short investigation times, non-invasiveness and less corruption by patients movements, will further promote the use of TCS for the intra- and post-operative monitoring of deep brain implants, especially in patients with movement disorders [9]. The major current limitation of TCS application is, beside its dependence on the quality of transtemporal acoustic bone windows, the necessity of a highly qualified investigator. The investigator performing intra-operative TCS for guiding therapeutic decisions needs to be well trained beforehand in the pre- and post-operative routine setting [9]. Moreover, the applied TCS system as well as the assessed brain implant should be studied in advance for the exact size of their imaging artifacts using a skull phantom as described earlier [8,10].

The upcoming technologies allowing the in-time fusion of intra- and post-operative TCS images with pre-operative MRI images may facilitate an easier and less investigator-dependent application of intra-operative TCS.

Currently, an international multi-center study is being planned to further prove the value of TCS in the post-operative monitoring of STN DBS electrode position which is intended to start in summer 2012. Centers with both, experience in TCS and DBS, are invited to join this trial. For more details regarding this study, interested colleagues may contact the author of this article via email.

References

[1] Machado HR, Martelli N, Assirati Júnior JA, Colli BO. Infantile hydrocephalus: brain sonography as an effective tool for diagnosis and follow-up. Childs Nerv Syst 1991;7:205—10.

[2] Babcock DS. Sonography of the brain in infants: role in evaluating neurologic abnormalities. AJR Am J Roentgenol 1995;165:417—23.

[3] Mursch K, Behnke J, Christen HJ, Markakis E. Use of transcranial real-time ultrasonography for programming a shunt valve system. Childs Nerv Syst 1996;12:392—5.

[4] Wijnhoud AD, Franckena M, van der Lugt A, Koudstaal PJ, Dippel ED. Inadequate acoustical temporal bone window in patients with a transient ischemic attack or minor stroke: role of skull thickness and bone density. Ultrasound Med Biol 2008;34:923—9.

[5] Walter U, Behnke S, Eyding J, Niehaus L, Postert T, Seidel G, et al. Transcranial brain parenchyma sonography in movement disorders: state of the art. Ultrasound Med Biol 2007;33:15—25.

[6] Berg D, Godau J, Walter U. Transcranial sonography in movement disorders. Lancet Neurol 2008;7: 1044—55.
[7] Walter U, Kanowski M, Kaufmann J, Grossmann A, Benecke R, Niehaus L. Contemporary ultrasound systems allow high-resolution transcranial imaging of small echogenic deep intracranial structures similarly as MRI: a phantom study. Neuroimage 2008;40:551—8.
[8] Walter U, Wolters A, Wittstock M, Benecke R, Schroeder HW, Müller JU. Deep brain stimulation in dystonia: sonographic monitoring of electrode placement into the globus pallidus internus. Mov Disord 2009;24:1538—41.
[9] Walter U. Transcranial sonography-assisted stereotaxy and follow-up of deep brain implants in patients with movement disorders. Int Rev Neurobiol 2010;90:274—85.
[10] Walter U, Kirsch M, Wittstock M, Müller JU, Benecke R, Wolters A. Transcranial sonographic localization of deep brain stimulation electrodes is safe, reliable and predicts clinical outcome. Ultrasound Med Biol 2011;37:1382—91.
[11] Comeau RM, Sadikot AF, Fenster A, Peters TM. Intraoperative ultrasound for guidance and tissue shift correction in image-guided neurosurgery. Med Phys 2000;27:787—800.
[12] Coenen VA, Krings T, Weidemann J, Hans FJ, Reinacher P, Gilsbach JM, et al. Sequential visualization of brain and fiber tract deformation during intracranial surgery with three-dimensional ultrasound: an approach to evaluate the effect of brain shift. Neurosurgery 2005;56(1 Suppl.):133—41.
[13] Letteboer MM, Willems PW, Viergever MA, Niessen WJ. Brain shift estimation in image guided neurosurgery using 3-D ultrasound. IEEE Trans Biomed Eng 2005;52:268—76.
[14] Lindner D, Trantakis C, Renner C, Arnold S, Schmitgen A, Schneider J, et al. Application of intraoperative 3D ultrasound during navigated tumor resection. Minim Invasive Neurosurg 2006;49:197—202.
[15] Rygh OM, Cappelen J, Selbekk T, Lindseth F, Hernes TA, Unsgaard G. Endoscopy guided by an intraoperative 3D ultrasound-based neuronavigation system. Minim Invasive Neurosurg 2006;49:1—9.
[16] White PJ, Whalen S, Tang SC, Clement GT, Jolesz F, Golby AJ. An intraoperative brain shift monitor using shear mode transcranial ultrasound: preliminary results. J Ultrasound Med 2009;28:191—203.
[17] Moringlane JR, Fuss G, Becker G. Peroperative transcranial sonography for electrode placement into the targeted subthalamic nucleus of patients with Parkinson disease: technical note. Surg Neurol 2005;63:66—9.
[18] Khan MF, Mewes K, Gross RE, Skrinjar O. Assessment of brain shift related to deep brain stimulation surgery. Stereotact Funct Neurosurg 2008;86:44—53.
[19] Hall WA, Truwit CL. Intraoperative MR-guided neurosurgery. J Magn Reson Imaging 2008;27:368—75.
[20] O'Gorman RL, Shmueli K, Ashkan K, Samuel M, Lythgoe DJ, Shahidiani A, et al. Optimal MRI methods for direct stereotactic targeting of the subthalamic nucleus and globus pallidus. Eur Radiol 2011;21:130—6.
[21] Mehrkens JH, Bötzel K, Steude U, Zeitler K, Schnitzler A, Sturm V, et al. Long-term efficacy and safety of chronic globus pallidus internus stimulation in different types of primary dystonia. Stereotact Funct Neurosurg 2009;87:8—17.
[22] Van den Munckhof P, Contarino MF, Bour LJ, Speelman JD, de Bie RM, Schuurman PR. Postoperative curving and upward displacement of deep brain stimulation electrodes caused by brain shift. Neurosurgery 2010;67:49—54.
[23] Rezai AR, Baker KB, Tkach JA, Phillips M, Hrdlicka G, Sharan AD, et al. Is magnetic resonance imaging safe for patients with neurostimulation systems used for deep brain stimulation. Neurosurgery 2005;57:1056—62.
[24] Kurth C, Steinhoff BJ. Sonographic imaging of foramen ovale electrodes. J Ultrasound Med 2002;21:555—7.
[25] Bor-Seng-Shu E, Fonoff ET, Barbosa ER, Teixeira MJ. Substantia nigra hyperechogenicity in Parkinson's disease. Acta Neurochir (Wien) 2010;152:2085—7.

Transcranial ultrasound in adults and children with movement disorders

Jan Liman[a,*], Mathias Bähr[a], Pawel Kermer[a,b]

[a] Department of Neurology, University of Göttingen, Robert-Koch-Str. 40, 37075 Göttingen, Germany
[b] Department of Neurology, Nordwestkrankenhaus Sanderbusch GmbH, Hauptstraße 1, 26452 Sande, Germany

KEYWORDS
Ultrasound;
Child;
Pediatric;
Movement disorder;
TCS

Summary Since the first discovery, that ultrasound can overcome the skull allowing examination of the intracranial blood-flow as well as the first description of substantia nigra (SN) signal alterations via B-mode sonography, a plethora of applications especially in the field of movement disorders have been fostered. Up to now, however, most studies investigated adult individuals, even though numerous of the diseases studied have their onset already during childhood or adolescence. This overview summarizes recent studies of transcranial B-mode sonography (TCS) within the movement disorder field and outlines potential implications for pediatric applications.
© 2012 Elsevier GmbH. All rights reserved.

History of transcranial ultrasound

For decades it was thought, that it is impossible to penetrate the intact scull by ultrasound for the visualization of intracranial structures and measurement of blood flow in the circle of Wilis. It was in the 1980s when Aaslid et al. could demonstrate that blood flow of the intracranial arteries can be analysed by transcranial Doppler sonography [1]. In following years a rapid development of ultrasound systems evolved until Becker et al. were able to display the substantia nigra (SN) reproducibly via B-Mode sonography in 1995. Moreover, they were able to demonstrate an enlargement and hyperechogenicity of the SN area patients suffering from Parkinson's disease (PD) [2]. Up to now, this finding was reproduced by many independent groups and transcranial B-mode sonography (TCS) developed into an expanding research field for a multitude of medical applications. Here, we will shortly highlight the different ultrasound implementations in the medical field and will focus on the most recent advances in the diagnosis of movement disorders especially in children.

Current applications in adults

Applications in Parkinson's disease

In recent years, TCS has become widely accepted and used in the early and differential diagnosis of Parkinson's disease. One hallmark of this method, besides its inexpensiveness and non-invasive character, is the ability to discriminate between essential tremor, Parkinson's disease related tremor and the differentiation of atypical Parkinson syndromes [3–5]. In PD, the typical finding is a hyperechogenicity of the SN, which is normally more pronounced contralateral to the clinically more affected side [6]. This hyperechogenicitiy seems to stay constant during the course of the disease and patho-anatomical investigations revealed that it most likely reflects increased iron content, as was

* Corresponding author. Tel.: +49 551 3914139;
fax: +49 551 3914302.
E-mail address: jliman@gwdg.de (J. Liman).

shown in animal experiments, as well as in post mortem of brains [7–10].

In patients with atypical signs in Parkinson syndromes TCS is useful for assignment to the idiopathic forms. Patients with multi system atrophy, or supranuclear palsy of the Richardson subtype do normally not display a hyperechogenic SN, but rather show increased echogenicity of the lenticular nucleus [5]. In contrast, patients with corticobasal degeneration commonly display a hyperechogenic SN in combination with hyperechogenicity in the lenticular nucleus [11].

Other movement disorders

In clinical practice, B-mode sonography proved also to be useful for discrimination of IPS from other movement or gait disorders, such as normal pressure hydrocephalus or other disorders associated with metal accumulation in the basal ganglia.

B-mode sonography allows the visualization of the ventricular system, especially the third ventricle and the side ventricles. Thus, in patients with an unclear gait disorder the differential diagnosis of a normal pressure hydrocephalus can be ruled out easily [12]. Due to the fact, that iron accumulation is proposed to be the anatomical correlation of the SN hyperechogenicity in Parkinson's disease, TCS was also studied in other movement disorders related to metal accumulation. For example, it was found, that the lenticular nucleus displays increased echogenic values in patients suffering from Wilson's disease, a disorder with copper accumulation in and outside the brain. The intensity of hyperechogenicity correlates with disease severity [13]. In patients with cervical and upper limb dystonia TCS displays increased lenticular nucleus echogenicity pronounced contra lateral to the clinically affected side [14,15]. As hyperechogenicity in the parenchymal sonography was believed to be due to metal accumulation, a post mortem analysis was performed in individuals suffering from dystonia. This study could rule out an increased copper and manganese content in the lenticular nucleus compared to controls [16]. Recently, our group was able to show, that patients suffering from neurodegeneration with brain iron accumulation (NBIA), a disease with childhood onset which is caused by mutations in enzymes dealing with iron metabolism in the brain, also shows increased echogenicity in the SN compared to healthy controls [17].

Taken together, TCS seems to be a valid tool in the differential diagnosis of movement disorders, especially if they are related to metal accumulation in the brain. In comparison to MRI findings especially in patients suffering from Wilson's disease and NBIA, it has to be critically noted that the sonographic findings do concur, but especially within the basal ganglia. MRI scans by far show more affected areas than sonography does [18] [19]. For example in Wilson's disease, T2-weighted MR images show decreased signal intensities in the globus pallidus, putamen, substantia nigra, and caudate nuclei, while TCS only verifies changes in the lenticular nucleus. Similar to Wilson's disease, T2*-weighted scans in NBIA show hypointensities within the globus pallidus, SN, putamen and the dentate nucleus. It is not clear so far, why not all signal abnormalities documented by MRI can be reproduced by TCS. One reason may be higher sensitivity of MRI in the detection of metal deposition. On the contrary, changes seen in the SN by TCS in PD in our experience occur earlier than those seen by MRI. In conclusion, one may speculate, that the sensitivity of TCS differs in various brain regions with some shortcomings within the basal ganglia region.

Movement disorders in children

In the pediatric field, besides CCT and cMRI, transcranial ultrasound is already used routinely for several years due to its advantages regarding radiation exposure and the ability to examine the children without sedation. The American Academy of Neurology and the Practice Committee of the Child Neurology Society thus recommend the use of TCS for neonates with an increased risk for intraventricular hemorrhage, preterm white matter injury or ventriculomegaly [20]. However until now routine use of ultrasound in children and adolescents with movement disorders is not widely applied. In light of the TCS findings gained from studies in adult patients with movement disorders we will highlight in the following three diseases displaying TCS abnormalities in adults with disease onset already during childhood or adolescence. As already mentioned above, Wilson's disease is a disorder with copper storage abnormalities throughout the body and also in the basal ganglia due to mutations in the copper transport ATPase [21]. Besides other symptoms, accumulation of copper in the brain leads to dystonia, tremor and akinetic-rigid symptoms with the age of manifestation ranging from 7 to 37 years of age. Some cases have been reported though with even earlier onset at preschool age [22,23]. The broad range of symptoms, which occur during disease course can cause difficulties in the early diagnosis. Prashanth et al. analysed the clinical data of Wilson's disease patients which were registered over 30 years and found a mean time delay from disease onset to diagnosis of two years with a range from 0.08–30 years [24]. Besides clinical experience and education, these data underline the need for diagnostic modalities in the early diagnosis of this disorder. As the MRI displays typical signs (e.g. ''face of the giant panda'' and the ''bright claustrum'') in this disease, it appears as one of the most important diagnostic tools in differential diagnosis. However, especially in children, MRI examination is laborious and most of the children need sedation [18]. This is, besides the costs, a limiting factor of this method and highlights the necessity for the implementation of a screening method. Walter et al. demonstrated typical changes in the lenticular nucleus by TCS with increasing echogenicity depending on the disease activity in Wilson's disease patients [13]. These results raise the hope, that TCS can be useful as a screening method in addition to copper and ceruloplasmin analysis in serum.

A second movement disorder with adolescent onset is Friedreich's ataxia. It is the most common among the inherited ataxias in Europe. The main clinical features are dysarthria, pyramidal tract damage and progressive ataxia [25]. The first clinical symptoms of Friedreich's ataxia normally appear during puberty, but also early and late onset variants exist [25]. To date, the diagnosis is based on clinical examination, supported by electrophysiological findings and proven by genetic analysis with confirmation of a GAA expansion within the first exon of the Frataxin gene [26]. Recently Synofzik et al. published their study, which examined TCS in patients suffering from Friedreich's ataxia. Interestingly they could show hyperechogenic changes in the dentate nucleus, which was present in 85% of all patients and already visible after short disease duration [27]. This finding was accompanied by a hypoechogenic SN. One possible explanation for the hyperechogenicity of the dentate nucleus as discussed by the authors is an increased iron content, which is also detectable on T2*-weighted MRI images [28]. The authors see TCS useful for assessment of patients suffering from ataxia. One shortcoming is, that dentate nucleus hyperechogenicity is not specific for Friedreich's ataxia, but was also found in patients suffering from spinocerebellar ataxia type 3 (SCA3) [29]. In contrast to Friedreich's patients though, the hyperechogenicity appeared less frequent (54%) and in combination with SN hyperechogenicity (40%). Taken together, these two studies provide evidence for the usefulness of TCS in the differential diagnosis of ataxias, but further studies are needed to validate these data, especially a direct comparison of patients with Friedreich's ataxia to those suffering from SCA3 are needed to rule out the real diagnostic potential of TCS.

Neurodegeneration with brain iron accumulation, formerly known as Hallervorden—Spatz syndrome is a movement disorder with early onset and a wide range of initial neurological symptoms. The estimated prevalence is 1—3 per million. Neuropathological hallmarks are abnormal iron accumulations especially in the globus pallidus and the substantia nigra pars reticulata. Recently, mutations in the pantothenate kinase 2 (PANK2) gene were identified as causative for up to 70% of all NBIA cases. Hence, this subtype of NBIA was designated pantothenate kinase-associated neurodegeneration (PKAN) [30,31]. The first symptoms usually occur during childhood and patients initially present with walking difficulties. Later the typical symptoms consisting of dysarthria, dystonia and visual problems occur [32]. To date, the diagnosis is obtained using MR imaging showing the pathognomonic hypointensity within the globus pallidus along with high signal intensity in the center of the globus pallidus internus also known as "eye-of-the-tiger-sign" (EOT-sign) on T2-weighted images [33]. The verification of the diagnosis is done by documentation of PANK2 mutation. As the clinical presentation of patients can be unspecific and the MR imaging implies sedation in children, we recently performed a study examining the diagnostic properties of TCS in the diagnosis of NBIA. In this small study, 7 patients were examined by transcranial ultrasound and the results were compared to age matched controls without any history of neurological disease [17]. Interestingly, we found a highly significant hyperechogenicity of the SN in NBIA patients. Surprisingly, we were not able to detect valid changes within the basal ganglia, which in MRI usually display the pathognomonic EOT sign. As already discussed for Wilson's disease, further studies and more experience are needed to evaluate this shortcoming of TCS in the area of the basal ganglia. Due to the limited size of our study the findings need to be reproduced in a bigger cohort of patients. Nevertheless, it provides good evidence for the usefulness of TCS especially in children with suspected movement disorders prior to genetic testing or MR imaging.

Conclusion

Since the initial finding by Becker and co-workers, that TCS is capable of displaying changes in the SN in PD patients, the application of this method in the early and differential diagnosis of Parkinson related movement disorders is already part of the basic diagnostics in the clinical setting. To date, intensive research is examining the properties of this method in various diseases, especially in those where metal accumulation is causative or a result of the disorder. Unfortunately, this research usually is performed and focussed on adults. Because of the simplicity of this method, the ability to use it in patients without sedation and the lack of side effects a broader application is desirable with special focus on the pediatric field.

References

[1] Aaslid R, Markwalder TM, Nornes H. Noninvasive transcranial Doppler ultrasound recording of flow velocity in basal cerebral arteries. J Neurosurg 1982;57:769—74.
[2] Becker G, Seufert J, Bogdahn U, Reichmann H, Reiners K. Degeneration of substantia nigra in chronic Parkinson's disease visualized by transcranial color-coded real-time sonography. Neurology 1995;45:182—4.
[3] Stockner H, Wurster I. Transcranial sonography in essential tremor. Int Rev Neurobiol 2010;90:189—97.
[4] Stockner H, Sojer M, KS K, Mueller J, Wenning GK, Schmidauer C. Midbrain sonography in patients with essential tremor. Mov Disord 2007;22:414—7.
[5] Bouwmans AE, Vlaar AM, Srulijes K, Mess WH, Weber WE. Transcranial sonography for the discrimination of idiopathic Parkinson's disease from the atypical parkinsonian syndromes. Int Rev Neurobiol 2010;90:121—46.
[6] Berg D, Merz B, Reiners K, Naumann M, Becker G. Five-year follow-up study of hyperechogenicity of the substantia nigra in Parkinson's disease. Mov Disord 2005;20:383—5.
[7] Berg D, Grote C, Rausch WD, Maurer M, Wesemann W, Riederer P, et al. Iron accumulation in the substantia nigra in rats visualized by ultrasound. Ultrasound Med Biol 1999;25:901—4.
[8] Godau J, Berg D. Role of transcranial ultrasound in the diagnosis of movement disorders. Neuroimaging Clin N Am 2010;20:87—101.
[9] Walter U, Dressler D, Wolters A, Wittstock M, Benecke R. Transcranial brain sonography findings in clinical subgroups of idiopathic Parkinson's disease. Mov Disord 2007;22:48—54.
[10] Berg D, Roggendorf W, Schroder U, Klein R, Tatschner T, Benz P, et al. Echogenicity of the substantia nigra: association with increased iron content and marker for susceptibility to nigrostriatal injury. Arch Neurol 2002;59:999—1005.
[11] Walter U, Dressler D, Wolters A, Probst T, Grossmann A, Benecke R. Sonographic discrimination of corticobasal degeneration vs progressive supranuclear palsy. Neurology 2004;63:504—9.
[12] Seidel G, Kaps M, Gerriets T, Hutzelmann A. Evaluation of the ventricular system in adults by transcranial duplex sonography. J Neuroimaging 1995;5:105—8.
[13] Walter U, Krolikowski K, Tarnacka B, Benecke R, Czlonkowska A, Dressler D. Sonographic detection of basal ganglia lesions in asymptomatic and symptomatic Wilson disease. Neurology 2005;64:1726—32.
[14] Naumann M, Becker G, Toyka KV, Supprian T, Reiners K. Lenticular nucleus lesion in idiopathic dystonia detected by transcranial sonography. Neurology 1996;47:1284—90.

[15] Becker G, Naumann M, Scheubeck M, Hofmann E, Deimling M, Lindner A, et al. Comparison of transcranial sonography, magnetic resonance imaging, and single photon emission computed tomography findings in idiopathic spasmodic torticollis. Mov Disord 1997;12:79—88.

[16] Becker G, Berg D, Rausch WD, Lange HK, Riederer P, Reiners K. Increased tissue copper and manganese content in the lentiform nucleus in primary adult-onset dystonia. Ann Neurol 1999;46:260—3.

[17] Liman J, Wellmer A, Rostasy K, Bahr M, Kermer P. Transcranial ultrasound in neurodegeneration with brain iron accumulation (NBIA). Eur J Paediatr Neurol 2011.

[18] da Costa Mdo D, Spitz M, Bacheschi LA, Leite CC, Lucato LT, Barbosa ER. Wilson's disease: two treatment modalities. Correlations to pretreatment and posttreatment brain MRI. Neuroradiology 2009;51:627—33.

[19] McNeill A, Birchall D, Hayflick SJ, Gregory A, Schenk JF, Zimmerman EA, et al. T2* and FSE MRI distinguishes four subtypes of neurodegeneration with brain iron accumulation. Neurology 2008;70:1614—9.

[20] Ment LR, Bada HS, Barnes P, Grant PE, Hirtz D, Papile LA, et al. Practice parameter: neuroimaging of the neonate: report of the Quality Standards Subcommittee of the American Academy of Neurology and the Practice Committee of the Child Neurology Society. Neurology 2002;58:1726—38.

[21] Shah AB, Chernov I, Zhang HT, Ross BM, Das K, Lutsenko S, et al. Identification and analysis of mutations in the Wilson disease gene (ATP7B): population frequencies, genotype-phenotype correlation, and functional analyses. Am J Hum Genet 1997;61:317—28.

[22] Machado A, Chien HF, Deguti MM, Cancado E, Azevedo RS, Scaff M, et al. Neurological manifestations in Wilson's disease: report of 119 cases. Mov Disord 2006;21:2192—6.

[23] Wilson DC, Phillips MJ, Cox DW, Roberts EA. Severe hepatic Wilson's disease in preschool-aged children. J Pediatr 2000;137:719—22.

[24] Prashanth LK, Taly AB, Sinha S, Arunodaya GR, Swamy HS. Wilson's disease: diagnostic errors and clinical implications. J Neurol Neurosurg Psychiatry 2004;75:907—9.

[25] Schulz JB, Boesch S, Burk K, Durr A, Giunti P, Mariotti C, et al. Diagnosis and treatment of Friedreich ataxia: a European perspective. Nat Rev Neurol 2009;5:222—34.

[26] Campuzano V, Montermini L, Molto MD, Pianese L, Cossee M, Cavalcanti F, et al. Friedreich's ataxia: autosomal recessive disease caused by an intronic GAA triplet repeat expansion. Science 1996;271:1423—7.

[27] Synofzik M, Godau J, Lindig T, Schols L, Berg D. Transcranial sonography reveals cerebellar, nigral, and forebrain abnormalities in Friedreich's ataxia. Neurodegener Dis 2011;8:470—5.

[28] Waldvogel D, van Gelderen P, Hallett M. Increased iron in the dentate nucleus of patients with Friedrich's ataxia. Ann Neurol 1999;46:123—5.

[29] Postert T, Eyding J, Berg D, Przuntek H, Becker G, Finger M, et al. Transcranial sonography in spinocerebellar ataxia type 3. J Neural Transm Suppl 2004:123—33.

[30] Zhou B, Westaway SK, Levinson B, Johnson MA, Gitschier J, Hayflick SJ. A novel pantothenate kinase gene (PANK2) is defective in Hallervorden—Spatz syndrome. Nat Genet 2001;28:345—9.

[31] Hayflick SJ, Westaway SK, Levinson B, Zhou B, Johnson MA, Ching KH, et al. Genetic, clinical, and radiographic delineation of Hallervorden—Spatz syndrome. N Engl J Med 2003;348:33—40.

[32] Gordon N. Pantothenate kinase-associated neurodegeneration (Hallervorden—Spatz syndrome). Eur J Paediatr Neurol 2002;6:243—7.

[33] Sethi KD, Adams RJ, Loring DW, el Gammal T. Hallervorden—Spatz syndrome: clinical and magnetic resonance imaging correlations. Ann Neurol 1988;24:692—4.

Possibilities of transcranial color-coded sonography in pathology of deep brain veins in children

Marina Abramova*, Irina Stepanova, Svetlana Shayunova

Russian National Research, Medical University Named After N.I. Pirogov, Pediatric Faculty, Neurology, Neurosurgery and Medical Genetics Department, Laboratory of Child Cerebrovascular Disorders, Russia

KEYWORDS
Children;
Cerebral venous hemodynamic;
Chiari abnormalities;
Hypoplasia of cerebral venous sinuses;
Sinus cavernous;
Ultrasonic methods

Abstract   A study in children with headaches associated mainly with venous hemodynamic disturbances has been performed. The role of cerebral venous disturbances has been defined in children with structural cerebral abnormalities: craniovertebral junction anomalies (Chiari abnormalities I) and hypoplasia of cerebral venous sinuses. Disturbances of cerebral hemodynamics revealed by ultrasonic methods determine the management of patients with different cerebral venous abnormalities.
© 2012 Published by Elsevier GmbH.

Introduction

The estimation of cerebral venous hemodynamic disturbances in literature is described mainly in adults. Diagnosis of such disturbances in children is not detected in time, though they often turn out to be one of the main evidence of cerebrovascular pathology. Venous outflow in deep brain veins (straight sinus, cavernous sinus, great cerebral vein of Galen) was registered by ultrasonic Doppler and duplex methods. Cavernous sinus is described in literature basically in case of craniocerebral trauma with formation of carotid-cavernous fistulas. Cavernous sinus actively participates in regulation of venous brain outflow from a cranial cavity. The internal carotid artery is located in the center of the cavernous sinus which changes the volume of sinus by its pulse fluctuations. Thus a venous outflow is stimulated and makes influence on intracranial venous circulation. Therefore, the cavernous sinus is often designated as a ''venous heart''. Hemodynamic disturbances in the cavernous sinus are ''markers'' of cerebral venous hemodynamic dysfunction. Thus research of cavernous sinus hemodynamics presents new possibilities for revealing the disturbances of cerebral venous blood circulation in the complex investigation of deep brain veins.

It is difficult to assess the cavernous sinus in children by standard (transorbital) approach. We worked out a new approach of transcranial duplex scanning to visualize the cavernous sinus, with determination of structures and features of venous blood flow for subsequent elaboration of diagnosis algorithm and possibility of conservative care of children, who have disturbances of venous cerebral hemodynamics.

Purpose

Cerebral hemodynamic features and the role of venous hemodynamic disturbances under structural cerebral abnormalities in children have been studied.

* Corresponding author at: Ostrovityanova str. 1, Moscow 117997, Russia. Tel.: +7 925 510 71 48.
E-mail address: de_mar@bk.ru (M. Abramova).

2211-968X/$ — see front matter © 2012 Published by Elsevier GmbH.
http://dx.doi.org/10.1016/j.permed.2012.04.002

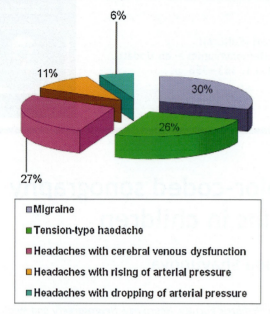

Fig. 1 Different types of children's headaches.

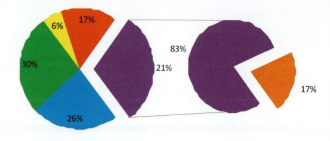

Fig. 3 Headaches in children. Structural cerebral abnormalities.

Materials and methods

1200 patients aged from 3 to 17 years who complained of headache have been examined. The control group consisted of 95 healthy children.

The examination of children has been performed by transcranial Doppler analyzer (TCD) "ANDIOGIN", "SONOMED-500" of "BIOSS" and "SPECTROMED" companies (Russia) equipped with a standard transducer (2 MHz). Transcranial color-coded duplex (TCCD) scanning of brain vessels has been carried out by "Logic P-5" device (Japan) with a sectoral transducer (5 MHz) in triplex mode (B + CF + PW; B + PDI + PW). Blood flow velocity and structure features of the cavernous sinus, carotid arteries, ophthalmic arteries and veins, the extracranial part of the internal jugular vein, the straight venous sinus and the great cerebral vein of Galen have been registered. We proposed a new technique of transcranial duplex scanning of the cavernous sinus. This approach provides a good overview of forms and peculiarities of the hemodynamics of the cavernous sinus.

Magnetic resonance imaging (MRI) has been performed as well.

Results

All children with headaches were separated into several groups according to the clinical and ultrasound findings: migraine headache (30%), tension type of headache (26%), headache with increase or reduction of arterial pressure (17%), headache caused by cerebral venous dysfunction (27%) (Fig. 1).

It is noted that children with different types of headache (migraine, tension headache, one with changing arterial pressure) had also cerebral venous hemodynamic disturbances with different intensity. This fact is usually not mentioned in literature regarding headache research (Fig. 2).

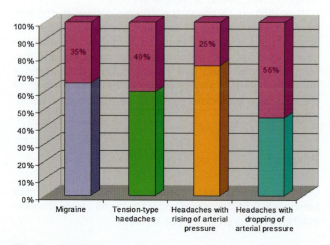

Fig. 2 Cerebral venous dysfunction in children with different types of headache.

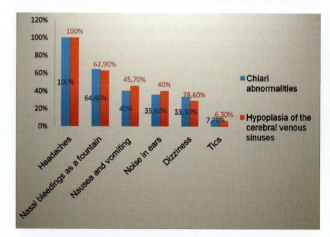

Fig. 4 Clinical manifestations in children with structure abnormalities.

Cerebral vessels	Chiari abnormality (%) / VPS cm/s	Hypoplasia of the cerebral venous sinuses (%) / VPS cm/s
vein of Galen	100% / 47 ± 9,4	100% / 61 ± 2,6
straight sinus	100% / 44 ± 5,6	100% / 60 ± 2,5
cavernous sinus	54% / 40 ± 2,1	76% / 48 ± 4,6
vertebral veins	50% / 51 ± 3,6	35% / 30 ± 2,3
basilar vein	32% / 71 ± 3,1	28% / 23 ± 2,4
Increase of VPS at basilar artery	68% / 110 ± 14,5	15% / 31 ± 3,6
blood flow asymmetry at vertebral arteries	39%	28%

Fig. 5 Structural cerebral abnormalities in children. Cerebrovascular hemodynamic parameters (TCD, TCCD).

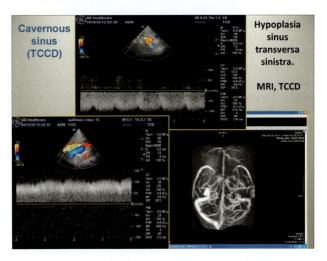

Fig. 7 Agreement between TCD, TCCD and MRI data.

In a group of children with headaches caused by cerebral venous dysfunction, 88 children had different structural abnormalities (confirmed by MRI): 46 of them had abnormalities of craniovertebral junction (Chiari abnormalities I).

42 children had abnormalities of deep brain veins. Hypoplasia of transverse sinuses combined with hypoplasia of sigmoid sinuses was revealed in 36 children, hypoplasia of the superior sagittal sinus in 3 children, and Chiari abnormality in 5 children (Fig. 3).

The clinical picture of children with structure abnormalities was characterized by headaches (100%), nasal bleeding (60%), sickness and vomiting (40%), noise in ears (35%), dizziness (30%), vegetative dysfunction, 1% of children had relative deafness, and 8% of children had tics (mostly of face muscles). All examined children complained of headaches localized in cervical and parietal regions, that arised while or after night/day sleeping. Increase of headaches occured after physical exercises, and lessons at school. 60% of children had typical nasal bleeding, mostly abundant and spontaneous as a "fountain" (Fig. 4).

As a result of the research we revealed an increase of velocity in deep brain veins (peak systolic velocity—VPS): in the straight sinus 56 ± 5.6 cm/s, and in the great cerebral vein of Galen 57 ± 9.4 cm/s (our normal values were 26 and 22 cm/s, respectively). An increase of blood flow velocity in vertebral venous plexus was also registered (not registered regularly) (Fig. 5).

Considering the difficulties of localizing the cavernous sinus using the transorbital access in children (especially in younger ones), we applied a new technology of evaluating the cavernous sinus by transcranial duplex scanning. This allows to determine the structure and features of the cavernous sinus and blood flow in eye veins. Disturbances of venous outflow in the cavernous sinus have been revealed in 68% of children by TCCD (Fig. 6).

Ultrasonic data in children with structural cerebral abnormalities was in accordance with MRI findings (Fig. 7).

The conservative treatment which has been performed under ultrasonographic control (TCD, TCCD) in children with disturbances of cerebral hemodynamics, led to subjective and objective improvement in 85% of children. We recommend ultrasonic methods not only for diagnostics of cerebral venous disturbances, but also for follow-up of the therapy. Clinically, the frequency and intensity of headache, nasal bleeding, dizziness, nausea and vomiting were reduced after the treatment (up to total disappearance of symptoms) (Fig. 8).

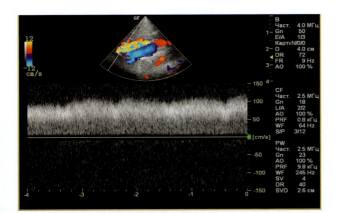

Fig. 6 Disturbances of venous outflow in the cavernous sinus.

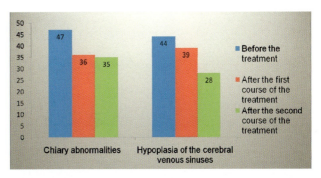

Fig. 8 Blood flow velocities (cm/s) in straight sinus measured by TCD after treatment.

Discussion

Features of cerebral hemodynamics causing disturbances of venous outflow are described in cases of abnormalities of craniovertebral junction and deep brain veins. These venous outflow disturbances are probably caused by obstacles to venous outflow (anomaly of craniovertebral junction, hypoplasia of cerebral venous sinuses) and increase of intracranial pressure. These disturbances are of great importance in clinical manifestations, especially in children. Nevertheless, there is a lack of sufficient information in literature concerning possibilities and necessity of carrying out TCD and TCCD investigations for diagnostics and therapy.

Conclusion

Clinical and ultrasound investigation of children with different types of headaches shows various dysfunctions in deep brain veins: great vein of Galen, cavernous and straight venous sinuses.

Venous disturbances most frequently occured in children with Arnold-Chiari I and deep brain vein abnormalities.

Hemodynamic findings in sinus cavernous revealed by TCD and TCCD in our patients were "markers" of disturbances in cerebral venous hemodynamics. An agreement between TCD, TCCD and MRI data was found.

The ultrasonographic examination of venous hemodynamics is necessary in complex diagnostics in children with cerebral abnormalities for prevention and treatment.

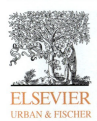

Transcranial sonography in psychiatric diseases

Milija D. Mijajlovic*

Neurology Clinic, Clinical Center of Serbia, School of Medicine University of Belgrade, Belgrade, Serbia

KEYWORDS
Transcranial sonography;
Basal ganglia;
Brainstem raphe;
Psychiatric diseases

Abstract Transcranial sonography (TCS) revealed reduced echogenicity of the brainstem raphe (BR) as a characteristic finding in unipolar depression and in depression associated with Parkinson's or Wilson's disease, but not in healthy adults, schizophrenia, multiple sclerosis with depression or Parkinson's disease without concomitant depression. Similar findings were shown also for adjustment disorder with depressed mood. In contrast to unipolar depression, sonographic findings of bipolar patients may generally indicate preserved structural integrity of mesencephalic raphe structures. If bipolar disorder is associated with hypoechogenic BR, depressive symptoms are more severe. BR hypoechogenicity could be caused by a modification of tissue cell density, the interstitial matrix composition or an alteration of fiber tracts integrity representing involvement of the basal limbic system in the pathogenesis of unipolar depression and depression associated with certain neurodegenerative diseases.

Recently it was shown that nigrostriatal dopaminergic system is abnormal in children with attention-deficit hyperactivity disorder which was expressed by significantly larger echogenicity of substantia nigra.

The increasingly broad application of TCS in the early and differential diagnosis of neurodegenerative and psychiatric disorders in many centers all over the world is probably the best evidence for the value of the method. Main advantages include the easy applicability, the fact that it is quick and repeatedly performable with no limitations as known from other neuroimaging techniques and that it is relatively cheap and side effect free.
© 2012 Elsevier GmbH. All rights reserved.

Transcranial sonography — historical overview and method in psychiatric diseases

Transcranial sonography (TCS) is a relatively new neuroimaging method which displays tissue echogenicity (intensity of reflected ultrasound waves) of the brain through the intact skull.

* Correspondence address: Neurology Clinic, Clinical Center of Serbia, School of Medicine University of Belgrade, Dr Subotica 6, 11000 Belgrade, Serbia. Tel.: +381 11 3064265; fax: +381 11 2684577.
  E-mail address: milijamijajlovic@yahoo.com

Besides the specific finding of the substantia nigra (SN) hyperechogenicity in Parkinson's disease (PD), first time described in 1995 by Becker et al. [1], a series of studies using TCS has reported another specific ultrasound feature: structural abnormality of the midbrain raphe depicted as reduced echogenicity or invisible brainstem raphe (BR) in patients with unipolar depression compared with healthy individuals [2,3]. The structural abnormality which was reported to occur in unipolar depressed patients, was unrelated to severity of current illness, and was absent in patients with schizophrenia [3]. The same structural abnormality has also been reported when depressed patients have been compared to non-depressed patients, having a variety of neurological diseases, for example, PD [4,5], dystonic syndromes [6] and Wilson's disease [7] but not multiple sclerosis with or without depression [8,9]. Modern clinical TCS systems display deep echogenic brain structures with a high image resolution of up to 0.7 mm × 1 mm which is even higher than that of magnetic resonance imaging (MRI) under clinical conditions [10]. Meanwhile, consensus guidelines for standardized procedure of TCS of midbrain structures, basal ganglia and ventricles have been established [11,12], allowing standardized scanning procedure and comparability of TCS findings between different research groups.

TCS of brain structures is performed through the temporal acoustic bone window, with preauricular position of the ultrasound probe parallel to the orbitomeatal line. Modern clinical ultrasound systems equipped with 2.0- to 3.5-MHz transducers can be applied [11,12]. The parameter settings of the TCS system should be chosen as follows: dynamic range 45—60 dB, insonation depth 14—16 cm, time gain compensation and image brightness are adapted as needed for the best visualization. When the brain structure of interest is clearly displayed, the image should be fixed and zoomed in two- to three-fold for further measurements [11]. The examination is performed at axial scanning planes through the midbrain and the thalami [11,12]. The mesencephalic brainstem can be depicted as a butterfly shaped structure of low echogenicity surrounded by the highly echogenic basal cisterns. The echogenicity of the ipsilateral SN, red nucleus (RN) and the BR could be evaluated (Fig. 1). The BR is usually seen as a highly echogenic continuous line with an echogenicity that is identical to that of the RN [13]. Echogenicity of BR is rated semiquantitatively, using either a 3-point (grade 1: raphe invisible; grade 2: slightly echogenic or interrupted BR; grade 3: high echogenicity identical to that of RN or basal cisterns) or, preferably, a 2-point (grade 0: invisible, hypoechogenic or interrupted BR; grade 1: highly echogenic BR as a continuous line) grading system [13]. It is important to scan the subject investigated from both sides, as the bone window may vary allowing sufficient visualization of the BR only if both sides are considered. Therefore, if the BR can be depicted as continuous line from one side, it is rated as a normal (grade 1) — that is, hyperechogenic, non-interrupted continuous line.

Changes in raphe echogenicity reflect changes in tissue impedance and point towards an alteration of the brainstem microarchitecture which could be due to a shift in tissue cell density, a change in interstitial matrix composition, or an alteration of fiber tract integrity [5,14]. Various anatomical, physiological, and biochemical findings underline the importance of the basal limbic system in the pathogenesis of affective disorders, and compelling evidence suggests that the nuclei, fiber tracts, and neurotransmitter systems associated with the basal limbic system are involved in the pathogenesis of primary depression and depression associated with some neurodegenerative diseases such as PD [15,16]. The change of acoustic impedance, which is recorded by TCS as reduced BR echogenicity, might be the result of microstructual changes, gliosis and disruption of fiber tract integrity [14].

TCS in unipolar depression

Numerous evidence from neuroimaging, biochemical and animal studies implicates basal limbic system and raphe

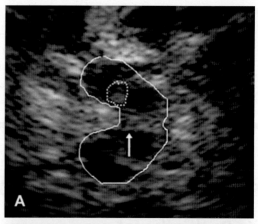
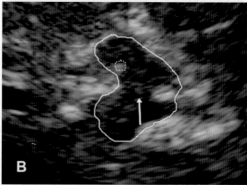
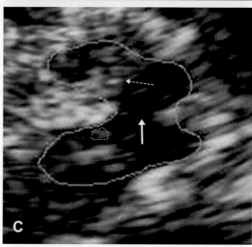

Figure 1 Sonographic images of corresponding midbrain axial sections in three subjects. The butterfly-shaped hypoechognic midbrain was encircled for better visualization (full line). Thick arrows indicate brainstem raphe; red nucleus is encircled with dotted line. (A) Mesencephalic brainstem of a healthy individual with normal, highly echogenic brainstem raphe as a continuous line which has the same echogenicity as the red nucleus. (B) Mesencephalic brainstem of a patient with unipolar depression with interrupted, reduced echogenicity of the brainstem raphe. (C) Mesencephalic brainstem of a PD patient with depression displays marked hyperechogenicity of the substantia nigra (thin dotted arrow) and invisible brainstem raphe (thick full arrow).

nuclei involvement in the pathogenesis of the mood disorders, particularly depression. Typical ultrasound marker that can be of value in the diagnosis and differential diagnosis of depression is the low echogenicity or interrupted BR. Raphe hypoechogenicity is a common finding in 50—70% of patients with unipolar depression [2,17] and is associated with responsivity to serotonin-reuptake inhibitors (SSRI) [18]. In a pioneer study, echogenicity of the BR was examined by TCS in 20 patients with unipolar depression and 20 healthy adult controls. A marked reduction of raphe echogenicity in depressed patients was found [2]. This finding was confirmed a year later on larger number of patients in the study which compared echogenicity of the BR between 40 patients with unipolar depression, 40 patients with bipolar disorder and 40 healthy controls. Raphe echogenicity in patients with unipolar depression was found to be distinctly reduced as compared with healthy adults and patients with bipolar affective disorder. BR echogenicity, on average, was halved in the unipolar depressed group. No correlation was found between BR echogenicity and age, sex or disease severity [3]. Reduced brainstem midline echogenicity of depressed patients was interpreted as a structural alteration of the dorsal raphe nucleus or fiber tracts in this region [14]. Increased T2-relaxation time in a pontine brainstem in patients with major depression could be in line with previous reports of brainstem pathology in these patients [14]. The observation might indicate a subtle tissue alteration, which cannot be identified by visual inspection of the images. T2-relaxation time depends on physical tissue characteristics and is influenced by hydration status or iron content. Differences in T2-relaxation time of specific brain areas between patients with major depression and healthy controls may indicate different tissue composition caused by histological changes.

Several further studies confirmed the finding of reduced echogenicity of the BR in unipolar depression. In the study of Walter [17] the frequency of patients with reduced echogenicity of BR was higher in unipolar depression compared with healthy individuals and in depressed PD patients compared with non-depressed. The frequency of reduced echogenicity of BR was the highest in patients with unipolar depression. In this study, reduced echogenicity of the BR was more frequent in depressed than in non-depressed patients, irrespective of presence of PD.

TCS findings of another study [19], showed that reduced echogenicity of pontomesencephalic BR is frequent in depressive states, irrespective of diagnostic category of depression, but only rare in healthy subjects without any history of psychiatric disorder. BR echogenicity could not discriminate between major depressive disorder and adjustment disorder with depressed mood. BR echogenicity scores showed in this study were significantly lower in SSRI responders compared with SSRI non-responders. Reduced BR echogenicity indicated SSRI responsivity with a positive predictive value of 88%.

Recently, reduced raphe echogenicity was found in 47% of the patients with major depressive disorder but only in 15% of healthy controls. In patients with suicidal ideations that finding was even more pronounced (86%) with the highest frequency of completely not visible TCS raphe finding (72%). Data showed that altered echogenicity of the BR is frequent in patients with suicidal ideation. Normal raphe echogenicity in patients with major depression was associated with less severe depressive symptoms and rarely with the presence of suicidal ideations [20].

Although there are several reports of MRI signal alteration of BR in depression, a characteristic neuroimaging pattern of BR abnormality has not yet been found [21].

Ultrasound investigations have been supplemented by T2-weighted MRI studies in order to investigate pathomorphological pattern of the BR in depression. Increased intensity of the midline has been reported for unipolar depressed patients when compared to bipolar patients and controls in a retrospective study using T2-weighted MRI [22]. A difference between patients with major depression and control subjects for T2-relaxation times was found in a region of interest located along the midline of the pons. No difference was found between patients with bipolar disorder and control subjects. Alterations of T2-relaxation times might indicate subtle tissue changes [23]. These findings are in line with the results of pathoanatomic and PET studies demonstrating morphological and functional alteration of the dorsal raphe nucleus in major depression, with decreased serotonin type 1A receptor binding and fewer neurons expressing serotonin transporter mRNA compared with findings in controls [24]. The relationship of BR echogenicity and SSRI responsivity which was found in the study of Walter [19] further supports the idea that reduced BR echogenicity reflects an alteration of the serotonergic system.

In contrast with previous reports, no difference in echogenicity of the BR of unipolar depressed patients was found in the study of Steele, the only one which investigated possible structural changes of the BR in unipolar depression using diffusion tensor imaging, did not confirm structural changes of the BR in unipolar depressive patients using this method [25]. One of the important advantages of TCS is that it could also detect a subgroup of patients with depression characterized by mild clinical signs of parkinsonism who are possibly at an elevated risk of developing definite PD.

TCS data in a recent study showed that the finding of SN hyperechogenicity, which is characteristic for idiopathic PD, was related to motor asymmetry and reduced verbal fluency in patients with depressive disorders. This relationship was even stronger in younger patients (<50 years) and independent from age, in patients who had reduced BR echogenicity [21]. Since, both liability for developing PD and frequency of PD-like TCS findings were found to be increased in depression, patients with depressive disorders might be an important population to screen for sonographic and clinical signs of early PD.

TCS in adjustment disorder with depressed mood (ADDM)

Major depressive disorder (MDD) and adjustment disorder with depressed mood (ADDM) are currently regarded as distinct disease entities [26]. Especially, DSM axis-II comorbidity and suicidal behavior have been reported to differ between MDD and ADDM. Following the Structured Clinical Interview for DSM-IV Axis-I Disorders [27], in the study performed by Walter et al. [18], 15 patients with single episode of MDD (MDDs), 22 with recurrent MDD (MDDr) and 15 with ADDM. Reduced BR echogenicity was found in 54% of the patients with MDD and ADDM, but only in four (8%) of the healthy subjects. BR echogenicity scores did not differ among patients with MDDs, MDDr, or ADDM, and pair-wise group comparisons failed to show differences between diagnostic groups with respect to frequency of reduced BR echogenicity. TCS findings of this study showed that reduced echogenicity of pontomesencephalic BR is frequent in depressive states, irrespective of diagnostic category. As a result of the present study, the hypothesis that BR echogenicity might distinguish patients with MDD and patients with ADDM had to be rejected. Reduced BR echogenicity is found with similar frequency in MDDs, MDDr, and ADDM. This is in agreement with results of clinical and neurophysiological studies suggesting common pathophysiological mechanisms in MDD and ADDM [28].

TCS in bipolar disorder

Bipolar affective disorders are characterized by recurrent episodes of depression as well as mania or hypomania [26]. In histological studies, subtle structural deficits in the dorsal raphe with a regional reduction in the synthesis of noradrenalin have been described in patients with bipolar disorder. The first TCS study evaluated BR alterations in patients with bipolar affective disorders, revealed normal or even increased echogenicity of BR in bipolar disorder, irrespective of the existing disease conditions. This observation led to the assumption that reduced echogenicity of BR may be specific to unipolar depression [3]. Recently, Krogias et al. found the BR hypoechogenicity in 36.1% of the 36 patients with bipolar I disorder (14 depressed, 8 manic, 14 euthymic) and in 20% of the 35 healthy controls. Compared to the control group, frequency of altered BR echogenicities did not reach statistical significance. Hypoechogenicity of BR was depicted in six (42.9%) of the depressed, in three (37.5%) of the manic and in four (28.6%) of the euthymic bipolar patients, with no significant difference between the three subgroups [29].

The width of third ventricle was significantly larger in the patient group (3.8 ± 2.1 mm vs. 2.7 ± 1.2 mm). Depressed bipolar patients with reduced BR echogenicity showed significantly higher scores on the Hamilton Depression Rating Scale as well as the Montgomery-Åsberg Depression Rating Scale [29].

Relating to echogenicity of SN, a strong trend of more frequent SN hyperechogenicities in the depressed subgroup was identified. Hyperechogenic SN was seen in six patients (16.7%): five (35.7%) of the depressed, in none (0%) of the manic and in one (7.1%) of the euthymic patients, indicating cyclical dysregulation in quantitative dopaminergic transmission as one of the underlying pathologies in the pathogenesis of bipolar disorder.

One of the main conclusions to be drawn from the study is that sonographic findings do not differ in different mood states of bipolar I disorder. Regarding the brainstem raphe, hypoechogenicity is correlated to the severity of symptoms in bipolar depression. Furthermore, bipolar patients in general showed significantly larger widths of the third ventricle than the control group in this study [29].

TCS in attention-deficit hyperactivity disorder

Attention-deficit hyperactivity disorder (ADHD) is frequent neuropsychiatric disorder characterized by excessive motor activity, increased impulsivity and attention deficits. Hypotheses about its pathophysiology implicate various neurotransmitters including dopamine [30]. One recent study investigated echogenicity of the SN as a potential structural marker for dysfunction of the nigrostriatal dopaminergic system in children with ADHD. Echogenicity of the SN in this study was determined in 22 children with DSM-IV diagnosis of ADHD and 22 healthy controls matched for age and sex. The echogeniciity of SN was significantly larger in ADHD patients than in healthy controls ($F_{1,42} = 9.298$, $p = 0.004$, effect size = 0.92, specificity was 0.73 and sensitivity 0.82) without effects of age or sex. The study showed that nigrostriatal dopaminergic system is abnormal in children with ADHD. Increased SN echogenicity in ADHD patients relative to healthy controls might be explained by a developmental delay. Although most findings with regard to a presumptive developmental delay in ADHD relate to diminished growth of cortical thickness, recent studies have reported structural alterations in the basal ganglia of patients with ADHD. It remains unclear whether an enlarged echogenic SN area in ADHD patients can be attributed to a primary disturbance of nigral iron metabolism, whether it is related to a primary developmental delay of brain structure, or whether it indicates a general structural marker for dysfunction of the dopaminergic system [31].

Conclusion

The increasingly broad application of TCS in the early and differential diagnosis of psychiatric and neurodegenerative diseases in many centers all over the world is probably the best evidence for the value of the method. The main advantages include the easy applicability, even in moving (e.g. tremulous or agitated) patients, the fact that it is quick and repeatedly performable with no limitations as known from other neuroimaging techniques (metal in the body as a limitation for MRI imaging, specific medication as a limitation for many forms of functional neuroimaging), and that it is relatively cheap and side effect free.

It is a reliable method to investigate, diagnose and follow-up patients with unipolar depression, bipolar disorder, ADHD and depression associated with some neurodegenerative diseases.

References

[1] Becker G, Seufert J, Bogdahn U, Reichmann H, Reiners K. Degeneration of substantia nigra in chronic Parkinson's disease visualized by transcranial color-coded real-time sonography. Neurology 1995;45:182—4.
[2] Becker G, Struck M, Bogdahn U, Becker T. Echogenicity of the brainstem raphe in patients with major depression. Psychiatry Res 1994;55:75—84.
[3] Becker G, Becker T, Struck M, Lindner A, Burzer K, Retz W, et al. Reduced echogenicity of brainstem raphe specific to unipolar depression: a transcranial color-coded real-time sonography study. Biol Psychiatry 1995;38:180—4.

[4] Becker T, Becker G, Seufert J, Hofmann E, Lange KW, Naumann M, et al. Parkinson's disease and depression: evidence for an alteration of the basal limbic system detected by transcranial sonography. J Neurol Neurosurg Psychiatry 1997;63:590—6.

[5] Berg D, Supprian T, Hofmann E, Zeiler B, Jager A, Lange KW, et al. Depression in Parkinson's disease: brainstem midline alteration on transcranial sonography and magnetic resonance imaging. J Neurol 1999;246:1186—93.

[6] Naumann M, Becker G, Toyka KV, Supprian T, Reiners K. Lenticular nucleus lesion in idiopathic dystonia detected by transcranial sonography. Neurology 1996;47:1284—90.

[7] Walter U, Krolikowski K, Tarnacka B, Benecke R, Czlonkowska A, Dressler D. Sonographic detection of basal ganglia lesions in asymptomatic and symptomatic Wilson disease. Neurology 2005;64:1726—32.

[8] Berg D, Supprian T, Thomae J, Warmuth-Metz M, Horowski A, Zeiler B, et al. Lesion pattern in patients with multiple sclerosis and depression. Mult Scler 2000;6:156—62.

[9] Berg D, Mäurer M, Warmuth-Metz M, Rieckmann P, Becker G. The correlation between ventricular diameter measured by transcranial sonography and clinical disability and cognitive dysfunction in patients with multiple sclerosis. Arch Neurol 2000;57:1289—92.

[10] Walter U, Kanowski M, Kaufmann J, Grossmann A, Benecke R, Niehaus L. Contemporary ultrasound systems allow high-resolution transcranial imaging of small echogenic deep intracranial structures similarly as MRI: a phantom study. Neuroimage 2008;40:551—8.

[11] Walter U, Behnke S, Eyding J, Niehaus L, Postert T, Seidel G, et al. Transcranial brain parenchyma sonography in movement disorders: state of the art. Ultrasound Med Biol 2007;33:15—25.

[12] Berg D, Godau J, Walter U. Transcranial sonography in movement disorders. Lancet Neurol 2008;7:1044—55.

[13] Mijajlovic MD. Transcranial sonography in depression. Int Rev Neurobiol 2010;90:259—72.

[14] Becker G, Berg D, Lesch KP, Becker T. Basal limbic system alteration in major depression: a hypothesis supported by transcranial sonography and MRI findings. Int J Neuropsychopharmacol 2001;4:21—31.

[15] Ball WA, Whybrow PC. Biology of depression and mania. Curr Opin Psychiatry 1993;6:27—34.

[16] Mayberg HS, Solomon D. Depression in Parkinson's disease: a biochemical and organic viewpoint. Adv Neurol 1995;65:49—60.

[17] Walter U, Hoeppner J, Prudente-Morrissey L, Horowski S, Herpertz SC, Benecke R. Parkinson's disease-like midbrain sonography abnormalities are frequent in depressive disorders. Brain 2007;130:1799—807.

[18] Walter U, Prudente-Morrissey L, Herpertz SC, Benecke R, Hoeppner J. Relationship of brainstem raphe echogenicity and clinical findings in depressive states. Psychiatry Res 2007;155:67—73.

[19] Walter U, Horowski S, Benecke R, Zettl U. Transcranial brain sonography findings related to neuropsychological impairment in multiple sclerosis. J Neurol 2007;254(Suppl. 2): 49—52.

[20] Budisic M, Karlovic D, Trkanjec Z, Lovrencic-Huzjan A, Vukovic V, Bosnjak J, et al. Brainstem raphe lesion in patients with major depressive disorder and in patients with suicidal ideation recorded on transcranial sonography. Eur Arch Psychiatry Clin Neurosci 2010;260(3):203—8.

[21] Hoeppner J, Prudente-Morrissey L, Herpertz SC, Benecke R, Walter U. Substantia nigra hyperechogenicity in depressive subjects relates to motor asymmetry and impaired word fluency. Eur Arch Psychiatry Clin Neurosci 2009;259: 92—7.

[22] Becker T, Becker D, Berg D, Hofmann E, Lange K, Struck M. Pathological findings in neuropsychiatric diseases. In: Bogdahn U, Becker G, Schlachetzki F, editors. Echoenhancers and transcranial color duplex sonography. London: Blackwell Science; 1998. p. 359—73.

[23] Supprian T, Reiche W, Schmitz B, Grunwald I, Backens M, Hofmann E, et al. MRI of the brainstem in patients with major depression, bipolar affective disorder and normal controls. Psychiatry Res 2004;131:269—76.

[24] Meltzer C, Price J, Mathis C, Butters MA, Ziolko S, Moses-Kolko E, et al. Serotonin 1A receptor binding and treatment response in late-life depression. Neuropsychopharmacology 2004;29:2258—65.

[25] Steele JD, Bastin ME, Wardlaw JM, Ebmeier KP. Possible structural abnormality of the brainstem in unipolar depressive illness: a transcranial ultrasound and diffusion tensor magnetic resonance imaging study. J Neurol Neurosurg Psychiatry 2005;76:1510—5.

[26] American Psychiatric Association. Diagnostic and statistical manual of mental disorders. 4th ed. Washington, DC: American Psychiatric Press; 1994.

[27] First MB, Spitzer RL, Gibbon M, Williams JBW. Structured Clinical Interview for DSM-IV Axis I Disorders Clinician Version (SCID-CV). Washington, DC: American Psychiatric Press; 1996.

[28] Bar KJ, Brehm S, Boettger MK, Wagner G, Boettger S, Sauer H. Decreased sensitivity to experimental pain in adjustment disorder. Eur J Pain 2005;10:467—71.

[29] Krogias C, Hoffmann K, Eyding J, Scheele D, Norra C, Gold R, et al. Evaluation of basal ganglia, brainstem raphe and ventricles in bipolar disorder by transcranial sonography. Psychiatry Res 2011;194(November (2)):190—7.

[30] Biederman J, Faraone SV. Attention-deficit hyperactivity disorder. Lancet 2005;366:237—48.

[31] Romanos M, Weise D, Schliesser M, Schecklmann M, Löffler J, Warnke A, et al. Structural abnormality of the substantia nigra in children with attention-deficit hyperactivity disorder. J Psychiatry Neurosci 2010;35(1):55—8.

The role of color duplex sonography in the brain death diagnostics

Igor D. Stulin[a], Denis S. Solonskiy[a,*], Mikhail V. Sinkin[b], Rashid S. Musin[a], Alexandr O. Mnushkin[a], Alexey V. Kascheev[a], Leonid A. Savin[a], Mikhail A. Bolotnov[c]

[a] Moscow State University for Medicine and Dentistry, Department of Neurology, Russia
[b] Moscow Clinical Hospital 11, Russia
[c] Moscow Clinical Hospital 13, Russia

KEYWORDS
Brain death;
Transcranial Doppler sonography;
Cerebral blood arrest;
Confirmatory test

Summary In Russia brain death diagnostic is still under great public attention. In such environment confirmatory tests are absolutely necessary. Aim of our study is to investigate the cerebral blood flow in brain death using color-coded duplex sonography. The sonographic study of 20 patients with brain death was performed and included transcranial and extracranial color duplex sonography. All patients were untrepanized. The following parameters were measured — presence of reverberating flow, Vmax ranges.

Results: At baseline TCDS revealed both MCA in all patients, and the BA in 18 patients. Oscillating flow with Vmax -32 ± 12 sm/s in MCA was found. Reverberating flow in the proximal segment of ICA and in the V2 segment of VA was found in all patients. Vmax ranges were 96 ± 27 sm/s in ICA and 58 ± 17 sm/s in VA. After 6 h TCDS was successful in 16 patients. In all of 16 cases blood flow in the MCA as a systolic peak or reverberating flow was detected. Basilar system study was successful in 12 cases. In all vessels blood flow was as systolic peaks.

Extracranial ICA and VA were visualized in all cases. In the ICA and V2, V3 segments of the VA reverberating flow were detected. Vmax was 47 ± 25 sm/s in ICA and 35 ± 17 sm/s in VA. In BD color duplex scanning reveals oscillating flow or systolic spikes in distal ICA, VA, intracranial vessels. In TCDS, the most common finding is MCA with reverberating flow. The optimum combination is extracranial and intracranial scanning in the early stages of BD.
© 2012 Elsevier GmbH. All rights reserved.

Introduction

The brain death (BD) is defined as the irreversible loss of function of the brain, including the brainstem, developing on the assumption of pulmonary ventilation and heart beating. The BD is diagnosed in intensive care units (ICU) as a result of severe brain damaging and causes at least 10% of mortality in ICU in developed countries. Traumatic brain injury, malignant stroke, tumor, diffuse hypoxic–ischemic brain damage are supposed to be the main causes of BD. All these factors affect the brain and lead to brain edema and swelling, intracranial pressure increase, gradual reduction of cerebral perfusion pressure, decrease and termination of intracranial blood flow and necrosis of brain parenchyma up to 2nd cervical segment [1–3].

* Corresponding author. Tel.: +7 9175878262.
E-mail address: dsolonsky@hotmail.com (D.S. Solonskiy).

According to the Russian National Guidelines of BD there are Diagnostic criteria for clinical diagnosis of BD [4]:

1. Defined cause irreversible deep coma.
2. Exclusion of complicating medical conditions that may confound clinical assessment (absence of hypothermia, drug intoxication, severe electrolyte and endocrine disturbance).
3. Systolic blood pressure ≥ 90 mm Hg.
4. Absence of brainstem reflexes.
5. Mydriasis with no response to the bright light.
6. Apnea with arterial $pCO_2 \geq 60$ mm Hg.
7. The observation period of 6 and 24 h with the primary and secondary brain injury respectively.

In general, these criteria correspond to neurologic criteria for the diagnosis of brain death of American Academy of Neurology [2,5].

The following two confirmatory tests are approved for BD diagnosis in Russia:

1. Electroencephalography (EEG) — reveals no electrical activity of brain in BD patients.
2. Cerebral angiography — detects cerebral blood arrest in BD patients.

Angiography is believed to reduce the observational period only and does not substitute to any clinical criteria of BD. According to the Russian National Guidelines on Diagnostics of Brain Death, ultrasound confirmatory tests are being investigated and can not be recommended for BD diagnosis, at the same time, all over the world ultrasound tests are the 3rd in order of sensitivity and frequency for BD diagnostics [6,7]. Transcranial Doppler (TCD) is notably desirable in patients in whom specific components of clinical testing cannot be reliably performed or evaluated such as barbiturate brain protection, hypothermia or face trauma [8—10].

Our department has gained experience in ultrasonography in clinical and confirmatory tests, 438 cases of BD were diagnosed since January 1995 to December 2010 [11]. The diagnosis of BD was confirmed by TCD and EEG. Color duplex sonography (CDS) was started to be performed in 2009.

We initiated a prospective observational study of the extra- and intracranial artery CDS in BD diagnostics in 2009. 20 patients with BD have been enrolled in the study up to December 2010. The study was approved by Local Ethic Committee of Moscow State University for Medicine and Dentistry in 2008.

The aim of the study was

- to investigate whether CDS of both extra- and intracranial arteries increases sensitivity of the test in patients with BD compared with CDS of intracranial arteries alone;
- to clarify CDS criteria of circulatory blood arrest.

Materials and methods

The study was started in Moscow hospital intensive care units in 2009 and has still been going on.

20 patients with BD due to traumatic brain injury and intracranial hemorrhage were included in the study and underwent a sonographic study which included color duplex sonography (CDS) of extracranial and intracranial arteries.

BD was diagnosed according to the Russian National Guidelines of BD. The average age of patients was 25 ± 5.4 years. The average time from ICU admission to BD development was 27 ± 6.5 h. The diagnosis of traumatic brain injury and intracranial hemorrhage was detected by computer tomography at the admission. All the patients had severe diffuse brain injury with the transverse and axial dislocation. Craniotomy was not carried on.

The sonographic study was performed according to the Rules of Task Force Group on Cerebral Death of Neurosonology Research Group of the World Federation of Neurology [12].

The following criteria of the test were mandatory:

1. The investigation of anterior and posterior circulation.
2. Bilateral visualization of intracranial internal carotid artery branches.

The study was conducted on a portable device Sonosite Micromaxx (USA) with broadband transducers L5—10 mHz, P1—5 mHz twice: at baseline after assessment of clinical criteria of BD and 6 h later. Presence of reverberating flow, Vmax ranges, presence of midline shift in B mode were also measured.

Results

At baseline CDS revealed both MCA (right and left) in all 20 patients, both ACA in 16 patients and BA in 18 patients. Oscillating flow with Vmax -32 ± 12 sm/s in MCA was found.

Data of extra- and intracranial artery and blood flow rates are presented below (Tables 1 and 2).

A midline shift 4—10 mm in B-mode was noted in 13 patients and it made artery differentiation difficult.

Reverberating flow in the proximal segment of ICA and in the V2 segment of VA was found in all patients.

Vmax ranges were 96 ± 27 sm/s in ICA and 58 ± 17 sm/s in VA respectively.

Reverberating and oscillating flow of intracranial and extracranial artery are presented in Figs. 1—4.

Table 1 Systolic velocity ranges in extra- and intracranial arteries.

Systolic velocity	ICA (sm/s)	VA (sm/s)	MCA (sm/s)	BA (sm/s)
1ast exam	96 ± 27	58 ± 17	32 ± 12	38 ± 9
2nd exam	47 ± 25	35 ± 17	15 ± 8	21 ± 7

Table 2 Visualization frequency of extra- and intracranial arteries (n = 20).

N = 20	MCA	ACA	PCA	BA	VA V2	ICA prox
1st exam	20	16	15	18	20	20
2nd exam	16	11	5	12	20	20

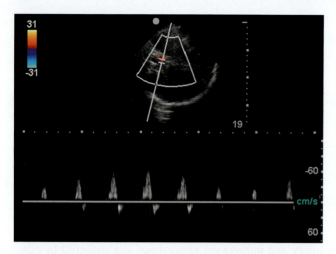

Figure 1 Reverberating flow in MCA in case of brain death.

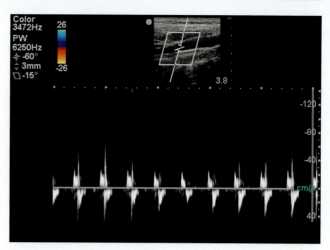

Figure 3 Reverberating flow in ICA (extracranial) in case of brain death.

After 6 h TCCS was successful in 16 patients. In all of 16 cases blood flow in the MCA as a systolic peak or reverberating flow was detected.

Extracranial ICA and VA were visualized in all cases. In the ICA and V2, V3 segments of the VA reverberating flow were detected. Vmax was 47 ± 25 sm/s in ICA and 35 ± 17 sm/s in VA. Spontaneous echo contrast in ICA and bulb was observed in 14 cases.

Thus, the sensitivity of the method in extra and intracranial study was 100%. The separate holding TCD in early sensitivity was 90%, at a later date from the time of clinical brain death sensitivity decreased to 80%.

Discussion

Brain death is a clinical diagnosis and neurologic criteria are still the main valid in BD diagnosis. However BD diagnosis has a comprehensive ethic value and on the one hand, there are some patients in whom specific components of clinical testing cannot be reliably performed or evaluated. Thus new maximal accurate, fast and safe test for BD diagnosis are required. On the other hand, frequently spontaneous and reflex movements, face trauma make difficulties of the BD diagnostics that is why additional confirmatory tests are considered to trend in unclear cases. Moreover, significant restriction of observational period or complete rejection of re-examination for BD diagnosis is discussed when confirmatory tests are performed [2,8,13].

All the tests for BD diagnosis perfectly have to be:

(a) feasible at the bedside;
(b) survey should not take much time;
(c) should be safe for the examinee, and a potential recipient of donor organs as well as performing their medical staff;
(d) to be sensitive, specific, reproducible and protected from external factors.

Color duplex scanning is the test which satisfies better than others to the requirements listed above. The great advantage of duplex scanning compared with the blind Doppler in BD is an opportunity of direct visualization of the lumen, which facilitates the diagnostics.

The most important is the qualitative analysis of the spectrograms with the definition of specific patterns of oscillating or reverberating flow, indicating the development of circulatory blood arrest. Quantitative parameters, including

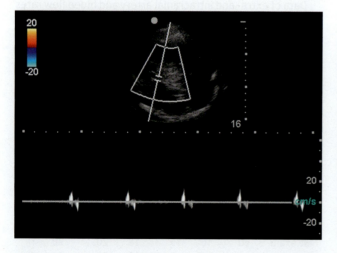

Figure 2 Systolic spikes in MCA in case of brain death.

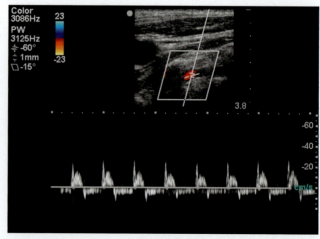

Figure 4 Reverberating flow in VA (V2 extracranial) in case of brain death.

systolic velocity, the index of Gosling, volumetric flow rate are more unsteady than qualitative ones and in patients with BD depend generally on two factors — level of systolic blood pressure and intracranial pressure during the investigation [6,14—16]. Although there are some reports that showed that a decrease in the total volume of cerebral blood flow below 100 ml/min is in line with 100% mortality [17,18].

As it was shown in our study, the combination of intracranial and extracranial tests increased the sensitivity of the study up to 100%. The sensitivity of isolated transcranial color duplex scanning was lower and depended on the time when the test was carried on in patients who had their clinical symptoms developed. The maximum sensitivity was 90% when the test was performed in the early period and decreased to 80% when the investigation was done 6 h after the symptom manifestation.

In addition, another factor which makes difficulty in interpretation of ultrasound data is previous extensive resection craniotomy in neurosurgical patients. In this case, the intracranial pressure is usually much lower. Here TCD is supposed to prolong the period when diagnosis of BD will be established. Although in any case, the typical ultrasound picture of circulatory blood arrest is developed with the lapse of time [19].

Cerebral angiography remains a "gold standard" of diagnostics in angiology. It should be noted that in cases with craniotomy, even when cerebral angiography was performed, there is flow of contrast into the cranial cavity, which makes the interpretation of the clinical data difficult [20—23].

BD is a clinical diagnosis and any confirmatory tests are auxiliary. The diagnosis of BD cannot be based only on confirmatory tests and neurologic criteria assessment is required.

Conclusions

CDS of patients with BD reveals oscillating flow or systolic spikes in distal ICA, VA, intracranial vessels and spontaneous echo contrast in proximal ICA. In TCD, the most common finding is MCA with reverberating flow. There are some difficulties in detection of basilar system and it depends on the time of BD manifestation.

The optimum combination is extracranial and intracranial scanning in the early stages of BD.

References

[1] A definition of irreversible coma: report of Ad Hoc Committee of the Harvard Medical School to Examine the Definition of Brain Death. JAMA 1968;205:337—40.

[2] American Academy of Neurology Practice Parameters for Determining Brain Death in Adults (summary statement) (current guideline-reaffirmed on 01/13/2007 and 10/18/2003). Neurology 1995;45:1012—4.

[3] Wijdicks EFM. Brain death. Philadelphia: Lippincott Williams & Wilkins; 2001.

[4] Stulin ID, Khubutiia ASh, Sinkin MV, Solonskiy DS, Musin RS, Vlasov PN, et al. The analysis of an instruction of the diagnosis of brain death. Zhurnal nevrologii i psikhiatrii imeni S.S. Korsakova/Ministerstvo zdravookhraneniia i meditsinskoĭ promyshlennosti Rossiĭskoĭ Federatsii, Vserossiĭskoe obshchestvo nevrologov i Vserossiĭskoe obshchestvo psikhiatrov 2010;110(12):82—90.

[5] Wijdicks EFM, Varelas PN, Gronseth GS, Greer DM. Evidence-based guideline update: determining brain death in adults: report of the Quality Standards Subcommittee of the American Academy of Neurology. Neurology 2010;74(June (23)):1911—8.

[6] Ducrocq X, Braun M, Debouverie M, Junges C, Hummer M, Vespignani H. Brain death and transcranial Doppler: experience in 130 cases of brain dead patients. J Neurol Sci 1998;160:41—6.

[7] Monteiro LM, Bollen CW, Van Huffelen AC, Ackerstaff RG, Jansen NJG, Van Vught AJ. Can transcranial Doppler ultrasonography confirm the diagnosis of brain death? Intensive Care Med 2005;31:S1—174.

[8] Marrache F, Megarbane B, Pirnay S, Rhaoui A, Thuong M. Difficulties in assessing brain death in a case of benzodiazepine poisoning with persistent cerebral blood flow. Hum Exp Toxicol 2004;23:503—5.

[9] Petty GW, Mohr JP, Pedley TA, Tatemichi TK, Lennihan L, Duterte DI, et al. The role of transcranial Doppler in confirming brain death: sensitivity, specificity, and suggestions for performance and interpretation. Neurology 1990;40:300—3.

[10] Segura T, Jimenez P, Jerez P, Garcia F, Corcoles V. Prolonged clinical pattern of brain death in patients under barbiturate sedation: usefulness of transcranial Doppler. Neurologia 2002;17:219—22.

[11] Stulin ID, Sinkin MV, Shibalev AL, Musin RS, Vlasov PN, Mnushkin AO. Diagnosis of brain death in Russia: experience of mobile neurodiagnostic group. In: Abstr. of the 8th Congress of the European Federation of Neurological Societies. 2004.

[12] Ducrocq X, Hassler W, Moritake K, Newell DW, von Reutern GM, Shiogai T, et al. Consensus opinion on diagnosis of cerebral circulatory arrest using Doppler-sonography: Task Force Group on Cerebral Death of the Neurosonology Research Group of the World Federation of Neurology. J Neurol Sci 1998;159:145—50.

[13] Lustbader D, O'Hara D, Wijdicks EF, MacLean L, Tajik W, Ying A, et al. Second brain death examination may negatively affect organ donation. Neurology 2011;76(January (2)):119—24.

[14] Feri M, Ralli L, Felici M, Vanni D, Capria V. Transcranial Doppler and brain death diagnosis. Crit Care Med 1994;22:1120—6.

[15] Hadani M, Bruk B, Ram Z, Knoller N, Spiegelmann R, Segal E. Application of transcranial Doppler ultrasonography for the diagnosis of brain death. Intensive Care Med 1999;25:822—8.

[16] Newell DW, Grady MS, Sirotta P, Winn HR. Evaluation of brain death using transcranial Doppler. Neurosurgery 1989;24:509—13.

[17] Payen DM, Lamer C, Pilorget A, Moreau T, Beloucif S, Echter E. Evaluation of pulsed Doppler common carotid blood flow as a noninvasive method for brain death diagnosis: a prospective study. Anesthesiology 1990;72:222—9.

[18] Schöning M, Scheel P, Holzer M, Fretschner R, Will BE. Volume measurement of cerebral blood flow: assessment of cerebral circulatory arrest. Transplantation 2005;80(3):326—31.

[19] Dosemeci L, Dora B, Yilmaz M, Cengiz M, Balkan S, Ramazanoglu A. Utility of transcranial Doppler ultrasonography for confirmatory diagnosis of brain death: two sides of the coin. Transplantation 2004;77(January (1)):71—5.

[20] Alvarez LA, Lipton RB, Hirschfeld A, Salamon O, Lantos G. Brain death determination by angiography in the setting of a skull defect. Arch Neurol 1988;45:225—7.

[21] Bergquist E, Bergstorm K. Angiography in cerebral death. Acta Radiol 1972;12:283—8.

[22] Kricheff II, Punto RS, George AE, Braunstein P, Korein J. Angiographic findings in brain death. Ann NY Acad Sci 1978;315:168—83.

[23] Spittler JF, Langenstein H. Diagnosis of brain death: limitations of angiography after osteoclastic trepanation. Dtsch Med Wochenschr 1991;116:1828—31.

10. Cerebral and Cervical Venous Ultrasonography

Ultrasound examination techniques of extra- and intracranial veins

Erwin Stolz*

Head of the Department of Neurology, CaritasKlinikum Saarbruecken, St. Theresia, Rheinstrasse 2, 66113 Saarbruecken, Germany

KEYWORDS
Duplex sonography;
Internal jugular vein;
Intracranial veins;
Dural sinus

Summary While arterial ultrasonography is an established and widely used method, the venous side of circulation has long been neglected. Reasons for this late interest may be the relatively lower incidence of primary venous diseases.

It was not until the mid 1990s that venous transcranial ultrasound in adults was systematically developed. This paper reviews the extra- und intracranial examination techniques of the cranial venous outflow.
© 2012 Elsevier GmbH. All rights reserved.

Examination of the internal jugular vein

The internal jugular vein (IJV) forms as an extension of the sigmoid sinus and leaves the cranial cavity through the jugular foramen. Similar to the distal part of the internal carotid artery, the slight dilatation at the origin of the IJV, called the superior bulb, and the proximal part of the vessel cannot be insonated due to lack of access because of the mandible. The IJV takes a course vertically down the side of the neck, lying at first lateral to the internal carotid artery, and then lateral to the common carotid. In the venous angle of the neck it unites with the subclavian vein to form the brachiocephalic vein. Above its termination it forms a second dilatation, the inferior bulb, in which on each side valves are present. While on the left side the valve is tricuspid in more than 60% of cases, it is bicuspid in approximately 50% and monocuspid in approximately 35% on the right side [1]. These anatomical differences are of importance because the right side is more frequently affected by incompetent valve closure than the left.

The ultrasound examination as such is not very demanding using the internal and common carotid artery as a landmark structure. The equipment and machine settings are similar to the examination of the carotid artery. However, the pulse repetition frequency (PRF) may need adjustment.

Care has to be taken because the vessel can easily be compressed even by applying slight pressure on the probe and hence mimic stenosis and induce changes of the Doppler waveform. On the other hand lack of compressibility is one of the diagnostic criteria for IJV thrombosis. Turning the head also leads to caliper changes mimicking stenosis [2]. Therefore, a fairly straight head position should be used to avoid artifacts and to increase reproducibility.

The walls of the vessel exhibit movements dependent on the respiration; the maximum extension occurs during expiration, the minimum during inspiration. On the respiratory wall movements faster wall movements caused by

Abbreviations: BV, basal vein; dMCV, deep middle cerebral vein; GCV, great cerebral vein; ICV, internal cerebral vein; IJV, internal jugular vein; MCA, middle cerebral artery; PCA, posterior cerebral artery; PRF, pulse repetition frequency; SPaS, sphenoparietal sinus; SPS, superior petrosal sinus; SRS, straight sinus; SSS, superior sagittal sinus; TCCS, transcranial color coded duplex sonography; TS, transverse sinus.

* Corresponding author. Tel.: +49 681 4063101; fax: +49 681 4063103.
  E-mail address: e.stolz@caritasklinikum.de

the valves and by the right heart function are superimposed.

By following the IJV to the venous angle the valvular plane is reached. Movement of the valve leaflets can be observed in a longitudinal and transverse examination plane in B-mode (Fig. 1). The movement of the valve leaflets is heart circle dependent. The valve closes during diastole when the right atrium transmits pressure to the superior vena cava. During closure the valve bulges cranially into the lumen of the IJV causing a short transient spontaneous retrograde flow in the Doppler spectrum. Cranial to the valve plane the vessel is slightly dilated and flow is slow, so that cloud-like currents of slowly flowing venous blood can be observed on B-mode imaging without being pathological. Not in all persons the IJV valves can be imaged sufficiently because they may be located quite distally behind the clavicle. Of course, a trapezoid transducer design is of help.

Effect of body position on the extracranial venous system

The body position has a profound influence on the IJVs cross-sectional area and flow velocities [3]. In the supine position the IJVs constitute the major cranial venous outflow route, however, in sitting or standing position the IJVs collapse following the hydrostatic pressure drop [4]. Then cranial blood is drained predominantly via the vertebral venous plexus [5]. As a consequence, the cross-sectional area of the IJV decreases from the lying to the upright position.

Internal jugular vein valve incompetence

The strongest connection of IJV incompetence has so far been reported with transient global amnesia [6]. All methods for assessment of IJV valve competence have in common that valve function is examined using a short Valsalva maneuver. This has to be strong enough to induce a complete closure of the investigated valve. Sander et al. described a method which is based on the observation of retrograde flow in color-mode during a Valsalva maneuver [7]. A second method is based on the detection of air bubbles in the jugular vein that had been administered intravenously just prior to the maneuver by injecting agitated saline into an antecubital vein [8].

The most wide spread method utilizes the detection of a retrograde flow in the Doppler spectrum (Fig. 2) [9]. Even in competent valves, a Valsalva maneuver leads to a short reflux during valve closure (Fig. 2A). This physiological reflux, with a duration corresponding to the valve closing time, has to be differentiated from an ongoing retrograde flow component in insufficient valves. Nedelmann et al. evaluated a cut-off time of 0.88 ms which differentiates normal valve closure from valve incompetence with reflux with a sensitivity and specificity of 100% [9]. Using this method, care has also to be taken to increase the sample volume size to the size of the IJV because retrograde jet streams along the venous wall might otherwise be missed.

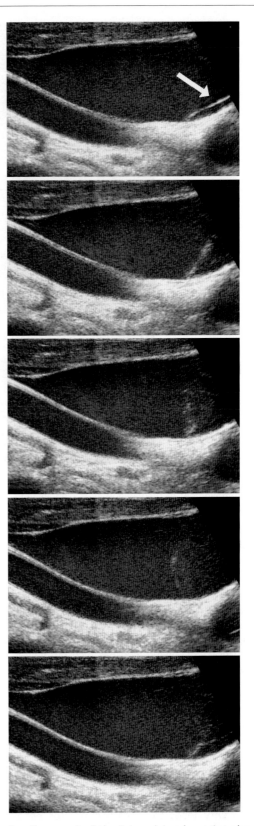

Figure 1 Movement of the internal jugular vein valve. The figure shows a movement sequence of a valve leaflet in the internal jugular vein. Please note the relatively large movement span.

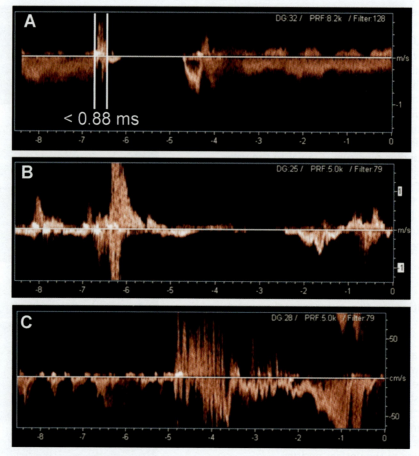

Figure 2 Internal jugular vein valve incompetence. (A) Normal finding. The short reflux lasts less than 0.88 ms and is caused by a cranial movement of the valve leaflets (see also Fig. 1). (B) Slight, (C) marked valve incompetence.

Examination of the vertebral veins

The vertebral veins are part of the outer vertebral venous plexus. The veins themselves largely follow the course of the vertebral artery and descent through the first to the sixths vertebral transverse processes, then run free down the neck to enter the brachiocephalic vein. The opening of the veins into the brachiocephalic vein has bicuspid valves [10]. In principal, valve function can be assessed similar to the IJV. However, no evaluated criteria exist so far.

Examination of intracranial veins and sinuses

Other than in the extracranial venous system, intracranial veins and dural sinuses lack any valves. As a consequence, their flow direction is governed solely by the current pressure gradient and flow resistance. The location within the cranial cavity leads to a Starling resistor behavior, i.e. intracranial veins and sinuses show a constant outwards flow as long as the ICP is lower than the arterial inflow pressure.

Only those venous structures located in proximity of the cranial base and in the posterior fossa can be examined by ultrasound techniques. The most important limitation of venous ultrasound is the inability to visualize cortical veins and the superior sagittal sinus (SSS) in its frontal, mid, and posterior part, except for the portion adjacent the confluens sinuum [11].

For venous transcranial color coded duplex sonography (TCCS) examinations adjustments in the machine settings are necessary: a low-flow sensitive color program with a low wall filter setting has to be used, the PRF needs to be reduced, and the color gain has to be increased to the artifact threshold.

TCCS examination usually starts in the mesencephalic examination plane with the butterfly-shaped mesencephalon as a landmark. Adjacent the middle cerebral artery (MCA) the deep middle cerebral vein (dMCV) is constantly found and is best insonated in the transition of the M1- to the M2-segments (Fig. 3A). Flow is directed away from the probe to the center of the brain.

For imaging of the cavernous sinus inflow the transducer is tilted to the cranial base. Landmark structures for insonation of the sphenoparietal sinus (SPaS) is the echogenic lesser wing and for the superior petrosal sinus (SPS) the echogenic pyramid of the sphenoid bone (Fig. 3B). Normal flow direction of both sinuses is directed away from the probe towards the cavernous sinus. For depiction of the basal vein (BV) the transducer is angulated upwards from the mesencephalic towards the diencephalic plane. The BV is found slightly cranial from the P2-segment of the posterior cerebral artery (PCA) which both display a flow away

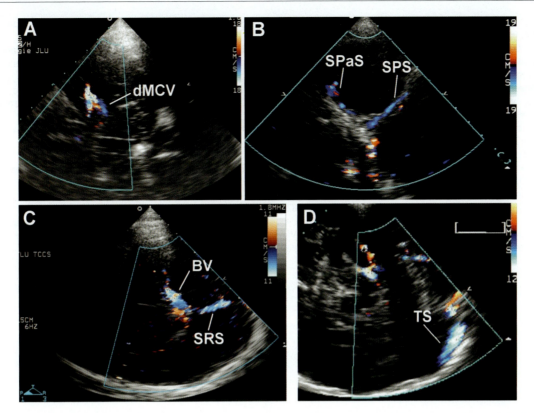

Figure 3 Ultrasound examination of intracranial veins and sinuses. *Abbreviations*: dMCV, deep middle cerebral vein; SPaS, sphenoparietal sinus; SPS, superior petrosal sinus; BV, basal vein; SRS, straight sinus; TS, transverse sinus.

Table 1 Normal values of flow velocities of intracranial veins and sinuses. Flow velocities (FV) are given as range of systolic/diastolic values in [cm/s]. dMCV, deep middle cerebral vein; BV, basal vein; GCV, great cerebral vein (of Galen); ICV, internal cerebral vein; SRS, straight sinus; ST, transverse sinus; SSS, superior sagittal sinus; SPaS, sphenoparietal sinus; SPS, superior petrosal sinus.

dMCV	FV	4–15/3–11	SRS	FV	6–39/4–27
BV	FV	7–20/5–15	ST	FV	6–56/5–38
GCV	FV	6–32/4–25	SSS	FV	6–20/3–14
SPaS + SPS	FV	27 ± 17	ICV	FV	7–22/4–16

from the probe (Fig. 3C). The vein can easily be identified by its low pulsatile Doppler spectrum.

By increasing the B-mode depth the contralateral skull becomes visible. Prominent midline structures of the diencephalic insonation plane are the echogenic double reflex of the third ventricle and the echogenic pineal gland. The great cerebral vein (GCV) is found immediately behind the pineal gland with a flow away from the transducer. In this examination plane the rostral part of the SSS may be visible. In order to examine the straight sinus (SRS) the anterior tip of the transducer needs to be rotated upwards to align the insonation plane with the plane of the apex of the cerebellar tentorium which possesses an increased echogenicity (Fig. 3C). The course of the SRS is directed away from the transducer towards the confluens sinuum. Proceeding from this transducer position the probe is angulated downwards again to depict the contralateral transverse sinus (TS) (Fig. 3D). The frontal and occipital acoustic bone windows can be used to examine the midline venous vessels (ICV, GCV, SRS).

Normal values and reproducibility

Normal values for venous flow of intracranial veins and sinuses velocities are summarized in Table 1. In healthy controls the detection rates of the deep cerebral veins (dMCV, BV, GCV) is high, however, variable insonation rates have been reported for the posterior fossa sinuses [12]. The reproducibility and interobserver reliability of venous measurements are comparable to those in the arterial system [13].

References

[1] Sanchez-Hanke F, Püschel K, Leuwer R. Zur Anatomie der Venenklappen der V. jugularis interna. Laryngo Rhino Otol 2000;79:332—6.

[2] Gooding CA, Stimac GK. Jugular vein obstruction caused by turning of the head. Am J Roentgenol 1984;142:403—6.

[3] Valdueza JM, von Münster T, Hoffman O, Schreiber S, Einhäupl KM. Postural dependency oft he cerebral venous outflow. Lancet 2000;355:200—1.
[4] Epstein HM, Linde HW, Crampton AR, Ciric IS, Eckenhoff JE. The vertebral venous plexus as a major cerebral venous outflow tract. Anesthesiology 1970;32:332—7.
[5] Gisolf J, van Lieshout JJ, van Heusden K, Pott F, Stok WJ, Karemaker JM. Human cerebral venous outflow pathway depends on posture and central venous pressure. J Physiol 2004;560:317—27.
[6] Chung CP, Hu HH. Jugular venous reflux. J Med Ultrasound 2008;16:210—22.
[7] Sander D, Winbeck K, Etgen T, Knapp R, Klingelhöfer J, Conrad B. Disturbance of venous flow patterns in patients with transient global amnesia. Lancet 2000;356:1982—4.
[8] Akkawi NM, Agosti C, Borroni B, Rozzini L, Magoni M, Vignolo LA, et al. Jugular valve incompetence. A study using air contrast ultrasonography on a general population. J Ultrasound Med 2002;21:747—51.
[9] Nedelmann M, Eicke B, Dieterich M. Functional and morphological criteria of internal jugular valve insufficiency as assessed by ultrasound. J Neuroimaging 2005;15:70—5.
[10] Chou CH, Chao AC, Hu HH. Ultrasonographic evaluation of vertebral venous valves. AJNR Am J Neuroradiol 2002;23:1418—20.
[11] Schreiber SJ, Stolz E, Valdueza JM. Transcranial ultrasonography of cerebral veins and sinuses. Eur J Ultrasound 2002;16:59—72.
[12] Stolz E. Cerebral veins and sinuses. In: Baumgartner RW, editor. Handbook on neurovascular ultrasound, 21. Basel: Karger; 2006. p. 182—93 [Front Neurol Neurosci].
[13] Stolz E, Babacan SS, Bödeker RH, Gerriets T, Kaps M. Interobserver and intraobserver reliability of venous transcranial color-coded flow velocity measurements. J Neuroimaging 2001;11:385—92.

Fact or fiction: Chronic cerebro-spinal insufficiency

Claudio Baracchini*, Paolo Gallo

Department of Neurological Sciences, University of Padua, Via Giustiniani 5, 35128 Padova, Italy

KEYWORDS
CCSVI;
Ultrasound;
Multiple sclerosis

Summary Multiple sclerosis (MS) is a chronic inflammatory and neurodegenerative disease of the central nervous system (CNS). Its autoimmune origin has been recently challenged by a substantially different mechanism termed chronic cerebrospinal venous insufficiency (CCSVI), which has attracted worldwide attention in the scientific community, in the media and among MS patients. According to this hypothesis, a congestion of cerebrovenous outflow induces an increased intracranial pressure and a disintegration of the blood—brain barrier in perivenular regions promoting local iron deposition and activation of pro-inflammatory factors, ultimately leading to MS. After the initial report of a perfect association between CCSVI and MS, different independent groups were not able to replicate these results, casting doubts on the credibility of the CCSVI concept in MS. In spite of this, interventional procedures like venous angioplasty named the ''liberation'' treatment have been claimed as a cure of MS or at least as a major improvement of MS symptoms. As a result, an increasing number of MS patients are undergoing endovascular treatment, in spite of a lack of an evidenced-based benefit and recent reports of serious adverse events. This review represents a critical appraisal of the CCSVI hypothesis, discusses its basis, the diagnostic criteria and its relationship with MS.
© 2012 Elsevier GmbH. All rights reserved.

Introduction

Multiple sclerosis (MS) is a chronic inflammatory, neurodegenerative disease of the central nervous system (CNS). Its autoimmune origin is supported by immunological, genetic, histopathological, and therapeutic observations, even though the mechanisms that initiate this autoimmune attack are still unknown [1—4]. A disorder of cerebrospinal blood flow named ''chronic cerebrospinal venous insufficiency'' (CCSVI) has been proposed by Zamboni to play a possible etio-pathogenetic role in multiple sclerosis [5,6]. This ''big idea'', a term used by Zamboni himself to define his theory, rises from observations on systemic venous diseases and the possible parallels between these and brain inflammation [5]. Zamboni's working hypothesis is that brain inflammation is iron-dependent [7]: he postulated that multiple extracranial venous anomalies of the internal jugular and/or azygos veins [8] cause a venous reflux into the cerebrospinal compartment, determining an increased intra-venous pressure that disaggregates the blood—brain barrier, thus causing the deposition of iron in brain tissue and evoking a local inflammatory response. By applying five parameters of abnormal venous outflow, indicative of CCSVI, Zamboni and co-workers were able to demonstrate a strong relationship between CCSVI and MS. Indeed, in their pivotal study, they analyzed 109 patients with clinically definite MS and 177 control subjects by means of transcranial and extracranial color Doppler sonography and found that all patients with MS had abnormal venous parameters: the presence of at least 2 of those 5 parameters was

* Corresponding author. Tel.: +39 049 8213600;
fax: +39 049 8751770.
 E-mail addresses: claudiobaracchini@tin.it (C. Baracchini),
paolo.gallo@unipd.it (P. Gallo).

Table 1 Ultrasound CCSVI criteria.

1. Reflux ($t > 0.88$ s) in the IJVs and/or in the VVs in sitting and supine position
2. Reflux ($t > 0.5$ s) in the DCVs
3. High-resolution B-mode evidence of proximal IJV stenoses (local reduction of CSA $\geq 50\%$ in the recumbent position or CSA ≤ 0.3 cm^2)
4. Flow not Doppler-detectable in the IJVs and/or VVs despite numerous deep inspirations with the head at 0° and +90°
5. Reverted postural control of the main cerebral venous outflow pathways: negative ΔCSA in the IJV

CSA, cross-sectional area of the internal jugular vein; IJV, internal jugular vein; VV, vertebral vein; DCVs, deep cerebral veins; ΔCSA = CSA$_{sitting}$ − CSA$_{supine}$.

observed as being diagnostic of MS with 100% specificity, 100% sensitivity, and positive and negative predictive values for MS of 100%. Zamboni and co-workers went on to perform unblinded selective venography in 65 patients with MS as well as in some control subjects, and reported that patients with MS had multiple severe extracranial stenoses, while these abnormalities were never found in normal controls [9]. Furthermore, in a retrospective study, the same authors found that the distribution of the pathological hemodynamic patterns was highly predictive of the symptoms at onset and of the following clinical course [10]. In this review, we try to analyze critically the various aspects of Zamboni's theory and address several questions not only on the relationship between CCSVI and MS, but also on the scientific basis of CCSVI and thus, on its real existence.

The ultrasound puzzle

The diagnosis of CCSVI is based on five ultrasonographic criteria (Table 1), four extracranial and one intracranial [11]. According to Zamboni's initial findings the presence of at least two of these criteria provides indirect evidence of impaired cerebral venous drainage and should be consistent with the diagnosis of MS. Several independent investigators have tried to reproduce — with various methodological approaches — the striking results obtained by Zamboni, but none have succeeded [12—19]. In particular, we performed two large studies. In the first study, we aimed at analyzing the occurrence of CCSVI at MS onset, to elucidate the possible causative role of CCSVI in MS as suggested by Zamboni, who surprisingly did not study these patients. Fifty patients presenting a clinically isolated syndrome (CIS) and having evidence of dissemination in space of the inflammatory lesions underwent a comprehensive diagnostic workup, including extracranial and transcranial venous echo-color Doppler sonography. Patients who showed evidence of CCSVI were further evaluated by selective venography. Fifty MS-matched normal controls (NC), 60 patients with transient global amnesia (TGA), and 60 TGA-matched NC were studied. Transcranial venous echo-color Doppler was normal in all patients with CIS. One or more abnormal extracranial venous echo-color Doppler findings were observed in 26 of 50 (52.0%) of the patients with CIS, 35 of 110 (31.8%) of the controls and 41 of 60 (68.3%) of the patients with TGA. The eight (16%) patients with CIS who fulfilled the diagnosis of CCSVI were further evaluated blindly by selective venography, which did not disclose any venous anomalies. Thus, we could not demonstrate any causative effect of CCSVI on MS [14]. The second study was focused on the progressive forms of MS, to investigate whether CCSVI could play a role in determining disease progression. We analyzed 60 patients with chronic progressive forms of MS (35 SP, 25 PP) and 60 age-/gender-matched NC. TCDS was normal in all patients. ECDS showed one or more abnormal findings in 9/60 (15.0%) patients [7/35 (20.0%) SPMS, 2/25 (8.0%) PPMS] and in 14/60 (23.3%) NC (p not significant for all comparisons). CCSVI criteria were fulfilled in 0 NC and 4 (6.7%) MS patients: 3 SPMS and 1 PPMS. VGF, performed blindly in 6/9 patients, was abnormal only in one case that had bilateral internal jugular vein (IJV) stenosis [17]. These findings indicate that CCSVI is not a late secondary phenomenon of MS and is not responsible for disability progression.

The ultrasound method

On the basis of these contradictory results, it is absolutely necessary to question the validity of the five ultrasound criteria proposed by Zamboni for the diagnosis of CCSVI. In the first criterion, Zamboni et al. used the threshold value of 0.88 s to discriminate IJV and vertebral vein (VV) physiological back flow due to valve closure from pathological reflux without performing the Valsalva maneuver (VM) [8] and they found that 71% of MS patients had a pathological reflux vs. 0% of controls. This threshold value comes from a totally different study on IJV valve insufficiency during a controlled VM [20] where it was chosen to differentiate VM-induced insufficiency through insufficient valves lasting >1.23 s, from physiological backward flows during normal valve closure, lasting 0.22—0.78 s. In this study it was found that about 30% of normal subjects have a physiological ($t < 0.88$ s) back flow during normal valve closure. Furthermore, the utilization of this threshold by Zamboni for assessing reflux in other vessels (i.e. VVs) other than IJV valve insufficiency is also scientifically incorrect.

For the second criterion, the intracranial veins and sinuses were not examined through the transtemporal bone window for which there are published ultrasound criteria and velocity data [21,22]. Zamboni et al. used a new bone window (supracondylar) for which there are neither accepted published criteria nor normative data, and the figures published are not compatible with normal anatomy [8,11]. With regard to venous reflux, this evaluation requires a Doppler spectrum analysis, because a color-based approach is inadequate and can easily lead to the misinterpretation of flow direction. More importantly, the rationale of adopting a threshold value of 0.5 s to discriminate pathological reflux in the deep cerebral veins is unclear. This value was derived from studies in the veins of the leg where it served to quantify venous valve insufficiency following deflation of a tourniquet [23,24]. The rationale for transferring this value from the legs to the brain is very questionable since it has never been validated for deep cerebral veins. The validity and significance of data collected by this method are therefore unclear especially if it is used to diagnose CCSVI, where cerebral reflux is not described by the same author as associated with valve incompetence.

The third criterion defines a stenosis of the IJV as a local reduction of the cross sectional area (CSA) $\geq 50\%$ in the recumbent position or CSA $\leq 0.3\,cm^2$ [8]. This latter cut-off value was derived from a study on intensive care patients [25], with possible confounders such as mechanical ventilation and hypovolemia. It can, therefore, not be used as a reference point in healthy subjects. Furthermore, it is difficult to decide where to measure the diameter of the vein since IJVs are normally tortuous and the most proximal and distal parts near the superior and inferior bulb are physiologically dilated more than others. It is important to stress that even mild pressure exerted by the ultrasound probe or by a contraction of the cervical musculature itself can alter the diameter of the vein leading to false-positive results.

The fourth criterion, which is the inability to detect flow in the IJVs and/or in the VVs during deep inspiration, according to Zamboni et al., provides indirect evidence of venous obstruction [8]. This criterion has never been validated. A lack of flow is not necessarily due to obstruction since it can occur, e.g. at 15° in both IJVs in healthy subjects [22]. In the upright position, there is a dramatic reduction and frequently a complete cessation of blood flow in the IJV. In the supine position there may also be no flow in the VVs [26]. Furthermore, an inadequate setting of ultrasound indices such as pulse repetition frequency might lead to an apparent absence of color-coded signal and a misinterpretation of no-flow.

The fifth criterion examines the presence of a physiological shift of cerebral venous drainage from the jugular venous system to the vertebral plexus with postural change: from the supine to the sitting position. In normal subjects, subtracting the CSA measured in the supine position from that in a sitting position (ΔCSA) is usually negative [22]. Instead, Zamboni wrongly considered that a negative ΔCSA value would represent a reverted postural control of the main cerebral venous outflow pathways [8]. Furthermore, similarly to criterion three, a mild pressure exerted by the ultrasound probe or by a contraction of the cervical muscles may alter the diameter of the vein possibly leading to false-positive results. A more correct method would be to calculate the difference of blood flow (CSA $\times$ velocity) in the two positions (supine and sitting) as has been recently performed [12], not confirming the hypothesis of Zamboni and co-workers.

A very important issue is the cut-off point of these criteria to diagnose CCSVI. In fact, it is unclear how Zamboni decided that two or more of the five ultrasound criteria may be used to diagnose CCSVI. Diagnostic criteria using a new alternative method (i.e. ultrasound) are usually compared with a validated gold-standard investigation (venography according to Zamboni et al.). However, Zamboni et al.'s comparison of venography in 65 CCSVI ultrasound-positive MS patients was not blinded and is therefore open to bias. There was also no validation of the CCSVI-criteria by different and independent observers. Finally, subsequent studies using MR-venography could not confirm differences regarding cerebrospinal drainage in MS patients and controls [27–30].

Conclusions

Ultrasound investigation of intracranial and cervical veins is highly operator dependent owing to the wide anatomic and physiological variability of these vessels. Therefore a study of cerebral venous drainage requires very experienced neurosonographers, but most importantly, blinding algorithms are mandatory in assessing MS patients especially during venographic verification of ultrasound findings; these were completely omitted in Zamboni's studies. To this day, a scientifically sound validation of each of the five criteria proposed by Zamboni for the diagnosis of CCSVI is missing, not to mention their combined application. Concurrently, there is growing evidence which rejects the role of CCSVI in the pathogenesis of MS and which suggests that the proposed CCSVI criteria are questionable due to miscitation, manipulation of known data and methodological flaws. Thus, any potentially harmful interventional treatment such as transluminal angioplasty and/or stenting should be strongly discouraged, not only for the lack of any evidence, but also for the risk of serious peri-procedural complications.

Author contributions

Claudio Baracchini: Conception, organisation and execution of the research project; writing and review of the manuscript.

Paolo Gallo: Conception, organisation and execution of the research project; writing and review of the manuscript.

Disclosures

Dr. Baracchini serves on the executive committee of the European Society of Neurosonology and Cerebral Hemodynamics; has received funding for travel and speaker honoraria from Pfizer, Sanofi-Aventis, Laboratori Guidotti and Novartis; serves as Associate Editor for *BMC Neurology*; and has given expert testimony in a medico-legal case.

Dr. Gallo serves on scientific advisory boards, as a consultant, and on speakers' bureaus for and has received funding for travel and speaker honoraria from Novartis, Biogen Idec/Elan Corporation, Merck Serono, Sanofi-Aventis, and Bayer Schering Pharma; and receives research support from Novartis, Biogen Idec/Elan Corporation, Merck Serono, Sanofi-Aventis, and Bayer Schering Pharma, the Veneto Region of Italy, the University of Padova, and the Ministry of Public Health of Italy.

References

[1] Frischer JM, Bramow S, Dal-Bianco A, Lucchinetti CF, Rauschka H, Schmidbauer M, et al. The relation between inflammation and neurodegeneration in multiple sclerosis brains. Brain 2009;132:1175–89.

[2] Trapp BD, Nave KA. Multiple sclerosis: an immune or neurodegenerative disorder? Annu Rev Neurosci 2008;31:247–69.

[3] Lassmann H, Bruck W, Lucchinetti CF. The immunopathology of multiple sclerosis: an overview. Brain Pathol 2007;17:210–8.

[4] Compston A, Coles A. Multiple sclerosis. Lancet 2008;372:1502–17.

[5] Zamboni P. The big idea: iron-dependent inflammation in venous disease and proposed parallels in multiple sclerosis. J R Soc Med 2006;99:589—93.
[6] Zamboni P, Menegatti E, Bartolomei I, Galeotti R, Malagoni AM, Tacconi G, et al. Intracranial venous hemodynamics in multiple sclerosis. Curr Neurovasc Res 2007;4:252—8.
[7] Singh AV, Zamboni P. Anomalous venous blood flow and iron deposition in multiple Sclerosis. J Cereb Blood Flow Metab 2009;29:1876—8.
[8] Zamboni P, Galeotti R, Menegatti E, Malagoni AM, Tacconi G, Dall'Ara S, et al. Chronic cerebrospinal venous insufficiency in patients with multiple sclerosis. J Neurol Neurosurg Psychiatry 2009;80:392—9.
[9] Zamboni P, Galeotti R, Menegatti E, Malagoni AM, Gianesini S, Bartolomei I, et al. A prospective open-label study of endovascular treatment of chronic cerebrospinal venous insufficiency. J Vasc Surg 2009;50:1348—58, e1341—3.
[10] Bartolomei I, Salvi F, Galeotti R, Salviato E, Alcanterini M, Menegatti E, et al. Hemodynamic patterns of chronic cerebrospinal venous insufficiency in multiple sclerosis. Correlation with symptoms at onset and clinical course. Int Angiol 2010;29(April (2)):183—8.
[11] Zamboni P, Menegatti E, Galeotti R, Malagoni AM, Tacconi G, Dall'Ara S, et al. The value of cerebral Doppler venous haemodynamics in the assessment of multiple sclerosis. J Neurol Sci 2009;282:21—7.
[12] Doepp F, Paul F, Valdueza JM, Schmierer K, Schreiber SJ. No cerebrocervical venous congestion in patients with multiple sclerosis. Ann Neurol 2010;68:173—83.
[13] Krogias C, Schröder A, Wiendl H, Hohlfeld R, Gold R. ''Chronic cerebrospinal venous insufficiency'' and multiple sclerosis: critical analysis and first observation in an unselected cohort of MS patients. Nervenarzt 2010;81:740—6.
[14] Baracchini C, Perini P, Calabrese M, Causin F, Rinaldi F, Gallo P. No evidence of chronic cerebrospinal venous insufficiency at multiple sclerosis onset. Ann Neurol 2011;69:90—9.
[15] Mayer CA, Pfeilschiffer W, Lorenz MW, Nedelmann M, Bechmann I, Steinmetz H, et al. The perfect crime? CCSVI not leaving a trace in MS. J Neurol Neurosurg Psychiatry 2011;82:436—40.
[16] Centonze D, Floris R, Stefanini M, Rossi S, Fabiano S, Castelli M, et al. Proposed CCSVI criteria do not predict MS risk or severity. Ann Neurol 2011;70(July (1)):52—9.
[17] Baracchini C, Perini P, Causin F, Calabrese M, Rinaldi F, Gallo P. Progressive multiple sclerosis is not associated with chronic cerebrospinal venous insufficiency. Neurology 2011;77(August (9)):844—50.
[18] Tsivgoulis G, Mantatzis M, Bogiatzi C, Vadikolias K, Voumvourakis K, Prassopoulos P, et al. Extracranial venous hemodynamics in multiple sclerosis: a case—control study. Neurology 2011;77(September (13)):1241—5.
[19] Auriel E, Karni A, Bornstein NM, Nissel T, Gadoth A, Hallevi H. Extra-cranial venous flow in patients with multiple sclerosis. J Neurol Sci 2011;309(October (1—2)):102—4.
[20] Nedelmann M, Eicke BM, Dieterich M. Functional and morphological criteria of internal jugular valve insufficiency as assessed by ultrasound. J Neuroimaging 2005;15:70—5.
[21] Stolz E, Kaps M, Dorndorf W. Assessment of intracranial venous hemodynamics in normal individuals and patients with cerebral venous thrombosis. Stroke 1999;30:70—5.
[22] Valdueza JM, von Münster T, Hoffmann O, Schreiber S, Einhäupl KM. Postural dependency of the cerebral venous outflow. Lancet 2000;355:200—1.
[23] van Bemmelen PS, Bedford G, Beach K, Strandness DE. Quantitative segmental evaluation of venous valvular reflux with duplex ultrasound scanning. J Vasc Surg 1989;10: 425—31.
[24] Sarin S, Sommerville K, Farrah J, Scurr JH, Coleridge Smith PD. Duplex ultrasonography for assessment of venous valvular function of the lower limb. Br J Surg 1994;81:1591—5.
[25] Lichtenstein D, Saifi R, Augarde R, Prin S, Schmitt JM, Page B, et al. The Internal jugular veins are asymmetric. Usefulness of ultrasound before catheterization. Intensive Care Med 2001;27:301—5.
[26] Hoffmann O, Weih M, Einhäupl KM, Valdueza JM. Normal blood flow velocities in the vertebral veins. J Neuroimaging 1999;9:198—201.
[27] Wattjes MP, Oosten BW, de Graaf W, Seewann A, Bot JC, van den Berg R, et al. No association of abnormal cranial venous drainage with multiple sclerosis: a magnetic resonance venography and flow-quantification study. J Neurol Neurosurg Psychiatry 2011;82:429—35.
[28] Sundstrom P, Wahlin A, Ambarki K, Birgander R, Eklund A, Malm J. Venous and cerebrospinal fluid flow in multiple sclerosis: a case—control study. Ann Neurol 2010;68:255—9.
[29] Zivadinov R, Lopez-Soriano A, Weinstock-Guttman B, Schirda CV, Magnano CR, Dolic K, et al. Use of MR venography for characterization of the extracranial venous system in patients with multiple sclerosis and healthy control subjects. Radiology 2011;258:562—70.
[30] Doepp F, Wuerfel JT, Pfueller CF, Valdueza JM, Petersen D, Paul F, et al. Venous drainage in multiple sclerosis: a combined magnetic resonance venography and duplex ultrasound study. Neurology 2011;77(19):1745—51.

Chronic cerebrospinal venous insufficiency in patients with multiple sclerosis: A case-control study from Iran

Masoud Mehrpour [a,*], Neda Najimi [b], Seyed-Mohammad Fereshtehnejad [b,c], Fatemeh Naderi Safa [d], Samira Mirzaeizadeh [d], Mohammad Reza Motamed [a], Masoud Nabavi [e], Mohammad Ali Sahraeian [f]

[a] *Firoozgar Clinical Research Development Center (FCRDC), Neurology Department, Tehran University of Medical Sciences, Tehran, Iran*
[b] *Firoozgar Clinical Research Development Center (FCRDC), Tehran University of Medical Sciences, Tehran, Iran*
[c] *Karolinska Institutet, Department of Neurobiology & Health Care Sciences, Stockholm, Sweden*
[d] *Student Scientific Research Center (SSRC), Tehran University of Medical Sciences, Tehran, Iran*
[e] *Neurology Department, Shahed University of Medical Sciences, Tehran, Iran*
[f] *Neurology Department, Tehran University of Medical Sciences, Tehran, Iran*

KEYWORDS
Chronic cerebrospinal venous insufficiency (CCSVI);
Multiple sclerosis (MS);
Internal cerebral vein;
Internal jugular vein (IJV)

Summary

Introduction: Chronic cerebrospinal venous insufficiency (CCSVI) is a newly suggested cause for multiple sclerosis (MS) detected by color-coded Doppler sonography. Our aim was to evaluate the relationship between CCSVI and MS compared to the control group.
Methods: The study was performed on 84 MS patients and 115 healthy subjects. The presence of at least two of the extra- and/or intra-cranial Zamboni's criteria was considered positive for evidence of CCSVI.
Results: Although the total number of MS patients with any detectable CCSVI criterion was significantly higher than the controls (22.6% vs. 10.4%, $P=0.019$), only one out of 84 patients fulfilled the Zamboni's criteria (1.2% vs. none, $P=0.422$).
Conclusion: Our results do not support the presence of a relationship between MS and CCSVI criteria defined by Zamboni.
© 2012 Elsevier GmbH. All rights reserved.

* Corresponding author. Tel.: +98 21 82141367; fax: +98 21 82141321; mobile: +98 9121222956.
E-mail addresses: m-mehrpour@tums.ac.ir (M. Mehrpour), neda_najimi@yahoo.com (N. Najimi), sm.fereshtehnejad@ki.se (S.-M. Fereshtehnejad), safa_3318@yahoo.com (F.N. Safa), smr.mirzaei@gmail.com (S. Mirzaeizadeh), mrmotamed2005@yahoo.com (M.R. Motamed), smf681@yahoo.com (M. Nabavi), m.sahrai@sina.ac.ir (M.A. Sahraeian).

Introduction

Multiple sclerosis (MS) is an autoimmune and neurodegenerative disease of the Central Nervous System (CNS) with the exact cause still being unknown [1]. Chronic cerebrospinal venous insufficiency (CCSVI) has recently been suggested as a probable cause for MS. Zamboni first described this syndrome after observing reflux in internal jugular vein (IJV) as a result of valsalva maneuver in an MS patient which was followed by more researches [2]. He also defined a set of criteria for the diagnosis of CCSVI, which is detected by transcranial and extracranial color coded Doppler sonography [3].

The presumed mechanism behind this theory is the presence of a vein in the center of MS lesions in the CNS and parenchymal iron deposition as the result of venous stasis and occurrence of neurodegeneration afterwards as a result of an autoimmune reaction [2].

As the pathogenesis of MS is multifactorial and is not clearly defined, this hypothesis attracted a lot of attention because of the known treatment for venous insufficiency and reversible nature of it that could also be applied to MS [3].

Many studies have been performed on the subject since the hypothesis was introduced that have debating results. Some of them claim a strong relationship between CCSVI and MS [3], while others report that there's no relationship between these two conditions [4—6]. Even systematic reviews carried out on the subject admit that more studies with similar methods are needed [7]. This need becomes more important when endovascular interventions are being offered to MS patients as a treatment for their venous insufficiency [8].

The aim of this study was to evaluate the relationship between CCSVI and MS with a comparison to the control group in order to fill a small gap in this field. For the first time, the study was performed on Iranian MS subjects.

Methods and subjects

Subjects and clinical assessments

This was an analytical cross-sectional study, which was conducted in Firoozgar general hospital, Tehran, Iran, from September 2010 to 2011. All of the clinically definite MS (CDMS) patients diagnosed using revised McDonald criteria 2010 [9] who attended Firoozgar hospital's neurology clinic or were admitted in neurology ward were recruited into the study. A total of 84 patients were studied, 2 patients with primary progressive MS (PPMS), 16 patients with secondary progressive MS (SPMS), 46 patients with relapsing-remitting MS (RRMS) and 20 patients with clinically isolated syndrome (CIS). One hundred and fifteen subjects with no neurological or other pertinent diseases were matched by age and sex distribution with MS patients. Subjects with vasculitis or any vascular malformations were excluded from the study. No invasive study was performed on the patients and controls, informed consent was obtained from all of the subjects and they were not charged for the evaluations.

Demographic data of the patients, MS duration and organ system dysfunctions (including GI, urinary, memory, visual, motor, sensory, etc.) were also recorded at the visit or by calling the patients in case they were not able to attend the clinics. The Kurtzke expanded disability status scale (EDSS) method was used to quantify disability of MS patients [10]. Measuring EDSS was done by one neurologist to decrease probable interpersonal errors.

Ultrasound assessment

All of the studied subjects underwent color-coded sonographic evaluation of intracranial [deep middle cerebral vein (DMCV)] and extracranial [bilateral jugular] veins.

For bilateral jugular veins assessment, a 6.0 MHz linear probe and for intracranial veins, a 2.0 MHz phase array probe was used (MyLab™ 40, Esaote, Italy). Each subject underwent ultrasound evaluations twice. The first time was in supine position and then in upright (90°, sitting) position. Velocity of intra- and extracranial veins was recorded. The diameter of bilateral internal jugular veins was also measured using B mode imaging in horizontal plane. When measuring veins' diameter, special attention was paid not to compress the veins by the probe.

The mentioned indices were measured in patients and controls in supine and upright positions, on an identical point and the differences between these 2 measures were calculated.

Cerebrospinal venous return was also assessed in subjects while they were positioned on a tilt bed. The blood flow to the opposite of physiologic direction for more than 0.88 s in extracranial and more than 0.5 s in intracranial veins were considered as reflux in the subjects [11].

To decrease interpersonal measurement errors, one specialist performed all of the assessments. If there was a significant respiratory variation in the blood flow velocity and the diameter in the assessed veins within subjects, we asked the patient to hold his breath for a short time after a normal exhalation, and the assessments were performed in these breathless times. If there was a local narrowing in the vein, all of the available length of the vein was studied in sagittal plane for more accurate measurements.

The vein diameter less than $0.4\,cm^2$ in supine position was considered stenosis.

The presence of 2 or more of the following criteria was known as CCSVI in studied patients:

1. A reflux in right or left internal jugular veins.
2. A reflux in deep middle cerebral vein.
3. An evidence of internal jugular vein stenosis.
4. Increase in the diameter of internal jugular vein in the sitting position, rather than decreasing [3].

Statistical analysis

The data were analyzed using SPSS software v.16 for windows. One sample K—S test was used to check the distribution of quantitative variables. To compare normally distributed variables between the 2 groups Independent Samples T-test was used and in skewed variables Mann—Whitney U test was performed. In qualitative data, chi-square test was used. In order to evaluate the relationship between 2 continuous variables we used correlation test, Pearson r in normally distributed and Spearman's r

Table 1 Baseline characteristics of the recruited MS patients (n = 84).

Baseline variable	Description
Age (yr)	
Mean ± SD	36.44 ± 11.44
Gender (%)	
Female	61 (72.6%)
Male	23 (27.4%)
Disease duration (yr)	
Mean ± SD	8.94 ± 8.56
MS type (%)	
RRMS	54.8%
PPMS	2.4%
SPMS	19%
CIS	23.8%
EDSS score	
Mean ± SD	3.95 ± 2.75
Symptoms (%)	
Sensory dysfunction	78.8%
Visual dysfunction	72.3%
Motor dysfunction	66.2%
Pain	38.5%
Memory dysfunction	53.8%
facial palsy	20%
Urinary dysfunction	40.6%
Balance disturbance	64.6%
Gastrointestinal disturbance	32.3%
Interferon therapy (%)	80%

in skewed data are reported. P-Value less than 0.05 was considered statistically significant.

Results

Baseline characteristics

Eighty four multiple sclerosis (MS) patients and 115 healthy controls were recruited in this prospective study. The patients group consisted of 61 (72.6%) female and 23 (27.4%) male with the mean age of 36.44 ± 11.44 yr which was matched with the control group involving 78 (67.8%) female and 37 (32.2%) male with the mean age of 35.92 ± 10.73 ($P = 0.467$ and 0.754 for gender and age, respectively).

All of the demographic and disease characteristics of the patients are listed in Table 1. As it is shown, the mean duration of disease and EDSS score were 8.94 ± 8.56 yr and 3.95 ± 2.75, respectively. Sensory dysfunction was the most common symptom among MS cases (78.8%).

Transcranial color-coded Doppler (TCCD) assessment

TCCD evaluations of right and left internal jugular veins (IJVs) and deep middle cerebral vein (DMCV) were performed for all of the patients and healthy controls in two positions — supine and sitting. The mean of blood flow velocities (BFV) and cross-sectional diameters or areas (CSA) of evaluated cerebral veins are reported and compared between the two groups of study in Table 2. The mean BFV of the right IJV was 54.07 ± 22.71 cm/s and 53.74 ± 20.39 cm/s in MS patients and controls, respectively. Although the mean changes (Δ) of BFV of the right IJV after altering to the sitting position was lower in patients' group, the difference was not statistically significant (7.48 ± 5.45 cm/s vs. 14.38 ± 4.02 cm/s, $P = 0.301$). A similar finding was observed for the left IJV, too (6.24 ± 5.10 cm/s vs. 14.68 ± 3.63 cm/s, $P = 0.168$).

The mean CSA of the right IJV in the supine position was significantly lower in MS group compared with the healthy controls (1.02 ± 0.55 cm^2 vs. 1.17 ± 0.50 cm^2, $P = 0.038$). While the mean CSA changes were not statistically significant either in the right or the left IJV between the two study groups ($P = 0.109$ and 0.943). Moreover, the mean BFV of the DMCV was not significantly different between patients group and the healthy controls (64.25 ± 23.48 cm/s vs. 60.98 ± 15.85 cm/s, $P = 0.337$).

Table 3 shows the qualitative comparison of the postural changes in BFV of IJVs between two groups. Both in the MS patients group and healthy controls, the BFVs of IJVs were increased in the majority of evaluated cases following sitting position. Even though this increase occurred more in the control group, the difference could not meet the significant level ($P = 0.334$ and 0.199 for the right and left IJV, respectively).

Chronic cerebrospinal venous insufficiency (CCSVI) criteria

More TCCD assessment was performed to evaluate other CCSVI criteria. As summarized in Table 4, the results of Fishers' exact test show that IJVs' reflux was significantly more frequent in MS patients (8.3% vs. 1.7%, $P = 0.038$). On the other hand, no DMCV reflux was detected either in MS patients or healthy controls. Evidence of proximal IJV stenosis was observed in 10 (12%) patients and 7 (6.1%) healthy subjects which failed to show any significant difference ($P = 0.145$). Of 84 MS cases, only 3 (3.6%) were found with an increase in the diameter of IJVs in the sitting position which was not significantly different with the reported frequency percentage of 2.6% among the reference controls ($P = 0.695$).

Although the total number of MS patients with any detectable CCSVI criterion was significantly higher than the controls (22.6% vs. 10.4%, $P = 0.019$), only one out of 84 patients fulfilled the Zamboni's criteria for CCSVI with at least two mentioned criteria (1.2% vs. none, $P = 0.422$).

Disease characteristics and (CCSVI) criteria

More detailed analysis was performed to assess any probable relationship between MS characteristics and CCSVI criteria in patients group. Mean EDSS score and disease duration of the cases with at least one CCSVI criteria was higher than MS patients without any abnormal TCCD findings (EDSS: 4.72 ± 2.72 vs. 3.67 ± 2.73; disease duration: 10.81 ± 9.07 vs. 8.33 ± 8.38 yr). Nevertheless, these differences were not statistically significant ($P = 0.168$ and 0.269, respectively). Motor dysfunction (75% vs. 63.3%, $P = 0.546$), sensory dysfunction (93.85 vs. 74%, $P = 0.159$), pain (43.8 vs.

Table 2 Mean comparison of baseline characteristics, blood flow velocities (BFV) and cross-sectional vessel diameters or areas (CSA) of evaluated cerebral veins between MS patients and healthy controls.

Variable	Group of study		P-Value
	MS patients (n = 84)	Healthy controls (n = 115)	
Age (yr)			
Mean ± SD	36.44 ± 11.44	35.92 ± 10.73	0.754
Gender (%)			
Female	61 (72.6%)	78 (67.8%)	0.467
Male	23 (27.4%)	37 (32.2%)	
BFV of right IJV (cm/s)			
Mean ± SD			
Supine	54.07 ± 22.71	53.74 ± 20.39	0.918
Sitting	61.09 ± 39.38	69.03 ± 34.56	0.156
Δ	7.48 ± 5.45	14.38 ± 4.02	0.301
BFV of left IJV (cm/s)			
Mean ± SD			
Supine	47.73 ± 22.20	47.78 ± 21.73	0.872
Sitting	51.96 ± 37.15	59.52 ± 32.42	0.165
Δ	6.24 ± 5.10	14.68 ± 3.63	0.168
CSA of right IJV (cm^2)			
Mean ± SD			
Supine	1.02 ± 0.55	1.17 ± 0.50	0.038*
Sitting	0.12 ± 0.14	0.12 ± 0.10	0.179
Δ	0.92 ± 0.55	1.05 ± 0.52	0.109
CSA of left IJV (cm^2)			
Mean ± SD			
Supine	0.82 ± 0.60	0.76 ± 0.41	0.942
Sitting	0.16 ± 0.36	0.14 ± 0.19	0.334
Δ	0.68 ± 0.73	0.62 ± 0.40	0.943
BFV of DMCV (cm/s)Mean ± SD	64.25 ± 23.48	60.98 ± 15.85	0.337

Table 3 Qualitative comparison of postural changes in blood flow velocities (BFV) of internal jugular veins between MS patients and healthy controls.

Variable	Group of study		Chi-square	P-Value
	MS patients (n = 84)	Healthy controls (n = 115)		
BFV of right IJV (%)				
Increased	51.5%	62.9%		
Decreased	45.5%	35.2%	2.19	0.334
Unchanged	3%	1.9%		
BFV of left IJV (%)				
Increased	53.1%	61.6%		
Decreased	45.3%	33.3%	3.23	0.199
Unchanged	1.6%	5.1%		

36.7%, P = 0.617) and balance disturbance (81.3% vs. 59.2%, P = 0.139) were all reported to be more frequent in patients with any CCSVI criterion. However, these differences were not statistically significant.

Discussion

Zamboni, first reported reflux from the chest into the IJV using duplex scan during valsalva maneuver in MS patients [2] and based on previous reports about the relationship between dilated cerebral veins and inflammatory MS lesions [12,13], he presented the hypothesis that there may be a role for the venous system, following iron deposition in the pathogenesis of MS. Until now many studies have been performed on the subject with conflicting results.

The most prominent finding in our study was that our results do not support the presence of a relationship between MS and CCSVI criteria defined by Zamboni [3]. Only one MS patient fulfilled the Zamboni's definition for CCSVI. Statistically significant difference between the 2 groups was

Table 4 Comparison of chronic cerebrospinal venous insufficiency (CCSVI) criteria according to Zamboni description [3] between MS group and healthy controls.

Criterion	Group of study		Chi-square	P-Value
	MS patients (n = 84)	Healthy controls (n = 115)		
Reflux in right or left IJVs (%)	7 (8.3%)	2 (1.7%)	4.89	0.038*
Reflux in DMCV (%)	—	—	—	NS
Stenosis in right or left IJVs (%)	10 (12%)	7 (6.1%)	2.13	0.145
Increase in diameter of IJVs in the sitting position (%)	3 (3.6%)	3 (2.6%)	0.15	0.695
CCSVI (%)				
Any single criterion detectable	19 (22.6%)	12 (10.4%)	5.48	0.019*
Full criteria	1 (1.2%)	0	1.38	0.422

found in only one criterion (reflux in the IJV). Although, the total number of MS patients with any detectable CCSVI criterion was significantly higher than the controls. Doepp and colleagues also did not find a difference between the 2 groups based on the criteria but in 2 other venous indices [4]. We also detected the blood flow using Doppler in all of the MS patients with a direction toward the heart.

Although the mean changes of BFV of the bilateral IJVs after altering the position from supine to sitting was lower in patients' group, which means that the increase in velocity was smaller in MS patients, but this difference was not statistically significant. A larger proportion of MS patients had decreased velocity, and the percentage with increased velocity was more in healthy controls. These findings are not in accordance with Doepp et al.'s study that shows a decrease in velocity in reference group and an increase in the patients' group, which they relate to sympathetic chain involvement in MS patients [4].

No reflux was found in DMCV, which is in accordance with the results of Baracchini et al. [5].

Of 84 MS cases, 3.6% were found with an increase in the diameter of IJVs in the sitting position, which was not significantly different with the reported frequency percentage of 2.6% among the reference controls. But this is not as much as reported by Zamboni, showing the impaired postural regulation of the veins. The CSA of IJV typically decreases when changing the position from supine to sitting, because the vein collapses partially. Our study results are in accordance with Doepp et al. [3,4,14].

Mean EDSS score and disease duration of the cases with at least one CCSVI criteria was higher than MS patients without any abnormal TCCD findings, which also had a relationship with increasing age and the possible effect of aging on venous system.

Zivadinov and Wattjes compared extracranial venous system in MS patients and healthy controls, using MR venography and did not find any significant difference in IJV and vertebral veins blood flow between the 2 groups [15,16]. These reports are in agreement with our results that show no statistically significant difference between blood flow velocity in IJV of both sides between MS patients and healthy controls (Table 2). But is in disagreement with Simka [17] and Hojnacki's [18] studies. Simka et al. evaluated 70 MS patients using Doppler sonography and reported 90% of the patients with at least 2 of 4 extracranial criteria, being positive and also a high rate of reflux and IJV stenosis [17].

Hojnacki et al. assessed 10 MS patients and 7 healthy controls and observed CCSVI in all MS patients and none of the healthy controls, according to the Doppler sonography criteria [18].

Centonze and colleagues also did not find a relationship between CCSVI and MS, reporting that the tendency for CCSVI occurrence was the same in patients and control group and also suggest that any possible stricture in the IJV is for compensation of disease process in the patients [6]. As it's shown in our results, the mean CSA of the right IJV in the supine position was significantly lower in MS group compared with the healthy controls, but stenosis was not significantly more in MS patients.

In studies performed by other researchers on patients who underwent internal jugular vein resection for causes such as malignancies, none of them ended to MS [19,20]. It must be taken into account that the absence of a relationship between IJV resection (uni- or bilateral) and MS in these studies might be because of a short period of follow up. Actually, there are some other conditions that affect the venous drainage of the brain like cerebral venous thrombosis, idiopathic intracranial hypertension, and chronic obstructive pulmonary disease, but there is no evidence that these disorders are associated with an increased risk of developing MS [8] that brings the results of those studies into challenge and seeks more investigations.

Limitations and suggestions

One of the advantages of our study was the large number of participants in the study compared to previous researches, 84 patients with MS and 115 healthy controls.

Most of the participants in our study were RRMS and SPMS, with a small percentage of PPMS. We recommend future studies to include other types of MS in the evaluation to check for differences between all types of the disease.

As there is controversy between different studies assessing CCSVI criteria in MS patients and above-mentioned reports about IJV resection consequences, reconsidering the criteria may be an option. Another reason for these controversies might be differences in techniques, instruments, anatomical site and patient's position when performing sonography, which can be decreased by using the same method and mode of sonography.

The person who performed sonographic evaluations was not blind to patient's group in our study. Blinding the assessors also can decrease the bias in the future studies.

Acknowledgments

The authors would like to thank Dr. Jalil Kouhpayezadeh for his confidential supports in statistical procedures and sample size calculation. Also we would like to appreciate the staff of Firoozgar Clinical Research Development Center (FCRDC) for their technical supports and helps.

References

[1] Bar-Or A. The immunology of multiple sclerosis. Semin Neurol 2008;28:29—45.
[2] Zamboni P. The big idea: iron-dependent inflammation in venous disease and proposed parallels in multiple sclerosis. J Roy Soc Med 2006;99:589—93.
[3] Zamboni P, Galeotti R, Menegatti E, Malagoni AM, Tacconi G, Dall'Ara S, et al. Chronic cerebrospinal venous insufficiency in patients with multiple sclerosis. J Neurol Neurosurg Psychiatry 2009;80(4):392—9.
[4] Doepp F, Paul F, Valdueza JM, Schmierer K, Schreiber SJ. No cerebrocervical venous congestion in patients with multiple sclerosis. Ann Neurol 2010;68:173—83.
[5] Baracchini C, Perini P, Calabrese M, Causin F, Rinaldi F, Gallo P. No evidence of chronic cerebrospinal venous insufficiency at multiple sclerosis onset. Ann Neurol 2011;69:90—9.
[6] Centonze D, Floris R, Stefanini M, Rossi S, Fabiano S, Castelli M, et al. Proposed chronic cerebrospinal venus insufficiency criteria do not predict MS risk nor MS severity. Ann Neurol 2011;70:51—8.
[7] Laupacis A, Lillie E, Dueck A, Straus Sh, Perrier L, Burton JM, et al. Association between chronic cerebrospinal venous insufficiency and multiple sclerosis: a meta-analysis. CMAJ 2011;183(16):E1203—12.
[8] Petrov I, Grozdinski L, Kaninski G, Iliev N, Iloska M, Radev A. Safety profile of endovascular treatment for chronic cerebrospinal venous insufficiency in patients with multiple sclerosis. J Endovasc Ther 2011;18:314—23.
[9] Polman CH, Reingold SC, Banwell B, Clanet M, Cohen JA, Filippi M, et al. Diagnostic criteria for multiple sclerosis: 2010 revisions to the McDonald criteria. Ann Neurol 2011;69(2):292—302.
[10] Kurtzke JF. Rating neurologic impairment in multiple sclerosis: an expanded disability status scale (EDSS). Neurology 1983;33(11):1444—52.
[11] Menegatti E, Zamboni P. Doppler haemodynamics of cerebral venous return. Curr Neurovasc Res 2008;5(November (4)):260—5.
[12] Fog T. The topography of plaques in multiple sclerosis with special reference to cerebral plaques. Acta Neurol Scand 1965;15(Suppl.):1—161.
[13] Tan IL, van Schijndel RA, Pouwels PJ, van Walderveen MA, Reichenbach JR, Manoliu RA, et al. MR venography of multiple sclerosis. AJNR Am J Neuroradiol 2000;21(June—July (6)):1039—42.
[14] Zivadinov R, Galeotti R, Hojnacki D, Menegatti E, Dwyer MG, Schirda C, et al. Value of MR venography for detection of internal jugular vein anomalies in multiple sclerosis: a pilot longitudinal study. AJNR Am J Neuroradiol 2011 May;32(5):938—46.
[15] Zivadinov R, Lopez-Soriano A, Weinstock-Guttman B, Schirda CV, Magnano CR, Dolic K, et al. Use of MR venography for characterization of the extracranial venous system in patients with multiple sclerosis and healthy control subjects. Radiology 2011;258(February (2)):562—70.
[16] Wattjes MP, van Oosten BW, de Graaf WL, Seewann A, Bot JC, van den Berg R, et al. No association of abnormal cranial venous drainage with multiple sclerosis: a magnetic resonance venography and flow-quantification study. J Neurol Neurosurg Psychiatry 2011;82(April (4)):429—35.
[17] Simka M, Kostecki J, Zaniewski M, Majewski E, Hartel M. Extracranial Doppler sonographic criteria of chronic cerebrospinal venous insufficiency in the patients with multiple sclerosis. Int Angiol 2010;29(April (2)): 109—14.
[18] Hojnacki D, Zamboni P, Lopez-Soriano A, Galleotti R, Menegatti E, Weinstock-Guttman B, et al. Use of neck magnetic resonance venography, Doppler sonography and selective venography for diagnosis of chronic cerebrospinal venous insufficiency: a pilot study in multiple sclerosis patients and healthy controls. Int Angiol 2010;29(April (2)):127—39.
[19] Doepp F, Hoffmann O, Schreiber S, Lammert I, Einhäupl KM, Valdueza JM. Venous collateral blood flow assessed by Doppler ultrasound after unilateral radical neck dissection. Ann Otol Rhinol Laryngol 2001;110(November (11)):1055—8.
[20] Gius JA, Grier DH. Venous adaptation following bilateral radical neck dissection with excision of the jugular veins. Surgery 1950;28(August (2)):305—21.

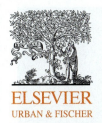
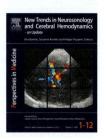

Ultrasound findings of the optic nerve and its arterial venous system in multiple sclerosis patients with and without optic neuritis vs. healthy controls

Nicola Carraro [a,*], Giovanna Servillo [a], Vittoria M. Sarra [a], Angelo Bignamini [b], Gilberto Pizzolato [a], Marino Zorzon [a]

[a] Department of Medical Sciences, University of Trieste, Italy
[b] School of Specialization in Hospital Pharmacy, University of Milan, Italy

KEYWORDS
Optic Neuritis;
Ophthalmic venous flow;
Optic Nerve atrophy;
Doppler ultrasound imaging

Summary

Background: Optic Neuritis (ONe) is common in Multiple Sclerosis (MS). The aim of this study was to evaluate the Optic Nerve (ONr) and its vascularisation in MS patients with and without previous ONe and in Healthy Controls (HC).

Methods: We performed high-resolution echo-color ultrasound examination in 50 subjects (29 MS patients and 21 HC). By a suprabulbar approach we measured the ONr diameter at 3 mm from the retinal plane and at another unfixed point. We assessed the flow velocities of Ophthalmic Artery (OA), Central Retinal Artery (CRA) and Central Retinal Vein (CRV) measuring the Peak Systolic Velocity (PSV) and the End Diastolic Velocity (EDV) for the arteries and the Maximal Velocity (MaxV), Minimal Velocity (MinV) and mean Velocity (mV) for the veins. The Pulsatility Index (PI) and the Resistive Index (RI) were also calculated.

Results: No significant variation for OA supply was found as well as no significant variation for CRA supply, while significant higher PI in the CRV of non-ONe MS eyes vs. both HC and ONe MS eyes was measured. We found that ONr diameter was decreased significantly from HC to non-ONe MS eyes and ONe MS eyes.

Conclusions: Ultrasound examination of ONr and its vascularisation is feasible and can demonstrate ON atrophy. The increase of CRV PI in unaffected eyes of MS patients is intriguing and seems not associated to ONr atrophy. Larger studies are needed to confirm these results.
© 2012 Elsevier GmbH. All rights reserved.

Introduction

Optic Neuritis (ONe) is a common feature of Multiple Sclerosis (MS) both in the early phase and during the disease course [1].

MS and ONe are due to demyelination [2], but it has been postulated that vascular mechanisms may have a role in MS and ONe pathogenesis [3–6].

* Corresponding author. Tel.: +39 040 421712; fax: +39 040 910861.
E-mail address: n.carraro@fmc.units.it (N. Carraro).

According to a recent hypothesis, cerebrospinal venous system alterations may contribute to the development of the disease and may drive its clinical course [7,8]. As a matter of fact, a correlation between the hemodynamic pattern of Chronic Cerebrospinal Venous Insufficiency (CCSVI) and the clinical features in patients with MS has been described [9]. In particular, ONe at onset seems to be associated with Internal Jugular Veins (IJV) and/or of proximal Azygous Vein (AV) high grade stenosis, with consequent reflux in the deep cerebral veins. The blood then flows to the pterygoid plexus, and from there to the facial veins via the deep facial vein, to the cavernous sinus and to the ophthalmic veins.

While changes in the hemodynamics of the eye's arterial system, detected by Doppler ultrasound sonography, have been previously described in MS patients with both acute and chronic ONe [10—13], the venous flow has not been studied yet, as far as we know.

Taking into account the peculiar environment of the arterial-venous system supplying and draining the Optic Nerve, we have considered it as a representative site for studying the relationship between veins and nervous parenchyma. For this purpose we investigated if any blood flow alteration, possibly contributing to MS disease process, could be recorded.

Aim of the study was to evaluate the vascularisation of the Optic Nerve (ONr) by means of color Doppler ultrasonography in MS patients with and without previous ONe. Furthermore, the possibility to measure the ONr thickness by ultrasound sonography was assessed. We compared Optic Nerve anatomical and vascular features of MS patients with those of age- and gender-matched Healthy Controls (HC).

Methods

With a high-resolution echo-color duplex ultrasound equipment we studied the ONr and its vascularisation [i.e. Ophthalmic Artery (OA), Central Retinal Artery (CRA), Central Retinal Vein (CRV)] in 29 Relapsing—Remitting (RR) clinically definite MS patients [14] and 21 age- and gender-matched HC, volunteers. Table 1 shows the characteristics of the subjects studied. Seventeen MS patients have had an ONe at least one year before examination (5 have had a right ONe, 7 a left ONe and five a bilateral ONe) while 12 MS patients have not suffered from ONe. All MS patients underwent a Visual Evoked Potentials Examination to confirm the ONe diagnosis.

By means of a Toshiba Aplio XG, equipped with a linear probe (PLT-1204AX: 7.2-14 MHz), we insonated the ONe

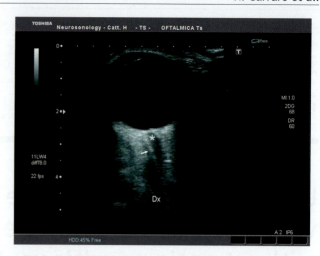

Figure 1 Sagittal B-mode ultrasound scan of a right eye: Optic Nerve (asterisk) with its meningeal sheath (arrow).

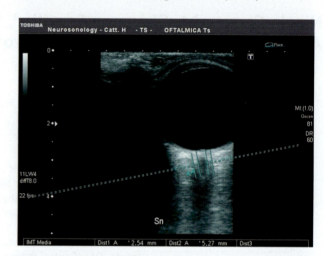

Figure 2 Sagittal B-mode ultrasound scan of a left eye: measure of the Optic Nerve diameter, with and without the meningeal sheath, in an unfixed site where the maximum nerve diameter is detectable.

(Fig. 1) and measured the diameter of ONr, with and without the meningeal sheaths, at two distances, the first at 3 mm from the retinal plane (Fig. S1, online supplementary file) and the second at an unfixed point where the nerve structures were best recognised (maximum diameter), through the usual suprabulbar approach (Fig. 2). We detected the OA (Fig. 3) and CRA (Fig. S2, online supplementary file) flow velocities [Peak Systolic Velocity (PSV), End

Table 1 Charateristics of study subjects.

Variable		Controls (N=21)	MS (N=29)	Total (N=50)	p
Sex	Females, n (%)	15 (71.4%)	26 (89.7%)	41 (82.0%)	0.098[a]
	Males, n (%)	6 (28.6%)	3 (10.3%)	9 (18.0%)	
Age	Mean ± SD	34.0 ± 7.5	34.8 ± 7.5	34.4 ± 7.4	0.697[b]
	Median [RIQ]	31 [29—38]	36 [28—40]	35 [29—40]	

[a] Chi-square test.
[b] Independent samples t-test.

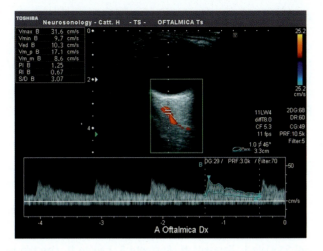

Figure 3 Color Doppler and velocity waveforms of a right Ophthalmic Artery. Measurement of the PSV (indicated as Vmax), EDV (indicated as Ved), mV (indicated as Vm_p: mean of peak velocities) and Vm_m (mean of mean velocities), PI and RI.

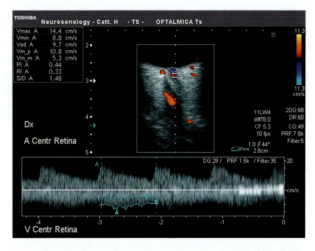

Figure 4 Color Doppler and velocity waveforms of right Central Retinal Vein. Measurement of the MV (indicated as Vmax), MinV (indicated as Vmin), mV (indicated as Vm_p: mean of peak velocities) and Vm_m (mean of mean velocities), PI and RI.

Diastolic Velocity (EDV), mean Velocity (mV)], and the CRV flow velocities [(Maximum Velocity (MV), Minimum Velocity (MinV), mean Velocity (mV)] and calculated, for each blood vessel, the Pulsatility Index (PI) and the Resistive Index (RI) (Fig. 4).

Overall, we examined and compared 42 eyes of HC with 36 unaffected and 22 affected eyes of RR MS patients.

The study was approved by the local Ethics Committee. Written informed consent was obtained from all patients and HC.

Table 2 Arterial and Venous flow variables of the Optic Nerve Vascularization, measured in Multiple Sclerosis Patients with and without previous Optic Neuritis and Healthy Controls.

Variable	Controls (N = 42)	MS, not affected eyes (N = 36)	MS, affected eyes (N = 22)	p ANOVA	p[a]	p[b]
OA						
PSV	48.20 ± 12.93	48.71 ± 12.81	42.03 ± 13.83	ns	ns	ns
EDV	12.84 ± 4.22	12.58 ± 3.56	11.64 ± 6.54	ns	ns	ns
mV	23.01 ± 7.37	23.16 ± 6.02	20.76 ± 9.59	ns	ns	ns
RI	0.73 ± 0.05	0.74 ± 0.06	0.73 ± 0.09	ns	ns	ns
PI	1.58 ± 0.28	1.59 ± 0.37	1.60 ± 0.54	ns	ns	ns
CRA						
PSV	14.37 ± 3.71	16.20 ± 5.75	13.64 ± 4.80	ns	ns	ns
EDV	4.60 ± 1.78	4.97 ± 2.54	4.19 ± 2.33	ns	ns	ns
mV	7.88 ± 2.48	8.95 ± 3.73	7.47 ± 3.22	ns	ns	ns
RI	0.70 ± 0.14	0.70 ± 0.09	0.70 ± 0.12	ns	ns	ns
PI	1.29 ± 0.42	1.32 ± 0.39	1.37 ± 0.48	ns	ns	ns
CRV						
MV	8.20 ± 2.74	9.01 ± 3.60	7.73 ± 4.37	ns	ns	ns
MinV	5.76 ± 2.03	5.99 ± 2.28	5.42 ± 2.83	ns	ns	ns
mV	6.80 ± 2.22	7.34 ± 2.63	6.41 ± 3.30	ns	ns	ns
RI	0.30 ± 0.09	0.36 ± 0.14	0.30 ± 0.12	0.047	0.046	ns
PI	0.26 ± 0.08	0.29 ± 0.09	0.25 ± 0.08	ns	ns	ns
ONr 3 mm	2.95 ± 0.44	2.86 ± 0.42	2.73 ± 0.31	ns	ns	ns
ONr + sheath 3 mm	5.19 ± 0.84	5.09 ± 0.65	5.08 ± 0.52	ns	ns	ns
MONr	3.38 ± 0.45	3.11 ± 0.37	2.92 ± 0.57	<0.001	0.016	<0.001
ONr + sheath	5.92 ± 0.70	5.58 ± 0.63	5.37 ± 0.84	0.010	ns	0.008

OA, Ophthalmic Artery; CRA, Central Retinal Artery; CRV, Central Retinal Vein; ONr, Optical Nerve; MONr, maximum ONr diameter; PSV, Peak Systolic Velocity; EDV, End Diastolic Velocity; mV, mean Velocity; MV, Maximum Velocity; MinV, Minimal Velocity; RI, Resistive Index; PI, Pulsatility Index.
[a] 2-Sided Dunnett t-test vs. controls, MS not affected eyes.
[b] 2-Sided Dunnett t-test vs. controls, MS affected eyes.

The data were analysed by SPSS 17.0. Demographic data were compared by independent samples t-test and chi square test, as appropriate. Data are reported as mean with standard deviation (SD) and as median and range interquartile (RIQ), when appropriate. Comparisons of the other variables were performed with the analysis of variance (ANOVA) complemented with the pairwise comparison vs. HC according to Dunnett. Statistical significance was set at $p < 0.05$.

Results

All the results are shown in Table 2. For the OA and the CRA we found no difference for all variables. For the CRV no detectable variation in velocities was found, while there was a significant difference in PI, that is greater in MS patients' eyes not affected by ONe vs. both HC and MS patients' eyes affected by ONe. ONr diameter measurement at 3 mm shows no difference between the three groups, while maximum ONr diameter is significantly smaller in MS patients' both affected and unaffected eyes, compared to HC.

Discussion and conclusions

As far as the arterio-venous ophthalmic system is concerned, our data did not show any arterial abnormality or any major venous flow alteration (i.e. absence, blocked or reversed flow). Recently, in MS patients with CCSVI, an association has been reported between ONe and Internal Jugular Vein (IJV) and Azygous Vein stenoses, with reflux in the deep cerebral veins. These findings suggest that the veins of the ONr might be involved in a compensatory outflow circle towards the IJV.

In our sample of MS patients we did not observe any alteration, in the ONr venous flow that supports this hypothesis. The increased CRV PI in MS patients' unaffected eyes is intriguing and seems not associated to ONr atrophy. This could suggest a venous drainage impairment, but at present we cannot confirm this hypothesis and larger studies are needed to confirm it.

The analysis of the diameter of the ONrs showed that it is possible to detect ONr atrophy in affected eyes and, at a lesser degree, also in unaffected eyes of MS patients. Maximum ONr diameter measurement seems to be more reliable than 3 mm measurement, probably because of the progressive ONr myelination.

In conclusion, ultrasound examination of ONr and its vascularisation is an easy, feasible, safe and low cost procedure and the measurement of ONr thickness can detect ONr atrophy.

Appendix A. Supplementary data

Supplementary data associated with this article can be found, in the online version, at http://dx.doi.org/10.1016/j.permed.2012.04.008.

References

[1] Ebers GC. Optic neuritis and multiple sclerosis. Arch Neurol 1985;42:702—4.
[2] Hauser SL, Oksenberg JR. The neurobiology of multiple sclerosis: genes, inflammation, and neurodegeneration. Neuron 2006;52:61—76.
[3] D'haeseleer M, Cambron M, Vanopdenbosch L, De Keyser J. Vascular aspects of multiple sclerosis. Lancet Neurol 2011;10:657—66.
[4] Speciale L, Sarasella M, Ruzzante S, Caputo D, Mancuso R, Calvo MG, et al. Endothelin and nitric oxide levels in cerebrospinal fluid of patients with multiple sclerosis. J Neurovirol 2000;(Suppl. 2):S62—6.
[5] Haufschild T, Shaw SG, Kaiser HJ, Flammer J. Transient raise of endotelin-1 plasma levels in patients with multiple sclerosis. Ophthalmologica 2003;217:451—3.
[6] Pache M, Kaiser HJ, Akhaldebashvili N, Lienert C, Dubler B, Kappos L, et al. Extraocular blood flow and endothelin-1 plasma levels in patients with multiple sclerosis. Eur Neurol 2003;49:164—8.
[7] Zamboni P, Menegatti E, Galeotti E, Malagoni AM, Sacconi G, Dall'Ara S, et al. The value of cerebral Doppler venous hemodynamics in the assessment of multiple sclerosis. J Neurol Sci 2009;282:21—7.
[8] Zamboni P, Menegatti E, Galeotti E, Malagoni AM, Sacconi G, Dall'Ara S, et al. Chronic cerebrospinal venous insufficiency in patients with multiple sclerosis. J Neurol Neurosurg Psychiatry 2009;0:392—9.
[9] Bartolomei I, Salvi F, Galeotti R, Salviato E, Alcanterini M, Menegatti E, et al. Hemodynamic patterns of chronic crebrospinal venous insufficiency in multiple sclerosis. Correlation with symptoms at onset and clinical course. Int Angiol 2010;29:183—8.
[10] Karaali K, Senol U, Aydin H, Cevikol C, Apaydin A, Luleci E. Radiology 2003;226:355—8.
[11] Akarsu C, Tan FU, Kendi T. Color Doppler imaging in optic neuritis with multiple sclerosis. Graefes Arch Clin Exp Ophthalmol 2004;242:990—4.
[12] Modrzejewska M, Karczewicz D, Wilk G. Assessment of blood flow velocity in eyeball arteries in multiple sclerosis patients with past retrobulbar optic neuritis in color Doppler ultrasonography. Klin Ocza 2007;109:183—6.
[13] Hradilek P, Stourac P, Bar M, Zapletova O, Skoloudic D. Colour Doppler imaging evaluation of blood flow parameters in the ophthalmic artery in acute and chronic phases of optic neuritis in multiple sclerosis. Acta Ophtalmol 2009;87:65—70.
[14] Polman CH, Reingold SC, Edan G, Filippi M, Hartung HP, Kappos L, et al. Diagnostic criteria for multiple sclerosis: 2005 revisions to the ''McDonald Criteria''. Ann Neurol 2005;58:840—6.

Virtual Navigator study: Subset of preliminary data about cerebral venous circulation

Marialuisa Zedde[a,*], Giovanni Malferrari[a], Gianni De Berti[b], Massimo Maggi[b], Luca Lodigiani[c]

[a] *Neurology Unit, Department of Neuromotor Physiology, Azienda Ospedaliera ASMN, Istituto di Ricovero e Cura a Carattere Scientifico, Viale Risorgimento 80, 42100 Reggio Emilia, Italy*
[b] *Neuroradiology Unit, Department of Radiology, Azienda Ospedaliera ASMN, Istituto di Ricovero e Cura a Carattere Scientifico, Viale Risorgimento 80, 42100 Reggio Emilia, Italy*
[c] *Ultrasound Operational Marketing, ESAOTE SpA, Via A. Siffredi 58, 16153 Genova, Italy*

KEYWORDS
Virtual Navigator;
Fusion imaging;
Cerebral veins;
Transcranial;
TCCS;
Transverse sinus

Summary

Introduction: Neuroradiological techniques are known for their high spatial resolution in imaging of intracranial structures, in comparison with neurosonological techniques (TCCS), known for their high temporal resolution. An ideal study of intracranial circulation should combine the high temporal resolution of ultrasound with the high spatial resolution of Magnetic Resonance (MR) Imaging. This imaging fusion system is actually used for the ultrasound liver examination and it is known as Virtual Navigator. Therefore we implemented this system for the examination of the intracranial venous hemodynamics.

Patients and methods: Fifteen consecutive subjects (7 men and 8 women, mean age 51.5 ± 8.64 years) were chosen among patients who underwent standard TCCS examinations at our lab and had age >18 years, a suitable temporal acoustic window and a recently performed intracranial MR venography. The axial scanning approach was used from the temporal window and the standard TCCS examination was compared with the Virtual Navigator examination, for the insonation rate of the basal vein of Rosenthal (BVR), Galen vein (GV), Straight sinus (SRS) and Transverse sinus (TS).

Results and discussion: The insonation rates of the venous structures are only slightly improved for BVR (from 90% to 96.67%) but are substantially increased for SRS and TS (for this last one from 63.33% to 86.67%) with a statistically significant difference ($p < 0.05$).

Conclusions: The Virtual Navigator protocol can help to insonate the intracranial venous system.
© 2012 Elsevier GmbH. All rights reserved.

Abbreviations: BVR, Basal vein of rosenthal; CT, Computed tomography; GV, Galen vein; MRI, Magnetic Resonance Imaging; SRS, Straight sinus; TCCS, Transcranial color-coded sonography; TS, Transverse sinus.
* Corresponding author. Tel.: +39 0522 296494.
E-mail addresses: zedde.marialuisa@asmn.re.it, marialuisa.zedde@tiscali.it (M. Zedde).

2211-968X/$ — see front matter © 2012 Elsevier GmbH. All rights reserved.
doi:10.1016/j.permed.2012.02.008

Introduction

Ultrasound techniques have an high dynamicity and therefore a good temporal resolution.

Instead neuroradiological techniques have an high anatomic definition and therefore a good spatial resolution. The possibility of combining the ultrasound examination with a reference modality and to fuse this data set with the ultrasound scan could improve the understanding of the current scan situation in real time. This combination of two diagnostic modalities may result is a faster and more reliable procedure. The Virtual Navigator allows the real-time visualization of the ultrasound scan next to the corresponding virtual slices obtained from other modalities. Its purpose is to enhance the informative content of images produced by an ultrasound scanner by combining them with a second modality in real-time, so combining the high temporal resolution of ultrasound techniques and the high spatial resolution of CT/MR techniques.

This fusion imaging software has been used in extraneurological applications, as abdominal ultrasound and in this setting it demonstrated a good reliability and a great improvement of focal lesion monitoring and treatment and of their identification.

Neurovascular application is in a pioneering phase even for the brain arterial circulation. Ultrasound examination of cerebral veins is a harder challenge than the one of the cerebral arteries, both for the basal scanning and for the fusion imaging technique. Particularly straight sinus and transverse sinus have a relatively low insonation rate.

The insonation rates of the main cerebral veins reported in the literature by using TCCS are [1,2]:

- BVR 84—93%
- GV 66—91%
- SRS 48—86%
- TS 35—73%

We planned this preliminary approach with the Virtual Navigator system to verify the feasibility of this strategy to increase the insonation rate of the main basal cerebral veins.

Patients and methods

Fifteen consecutive subjects (7 men and 8 women, mean age 51.5 ± 8.64 years) were chosen among patients who underwent standard TCCS examinations at our lab and had

- age >18 years
- a suitable temporal acoustic window for the arterial examination
- a recently performed intracranial MR angiography with normal venous findings.

All subjects did not have a disease of the venous system and the reasons why they underwent MRI were mainly migraine or dizziness or a control examination of a previously known nonspecific lesion pattern in the white matter.

All patients underwent a basal TCCS examination and a subsequent TCCS examination with the Virtual Navigator system. The axial scanning approach was used by TCCS from the temporal window, according to the validated scanning planes for the venous study, for the insonation of the BVR, GV, SRS and TS [2—5]. According to the reference data from

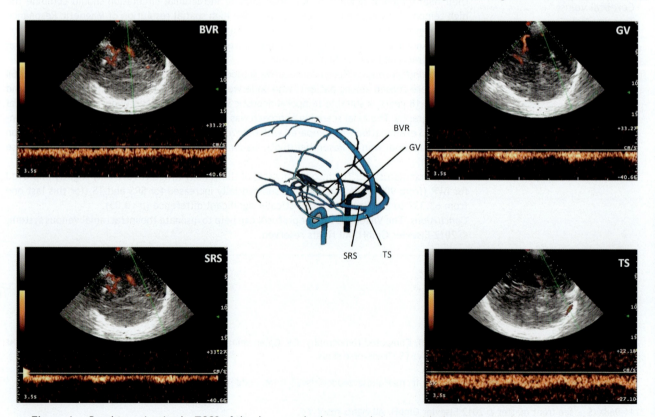

Figure 1 Basal examination by TCCS of the deep cerebral veins and sinuses with the corresponding anatomic drawing.

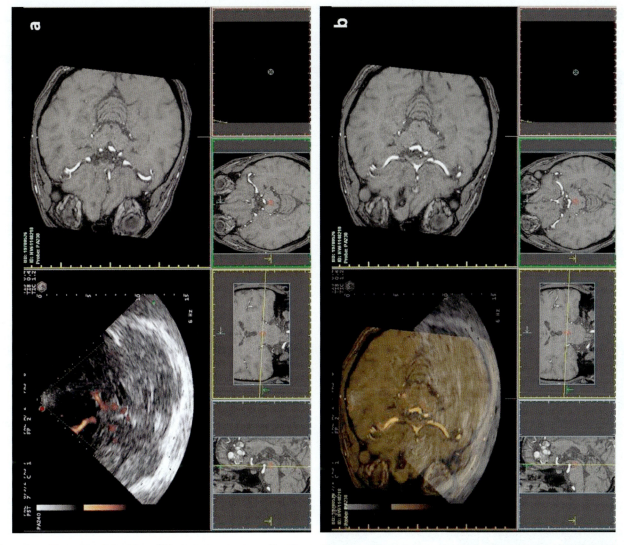

Figure 2 Example of the Virtual Navigator system application to the insonation of the main cerebral arteries. (a) The left side of the images shows the real time ultrasound examination, and the right side the corresponding MR oblique plane in a mesencephalic axial view. (b) Brain MR superimposed to the TCCS insonation image, showing the almost perfect correspondence of the anatomic structures, both vascular and parenchymal ones.

the literature, only the contralateral approach to the TS was used for this evaluation. A schematic drawing of the assessed cerebral veins and sinuses with the corresponding TCCS images is shown in Fig. 1.

The insonation rate of the BVR, GV, SRS and TS were registered both for the basal examination and for the Virtual Navigator system examination and they were compared by Mantel—Haenszel Chi-square for trend.

Experimental

Virtual Navigator is a MyLab optional license from Esaote, that provides additional image information from a second modality like CT or MR, during a clinical ultrasound session. By using the second modality the user gains security in assessing the morphology of the ultrasound image.

The Virtual Navigator system is inserted into a commercially available ultrasound machine and its use involved some sequential steps. First, the MR study was uploaded in the ultrasound platform and the Virtual Navigation software was activated. Second, the ultrasound examination was started and matched with the MR images by using a magnetic tracking system, solidary with the ultrasound probe, along a reference alignment plane. Third, the standard TCCS examination was compared with the Virtual Navigator examination, according to the validated scanning planes for the venous study, for the insonation rate of the BVR, GV, SRS and TS [2,5].

The exam steps are summarized as follows:

- CT/MR acquisition
- Data transferring and loading
- Automatic volume elaboration on the US
- Registration
- One scan plane
- Anatomical markers
- Real-time combined scanning

Step 1: matching and locking ultrasound scanning planes and corresponding MR recontructed oblique planes

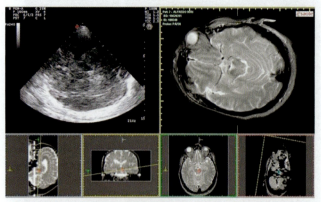

Step 2: verifying the TCCS-MR coupling by arterial imaging

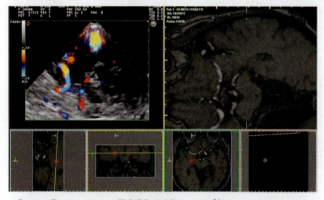

Step 3: venous TCCS-MR coupling

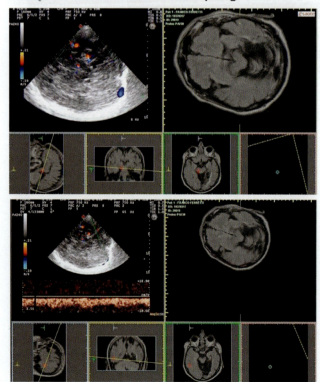

Table 1 Comparison of the insonation rates with basal TCCS and Virtual Navigator system.

Insonated veins	Insonation rate (%)		p-Value
	Basal examination	Virtual Navigator exam	
BVR	26/30 (90)	29/30 (96.67)	0.232
GV	13/15 (86.67)	15/15 (100)	0.150
SRS	10/15 (66.67)	15/15 (100)	0.016
TS	19/30 (63.33)	26/30 (86.67)	0.038

In Fig. 2 there is an example of the Virtual Navigator application for the arterial circulation and in Fig. 3 the practical steps of the examination are illustrated for the venous examination.

Results

For the purposes of the comparison between the basal and fusion imaging insonation rate of the BVR, GV, SRS, TS, few assumptions should be made: first, BVR and TS are paired structures, therefore the insonation rate take into account both sides of TCCS examination (30 TS); second, GV and SRS are unpaired structures, therefore 15 veins had to be insonated.

The basal and Virtual Navigator system insonation rate are reported in Table 1, with the p value of the Chi-square for trend. The comparison between the basal insonation rate and the Virtual Navigator insonation rate showed a significant difference for the SRS ($p=0.016$) and for the TS ($p=0.038$).

Discussion

The application of the Virtual Navigator system for brain imaging has been initially tried in neurosurgery, during the surgical procedure. In this condition the ultrasound study is easy, because of the removal of the skull bone, but the real-time ultrasound images without the skull bone are not always perfectly correspondent to the neuroradiological slices, achieved before skull removal. Moreover, TCCS gives access to a limited portion of the brain anatomy thought an intact skull, but the standard insonation planes are suitable for the imaging of main intracranial arteries and veins. Its main limitation is the quality of the temporal bone window; because a suboptimal window does not allow the visualization of all intracranial large vessels. Our hypothesis is that the use of a second imaging modality as a reference could increase the number of Doppler-sampled segments of the intracranial veins and sinuses in comparison with the basal insonation rate.

Instead of acquire brain MR with surface external magnetic landmarks, as in abdominal imaging, for a better

Figure 3 Description of the three main practical steps for the TCCS insonation of the cerebral veins with the Virtual Navigator system. The third step shows an example of the insonation of the con trilateral TS.

coupling between ultrasound and radiological study, a previously performed standard brain MRI was uploaded into the machine platform. The coupling of the ultrasound planes with the corresponding reconstructed oblique MR planes was manually performed in a reference plane and the sonologist checked it in real time in the axial scanning planes. The landmarks to be correspondent in the two imaging modalities were: the petrous edge in the pontine plane, the mesencephalon and the edge of sphenoid wing in the midbrain plane, and the third ventricle and the epiphysis in the diencephalic plane. The following step was to assess the correct locking of ultrasound and MRI in coronal scanning planes.

Our basal insonation data were similar to the insonation rates reported in the literature [1,2]. The insonation rate with the Virtual Navigator system improved for all examined segments, with a significant value for SRS and TS. The insonation rate of 96.67% for the BVR is in agreement with the anatomic data about 5.6% of BVR draining into the lateral mesencephalic vein [6].

The improvement of the insonation rate of the TS is good, although only the contralateral approach was used and it is possible that adding the ipsilateral approach could cause a further improvement of the insonation rate, particularly for hypoplasic sinuses.

Conclusions

The possibility of combining the ultrasound examination with a reference modality in real time can improve the identification of the main cerebral vein and sinuses, therefore increasing their insonation rate. The result is an increase in reliability of the ultrasound examination, also multiplying the scanning planes with the guide of the neuroradiological reconstructed planes.

References

[1] Stolz E, Kaps M, Kern A, Babacan SS, Dorndorf W. Transcranial color-coded duplex sonography of intracranial veins and sinuses in adults: reference data from 130 volunteers. Stroke 1999;30:1070–5.
[2] Baumgartner RW, Gönner F, Arnold M, Müri RM. Transtemporal power- and frequency-based color-coded duplex sonography of cerebral veins and sinuses. Am J Neuroradiol 1997;18:1771–81.
[3] Baumgartner RW, Mattle HP, Aaslid R. Transcranial color-coded duplex sonography, magnetic resonance angiography, and computed tomography angiography: methods, applications, advantages, and limitations. J Clin Ultrasound 1995;23:89–111.
[4] Valdueza JM, Schmierer K, Mehraein S, Einhäupl KM. Assessment of normal flow velocity in basal cerebral veins: a transcranial Doppler ultrasound study. Stroke 1996;27:1221–5.
[5] Schreiber SJ, Stolz E, Valdueza JM. Transcranial ultrasonography of cerebral veins and sinuses. Eur J Ultrasound 2002;16:59–72.
[6] Suzuki Y, Ikeda H, Shimadu M. Variations of the basal vein: identification using three-dimensional CT angiography. Am J Neuroradiol 2001;22:670–6.

Ipsilateral evaluation of the transverse sinus: Transcranial color-coded sonography approach in comparison with magnetic resonance venography

Marialuisa Zedde [a,*], Giovanni Malferrari [a], Gianni De Berti [b], Massimo Maggi [b]

[a] Neurology Unit, Department of Neuromotor Physiology, Azienda Ospedaliera ASMN, Istituto di Ricovero e Cura a Carattere Scientifico, Viale Risorgimento 80, 42100 Reggio Emilia, Italy
[b] Neuroradiology Unit, Department of Radiology, Azienda Ospedaliera ASMN, Istituto di Ricovero e Cura a Carattere Scientifico, Viale Risorgimento 80, 42100 Reggio Emilia, Italy

KEYWORDS
Transcranial;
Transverse sinus;
Cerebral veins;
Virtual Navigator;
TCCS;
Insonation rate

Summary

Introduction: The ultrasound examination of intracranial venous structures by transcranial color-coded sonography (TCCS) is a validated and standardized application. Similarly some intracranial venous sinuses are known for their relatively low insonation rate, as straight sinus (SRS) and transverse sinus (TS), ranging from 35% to 73%. The relatively high frequency of hypoplasia of TS can partially take account for these data. The aim of this study is to evaluate the feasibility of this approach in a standard TCCS examination, in comparison with magnetic resonance (MR) findings by using the Virtual Navigator system.

Patients and methods: The standardized approach to the TS was a contralateral insonation, starting to the SRS plane and angulating downwards the probe. In this way it is possible to insonate the proximal segment of the contralateral TS. We proposed a new approach with an extreme downwards tilting and a slow opposite angulation of the probe for examining the ipsilateral TS. Forty consecutive subjects were chosen among patients who underwent standard TCCS examinations at our lab and had a suitable temporal acoustic window, and a recently performed MR venography. The contralateral TS insonation rate was compared with the ipsilateral one.

Results and discussion: The insonation rate was 61/80 (76.25%) for the contralateral TS and 75/80 (93.75%) for the ipsilateral approach. Two of 5 not detectable TS were aplasic in MR venography and the others were not identified by a poor acoustic window.

Conclusions: The ipsilateral approach could be associated to the contralateral standard study for insonating the TS.
© 2012 Elsevier GmbH. All rights reserved.

Abbreviations: CT, computed tomography; MR, magnetic resonance; SPS, superior petrous sinus; SRS, straight sinus; SSS, superior sagittal sinus; SyS, sygmoid sinus; TCCS, transcranial color coded sonography; TS, transverse sinus.
* Corresponding author. Tel.: +39 0522 296494.
E-mail addresses: zedde.marialuisa@asmn.re.it, marialuisa.zedde@tiscali.it (M. Zedde).

2211-968X/$ — see front matter © 2012 Elsevier GmbH. All rights reserved.
doi:10.1016/j.permed.2012.02.007

Introduction

Neurosonology, mainly TCCS, has been recognized in the last years as a valuable technique to assess the intracranial venous hemodynamics, and to insonate the main deep cerebral veins and the dural sinuses. Reference data about normal subjects are available for several cerebral veins and sinuses, and there are some pathological situations for which the ultrasound examination of venous hemodynamics have a clear and recognized usefulness and rationale, as cerebral vein thrombosis, mainly for the monitoring of recanalization, transient global amnesia, space occupying lesions, etc.

One of the main limitations of the neurosonological study is the relatively low insonation rate of some intracranial venous structures that make virtually impossible the differential diagnosis between hypo-aplasia and obstruction for paired structures only by using TCCS, and without the presence of indirect signs. Indeed, if some veins are almost constantly present, as the paired basal vein of Rosenthal and the Galen vein, other veins are characterized by frequent side-by-side variability for hypoplasia or aplasia on one side, as the TS. Another limitation is the wide variability of communicating channels between the deep venous system, the dural sinuses and the cavernous sinus pathway, besides a complex anastomotic system between the intracranial and extracranial venous circulation.

For these aspects, the more problematic vein could be the TS, because of its relevance, as part of the jugular outflow system, and the side-by-side variability. Right and left TS arise at the torcularis herophyli and run laterally from the internal occipital protuberance in a bone groove within the insertion of the tentorium. At the lateral head of the petrous bone edge the TS leaves the tentorial course and it becomes SyS, after receiving the SPS. The right TS is usually larger than the contralateral one and it drains mainly the SSS. The size of the left TS is usually lesser than the contralateral one the left TS drains mainly the SRS.

The insonation rate of the TS in the sonological literature using TCCS is variable and substantially poor, if compared with other intracranial veins, as the basal vein of Rosenthal, ranging from 35% [1] to 73% [2]. The conventional approach at the insonation of the TS is a contralateral one and the reported data are derived from this approach, as described in [3]. But the contralateral approach to the TS has some limitations, because of its limited field of view; another known difficulty is the insonation of hypoplasic veins.

Therefore, an ipsilateral approach with a slightly different access could represent an alternative possibility and increase the insonation rate of TS. Moreover it can allow to insonate a longer segment of the TS.

For the validation of this new approach a comparison between the TCCS insonation planes and the corresponding neuroradiological oblique images of the same person is desirable, and a real time comparison while the sonological examination is performed would be also useful, but not yet codified and implemented for the intracranial circulation study. Indeed ultrasound techniques have a high dynamicity, and therefore a good temporal resolution and neuroradiological techniques have a high anatomic definition, and therefore a good spatial resolution. The possibility of combining the ultrasound examination with a reference modality in real time allows confirming the anatomical assumption of a new approach. Moreover the identification of vessel segments (TS in this case) is faster and more reliable. This system is a Virtual Navigator software, already used in other body districts.

Therefore, after the identification and the proposal of an extended ipsilateral insonation for the TS an imaging fusion system was implemented and tested validating it.

Patients and methods

Forty consecutive subjects (28 men and 12 women, mean age 55.63 ± 7.61 years) were chosen among patients who underwent standard TCCS examinations at our lab and had

- age >18 years;
- a suitable temporal acoustic window for the study of the arterial circulation;
- a recently performed intracranial MR angiography with normal venous findings (also patients with a marked hypoplasia of the TS were included).

All subjects have not a disease of the venous system and the reasons why they underwent brain MR were migraine or dizziness or a control examination of a previously known nonspecific lesion pattern in the white matter or previous ischemic stroke in the arterial circulation.

The basal TCCS examination was performed by using a MyLab 60 equipment and both the contralateral and the ipsilateral approach were used for the insonation of the TS.

The first 20 subjects underwent a further study with the Virtual Navigator software in order to validate the ipsilateral approach.

Fig. 1 shows an example of the contralateral and ipsilateral approach to the TS. It is notable that the proposed insonation plane for the ipsilateral TS, with a more anterior positioning of the probe and an opposite tilting, as compared to the contralateral approach, allows a larger field of view, and therefore an examination of a greater extent of TS.

The increased field of view led us to distinguish three segments of the TS through an ipsilateral approach, as shown in Fig. 2, because of the visualization of the entire course of the TS in the correspondent bone groove.

All segments were looked for during the basal TCCS and during the Virtual Navigator examination, and separated insonation rates were calculated.

Therefore, the global insonation rate of the TS is composed:

- for the contralateral approach by the insonation of the proximal segment;
- for the ipsilateral approach by the insonation of at least one of the proximal, middle and distal segment.

so potentially increasing the rate of success in the TCCS insonation of the TS. Considering both sides, 80 TS were insonated with both contralateral and ipsilateral approach.

Insonation rates were compared by using the Fisher exact test.

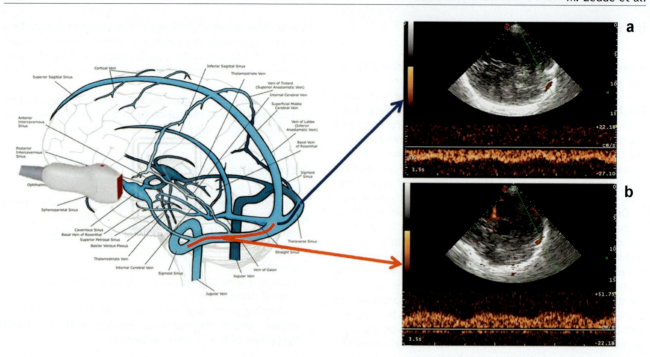

Figure 1 Overview of the classic contralateral (a) and ipsilateral (b) approach to the TS insonation over the schematic anatomical drawing (left side of the figure) with the ultrasound probe defining the side of the insonation. Contralateral TS has a flow direction away from to the probe and ipsilateral TS has a flow direction to the probe.

Experimental

The first 20 subjects underwent TCCS study with the Virtual Navigator system in order to confirm the anatomical correspondence of the new proposed insonation plane, and the identification of all segments of the ipsilateral TS, by using MR imaging of the same subject as a real time reference modality. The Virtual Navigation system is a software of imaging fusion between several techniques, neuroradiological techniques (CT or MRI) and real-time ultrasound examination, so improving the localization of predefined targets. This tool can combine the high time resolution of ultrasound with the high spatial resolution of MR or CT. The goal is to enhance the images produced

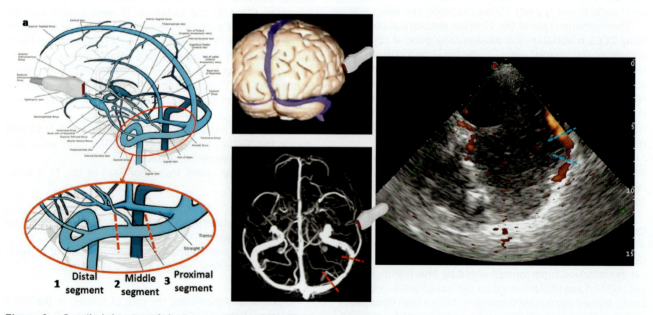

Figure 2 Detailed drawing of the segmentation of the TS into a proximal, middle and distal segment. (a) Anatomic schematic view. (b) Reconstructed ipsilateral insonation of the TS. (c) MR venography with corresponding TS segmentation. (d) TCCS from the temporal bone window in a posterior cranial fossa view in power mode with a similar segmentation. It is notable the visualization of the full course of the ipsilateral TS.

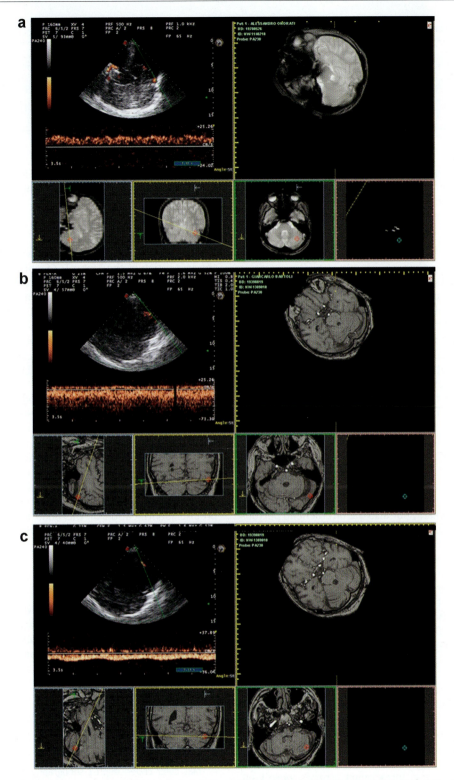

Figure 3 Virtual Navigator examination of the ipsilateral TS and its segmentation. In the right side of the images there is the corresponding oblique insonation plane of MR. (a) Proximal segment. (b) Middle segment. (c) Distal segment.

by an ultrasound scanner by combining them with a second modality (like CT or MR). The system consists of an ultrasound real time scanner equipped with an electromagnetic tracking device enabling the image fusion based on the geometry data and the content of the second modality dataset. Furthermore ultrasound images have a limited field of view and their quality can be affected by the physical and physiological conditions of the patient, but other methodologies, like CT and MR offer a wider field of view, are rather patient-independent. The first step of the examination is the

Table 1 Comparison of the insonation rates of the TS between contralateral and ipsilateral approach.

TS segments	Contralateral insonation (%)	Ipsilateral insonation (%)	P
Proximal segment	61/80 (76.25)	75/80 (93.75%)	0.0033
Middle segment	15/80 (18.75)	69/80 (86.25)	<0.0001
Distal segment	0/80	74/80 (92.5)	<0.0001
All segments	76/240 (31.67%)	218/240 (90.83)	<0.0001

matching and locking the MR reconstructed oblique plane with the TCCS examination for the main intracranial arteries. Therefore, the correspondence of the real-time moving insonation planes is assessed for the venous examination.

Results

The first 20 patients underwent the basal TCCS for the venous examination and the Virtual Navigator study in order to confirm the initial assumption of the ultrasound landmarks for the ipsilateral TS identification.

The Virtual Navigator examination and the anatomical matching were performed for the three segments of the TS though the ipsilateral scanning approach. Fig. 3 showed the examples of the corresponding TCCS MR planes for three segments of the TS. For the proximal segment of TS a posterior access to the transtemporal bone window was used (Fig. 3a), for the middle segment is used a slightly anterior approach under real time visual control of the corresponding moving plane of the MR (Fig. 3b); for the insonation of the distal segment both approaches along the temporal bone window, the anterior and the posterior one, can be used (Fig. 3c). In the anterior approach only the hyperechoic occipital bone is available as a landmark, but also the lateral head petrous bone is often identifiable during the insonation of the lateral segment of the TS.

The insonation rate was 61/80 (76.25%) for the contralateral TS, combining the classical approach with an oblique insonation in a posterior fossa plane.

19/80 (23.75%) of the TS were not identified by TCCS with a contralateral approach, and this result is according to the literature data. 10/80 (12.5%) of the non-visualized TS were hypoplasic at the neuroradiological evaluation, mainly on the left side.

75/80 (93.75%) TS were successfully insonated through the ipsilateral approach, considering at least one of the three segments; 69/80 (86.25%) TS were insonated in two segments.

Two of 5 (40%) not detectable TS were aplasic in MRA and the others 3 (60%) were hypoplasic and were not identified by a suboptimal temporal acoustic window for the venous examination (main intracranial arteries were well identifiable).

A comparison between controlateral and ipsilateral insonation rate is shown in Table 1. There was a statistical significant difference between contralateral and ipsilateral insonation in favor of the ipsilateral insonation, both for the global insonation rates and for segmental insonation rates.

Discussion

The challenge of this work was to find the way for improving the insonation of the TS by TCCS and the first step was the casual observation of the larger extent of the TS evaluable by an ipsilateral view. The direct comparison of TCCS images with the MRI reconstructed planes by the Virtual Navigator software helped to define and standardize the anatomical landmarks of this proposed approach. The insonation of the TS by an ipsilateral approach causes a higher success rate than the contralateral approach, mainly for severely hypoplasic TS.

The use of previously non-standardized approach for insonating cerebral vessels, particularly veins and sinuses, could be made easier by real time fusion imaging technologies, as Virtual Navigator. The proposed ipsilateral approach to the TS allows the arbitrary segmentation of its entire course, and it is not possible through the contralateral approach because of the lesser field of view. The standardization of this approach has been performed through the precise identification of the bone and parenchymal landmarks, comparing real time TCCS with MR angiography and brain MR imaging.

Conclusions

The ipsilateral approach could be even more successful than the contralateral one for the insonation of the TS, and the combination of both strategies could further increase the likelihood of successful insonation of the TS.

References

[1] Baumgartner RW, Nirkko AC, Müri RM, Gönner F. Transoccipital power-based color-coded duplex sonography of cerebral sinuses and veins. Stroke 1997;28:1319—23.
[2] Stolz E, Kaps M, Kern A, Babacan SS, Dorndorf W. Transcranial color-coded duplex sonography of intracranial veins and sinuses in adults. Reference data from 130 volunteers. Stroke 1999;30:1070—5.
[3] Stolz E. Cerebral vein and sinuses. In: Baumgartner RW, editor. Handbook on Neurovascular Ultrasound, vol. 21. Basel, Karger: Front Neurol Neurosci; 2006. p. 182—93.

Intraoperative color-coded duplex sonography of the superior sagittal sinus in parasagittal meningiomas

Vladimir B. Semenyutin*, Dmitriy A. Pechiborsch, Viktor E. Olyushin, Vugar A. Aliev, Vladislav Y. Chirkin, Alexander V. Kozlov, G.K. Panuntsev

Russian Polenov Neurosurgical Institute, Saint-Petersburg, Russia

KEYWORDS
Superior sagittal sinus;
Parasagittal meningioma;
Sonography;
Magnetic resonance venography;
Intraoperative

Summary

Background: Patency of the superior sagittal sinus (SSS) is a key factor in surgery of parasagittal meningiomas (PSM). The main and least invasive method of evaluation of the SSS is magnetic resonance venography (MR venography). However the efficacy of this method is limited in some cases especially in slow flow velocities.

Objective: Determine potentials of intraoperative color-coded duplex sonography (CCDS) for evaluation of the SSS in PSM comparing them with MR venography.

Methods: CCDS was conducted in 30 adult patients with PSM using linear ultrasound probe i12L-RS (Vivid E, GE) placed on the superior wall of the SSS after craniotomy. Intraoperative CCDS findings were compared with 2D time-of-flight MR venography.

Results: False-positive results of complete occlusion of the SSS by MR venography in our series were obtained in 7 out of 16 cases (for the anterior third of the SSS — 5 out of 6; middle third — 1 out of 8; posterior third — 1 out of 2). CCDS determined the degree of SSS invasion and differentiated invasion from compression or thrombosis of the SSS, which MR venography could not.

Conclusion: Intraoperative CCDS is safe and allows evaluation of SSS patency as well as venous lacunae, bridging veins and inferior sagittal sinus, classification according to degree of SSS invasion, and being more precise than MR venography it can be used to determine surgical strategy.
© 2012 Elsevier GmbH. All rights reserved.

Background

Patency of the superior sagittal sinus (SSS) is a key factor in surgery of parasagittal meningiomas (PSM) and, therefore, its determination is the standard of preoperative work-up [1]. Up to 50% of PSM invade the SSS lumen [2]. It is generally accepted that totally invaded SSS should be resected en bloc, but if the invasion is partial the SSS should be reserved even in cases with residual flow in it [3]. There are three methods of evaluation of the SSS — digital subtraction angiography (DSA), computed tomography (CT) and magnetic resonance venography (MR venography). DSA is the ''gold standard'' of cerebral angiography and cerebral venography in particular. It gives the most precise information about SSS patency, but it is invasive and costly, therefore its usage gradually declines. CT is believed to be slightly more accurate than MR venography in verification of SSS patency [4]. CT is less invasive than DSA yet requires irradiation and iodine contrast medium. MR venography is presently the method of choice for evaluation of SSS patency in patients with PSM due to its noninvasiveness [5]. There

* Corresponding author.
  E-mail address: lbcp@mail.ru (V.B. Semenyutin).

are three kinds of MR venography: 2D time-of-flight (TOF), phase-contrast and MR venography with contrast medium. They all differ by the method of revealing flowing blood [6]. 2D TOF MR venography is the most simple of all its three kinds, sensitive to slow flow (which is typical for venous blood flow) and does not even require contrast medium. Though 2D TOF MR venography is less precise than MR venography with contrast medium, it is widely used in preoperative evaluation of the SSS in patients with PSM [6—9]. However, the efficacy of this method is limited in low blood flow velocities that occur in substantial invasion and/or compression of the SSS by PSM [9]. As a result there is a dilemma — the more precise method we use the more it is invasive. Search of the altogether noninvasive and precise method leads us to sonography, but transcranial sonography is impossible for investigation of the SSS because of deep location and an inappropriate angle [10,11]. The method of intraoperative color-coded duplex sonography (CCDS) is known but information about it is scant and ambiguous, so we decided to study this method ourselves.

Objective

Determine potentials of CCDS for intraoperative evaluation of SSS patency in PSM and compare them with MR venography.

Methods

30 patients (20—67 years, mean age 55) with PSM were studied. Intraoperative CCDS (anterior third of the SSS — 7 patients; middle third — 20; posterior third — 3) was conducted with linear ultrasound probe i12L—RS (Vivid E, GE, USA) placed on the superior wall of the SSS after craniotomy. Intraoperative CCDS findings were compared with 2D time-of-flight MR venography (Signa Infinity, GE, USA).

There are some important points that we want to mention. First, the superior wall of the SSS should be free from bone. This can be achieved by bilateral craniotomy or unilateral craniotomy with additional resection of overlying bone with rongeurs. Our attempts to evaluate the SSS through its lateral wall were not successful. Second, hemostatic materials (Surgicel, collagen sponge) should not be used during sonography of the SSS as they hinder propagation of the ultrasound and therefore the quality of the image will be significantly worse. Small bleedings from the SSS were stopped by cauterization, while more significant ones were terminated by applying hemostatic material and then removing it before CCDS. The probe was placed on the superior wall of the SSS and CCDS was performed in two planes — frontal (transverse) and sagittal. In B-mode in the frontal plane the presence, location and degree of intraluminal invasion was evaluated. We used color flow Doppler in the frontal plane only to confirm the presence of flow. In the sagittal plane we used color-mode only, because B-mode is not informative. We do not recommend to evaluate invasion of the SSS only in the sagittal plane since artifact from the lateral wall of the SSS may occur. Thus, in the sagittal plane we determined Doppler Spectrum, direction of flow and its quantitative characteristics — TAMEAN (time-averaged mean velocity) and TAMAX (time-averaged maximum velocity).

We performed CCDS of the SSS and the adjacent venous structures (lacunae, bridging veins) within the craniotomy window both before and after removal of PSM. It is important to apply on the SSS as little pressure as possible (up to the appearance of artifact due to air between the SSS and the probe) since the SSS is very easy to compress and blood flow velocity significantly increases.

Results

MR venography showed absence of blood flow in the SSS in 16 out of 30 cases, which was confirmed by intraoperative CCDS in 9 cases only (complete invasion in 7 cases, thrombosis in 2 cases). In the remaining 7 cases the SSS was patent (blood flow velocity in the SSS was 5—29 cm/s and flow index reached 40 ml/min). In 14 out of 30 patients MR venography revealed flow in the SSS and it was confirmed by CCDS. Thus, false-positive results of complete occlusion of the SSS according to MR venography in our series were obtained in 7 out of 16 cases (for the anterior third of the SSS — 5 out of 6; middle third — 1 out of 8; posterior third — 1 out of 2). CCDS additionally evaluated the degree of SSS invasion/compression with its hemodynamics and differentiated invasion from compression of the SSS. Examples of different types of SSS invasion by PSM obtained intraoperatively by CCDS, where consistency (Fig. 1) and discrepancy (Fig. S1 — to view the figure, please visit the online supplementary file in ScienceDirect) between CCDS and preoperative MR venography are presented.

B-mode in the frontal (transverse) plane allows verification of compression, partial invasion and complete invasion of the SSS. It helps to determine the limits of completely invaded SSS in order to resect it en bloc (Fig. S2 — to view the figure, please visit the online supplementary file in ScienceDirect). This data allows to classify PSM according to degree of SSS invasion according to classification by Sindou and Alvernia [3], which is the mostly widely used (Fig. 2). Nowadays CCDS seems to be the only method that allows doing this noninvasively (without excision of the SSS). However, this classification is not ideal and could not encompass all the cases we had like in Fig. S3 (to view the figure, please visit the online supplementary file in ScienceDirect), where all three walls of the SSS are invaded but the latter is still patent. B-mode can also visualize intrasinal structures like septum (Fig. S4 — to view the figure, please visit the online supplementary file in ScienceDirect). It should be noted that arachnoid granulations may mimic invasion of the SSS angle.

CCDS may also be used to visualize venous lacunae, bridging veins (Fig. S5 — to view the figure, please visit the online supplementary file in ScienceDirect) and inferior sagittal sinus (Fig. S6 — to view the figure, please visit the online supplementary file in ScienceDirect), which can be of significant help during operation. Inferior sagittal sinus usually becomes seen when the SSS is totally invaded and serves as collateral venous channel. Therefore visualization of the inferior sagittal sinus in order to preserve it may be important when PSM is large and encompasses the sinus.

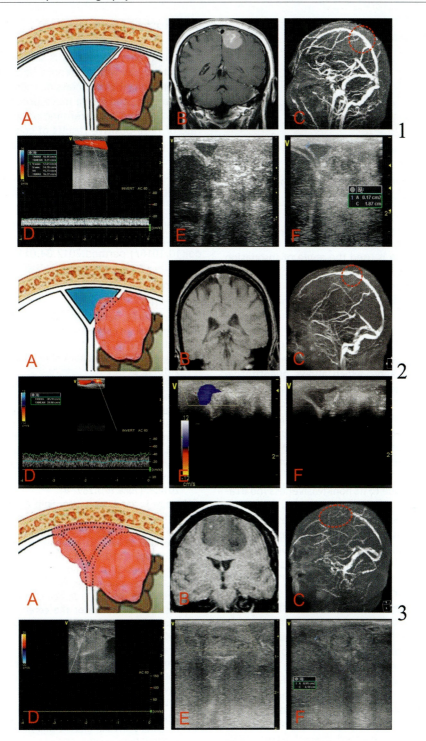

Figure 1 Examples of intraoperative CCDS: complete patency of SSS (1), partial invasion (2), complete invasion (3), (A) diagram of SSS invasion according to classification by Sindou and Alvernia [3]; (B and C) MRI and MR venography; (D—F) CCDS images ((D) sagittal plane, (E and F) frontal plane).

Discussion

Intraoperative sonography was first described by the American neurosurgeon B.W. Brawley in the Journal of Neurosurgery in 1969 [12]. There was a case with a 43-year-old female patient with PSM, in whom X-ray angiography (at that time it was the only method of preoperative evaluation of SSS patency) gave uncertain result and intraoperatively the SSS was evaluated with Doppler sonography revealing its patency. The PSM was therefore subtotally resected with SSS preserved.

It is obvious that since that time medical sonography has become much more sophisticated. Nowadays transcranial Doppler is considered to be the best noninvasive method

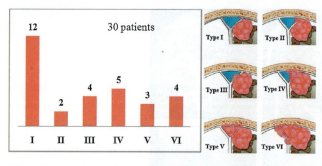

Figure 2 Diagram of patients' distribution (left) according to classification by Sindou and Alvernia [3] (right).

of quantitative evaluation of intracranial vessels. However, it is impossible to use it in adults for evaluation of the SSS. When the temporal window is used the angle of insonation is more than 60° and thus inappropriate [10]. It is possible to detect the posterior third of the SSS through the occipital window, but the detection rate is not more than 55% and even 38% for patients older than 60 years. In this case the flow velocity is 6—10 cm/s [11].

It is little known about the blood flow in the SSS. Aside from almost useless transcranial Doppler, there is phase-contrast MR venography, which allows quantitative evaluation of the SSS hemodynamics in patients with PSM. This method revealed that mean blood flow velocity in the SSS is 10—15 cm/s [13]. This method is rather approximate since it is operator dependent and based on several assumptions. There are no more methods of quantitative evaluation of blood flow velocity in the SSS in patients without cerebral pathology.

2D TOF MR venography due to its noninvasiveness (no irradiation, no contrast material) and simplicity and sensitivity to slow flow is the first-line method of preoperative evaluation of the SSS patency at our Institute and in many other clinics. However, this method has limitations, for example, artifactual signal loss resulting from in-plane vascular flow. To overcome this artifact, it is desirable to orient the acquisition plane perpendicular to the long axis of the vessel being imaged [9]. As a standard, frontal acquisition plane is used for SSS evaluation, therefore signal loss may occur in anterior and posterior parts of the SSS as these segments gradually become coplanar with the imaging plane. That is why in our study the rate of false-positive results of complete occlusion of the SSS according to 2D TOF MR venography is very high (83%) in anterior third of the SSS, and relatively low in its middle third (13%). According to the general opinion, anterior third of the SSS is not functionally significant and may be resected even if patent, 83% of false-positive results of complete occlusion do not discredit 2D TOF MR venography, but indicate that the method is useless for anterior third of the SSS. We would like to mention, that due to limited time of intraoperative study we did not use power Doppler, which is more sensitive to slow flow than color flow Doppler and could give even more accurate information about SSS patency.

CCDS is not invasive but requires removal of bone overlying the SSS which is not adequate in some cases like in small PSM. CCDS consumes little time (3—10 min) and is safe since neither one of our 30 patients had infectious or any other related complications.

Conclusion

Thus, intraoperative CCDS is safe and allows evaluation of SSS patency as well as venous lacunae, bridging veins and inferior sagittal sinus, classification according to degree of SSS invasion, and being more precise than MR venography it can be used to determine surgical strategy. The most rate of false-positive results of complete occlusion according to our study was observed in the anterior third of the SSS.

Appendix A. Supplementary data

Supplementary data associated with this article can be found, in the online version, at doi:10.1016/j.permed.2012.04.011.

References

[1] Connolly ES, McKhann G, Huang J, Choudhri T, Komotar R. Fundamentals of operative techniques in neurosurgery. 2nd edition Thieme; 2010. p. 421.
[2] Greenberg MS. Handbook of Neurosurgery. 7th edition Thieme; 2010. p. 614.
[3] DeMonte F, McDermott M. Al-Mefty's meningiomas. 2nd edition Thieme; 2011. p. 128.
[4] Khandelwal N, Agarwal A, Kochhar R, Bapuraj JR, Singh P, Prabhakar S, et al. Comparison of CT venography with MR venography in cerebral sinovenous thrombosis. American Journal of Roentgenology 2006;187(December (6)):1637—43.
[5] Lirng JF. Magnetic resonance venography of intracranial venous diseases. Journal of the Chinese Medical Association 2010;73(June (6)):289—91.
[6] Liauw L, van Buchem MA, Spilt A, de Bruïne FT, van den Berg R, Hermans J, et al. MR angiography of the intracranial venous system. Radiology 2000;214(March (3)):678—82.
[7] Glockner JF, Lee CU. Magnetic resonance venography. Applied Radiology 2010;39(June (6)), http://www.appliedradiology.com/Issues/2010/06/Articles/AR_06-10_Glockner/Magnetic-resonance-venography.aspx.
[8] Kirchhof K, Welzel T, Jansen O, Sartor K. More reliable noninvasive visualization of the cerebral veins and dural sinuses: comparison of three MR angiographic techniques. Radiology 2002;224(September (3)):804—10.
[9] Ayanzen RH, Bird CR, Keller PJ, McCully FJ, Theobald MR, Heiserman JE, et al. Cerebral MR venography: normal anatomy and potential diagnostic pitfalls. American Journal of Neuroradiology 2000;21(January (1)):74—8.
[10] Baumgartner RW, Gönner F, Arnold M, Müri RM. Transtemporal power- and frequency-based color-coded duplex sonography of cerebral veins and sinuses. American Journal of Neuroradiology 1997;18(October (9)):1771—81.
[11] Stolz E, Kaps M, Kern A, Babacan SS, Dorndorf W. Transcranial color-coded duplex sonography of intracranial veins and sinuses in adults. Reference data from 130 volunteers. Stroke 1999;30(May (5)):1070—5.
[12] Brawley BW. Determination of superior sagittal sinus patency with an ultrasonic Doppler flow detector in parasagittal meningioma. Technical note. Journal of Neurosurgery 1969;30(March (3)):315—6.
[13] Jordan JE, Pelc NJ, Enzmann DR. Velocity and flow quantitation in the superior sagittal sinus with ungated and cine (gated) phase-contrast MR imaging. Journal of Magnetic Resonance Imaging 1994;4(January—February (1)):25—8.

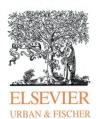
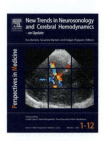

Bartels E, Bartels S, Poppert H (Editors):
New Trends in Neurosonology and Cerebral Hemodynamics — an Update.
Perspectives in Medicine (2012) 1, 399—403

journal homepage: www.elsevier.com/locate/permed

Italian multicenter study on venous hemodynamics in multiple sclerosis: Advanced Sonological Protocol

Giovanni Malferrari[a], Massimo Del Sette[b], Marialuisa Zedde[a,*], Sandro Sanguigni[c], Nicola Carraro[d], Claudio Baracchini[e], Marcello Mancini[f], Erwin Stolz[g,h]

[a] Neurology Unit, Department of Neuromotor Physiology, Azienda Ospedaliera ASMN, Istituto di Ricovero e Cura a Carattere Scientifico, Viale Risorgimento 80, 42100 Reggio Emilia, Italy
[b] Neurology Unit, Ospedale Sant'Andrea, Via Vittorio Veneto 197, 19100 La Spezia, Italy
[c] Neurology Unit, Ospedale Madonna del Soccorso, Via Silvio Pellico 68, 63039 San Benedetto del Tronto, Italy
[d] Neurology Unit, Ospedala Cattinara, via Farneto 3, 34142 Trieste, Italy
[e] Neurology Unit, Azienda Ospedaliera di Padova, Via Nicolò Giustiniani 2, 35121 Padova, Italy
[f] Consiglio Nazionale delle Ricerche, Istituto di Biostrutturee Bioimmagini, University Federico II, via Pansini 5, 80131 Napoli, Italy
[g] Justus-Liebig University, Giessen, Germany
[h] Caritasklinik St. Theresia, Neurologische Klinik, Universisty of Saarlands, Germany

KEYWORDS
Cerebral venous hemodynamics;
Transcranial;
CCSVI;
Internal jugular vein;
Multiple sclerosis;
Transient global amnesia

Summary Because of the recent hypothesis of involvement of the venous hemodynamics in multiple sclerosis (MS), and because of the pitfalls of these studies, there is the need to achieve a definite conclusion from a large sample of subjects by using a strict and controlled neurosonological protocol. The aim of the advanced protocol, designed for a subgroup of the FISM study, is to analyze several items of the venous hemodynamics in order to obtain more pathophysiological data on venous circulation. *Advanced Ultrasound Protocol*: This is a multicenter, observational study. From a pool of about 1200 adults with MS, 400 healthy subjects and 400 subjects with other neurodegenerative disorders (2000 subjects in total) will be selected a population able to be examined by the advanced protocol. The examiner will always be blind on the clinical diagnosis, and the exams will be performed according to a standard protocol, whose measurements are mandatory for all participating centers. The advanced protocol is on a voluntary basis and it is optional. It includes, besides the basic one, measurements of blood flow volumes in carotid and vertebral arteries and in jugular and vertebral veins (inflow and outflow), with the definition of the drainage pattern. The ultrasound examination at each clinical site will

Abbreviations: BF, blood flow; BVR, basal vein of rosenthal; CCSVI, chronic cerebro spinal venous insufficiency; CSA, cross-sectional area; ΔCSA, difference between J2 IJV CSA in upright position and J2 IJV CSA in supine position; FISM, Italian Foundation on Multiple Sclerosis; ICA, internal carotid artery; IJV, internal jugular vein; MRI, magnetic resonance imaging; MS, multiple sclerosis; SRS, straight sinus; TAV, time averaged velocity; TCCS, transcranial color-coded duplex sonography; TS, transverse sinus; VA, vertebral artery; VV, vertebral vein.
* Corresponding author. Tel.: +39 0522 296494.
  E-mail addresses: zedde.marialuisa@asmn.re.it, marialuisa.zedde@tiscali.it (M. Zedde).

2211-968X/$ — see front matter © 2012 Elsevier GmbH. All rights reserved.
http://dx.doi.org/10.1016/j.permed.2012.03.013

be followed by a second centralized blinded evaluation. The prevalence of CCSVI in MS will be estimated, with confidence intervals at 95%, and compared with the prevalence in other groups. Moreover, multiple analysis will be done comparing venous hemodynamics in the three different groups.
© 2012 Elsevier GmbH. All rights reserved.

Introduction

Recently a vascular hypothesis about the cause of MS was proposed [1,2], pursuing the impairment of the cerebral venous drainage as a main factor in determining the manifestation of the disease and the disability, through the combination of multiple site venous lesions, mainly in the extracranial location. Five criteria were elaborated for the ultrasound identification of the more significant venous abnormalities (four criteria for the extracranial veins and one criterion for the intracranial veins), and the authors proposed that the presence of two or more positive criteria are diagnostic for a congenital malformation of the venous outflow, called by them CCSVI [2,3]:

1. reflux constantly present in IJV or vertebral veins (VVs) with the head at 0° and 90° assessed as flow reversal from its physiologic direction for a duration of >0.88 s during a short period of apnea following a normal exhalation
2. reflux in deep cerebral veins assessed as the presence of flow reversal for a duration of >0.50 s during normal breathing
3. high-resolution B-mode ultrasound evidence of proximal stenosis of the internal jugular vein (CSA < 0.3 cm^2)
4. flow not Doppler detectable in the IJVs or VVs despite numerous deep inspirations with the head positioned at 0° and 90°
5. reverted postural control of the main cerebral venous outflow (negative ΔCSA)

Both the careful reading and analysis of the ultrasound protocol described and applied by the proposing authors [1,2] and the negative findings of standardized ultrasound studies from other groups [4—7], raised many doubts about the ability of these criteria to provide a reliable evaluation of the cerebral venous hemodynamics. These considerations suggested to make efforts for identifying, applying and validating other ultrasound-assessable items for describing the venous hemodynamics.

FISM, a non-profit organization, is the promoter of a multicentre study, with the aim of obtaining the best response about the proposed hypothesis of a venous involvement in for people with MS worldwide. It will be possible through a study of large sample size to estimate the prevalence of venous abnormalities in MS, compared with the observed rate in normal controls and in patients affected by other neurologic diseases.

In this context, the distinctive features of the present study and previous studies comparing the current state of knowledge are as follows:

1. multicenter observational study with blinded ultrasound examination;
2. sample size of at least 1200 MS people

3. assessment of the prevalence of CCSVI and other forms of changes of venous hemodynamics in clinically isolated syndrome, relapsing-remitting, primary progressive and secondary progressive MS, using a larger sample than the one used to date.

A standardized ultrasound examination protocol was designed and implemented in a detailed training phase of the sinologist of the participating centres. The ultrasound protocol was distinguished in a basic protocol and an advanced protocol. The proposal of an advanced protocol came from the consideration that the assessment of the cerebral venous hemodynamics, both in intracranial and in extracranial pathways, does not mean only CCSVI, but it involves a global balance of the cerebral venous system (blood outflow patterns), validated measurement of valve function and a complete evaluation of the intracranial pathways and other items.

The topic of this paper is to provide some details about the advanced items of the ultrasound evaluation of the cerebral venous hemodynamics, starting from the critical evaluation of the five criteria proposed by Zamboni et al. for the diagnosis of CCSVI [1,2], with the aim of overcoming their limitations and finding the more proper items to evaluate the physiology and pathology of the cerebral venous hemodynamics.

Advanced ultrasound protocol

The definition of a more detailed and advanced study of the venous hemodynamics started from the highlight of the limitations and pitfalls of the proposed CCSVI criteria [1,2] and continued with the proposal of an alternative method to overcome them, considering the ultrasound methodological items from the literature.

Criterion 1

One of the main pitfalls of the criterion 1 is that the proposed temporal threshold for the jugular and vertebral reflux is validated only in other conditions, i.e. at the site of the valve leaflets of the IJV and with the Valsalva maneuver (Fig. 1), and not in other breath conditions and outside the valve level for the IJV and other veins [8,9].

Another doubtful aspect in the published studies with their description of the ultrasound protocol is the measurement of the reflux duration, because of the lack of mentioning and image documentation of the corresponding Doppler waveform.

Although breathing is a known factor affecting the venous hemodynamics, both in the neck and in the brain, there is not a validated "breathing activation maneuver", measurable, repeatable and reliable. Instead the Valsalva maneuver

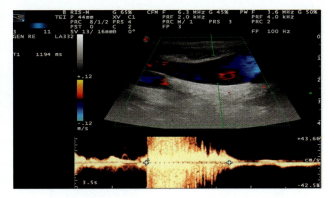

Figure 1 IJV valve incontinence lasting >0.88 s, elicited by a Valsalva maneuver.

is validated, executable in a measurable manner, with verifiable effects on IJV size and flow. Finally the threshold of 0.88 s is validated for diagnosing a significant valve incompetence of the IJV and it is not validated in other contexts and with other maneuvers.

Therefore, if the basic protocol contemplates the Valsalva maneuver as mandatory at the valve level, the advanced protocol added it along the extracranial course of IJV, at the level of its middle (J2) and distal (J3) segments. Outside the valve level there is not a validated threshold for a significant incontinence and maybe The inversion of the physiological flow direction during a Valsalva maneuver could not be called ''reflux'', but ''truncular incontinence''.

The execution of the Valsalva maneuver and its effects on volume and blood flow are well codified, also in mathematical models, both in supine and standing position, and both in the jugular and vertebral axis [10].

Fig. S1 shows the consequences of Valsalva maneuver also at middle (J2) and distal (J3) IJV segments of the IJV. But, why perform the Valsalva maneuver also in J2—J3 segments? The existence of a «truncular» jugular insufficiency is documented in patients with transient global amnesia with ultrasound techniques and the retrograde extent of this venous reflux into the sygmoid sinus has been found in this subgroup of patients by MRI [11—13].

Criterion 2

The main pitfall of this criterion is that Zamboni et al. [1,2] derived the threshold of >0.5 s from phlebological studies in CVI where it serves to quantify venous valve insufficiency following deflation of a tourniquet. Moreover the identification of the so-called intracranial reflux was performed by using a not validated window. In this study the known and validated temporal bone window will be used and in the advanced protocol also the TS is insonated, ipsi- or controlaterally.

The BVR is a virtually constant vein and it is very difficult to have abnormal flow patterns in it as a localized disease, outside cerebral vein thrombosis, particularly thrombosis of the SRS. The TS is characterized by a higher variability and it can be considered as a direct continuation to the IJV axis. Fig. S2 shows an abnormal flow direction in the Doppler waveform of the transverse sinus, as incidental finding in an asymptomatic subject.

Criterion 3

The main pitfalls of this criterion is that it was not defined consistently by Zamboni et al., because there are at least two different definition used in different papers:

- ΔCSA of <0.3 cm^2 [1]
- A local CSA reduction of >50% [2]

The first published studies of Zamboni et al. cited the paper of Lichtenstein et al. [14] as reference for the ultrasound diagnostic threshold of IJV stenosis, but the aim of the study was to assess the asymmetry of size of IJVs for selecting the best side to central venous catheterization, in 80 patients from Intensive Care Unit. Furthermore the asymmetry does not mean stenosis and the selected CSA for making the catheterization difficult is 0.4 cm^2. Moreover in angiographic studies of Zamboni et al. [15] there is not a pressure gradient across the venous stenosis.

In this protocol the threshold of CSA < 0.3 cm^2 was selected, coupled by a documentation of velocity parameters from a Doppler waveform.

In Fig. 2 there is an example of a positive criterion 3, but with a doubtful differential diagnosis between a so-called ''stenosis'' and a more physiological IJV hypoplasia.

Fig. 3 shows an ultrasound example of a real stenosis of the IJV at the valve level, in comparison with the MR venography of the same asymptomatic patient.

Criterion 4

The main pitfalls of this criterion derive from a general and nonspecific definition of this criterion. The authors [1,2] derived its validation from a study about extrajugular venous drainage pathways [16], comparing ultrasound and MRI and defining three types of venous drainage patterns: a total jugular volume flow of more than 2/3 (type 1), between 1/3 and 2/3 (type 2) and less than 1/3 (type 3) of the global arterial blood flow.

Moreover, in this study flow assessments were performed at rest and not during deep inspiration [17]. The documentation of a condition near to the ''blocked'' flow of the criterion 4 is provided in another pathological conditions, transient global amnesia, as a segmental IJV absence of flow with a reversed flow direction in IJV branches [12,13].

In Fig. 4, an example of this condition is shown in a patient with transient global amnesia. It is notable that the majority of so-called blocks are strictly positional conditions, often reversed by the ipsi- or contralateral tilting of the neck. For this reason in the present protocol, special attention was paid for avoiding to define a ''blocked'' flow in IJV if this condition was reversed by a minimal neck rotation.

It is also interesting to note that the situation described in Fig. 2 may gain two points, if the absence of flow is present in supine and upright positions, 1 for the criterion 3 and 1 for the criterion 4.

A global hemodynamics of the venous system rather than single segment evaluation is the aim; therefore a useful and validated tool is the calculation of the arterial blood flow and venous blood flow, as used in literature for distinguishing

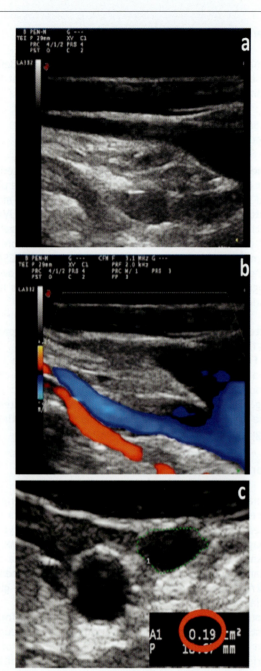

Figure 2 Example of the positivity of criterion 3. (a) B-mode ultrasound examination of the IJV in longitudinal scan. (b) Color-mode ultrasound examination of the IJV in longitudinal scan. (c) CSA measurement at J2 IJV level in transverse scan.

the cerebral drainage pattern in single subjects, because of the wide variability of the contribution of jugular, vertebral routes of both sides and extrajugular—extravertebral routes.

For this protocol the blood flow is calculated in both supine and standing position for IJV and VV for the outflow and for ICA and VA for the inflow (only in the supine position), by applying the formula BF = CSA × TAV [4,16,17].

Criterion 5

The definition of this criterion is that CSA of IJV in upright position is larger than the one in supine position, being the

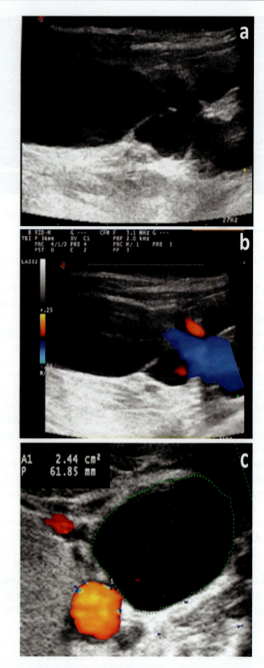

Figure 3 Example of an IJV stenosis at the valve level. (a) B-mode ultrasound examination of the IJV valve in their maximal opening position in longitudinal scan. (b) Color-mode ultrasound examination of the IJV valve in their maximal opening position in longitudinal scan. (c) CSA measurement at J2 IJV level in transverse scan.

normal condition the opposite one. Some authors questioned about a mistake for this criterion [4,7] and anyway a difference between right and left IJV in supine and upright position has been described in patients with transient global amnesia, because of the compression of the left brachiocephalic vein in the thoracic outlet [11].

This criterion has been proposed by Zamboni et al. [1,2] as a marker of the loss of venous compliance. In this protocol, considering the doubts expressed from other authors [4,7] also the deviation from the normal response to breath,

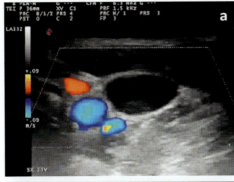
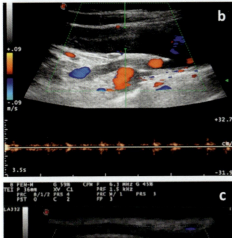
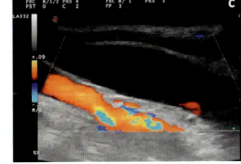

Figure 4 Example of the positivity of criterion 4. (a) Color-mode of the J2 IJV in transverse scan, showing the absence of color signal into the IJV lumen. (b) Corresponding Doppler waveform. (c) Color-mode of the J2 IJV in longitudinal scan, showing the absence of color signal into the IJV lumen.

with an increasing CSA during the inspirium phase and a decreasing CSA during the expirium phase, will be signaled, in order to better understand the global hemodynamic response.

Conclusions

The aim of the ultrasound study of the cerebral venous hemodynamics should be to understand the global hemodynamic responses and abnormalities, rather than to consider the alteration of the single segment of the single vein. For this aspect, it is possible that any criterion or combination of criteria cannot show this global view, but the blood flow study of inflow and outflow can help, in our opinion, to define a reliable and proper description of the global hemodynamics.

Appendix A. Supplementary data

Supplementary data associated with this article can be found, in the online version, at http://dx.doi.org/10.1016/j.permed.2012.03.013.

References

[1] Zamboni P, Galeotti R, Menegatti E, et al. Chronic cerebrospinal venous insufficiency in patients with multiple sclerosis. Journal of Neurology, Neurosurgery and Psychiatry 2009;80:392—9.

[2] Zamboni P, Menegatti E, Galeotti R. The value of cerebral Doppler venous haemodynamics in the assessment of multiple sclerosis. Journal of the Neurological Sciences 2009;282:21—7.

[3] Simka M, Kostecki J, Zaniewski M, Majewski E, Hartel M. Extracranial Doppler sonographic criteria of chronic cerebrospinal venous insufficiency in the patients with multiple sclerosis. International Angiology 2010;29:109—14.

[4] Doepp F, Paul F, Valdueza JM, Schmierer K, Schreiber SJ. No cerebrocervical venous congestion in patients with multiple sclerosis. Annals of Neurology 2010;68:173—83.

[5] Sundström P, Wåhlin A, Ambarki K, Birgander R, Eklund A, Malm J. Venous and cerebrospinal fluid flow in multiple sclerosis: a case-control study. Annals of Neurology 2010;68:255—9.

[6] Baracchini C, Perini P, Calabrese M, et al. No evidence of chronic cerebrospinal venous insufficiency at multiple sclerosis onset. Annals of Neurology 2011;69:90—9.

[7] Mayer CA, Pfeilschifter W, Lorenz MW, Nedelmann M, Bechmann I, Steinmetz H, Ziemann U. The perfect crime? CCSVI not leaving a trace in MS. Journal of Neurology, Neurosurgery and Psychiatry 2011;82:436—40.

[8] Nedelmann M, Eicke BM, Dieterich M. Functional and morphological criteria of internal jugular valve insufficiency as assessed by ultrasound. Journal of Neuroimaging 2005;15:70—5.

[9] Nedelmann M, Teschner D, Dieterich M. Analysis of internal jugular vein insufficiency — a comparison of two ultrasound methods. Ultrasound in Medicine and Biology 2007;33:857—62.

[10] Gisolf J, van Lieshout JJ, van Heusden K, Pott F, Stok WJ, Karemaker JM. Human cerebral venous outflow pathway depends on posture and central venous pressure. Journal of Physiology 2004;560:317—27.

[11] Chung CP, Hsu HY, Chao AC, et al. Detection of intracranial venous reflux in patients of transient global amnesia. Neurology 2006;66:1873—7.

[12] Chung CP, Hsu HY, Chao AC, Sheng WY, Soong BW, Hu HH. Transient global amnesia: cerebral venous outflow impairment-insight from the abnormal flow patterns of the internal jugular vein. Ultrasound in Medicine and Biology 2007;33:1727—35.

[13] Chung CP, Hsu HY, Chao AC, Wong WJ, Sheng WY, Hu HH. Flow volume in the jugular vein and related hemodynamics in the branches of the jugular vein. Ultrasound in Medicine and Biology 2007;33:500—5.

[14] Lichtenstein D, Saïfi R, Augarde R. The internal jugular veins are asymmetric. Usefulness of ultrasound before catheterization. Intensive Care Medicine 2001;27:301—5.

[15] Zamboni P, Galeotti R, Menegatti E, et al. A prospective open-label study of endovascular treatment of chronic cerebrospinal venous insufficiency. Journal of Vascular Surgery 2009;50:1348—58.

[16] Doepp F, Schreiber SJ, von Münster T, et al. How does the blood leave the brain? A systematic ultrasound analysis of cerebral venous drainage patterns. Neuroradiology 2004;46:565—70.

[17] Schreiber SJ, Lurtzing F, Gotze R. Extrajugular pathways of human cerebral venous blood drainage assessed by duplex ultrasound. Journal of Applied Physiology 2003;94:1802—5.

11. Nonvascular Neurosonography – Muscle, Nerve and Eye

B-mode sonography of the optic nerve in neurological disorders with altered intracranial pressure

Jochen Bäuerle*, Max Nedelmann

Department of Neurology, Justus-Liebig-University, Giessen, Germany

KEYWORDS
Optic nerve sheath diameter;
Optic nerve sonography;
Traumatic brain injury;
Idiopathic intracranial hypertension;
Spontaneous intracranial hypotension

Summary B-mode sonography of the optic nerve is a promising new technique in the field of neurology. It may serve as an additional diagnostic tool in different diseases with altered intracranial pressure. The aim of this article is to give an overview on this technique and on its possible clinical applications.
© 2012 Elsevier GmbH. All rights reserved.

Introduction

Over the past few decades the sonographic investigation of the eye and the adjacent structures in the orbit has become an important and well established tool in ophthalmology. It is crucial in the clinical work-up of patients suffering from a wide variety of ocular and orbital disorders.

Additionally, a growing body of literature demonstrates the usefulness of transbulbar B-mode sonography of the optic nerve for detecting raised intracranial pressure (ICP) in patients requiring neurocritical care. Therefore, neurologists increasingly take interest in this non-invasive and cost-effective bedside method. Even today ICP assessment continues to be a challenging task in critical care medicine. Invasive devices remain the cornerstone for measuring ICP in comatose or sedated patients but may not always be feasible due to a lack of neurosurgeons or contraindications such as coagulopathy or thrombocytopenia. Noninvasively, evaluation of pressure elevation relies on clinical symptoms or repeated CT or MR scanning to monitor for complications of raised ICP.

As part of the central nervous system the optic nerve is surrounded by cerebrospinal fluid and by meninges designated as optic nerve sheath. Hayreh shed light on the communication between the intracranial cerebrospinal fluid spaces and the subarachnoid space of the optic nerve sheath [1]. In his investigations in rhesus monkeys he described the development of papilledema in different situations of elevated ICP. Helmke and Hansen confirmed that ICP changes have an influence on the optic nerve sheath diameter (ONSD) [2]. In intrathecal infusion tests they found that the

Abbreviations: ICP, intracranial pressure; ONSD, optic nerve sheath diameter; IIH, idiopathic intracranial hypertension; CSF, cerebrospinal fluid.
* Corresponding author at: Department of Neurology, University of Freiburg, Breisacher Straße 64, D-79106 Freiburg, Germany.
Tel.: +49 761 27053060; fax: +49 761 27053100.
E-mail address: jochenbaeuerle@gmx.de (J. Bäuerle).

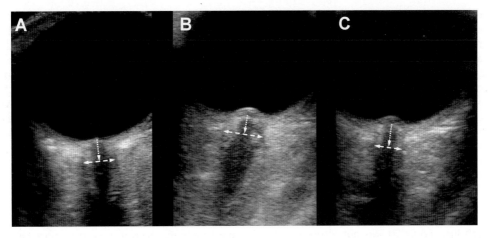

Figure 1 ONSD in IIH before and after lumbar puncture. (A) ONSD is measured 3 mm behind the base of the papilla (dotted arrow) in an axial plane showing the optic nerve in its longitudinal course. The dashed arrow denotes the ONSD. The picture for this figure was obtained from a healthy adult. Panel B shows the optic nerve sheath in a patient suffering from IIH. After lumbar puncture with therapeutic removal of CSF a normalization of the ONSD into the normal range could be observed without an apparent change of the optic disk elevation (C).

sonographic ONSD assessment is not suitable to evaluate exact ICP values, but may be used as surrogate variable of raised ICP. In contrast to the evolution of papilledema, ONSD changes correlated well with short-term ICP variations. This has been recently reproduced in an ultrasound-based study on brain injured patients [3]. Moreover, Helmke and Hansen developed a standardized transbulbar sonography technique for measuring the ONSD [4,5].

Transbulbar sonography

In our ultrasound laboratory we use a 9—3 MHz linear array transducer for transbulbar sonography of the optic nerve. Patients are examined in supine position with the upper part of the body and the head elevated to 20—30°. For safety reasons of biomechanical side effects we reduce the mechanical index to 0.2. The probe is placed on the temporal part of the closed upper eyelid using a thick layer of ultrasound gel. The retrobulbar part of the optic nerve can be depicted in an axial plane showing the papilla and the optic nerve in its longitudinal course. By convention the ONSD is assessed 3 mm behind the papilla. In order to gauge the ONSD, the distance between the external borders of the hyperechoic area surrounding the optic nerve should be quantified (Fig. 1).

Several studies reproduced a high intra- and interobserver reliability of the sonographic ONSD assessment [6—8]. However, data on normal values vary considerably, especially in former publications [9]. This may be explained by differing ultrasound equipments and their influence on sonographic findings and measurement criteria different from the ones stated above. Therefore, several authors emphasized the necessity of correctly used measuring points and clearly displayed optic nerve structures for reliable results [10,11].

In our study on this topic, using above criteria, the mean ONSD was 5.4 ± 0.6 mm in healthy adults that matches closely with results derived from two MRI studies [7]. Rohr et al. found a value of 5.3 ± 0.6 mm in patients with mental disorders but without intracranial lesions or signs of elevated ICP [12]. Geeraerts et al. indicated a mean ONSD of 5.1 ± 0.5 mm in healthy volunteers [13]. Accordingly, a cadaver study illustrated a good correlation between the evaluation of the ONSD by MRI and transbulbar sonography. Despite the unfavorable angle between the course of the optic nerve and the insonation direction in transbulbar sonography Steinborn et al. observed an acceptable agreement between MRI and the sonographic approach [11]. These results have been verified in an investigation of sixty-five children, recently [10].

Neurocritical care

In comatose or sedated patients with intracranial bleeding and traumatic head injury sonographic ONSD evaluation has been proven to be feasible in predicting raised ICP [3,14,15]. An MRI-based investigation confirmed this observation [13]. Geeraerts et al. found a mean ONSD of 6.3 ± 0.6 mm in brain injured adults using sonography [14]. By means of MRI they indicated a mean ONSD of 6.3 ± 0.5 mm [13]. The threshold of ONSD predicting an elevated ICP was proposed to be between 5.7 and 5.9 mm [3,13—15]. In a metaanalysis of six studies with data on a total of 231 patients with traumatic brain injury or intracranial hemorrhage the technique had a sensitivity of 90% and a specificity of 85% [16].

Furthermore, transbulbar ONSD assessment has been suggested for follow-up examinations of children with internal hydrocephalus and ventriculoperitoneal shunt systems [17]. Moreover, two sonographic investigations observed a correlation between the severity of acute mountain sickness and ONSD [18,19].

Idiopathic intracranial hypertension

Only few results were published on the sonographic ONSD evaluation in idiopathic intracranial hypertension (IIH) [20]. One MRI based retrospective study described a mean ONSD of 6.5 ± 0.9 mm in patients suffering from IIH and quote a cut-off value for raised ICP of 5.8 mm [21].

In a prospective study we examined the ONSD in ten adults with newly diagnosed IIH by transbulbar sonography before and after lumbar puncture [22]. Patients were recruited according to the updated diagnostic criteria of IIH and papilledema was documented in all subjects by an ophthalmological examination including funduscopy. Twenty-five individuals with other neurological disorders served as controls. Sonographic evaluation of the optic nerve was possible in all participants.

Compared to controls the ONSD was significantly enlarged among patients with IIH bilaterally [6.4 ± 0.6 mm vs. 5.4 ± 0.5 mm]. After lumbar puncture with a therapeutic removal of 30–50 ml of CSF we observed a significant decrease of the ONSD on both sides (right ONSD 5.8 ± 0.7 mm, left ONSD 5.9 ± 0.7 mm) (Fig. 1). However, in some patients with IIH, the ONSD was not altered or only slightly altered, e.g. a decline of 0.4 mm or more was only documented in five individuals. This may possibly be related to findings of a defective CSF circulation in the optic nerve sheath in this disorder, a state that is referred to as optic nerve compartment syndrome [23]. The ROC curve analysis revealed an optimal cut-off value for predicting raised ICP of 5.8 mm with a sensitivity of 90% and a specificity of 84%. The mean optic disk elevation in subjects with IIH was 1.2 ± 0.3 mm. Nevertheless, one patient showed no evidence of optic disk elevation in transbulbar sonography but had signs of papilledema in funduscopy. Corresponding to previous studies, we found no decrease of the optic disk elevation after lumbar puncture in the observation period of 24 h.

As a result sonographic ONSD evaluation may be useful in detecting raised ICP in patients with presumed IIH. Furthermore, our data suggest a potential usefulness of this technique for monitoring of treatment effects. In addition, ONSD values and optic disk levels were slightly asymmetric, reflecting the complex anatomy of the subarachnoidal space of the optic nerve and its possible influence on the cerebrospinal fluid dynamics. For this reason we recommend that each eye should be evaluated separately and mean ONSD values should be designated for both eyes.

Intracranial hypotension

Predominantly, the relationship of ONSD alterations and ICP changes was verified in clinical situations with raised ICP. One case series and one prospective study investigated the ONSD in spontaneous intracranial hypotension [24,25]. Examining the orbit with T2-weighted MRI techniques, they observed a collapsed optic nerve sheath.

Dubost et al. published an ultrasound study on ten patients with postdural puncture headache after lumbar puncture or epidural anesthesia [26]. Consistent with the mentioned MRI-results a small ONSD of 4.8 mm was detected before treatment. After successful therapy with a lumbar epidural blood patch a marked enlargement of the ONSD was found. Accordingly, in one patient in whom the intervention failed to resolve the headache they recorded no ONSD distension.

Recently, we examined a patient with spontaneous intracranial hypotension due to a cervical cerebrospinal fluid leakage in our ultrasound laboratory [27]. On admission transbulbar sonography revealed reduced ONSD of 4.1 mm on the right and 4.3 mm on the left side. After failure of medical treatment three consecutive targeted epidural blood patches were performed and a gradual extension of the ONSD was observed in both optic nerves [right 5.2 mm, left 5.3 mm]. In this article we documented changes of ONSD that were in line with initial clinical improvement and secondary worsening under conservative treatment and final improvement after occlusion of the cervical CSF leakage.

Limitations

Many studies on normal values found a relatively wide interindividual range of ONSD measurements [7,9,12]. Thus, as described previously absolute measurements of ICP will not be possible by transbulbar sonography [2]. Furthermore, with a false-negative rate of approximate 10%, ONSD values should only be interpreted in conjunction with clinical data and neuroimaging results.

Killer et al. found a decreased CSF circulation along the optic nerve in patients with IIH that seems to be a consequence of the complex trabecular architecture of the subarachnoid space of the optic nerve [23]. They proposed a compartment syndrome of the optic nerve sheath in sustained ICP elevation, as in IIH. In addition, Hayreh described varying degrees of communication between the intracranial subarachnoid space and the optic nerve sheath in different individuals [1]. This variety of the optic nerve sheath compliance and CSF fluid dynamics may limit the sonographic ONSD assessment in its value, especially for follow-up examinations, but on the other hand, may possibly allow to identify individual patients with continuing optic nerve compression albeit therapeutic lumbar puncture. Thus, studying long-term changes of the ONSD in different neurological disorders may be an interesting issue of future investigations.

With respect to the high variation of normal ONSD values published it is urgently necessary to determine consistent sonographic data in larger multicenter studies.

Conclusion

In summary, as a noninvasive and cost-effective bedside method transbulbar B-mode sonography is a promising technique for clinical neurologists. It may serve as an additional tool in neurocritical care medicine for detection of raised ICP. The method is of particular interest in situations when invasive ICP monitoring is contraindicated or when the expertise for invasive monitor placement is not immediately available.

Furthermore, it aids in the diagnostic work-up and in the follow-up of patients with IIH and in conditions of decreased ICP.

References

[1] Hayreh SS. Pathogenesis of oedema of the optic disc (papilloedema). A preliminary report. Br J Ophthalmol 1964;48:522–43.
[2] Hansen HC, Helmke K. Validation of the optic nerve sheath response to changing cerebrospinal fluid pressure: ultrasound findings during intrathecal infusion tests. J Neurosurg 1997;87(1):34–40.

[3] Geeraerts T, Merceron S, Benhamou D, Vigue B, Duranteau J. Non-invasive assessment of intracranial pressure using ocular sonography in neurocritical care patients. Intensive Care Med 2008;34(11):2062−7.

[4] Helmke K, Hansen HC. Fundamentals of transorbital sonographic evaluation of optic nerve sheath expansion under intracranial hypertension. I. Experimental study. Pediatr Radiol 1996;26(10):701−5.

[5] Helmke K, Hansen HC. Fundamentals of transorbital sonographic evaluation of optic nerve sheath expansion under intracranial hypertension. II. Patient study. Pediatr Radiol 1996;26(10):706−10.

[6] Ballantyne SA, O'Neill G, Hamilton R, Hollman AS. Observer variation in the sonographic measurement of optic nerve sheath diameter in normal adults. Eur J Ultrasound 2002;15(3):145−9.

[7] Bäuerle J, Lochner P, Kaps M, Nedelmann M. Intra- and interobsever reliability of sonographic assessment of the optic nerve sheath diameter in healthy adults. J Neuroimaging 2012;22(1):42−5.

[8] Shah S, Kimberly H, Marill K, Noble VE. Ultrasound techniques to measure the optic nerve sheath: is a specialized probe necessary? Med Sci Monit 2009;15(5):63−8.

[9] Lagreze WA, Lazzaro A, Weigel M, Hansen HC, Hennig J, Bley TA. Morphometry of the retrobulbar human optic nerve: comparison between conventional sonography and ultrafast magnetic resonance sequences. Invest Ophthalmol Vis Sci 2007;48(5):1913−7.

[10] Steinborn M, Fiegler J, Ruedisser K, Hapfelmeier A, Denne C, Macdonald E, et al. Measurement of the optic nerve sheath diameter in children: comparison between transbulbar sonography and magnetic resonance imaging. Ultraschall Med 2011 [Epub ahead of print].

[11] Steinborn M, Fiegler J, Kraus V, Denne C, Hapfelmeier A, Wurzinger L, et al. High resolution ultrasound and magnetic resonance imaging of the optic nerve and the optic nerve sheath: anatomic correlation and clinical importance. Ultraschall Med 2010 [Epub ahead of print].

[12] Rohr A, Riedel C, Reimann G, Alfke K, Hedderich J, Jansen O. Pseudotumor cerebri: quantitative in vivo measurements of markers of intracranial hypertension. Rofo 2008;180(10):884−90.

[13] Geeraerts T, Newcombe VF, Coles JP, Abate MG, Perkes IE, Hutchinson PJ, et al. Use of T2-weighted magnetic resonance imaging of the optic nerve sheath to detect raised intracranial pressure. Crit Care 2008;12(5):R114.

[14] Geeraerts T, Launey Y, Martin L, Pottecher J, Vigue B, Duranteau J, et al. Ultrasonography of the optic nerve sheath may be useful for detecting raised intracranial pressure after severe brain injury. Intensive Care Med 2007;33(10):1704−11.

[15] Soldatos T, Karakitsos D, Chatzimichail K, Papathanasiou M, Gouliamos A, Karabinis A. Optic nerve sonography in the diagnostic evaluation of adult brain injury. Crit Care 2008;12(3):R67.

[16] Dubourg J, Javouhey E, Geeraerts T, Messerer M, Kassai B. Ultrasonography of optic nerve sheath diameter for detection of raised intracranial pressure: a systematic review and meta-analysis. Intensive Care Med 2011;37(7):1059−68.

[17] Brzezinska R, Schumacher R. Diagnosis of elevated intracranial pressure in children with shunt under special consideration of transglobe sonography of the optic nerve. Ultraschall Med 2002;23(5):325−32.

[18] Sutherland AI, Morris DS, Owen CG, Bron AJ, Roach RC. Optic nerve sheath diameter, intracranial pressure and acute mountain sickness on Mount Everest: a longitudinal cohort study. Br J Sports Med 2008;42(3):183−8.

[19] Fagenholz PJ, Gutman JA, Murray AF, Noble VE, Camargo Jr CA, Harris NS. Optic nerve sheath diameter correlates with the presence and severity of acute mountain sickness: evidence for increased intracranial pressure. J Appl Physiol 2009;106(4):1207−11.

[20] Galetta S, Byrne SF, Smith JL. Echographic correlation of optic nerve sheath size and cerebrospinal fluid pressure. J Clin Neuroophthalmol 1989;9(2):79−82.

[21] Degnan AJ, Levy LM. Narrowing of Meckel's cave and cavernous sinus and enlargement of the optic nerve sheath in Pseudotumor cerebri. J Comput Assist Tomogr 2011;35(2):308−12.

[22] Bäuerle J, Nedelmann M. Sonographic assessment of the optic nerve sheath in idiopathic intracranial hypertension. J Neurol 2011;258(11):2014−9.

[23] Killer HE, Jaggi GP, Flammer J, Miller NR, Huber AR, Mironov A. Cerebrospinal fluid dynamics between the intracranial and the subarachnoid space of the optic nerve. Is it always bidirectional? Brain 2007;130:514−20.

[24] Rohr A, Jensen U, Riedel C, van Baleen A, Fruehauf MC, Bartsch T, et al. MR imaging of the optic nerve sheath in patients with craniospinal hypotension. AJNR 2010;31(9):1752−7.

[25] Watanabe A, Horikoshi T, Uchida M, Ishigame K, Kinouchi H. Decreased diameter of the optic nerve sheath associated with CSF hypovolemia. AJNR 2008;29(5):863−4.

[26] Dubost C, Le GA, Zetlaoui PJ, Benhamou D, Mercier FJ, Geeraerts T. Increase in optic nerve sheath diameter induced by epidural blood patch: a preliminary report. Br J Anaesth 2011;107(4):627−30.

[27] Bäuerle J, Gizewski ER, Stockhausen KV, Rosengarten B, Berghoff M, Grams AE, et al. Sonographic assessment of the optic nerve sheath and transorbital monitoring of treatment effects in a patient with spontaneous intracranial hypotension: case report. J Neuroimaging 2011, doi:10.1111/j.1552-6569.2011.00640.x.

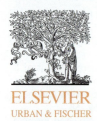

Bartels E, Bartels S, Poppert H (Editors):
New Trends in Neurosonology and Cerebral Hemodynamics — an Update.
Perspectives in Medicine (2012) 1, 408—413

journal homepage: www.elsevier.com/locate/permed

The retrobulbar spot sign in sudden blindness — Sufficient to rule out vasculitis?

Michael Ertl [a,*,1], Mathias Altmann [b,1], Elisabeth Torka [a], Horst Helbig [b], Ulrich Bogdahn [a], Anreea Gamulescu [b], Felix Schlachetzki [a]

[a] Department of Neurology, University of Regensburg, Bezirksklinikum Regensburg, Universitätsstraße 84, 93042 Regensburg, Germany
[b] Department of Opthalmology, University of Regensburg, Franz-Josef-Strauss-Allee 11, 93053 Regensburg, Germany

KEYWORDS
Vasculitis;
Stroke;
Blindness;
Diagnostic ultrasound;
Central retinal artery occlusion

Summary

Introduction: Sudden retinal blindness is a common complication of temporal arteritis (TA). Another common cause is embolic occlusion of the central retinal artery (CRA). The aim of this prospective study was to examine the diagnostic value of hyperechoic material in the CRA for exclusion of vasculitis as a cause. The authors used orbital color-coded sonography (OCCS) for the detection of hyperechoic material.

Materials and methods: Twenty-four patients with sudden visual loss were included in the study after opthalmoscopic exclusion of other causes (e.g. vitreous bleeding, retinal detachment). Parallel to routine diagnostic workup OCCS was performed in all patients.

Results: 7 patients with the diagnosis of TA presented with different degrees of hypoperfusion in the CRA without hyperechoic material (referred to as a ''spot sign'') detected by OCCS.

Diagnostic workup in the remaining 17 patients did not reveal any signs of TA. The hyperechoic spot sign was visible in 10 of 12 patients (83%) with embolic CRA occlusion. Altogether the frequency of the spot sign in this group was 59%.

Detection of embolic CRAO using the spot sign had a sensitivity of 83% and a specificity of 100%. The missing spot sign in patients with TA was a highly specific finding (*p*-value 0.01).

Conclusions: The ''spot sign'' is a highly specific finding, and its detection excludes the diagnosis of temporal arteritis in patients with sudden blindness. The finding of a spot sign helps prevent patients from receiving long-term steroid treatment, or an invasive temporal artery biopsy, with its immanent risks.
© 2012 Elsevier GmbH. All rights reserved.

Abbreviations: ACR, American College of Rheumatology; AFIB, Atrial fibrillation; AION, Anterior ischemic optic neuropathy; CRA, Central retinal artery; CRAO, Central retinal artery occlusion; DM 2, Diabetes mellitus type 2; ECST, European Carotid Surgery Trialists; ESR, Erythrocyte sedimentation rate; FA, Fluorescence angiography; ICA, Internal carotid artery; ION, Ischemic optic neuropathy; MI, Mechanical index; OCCS, Orbital color-coded sonography; OCT, Optic coherence tomography; PCA, Posterior ciliary artery; PION, Posterior optic neuropathy; TA, Temporal arteritis.
 * Corresponding author. Tel.: +49 941 941 0; fax: +49 941 941 3015.
   E-mail address: Michael.Ertl@medbo.de (M. Ertl).
 [1] Contributed equally.

2211-968X/$ — see front matter © 2012 Elsevier GmbH. All rights reserved.
doi:10.1016/j.permed.2012.02.048

Introduction

Sudden retinal blindness is a common complication of temporal arteritis (TA) due to ischemic optic neuropathy (ION) caused by vasculitic occlusion of the central retinal artery (CRA), the posterior ciliary artery (PCA) and other orbital arteries [1]. Depending on the affected arteries central retinal artery occlusion (CRAO), anterior optic neuropathy (AION) or posterior optic neuropathy (PION) are the results. In the elderly other common causes for hypoperfusion of the retina are thromboembolic events [2,3]. As a tool for the detection of TA, high-resolution ultrasonography of the superficial temporal artery has had a significant impact, with a high positive predictive value for the diagnosis of TA (specificity of 91%). However, a missing ''halo'' sign, suggestive for vessel wall inflammation seen on ultrasonography, does not sufficiently rule out presence of the disease (sensitivity 68%) and, therefore, superficial temporal artery biopsy remains the gold standard in the diagnosis of TA [4]. The differentiation of embolic versus arteritic occlusion remains a diagnostic challenge in elderly patients with ischemic optic neuropathy, because symptoms of TA, such as headache and elevation of inflammatory parameters, often coexist with significant cerebrovascular risk profiles. Additionally, depending on the cause of occlusion, different acute management strategies need to be applied quickly to improve long-term outcomes in these patients.

It is evident that we still need additional criteria with high negative predictive values to exclude the presence of vasculitis.

In a previously published series of patients with criteria for TA and sudden blindness, we found a hyperechoic embolic occlusion of the CRA in the area of the optic nerve head, which could be used to exclude TA; we called this a retrobulbar ''spot sign'' [5]. Foroozan et al. published a series of 29 patients with acute vision loss irrespective of the criteria for TA and observed this phenomenon in 9 patients with central retinal artery occlusion (CRAO) detected by retinal fluorescence angiography [6].

High-resolution color-coded ultrasonography can also be applied to the orbit since vitreous gel does not lead to any significant absorption of the incidental ultrasound beam. Orbital color-coded sonography (OCCS) allows detection of retrobulbar arteries and veins in addition to an assessment of orbital structures [7]. An analysis of Doppler flow spectra further aids the assessment and, to some degree the quantification, of retinal hypoperfusion due to CRA stenosis or occlusion. Normal flow velocity values within the CRA have been established previously [8].

This is the first prospective study in which patients suffering from acute vision loss due to either thromboembolic events or vasculitic changes in vessel walls were examined to identify the frequency of the ''spot sign'' in these specific disease patterns. We demonstrate that OCCS can be used to significantly discriminate embolic CRAO from arteritic causes of sudden ocular blindness in the elderly.

Materials and methods

Population and study protocol

The study protocol was approved by the local ethics committee at the University of Regensburg in accordance with the Declaration of Helsinki. Patients were first seen and screened at the Department of Ophthalmology of the University Hospital Regensburg. After exclusion of other reasons for visual loss, such as vitreous bleeding or retinal detachment, patients were referred to the Department of Neurology for OCCS and a routine neurovascular workup that included assessment of the superficial temporal artery. The funduscopic results were not disclosed before OCCS was performed. Before enrollment in the study, patients were made aware of the noninvasive and safe nature of OCCS and provided their written informed consent. In accordance with the study protocol, patients underwent routine diagnostic workups in the Departments of Ophthalmology and Neurology at our hospital, including registration of cerebrovascular risk factors, laboratory tests to detect criteria associated with TA (including the erythrocyte sedimentation rate [ESR]) according to American College of Rheumatology (ACR) criteria, a visual acuity test, retinal fundoscopy and color-coded sonography of brain-supplying arteries. All tests were performed within 24 h after admission.

Ultrasound equipment and data acquisition

For the visualization of retrobulbar structures, a high-resolution linear-array transducer with frequencies ranging from 8 to 15 MHz was used in combination with a Siemens Acuson system (Siemens AG, Erlangen, Germany) and a Toshiba XarioXG device (Toshiba, Tokyo, Japan). The acoustic output of the ultrasound systems was adjusted to the requirements of orbital sonography according to the ALARA principle (''as low as reasonably achievable'') to avoid damage to the lens and retina [9]. The settings for orbital sonography were the following: for B-mode, transmit frequency 14 MHz, mechanical index (MI) = 0.1, single focal zone at 2.5 cm, and bandwidth 74 dB; for C-mode, transmit frequency 10 MHz, MI = 0.2, color scale optimized for low velocities, and no wall filter; and for PW-mode, transmit frequency 2 MHz and MI < 0.44.

For OCCS the patients were placed supine with their eyes closed and asked to gaze forward. From above and slightly lateral, the transducer was placed with minimal pressure on the patient's orbit using plenty of contact gel. By definition the nasal side is depicted on the left image side.

Patient groups and statistical analysis

Depending on the final diagnosis and specific findings, patients were sorted into two different groups: (1) patients with a final diagnosis of TA; and (2) patients with visual loss on the basis of other pathologies. Patients were then further sorted depending on their funduscopic findings.

The frequency of the retrobulbar ''spot sign'' in patients with TA (group 1) was compared with that in patients without TA (group 2) by using a 2 × 2 table. A subgroup analysis was performed for patients with CRAO in funduscopy in both groups. Data analysis was performed using statistical software (IBM SPSS Statistics, Version 18, 2009, Armonk, USA). The independence of both variables (vasculitis and "spot sign") was tested using the exact Fisher test. Sensitivity and specificity were calculated including their respective confidence intervals.

Results

Between June 2010 and June 2011 we enrolled 24 patients with monocular blindness in this prospective study.

Group 1: 7 patients (3 male and 4 female) had retinal hypoperfusion due to TA. All 7 patients had 3 or more positive ACR criteria. In all but one patient, fundoscopic examination demonstrated AION with a blurred rim of the optic disc with optic disc edema and hyperemia with or without small splinter hemorrhages (Fig. 1d).

One patient had findings equivalent to CRAO, the diagnosis of TA was validated years before on the basis of ACR criteria by the Department of Rheumatology.

In 3 of the 7 patients we found a halo sign in the ipsilateral and/or contralateral superficial temporal artery during the ultrasound examination. The diagnosis was confirmed in 4 of 7 patients by means of temporal artery biopsy. In 1 patient, who was unable to undergo biopsy because of ongoing anticoagulation therapy with warfarin, a positive "halo" sign was identified in the left temporal artery. One patient had 4 out of 5 positive ACR-criteria but a negative finding in temporal artery biopsy. None of the patients in this group had a retrobulbar spot sign, but there was absent or pseudovenous flow in the CRA (Fig. 1a–c). Arterial hypertension was present in 4 patients, diabetes mellitus in 2 patients, hypercholesterolemia in 1 patient, and atrial fibrillation (AFIB) in a single patient who was treated with warfarin accordingly. One patient was a former smoker. The average number of risk factors per patient in this group was 2.

Group 2: 17 patients (8 male and 9 female) had sudden monocular blindness based on other pathologies than TA.

12 patients had CRAO in funduscopy. In 2 female patients we found typical fundoscopic findings of anterior ischemic optic neuropathy (AION). One male patient had small splinter hemorrhages in funduscopy but normal flow in both CRAs, probably as a result of recanalized CRAO. One male patient had an occlusion of a big retinal artery (CRA branch) with absent flow in the CRA, based on an ipsilateral ICA occlusion with collateralization from the contralateral ICA. One male patient with risk factors of hypertension, former tobacco use, and hyperuricemia, had a 90% stenosis (graded according to ECST criteria [10]) in the left ICA and visual loss in the left eye due to hypoperfusion of the left CRA; he was referred to vascular surgeons for carotid endarterectomy.

All of these patients had a maximum of 2 positive ACR criteria. On OCCS 10 (59%) of 17 patients had a visible hyperechoic plaque, known as "spot sign," at the tip of the CRA; taken in account only the patients with CRAO in funduscopy in this group, 10 of 12 patients (83%) had a visible "spot sign" and absent arterial flow (Fig. 2a and b). Moderate ipsilateral ICA stenosis (50–60% according to ECST criteria) was present in three patients (27%) and an additional 3 patients had contralateral ICA stenosis.

The average number of risk factors per patient in this group was 2.2. Arterial hypertension was present in 14 patients, AFIB in 2 and hypercholesterolemia in 7. Six patients had a history of smoking, 1 patient had hyperuricemia and 1 patient had comorbid migraine. Both of the patients with AFIB also had ICA stenosis on the ipsilateral side (both measuring 60% according to ECST criteria).

Summarizing, no patient with TA had a visible spot sign.

The spot sign was detectable in 10 out of 13 patients (73%) with CRAO. With the exception of one patient, CRAOs were not associated with TA. Taken in account only the patients with embolic CRAO (12 out of 13) the spot sign was present in 83% of the cases. No spot sign could be seen in patients with other forms of ischemic optic neuropathy (e.g. AION, retinal artery branch occlusion).

Statistical analysis

Using the exact Fisher test comparing the frequency of the spot sign in TA and non-TA patients we found a p-value of 0.01, the sensitivity of detecting embolic CRAO using the "spot sign" was 83% (95% CI: 65–99%). The specificity for embolic occlusions was 100% (95% CI: 65–100%).

Discussion

In this prospective study we demonstrate the diagnostic significance of retrobulbar ultrasonography for the differentiation of embolic and vasculitic causes of ischemic optic neuropathy.

The causes for ION can be subdivided into different groups, depending on the affected retinal arteries: CRAO, AION and PION [11]. TA, embolism or hypoperfusion are responsible for retinal ischemia in all subgroups. Reliable techniques to discriminate between the different forms are funduscopy and fluorescence angiography. Moreover FA can be helpful to show delayed filling or vascular leakage in choroidal vessels in AION for example. However, both methods cannot elicitate the underlying etiology because they lack sensitivity or depth penetration beyond the retina and thus cannot elucidate the underlying cause of ION.

Temporal arteritis (Horton disease or giant cell arteritis) and embolism from cerebrovascular disease require different acute and long-term therapeutic managements: for an embolic event, anticoagulation or platelet inhibition plus control of vascular risk factors should be initiated; whereas in TA, rapid initiation and long-lasting steroid therapy is essential. Due to the significant side effects of long-term steroid treatment, it is clear that a correct diagnosis is mandatory. So far, the only valid list of diagnostic criteria for TA has been established by the American College of Rheumatology. According to the ACR, 3 or more of the following criteria must be present for a diagnosis of TA: (1) age of 50 years or older; (2) new onset of localized headache; (3) temporal artery tenderness on palpation or decreased pulsation; (4) ESR of 50 mm/h or higher; (5) abnormal findings of a temporal artery biopsy. The sensitivity for this diagnosis was reported to be 93.5%, with a specificity of 91.2% for the discrimination of giant cell arteritis from other forms

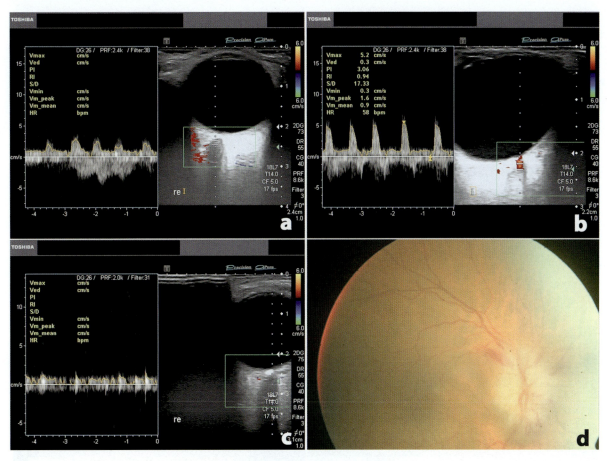

Figure 1 Ultrasound and funduscopic findings in patients with CRAO due to temporal arteritis. (a) Patient 1: a 84-year-old woman with visual loss for 2 days. Duplex- and color-mode OCCS images showing reduced flow in the affected CRA. (b) Patient 1: Duplex- and color-mode OCCS images showing normal flow in the unaffected contralateral CRA. (c) Patient 2: a 71-year-old man with visual loss for 2 weeks. Duplex- and color-mode OCCS images demonstrating zero flow in the affected CRA. (d) Patient 2: Funduscopic image showing a blurred rim of the optic disc, optic disc edema, and hyperemia, as well as a small splinter hemorrhage.

of vasculitis [12]. The main disadvantage of these criteria is that they were not developed and validated for diagnosis in the general population [13]. Secondly, a temporal artery biopsy with its immanent risks can provide false-negative results because of the possible ''skip lesion'' type of distribution of vasculitis-induced changes in the vessel wall. High-resolution ultrasonography of the superficial temporal artery has been proposed as an adjunct diagnostic tool in the workup of TA, and, indeed, an unequivocal finding of the halo sign has a high positive predictive value of > 90% [4]. Unfortunately, however, no halo finding does not sufficiently rule out presence of the disease.

Embolic artery occlusions are mainly due to atherosclerotic changes in the vessel wall, cardioembolism, or pathologies of the aortic arch [6]. Well-characterized risk factors for cerebral arterial occlusive diseases are hypertension, atrial fibrillation, coronary artery disease, diabetes mellitus, hypercholesterolemia, and tobacco use [14]. Within our patient groups an approximate mean of 2 of the aforementioned risk factors were present independent of the eventual cause of the occlusion. This underlines the inability to discriminate vasculitic from embolic causes of CRAO according to a specific risk profile.

The presence of the spot sign is highly suggestive for embolism, whereas vasculitic hypoperfusion is represented by absent or low-flow only. We found OCCS to be a highly specific tool in the further discrimination of these disease patterns in patients with sudden visual loss. The sensitivity of detecting embolic CRAO using the spot sign was 83% (95% CI: 65—99%), with a specificity of 100% (95% CI: 65—100%) to rule out vasculitic causes of ION. The missing spot sign in patients with TA was a highly significant finding ($p = 0.01$) despite the relatively small patient sample size. Thus, retrobulbar ultrasonography, an easy, safe, and rapid technique, should be considered in the workup in cases of sudden retinal blindness.

The only two retrospective studies of patients with sudden monocular blindness seem to have underestimated the frequency of the retrobulbar hyperechoic plaque, here referred to as the ''spot sign''. In the previously mentioned study by Foroozan et al. [6], the authors found the spot sign in 31% of patients using OCCS. In the second study, Ahuja et al. did not see any visible emboli in 18 patients with CRAO [14]. However, Ahuja et al. did not use OCCS in their study; they used only fundoscopy, a technique that visualizes typical signs of CRAO but no underlying pathological characteristics beyond the retinal level.

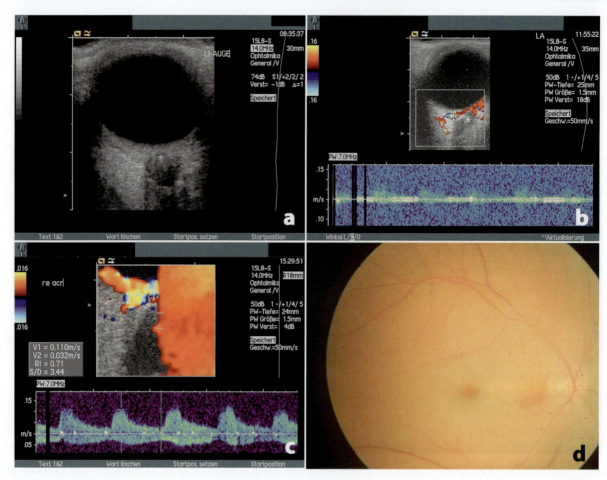

Figure 2 Ultrasound findings in a 77-year-old patient with embolic CRAO and visual loss for 3 days. (a) B-mode: hyperechogenic "spot sign" in the optic nerve head, representing an embolus in the distal CRA. (b) Duplex- and color-mode OCCS image depicting absent flow in the CRA. (c) Duplex- and color-mode OCCS image demonstrating normal flow in the unaffected contralateral CRA. (d) Funduscopic image showing a blurred rim of optic disc, the typical finding of a pale retina with a cherry-red macula (cherry-red spot) seen in patients with CRAO.

The presence of a spot sign on OCCS should lead to a detailed workup looking for sources of cardiac emboli (electrocardiography, echocardiography, long-term electrocardiography, and holter monitoring) and atherosclerosis (intima-media thickness measurements using carotid ultrasonography, presence of hemodynamically relevant carotid stenoses, and so forth). This may also prevent patients with a borderline diagnosis of giant cell arteritis (age >50 years, headache, elevated ESR due to other causes, or patients with ongoing steroid treatment obscuring the diagnosis) from receiving long-term steroid treatment with all its negative side effects or an invasive temporal artery biopsy with its immanent risks such as scalp necrosis [15] and facial nerve injury [16,17].

Conclusion

In summary, OCCS is a widely accessible method that can be used to discriminate different causes of sudden monocular blindness. Safety is ensured by the aforementioned technical modifications. Presence or absence of the "spot sign" helps to further discriminate embolic from vasculitic occlusion of the CRA. The expenditure of time for the examination is short and the technique is easily applied, even in the hands of less-experienced ultrasonographers.

Acknowledgments

We thank Florian Zeman of the Center for Clinical Studies, located at University Hospital Regensburg for his assistance in the statistical analysis. Further, we thank our collaborators in the Department of Pathology at the University Hospital Regensburg, especially Prof. Ferdinand Hofstätter, M.D., for providing fast results of the temporal artery biopsies. Special thanks go to our medical technical assistant, Beate Winheim, for conducting routine ultrasound diagnostic examinations of the brain-supplying arteries.

References

[1] McFadzean RM. Ischemic optic neuropathy and giant cell arteritis. Curr Opin Ophthalmol 1998;9(6):10—7.
[2] Brown GC, Magargal LE. Central retinal artery obstruction and visual acuity. Ophthalmology 1982;89(1):14—9.

[3] Gold D. Retinal arterial occlusion. Trans Sect Ophthalmol Am Acad Ophthalmol Otolaryngol 1977;83(3 Pt 1):OP392—408.

[4] Arida A, Kyprianou M, Kanakis M, Sfikakis P. The diagnostic value of ultrasonography-derived edema of the temporal artery wall in giant cell arteritis: a second meta-analysis. BMC Musculoskelet Disord 2010;11:44.

[5] Schlachetzki F, Boy S, Bogdahn U, Helbig H, Gamulescu MA. The retrobulbar ''spot sign'' — ocular sonography for the differential diagnosis of temporal arteritis and sudden blindness. Ultraschall Med 2010.

[6] Foroozan R, Savino PJ, Sergott RC. Embolic central retinal artery occlusion detected by orbital color Doppler imaging. Ophthalmology 2002;109(4):744—7 [discussion 747—8].

[7] Tranquart F, Bergès O, Koskas P, Arsene S, Rossazza C, Pisella P-J, et al. Color doppler imaging of orbital vessels: personal experience and literature review. J Clin Ultrasound 2003;31(5):258—73.

[8] Lieb WE, Cohen SM, Merton DA, Shields JA, Mitchell DG, Goldberg BB. Color Doppler imaging of the eye and orbit. Technique and normal vascular anatomy. Arch Ophthalmol 1991;109(4):527—31.

[9] Toms DA. The mechanical index, ultrasound practices, and the ALARA principle. J Ultrasound Med 2006;25(4):560—1.

[10] Arning C, Widder B, von Reutern GM, Stiegler H, Gortler M. Revision of DEGUM ultrasound criteria for grading internal carotid artery stenoses and transfer to NASCET measurement. Ultraschall Med 2010;31(3):251—7.

[11] Hayreh SS. Ischemic optic neuropathy. Prog Retin Eye Res 2009;28(1):34—62.

[12] Hunder GG, Bloch DA, Michel BA, Stevens MB, Arend WP, Calabrese LH, et al. The American College of Rheumatology 1990 criteria for the classification of giant cell arteritis. Arthritis Rheum 1990;33(8):1122—8.

[13] Watts RA, Scott DG. Classification and epidemiology of the vasculitides. Baillieres Clin Rheumatol 1997;11(2):191—217.

[14] Ahuja RM, Chaturvedi S, Eliott D, Joshi N, Puklin JE, Abrams GW. Mechanisms of retinal arterial occlusive disease in African American and Caucasian patients. Stroke 1999;30(8):1506—9.

[15] Dummer W, Zillikens D, Schulz A, Brocker EB, Hamm H. Scalp necrosis in temporal (giant cell) arteritis:implications for the dermatologic surgeon. Clin Exp Dermatol 1996;21(2):154—8.

[16] Slavin ML. Brow droop after superficial temporal artery biopsy. Arch Ophthalmol 1986;104(8):1127.

[17] Bhatti MT, Goldstein MH. Facial nerve injury following superficial temporal artery biopsy. Dermatol Surg 2001;27(1):15—7.

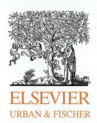
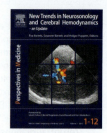

Bartels E, Bartels S, Poppert H (Editors):
New Trends in Neurosonology and Cerebral Hemodynamics — an Update.
Perspectives in Medicine (2012) 1, 414—416

journal homepage: www.elsevier.com/locate/permed

Ultrasonography of the optic nerve sheath in brain death

Arijana Lovrencic-Huzjan [a,*], Darja Sodec Simicevic [a], Irena Martinic Popovic [a], Marijana Bosnar Puretic [a], Vlasta Vukovic Cvetkovic [a], Aleksandar Gopcevic [b], Marinko Vucic [b], Bojan Rode [b], Vida Demarin [a]

[a] University Department of Neurology, University Hospital Center "Sisters of Mercy", Referral Center for Neurovascular Disorders of the Ministry of Health and Social Welfare of the Republic of Croatia, Referral Center for Headache of the Ministry of Health and Social Welfare of the Republic of Croatia, Zagreb, Croatia
[b] Department of Anesthesiology, University Hospital Center "Sisters of Mercy", Zagreb, Croatia

KEYWORDS
Optic nerve sheath diameter;
Ultrasonography;
Brain death;
Intracranial pressure

Summary Evaluation of optic nerve sheath by means of optic nerve ultrasonography (ONUS) is a reliable tool for assessment of patients with increased intracranial pressure. The aim of this study was to present the usefulness of optic nerve sheath ultrasonography in patients with brain death.

Ten patients with brain death as a result of traumatic or non-traumatic causes were evaluated by ONUS. Optic nerve sheath diameter (ONSD) was measured with a 12 MHz linear ultrasound probe (Terason T3000, Teratech Corporation, USA). The probe was adjusted to give a suitable angle for displaying the entry of the optic nerve into the globe, at the depth of 3 mm behind the globe. For each optic nerve four measurements were made, twice in transversal and twice in the sagittal plane, by rotating the probe clockwise. Mean ONSD for brain death patients were compared with mean ONSD of 17 healthy controls.

Ten individuals (7 males) with confirmed brain death (5 due to neurotrauma, 2 due to subarachnoid hemorrhage, 2 as a result of ischemic strokes and one of parenchymal hemorrhage), were evaluated. On the left side mean ONSD was 0.71 ± 0.06 cm on transversal plane and 0.72 ± 0.04 cm on sagittal plane. On the right side mean ONSD was 0.73 ± 0.05 cm on transversal plane and 0.73 ± 0.06 on sagittal plane. In controls left mean ONSD was 0.51 ± 0.05 cm on transversal plane and 0.55 ± 0.06 cm on sagittal plane. On the side right mean ONSD was 0.52 ± 0.05 cm on transversal plane and 0.54 ± 0.07 on sagittal plane. Mean ONSD in brain death was 0.72 ± 0.05 cm and 0.53 ± 0.06 cm in controls ($p < 0.01$).

Measurements of ONSD may be useful in distinguishing brain death persons from healthy controls.
© 2012 Elsevier GmbH. All rights reserved.

* Corresponding author at: University Department of Neurology, University Hospital Center "Sisters of Mercy", Vinogradska 29, Zagreb, Croatia. Tel.: +385 1 3768282; fax: +385 1 3768282.
E-mail address: arijana.lovrencic-huzjan@zg.htnet.hr (A. Lovrencic-Huzjan).

2211-968X/$ — see front matter © 2012 Elsevier GmbH. All rights reserved.
doi:10.1016/j.permed.2012.02.060

Introduction

Detection of increased intracranial pressure (ICP) is associated with poor outcome and therefore important in neurocritical care. Although invasive ventricular devices are the gold standard for continuous and reliable measurement of ICP, its placement could be challenging due to lack of immediate surgical availability, and their malfunction or obstruction has been reported. Transcranial Doppler sonography (TCD) is a suitable bedside method for daily assessment of the changes of ICP by continuous monitoring of the changes of blood flow velocities and pulsatility index, reflecting decreases in cerebral perfusion pressure due to increases in ICP [1]. However, its usage is restricted in patients with insufficient temporal bone windows. Noninvasive ocular ultrasonography has recently been proposed to detect elevated ICP, since the retrobulbar segment of the optic nerve is surrounded by a distensible subarachnoid space which can inflate during increase in cerebrospinal fluid pressure. Clinical studies have suggested that sonographic measurements of optic nerve sheath diameter correlate with clinical signs of increased intracranial pressure, and this technique could serve as a screening test in patients at risk for increased ICP, when invasive monitoring is not possible or is not clearly recommended [2—6].

Brain death is a clinical diagnosis developing after different pathological processes causing brain edema and raised ICP that finally lead to brain incarceration. As a result of extreme increased ICP, brain perfusion will cease, that is typically visualized as a stop of the contrast medium at the scull base on angiography. Several tests showing the cessation of brain perfusion are available like angiography, CT angiography, MR angiography and TCD [7,8].

The aim of this study was to present the usefulness of optic nerve sheath ultrasonography in patients with brain death.

Patients and methods

Ten patients with brain death as a result of traumatic or non-traumatic causes were evaluated by ONUS. Optic nerve sheath diameter (ONSD) was measured with a 12 MHz linear ultrasound probe (Terason T3000, Teratech Corporation, USA). The probe was adjusted to give a suitable angle for displaying the entry of the optic nerve into the globe, at the depth of 3 mm behind the globe (Fig. 1). For each optic nerve four measurements were made, twice in transversal and twice in the sagittal plane, by rotating the probe clockwise. Mean ONSD for brain death patients were compared with mean ONSD of 17 healthy controls (Fig. 2).

Data are presented as means and SD. Intergroup comparison was performed by Student's t-test.

Results

There were 10 patients (7 males) with confirmed brain death (5 due to neurotrauma, 2 due to subarachnoid hemorrhage, 2 as a result of ischemic stroke and one of parenchymal hemorrhage). Mean height was 163 ± 7 cm for females, and 179 ± 7 cm for males. Mean weight was 75 ± 13 kg in females

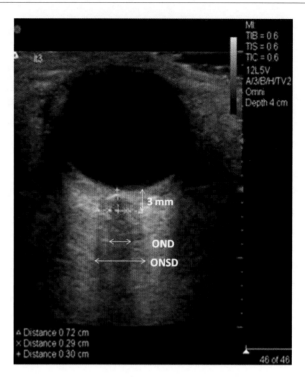

Figure 1 Measurement of optic nerve sheath diameter (ONSD) and optic nerve diameter (OND) in brain death.

and 86 ± 8 kg for males. Mean body mass index (BMI) was 26.7 ± 23.3.

There was no difference of measurements of mean ONSD between left and right eye in brain death persons or between measurements of mean ONSD between left and right eye in controls (Table 1). There was no difference of measurements

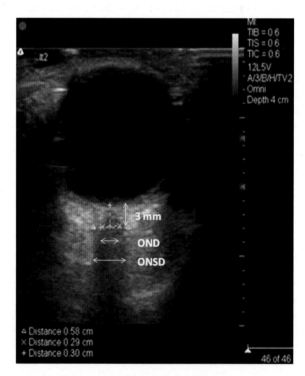

Figure 2 Measurement of optic nerve sheath diameter (ONSD) and optic nerve diameter (OND) in control.

Table 1 The comparison of mean optic nerve sheath diameter (ONSD) between brain death persons and controls.

	Brain death (N = 10)		Controls (N = 17)	
	Left (cm) mean ± SD	Right (cm) mean ± SD	Left (cm) mean ± SD	Right (cm) mean ± SD
Optic nerve sheath diameter transversal plane	0.71 ± 0.06	0.73 ± 0.0	0.51 ± 0.05	0.52 ± 0.0
Optic nerve sheath diameter sagittal plane	0.72 ± 0.0	0.73 ± 0.06	0.55 ± 0.06	0.54 ± 0.0
Mean optic nerve sheath diameter	0.72 ± 0.05		0.53 ± 0.06*	

* $p < 0.01$.

of mean ONSD either in left or right eye between measurement in transversal and sagittal plane in brain death persons or in between these two types of measurement of controls respectively (Table 1). Brain death persons have statistically significant wider mean ONSD measurements compared to measurements in controls with no overlapping of results (0.72 ± 0.05 vs 0.53 ± 0.06, $p < 0.01$) (Table 1).

Discussion

Brain death is a condition of extreme increase of intracranial pressure. Therefore we found statistically significant wider mean ONSD compared to controls. Up to now there was no report of ONSD in patients with brain death. Increased mean ONSD measurements were found in patients with increased ICP due to severe neurotrauma, or patients with spontaneous subarachnoid hemorrhage, intracranial hematoma or stroke. These patients had a mean ONSD of 5.99 ± 0.4 mm [6] and 6.3 ± 0.6 mm [4]. At the same time healthy controls had a mean ONSD of 5.1 ± 0.7 mm [4]. In our group of patients the same disease were the one leading to brain incarceration and finally to brain death. In our group we found a mean ONSD of 0.72 ± 0.05 cm. There was no difference if the measurement was performed in longitudinal or sagittal plain. Such measurements showed even wider ONSD compared to previously published results of patients with increased ICP [4–6]. At the same time, we found mean ONSD in controls 0.53 ± 0.05 cm, similar to previous published results of control subjects [4].

The optic nerve is a part of the central nervous system, surrounded by a subarachnoid space. The intraorbital part of the subarachnoid space is distensible and can therefore inflate if pressure in cerebrospinal fluid increases. Although there are limited reports on the values of OND and ONSD measurement by ultrasonography and no standardized values for healthy subjects, they usually have mean ONSD about 0.5 cm. In previous published results values of ONSD less than 5.8 mm were not likely to be associated with ICP increase above 20 mm Hg. Changes in ONSD are also strongly related to ICP changes. In patients with increased ICP mean ONSD were above 5.8 mm, and we found mean ONSD in brain death even higher, about 7.2 ± 0.5 mm. Such results are the consequence of extreme further increase of ICP in these persons due to brain incarceration.

The main limitation of this study was that all patients did not have invasive ICP monitoring to compare it with the results of ONSD. Also, some patients with neurotrauma had also ocular injury, disabling distinct demarcation of the optic nerve and optic nerve sheath, leading to some dispersion of results.

Conclusion

ONSD may be useful in distinguishing brain death persons from healthy controls.

References

[1] Hassler W, Steinmetz H, Gawlowski J. Transcranial Doppler ultrasonography in raised intracranial pressure and in intracranial circulatory arrest. J Neurosurg 1988;68:745–51.
[2] Geeraerts T, Duranteau J, Benhamou D. Ocular sonography in patients with raised intracranial pressure: the papilloedema revisited. Crit Care 2008;12:150.
[3] Girisgin AS, Kalkan E, Kocak S, Cander B, Gul M, Semiz M. The role of optic nerve ultrasonography in the diagnosis of elevated intracranial pressure. Emerg Med J 2007;24:251–4.
[4] Geeraerts T, Launey Y, Martin L, Pottecher J, Vigue B, Duranteau J, et al. Ultrasonography of the optic nerve sheath may be useful for detecting raised intracranial pressure after severe brain injury. Intensive Care Med 2007;33:1704–11.
[5] Blaivas M, Theodoro D, Sierzenski PR. Elevated intracranial pressure detected by bedside emergency ultrasonography of the optic nerve sheath. Acad Emerg Med 2003;10:376–81.
[6] Geeraerts T, Merceron S, Enhamou D, Vigue B, Duranteau J. Non-invasive assessment of intracranial pressure using ocular sonography in neurocritical care patients. Intensive Care Med 2008;34:2062–7.
[7] Lovrencic-Huzjan A, Vukovic V, Jergovic K, Demarin V. Transcranial Doppler as a confirmatory test in brain death. Acta Clin Croat 2006;45:365–73.
[8] Lovrencic-Huzjan A, Vukovic V, Gopcevic A, Vucic M, Kriksic V, Demarin V. Transcranial Doppler in brain death confirmation in clinical practice. Ultraschall Med/Eur J Ultrasound 2011;32:62–6.

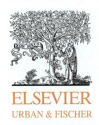

Ultrasonography of the peripheral nervous system

Henrich Kele*

Neurologie Neuer Wall, Neuer Wall 25, 20354 Hamburg, Germany

KEYWORDS
Nerve;
Sonography;
Compression;
Trauma;
Tumor;
Polyneuropathy

Summary With improvements in ultrasound (US) imaging equipment and refinements in scanning technique, an increasing number of peripheral nerves and related pathologic conditions can be identified. Modern US imaging supports the clinical examination and electrophysiologic testing in setting the diagnosis, and enhances this information by illuminating the morphological aspects and etiology of peripheral nerve pathology. US can readily be used for detection of nerve abnormalities caused by trauma, tumors, inflammation and a variety of nonneoplastic conditions, including compressive neuropathies. Well recognized advantages of the method such as the possibility of a dynamic examination, assessing long nerves segments in a short time, bed-side-availability, non-invasivity and low cost, make US the ideal imaging tool in peripheral nerve disease.
© 2012 Elsevier GmbH. All rights reserved.

Introduction

Diseases of the peripheral nerves are common in neurological practice. They are important differential diagnoses of nerve root lesions, and also of many musculoskeletal disorders in the fields of orthopaedy and rheumatology. The traditional diagnostics of peripheral nerve lesions is based on the clinical and electrophysiological findings. These methods reflect the functional status of the nerves and inform about the presence of nerve damage, its acuity, character (axonal / demyelinating) and regeneration processes. However, they do not inform about the morphological status of the nerves and their surroundings, especially in relation to the etiology of the disease. Ultrasonography visualizes these changes, so that it completes the information on nerve function and thus enhances the diagnostic information and contributes to the therapeutic decision. The contribution of the method in peripheral nerve diagnosis is comparable to diagnostic imaging (CT and MRI) in stroke or multiple sclerosis.

The first reports on nerve ultrasonography (NUS) were published already in the mid 1980s [1] detecting gross pathological changes, e.g. nerve tumors. But only the substantial improvement of ultrasound technology at the turn of the millennium enabled an accurate diagnostic visualization of the peripheral nerves. The following article gives an overview of the technical requirements, the examination technique and current applications of NUS in the diagnosis of peripheral nerve disease.

Technical requirements, equipment settings, and examination technique

For sonography of the peripheral nerves a high image quality and resolution are critical. For an optimal resolution a high-end ultrasound unit equipped with a high-resolution broadband linear-array probe (e.g. 5–17 MHz) and corresponding soft-tissue software are necessary. In the case of a 15 MHz transmission frequency, an axial resolution of up to 250 μm is achieved. Depending on the type of probe and

* Tel.: +49 40 3006876 0; fax: +49 40 3006876 40.
E-mail address: kele@neurologie-neuer-wall.de
URL: http://www.neurologie-neuer-wall.de/.

focusing, the highest resolution is achieved at a depth of approximately 0.5—1.5 cm from the skin [2]. The scanning frequency used is depending on the examined nerve and the clinical question. For superficial nerves (e.g. median nerve in the carpal tunnel or ulnar nerve at the elbow) the maximum frequency (up to 18 MHz) can be applied. Due to the limitation of the penetration depth of high frequencies, in deeper lying nerves or nerve segments (e.g. median nerve at the proximal forearm or sciatic nerve), lower frequencies (down to 5 MHz) are required. With low ultrasound frequencies, the resolution is worse and the differentiability of the nerves in the surrounding tissue as well as of their internal structure becomes difficult. Good ultrasonic devices allow up to a depth of about 2.5 cm also an assessment of subtle changes.

In addition to a high physical resolution, the soft-tissue contrast in particular, is decisive for optimal visualization of the peripheral nerves. Special software, e.g. "compound-imaging", "high-resolution-imaging", is very helpful in this process. Additional tools, e.g. extended field of view imaging, which create a panorama image from numerous individual images, can improve image documentation.

The application of color coded sonography (color Doppler or power Doppler) allows assessing the vascular situation of the nerves and their surroundings. This is particularly useful in inflammatory conditions, nerve tumors or compressive neuropathies. Color coded sonography is also helpful in localizing nerves that are often accompanied by vessels (e.g. radial nerve at the lateral upper arm accompanied by the profound brachial artery; sural nerve accompanied by a vein). For color Doppler, a small-flow-setting of the ultrasound device is recommended (pulse repetition frequency 500 Hz, band-pass filter 50 Hz). It is important to notice that an exploratory study, even without high-end ultrasound equipment, can detect major changes, such as severe nerve compression or a mass lesion. For the assessment of fine structures or complex changes, such as in post-operative conditions or nerve injuries, however, high-quality equipment is required. In addition to the apparative equipment a good knowledge of the regional topographic anatomy is important. Further, the examiner's expertise in diseases of the peripheral nervous system and electrophysiological knowledge facilitate the interpretation of NUS.

The typical examination of peripheral nerves begins with transverse sections. The nerve is initially visualized at a site with typical anatomical landmarks (e.g. median nerve in the carpal tunnel, ulnar nerve in the sulcus). After image optimization, the nerve can be followed further continuously in the proximal and distal directions, and in the area of suspected pathology. The site of underlying pathology is normally located in transverse sections, for a more precise information longitudinal scans and the examination of vascularization with color coded sonography are performed.

What nerves can be examined?

In normal-weight people, all major nerves of the extremities, e.g. the median, ulnar, radial, sciatic, tibial and peroneal nerves, can be visualized in their entire course at the extremities. Even smaller nerves, e.g. the interosseus posterior and the superficial radial nerve, are regularly

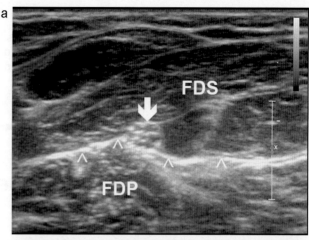

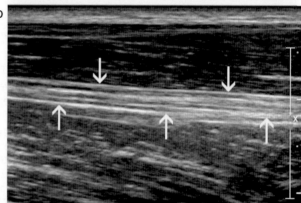

Figure 1 (a and b): Normal median nerve (arrows) in the mid of the forearm. Notice the echotexture in the transversal (honeycomb-like) and longitudinal (fascicular) scans. FDS = superficial finger flexor, FDP = deep finger flexor. Arrowheads = fascia between the muscles.

displayed. The spinal nerves C4-C8 and the supraclavicular brachial plexus can also be visualized, but especially the inferior trunk and the fascicles are not constantly imaged in good quality. The visualization of the infraclavicular and infrapectoral brachial plexus is restricted by the clavicle and the depth of the structures. Cranial nerves like the vagal and accessory nerves, can be visualized regularly. Particularly in obese patients, the examination of the sciatic nerve in the thigh and tibial nerve at the proximal lower leg is difficult or even impossible. In lean people, however, even small sensory nerves, such as the saphenous, sural and superficial peroneal nerve as well as the lateral femoral cutaneous nerve can be assessed.

Sonography of healthy peripheral nerves

The nerves are cable-like structures that appear on transverse sections as round to oval hyperechoic structures (Fig. 1a). They are surrounded by an echogenic rim representing the epifascicular epineurium and the perineurial fatty tissue. The sonographic echo pattern (echotexture) is called "honeycomb-shaped" [3]. The rounded hypoechoic areas correspond histologically to the nerve fascicles, and the echogenic septa to the interfascicular epineurium. In

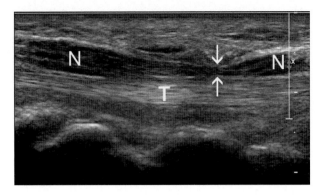

Figure 2 Longitudinal scan of median nerve compression (arrows) in the carpal tunnel. N = nerve, T = tendons. Left is proximal.

large nerves a clear cable-like fascicular echotexture can be seen (Fig. 1b). With color coded sonography the epineurial vasa nervorum can be displayed in some nerves (e.g. median nerve at the distal forearm).

Pathological findings

Compressive neuropathies

Nerve sonography is nowadays used in all disease categories of the peripheral nervous system. The compressive neuropathies, and in particular entrapment syndromes, are the most common illnesses. NUS allows examination of the most frequent entrapment sites in the upper extremities, e.g. the carpal tunnel (median nerve), the cubital tunnel and the Guyons canal (ulnar nerve), and the supinator tunnel (interosseus posterior nerve). In the lower extremities, peroneal nerve at the fibular head, tibial nerve in the tarsal tunnel, the interdigital nerves (Morton-Metatarsalgia) and the lateral femoral cutaneous nerve can be examined. The basic diagnostic criterion is the visualization of nerve compression, which appears regardless of anatomic location on longitudinal scans as an abrupt flattening (notching) at the site of nerve compression and a fusiform swelling proximal and distal to it (Fig. 2). The swelling is accompanied, depending on the degree of compression, by a hypoechogenicity and a reduction of visibility or extinction of the typical fascicular echotexture resulting of nerve edema. Correspondingly, the transverse sections show an enlargement of the nerve cross-sectional area of a hypoechoic nerve. The sonographic findings thus reflect the pathomorphological changes in terms of nerve constriction at the site of compression and the pseudoneuroma formation. In addition, NUS allows evaluation of the surrounding structures and finding nerve compression etiology, e.g. compression by a mass lesion. Anatomical variations can be evaluated as well. Thus, NUS helps in planning and timing of further therapy (conservative / operative, e.g. in case of compression by a mass lesion early surgical therapy).

Carpal Tunnel syndrome

Carpal tunnel syndrome (CTS) is the most common peripheral nerve disorder with a lifetime prevalence of about 15%. In typical cases the longitudinal scans show a nerve compression under the flexor retinaculum with the formation of a pseudoneuroma proximally and (often to a lesser extent) distally to the retinaculum. The transversal scans show a nerve enlargement at the site of pseudoneuroma, which is quantified by cross-sectional area measurements at the level of the carpal tunnel inlet (pisiform bone). In seldom cases, an enlargement at the carpal tunnel outlet only can be seen. NUS has a sensitivity (from 73% to 92%) and specificity comparable to electrophysiological methods [4]. Further, NUS represents a complementary method to the electrophysiological evaluation. Even with normal electrophysiology NUS can detect pathological findings, and vice versa. An even more important contribution of NUS is to rule out secondary CTS that includes tenosynovitis of the flexor tendons, ganglia, arthritic changes, amyloid deposits, accessory muscles or median artery thrombosis [5,6]. Furthermore, anatomical variants such as prolonged muscle bellies of the finger flexors reaching into the tunnel, can be detected. More important are nerve variants such as bifid median nerve divided into two strands already in the carpal tunnel or variants of the thenar branch (subligamentary or transligamentary course). Also, vessel variants like a persisting median artery or atypical course of the ulnar artery, can be seen. The detection of such normal variants can be significant especially for the endoscopic surgeon. In every third patient with CTS, sonography found one of the above-mentioned structural abnormalities [6]. Therefore, contrary to the prevailing opinion, CTS cannot be regarded as an idiopathic condition. NUS plays a very important role in postoperatively persisting or recurrent CTS. It allows visualization of surgically treatable causes like incomplete retinaculum transection with persistent nerve compression or surgery complications such as abnormal scarring or iatrogenic nerve injury. Based on personal experience, sonography can reveal a false preoperative diagnosis showing conditions mimicking CTS like nerve tumor [7] or neuritis.

Ulnar neuropathy at the elbow

Ulnar neuropathy in the elbow region (UNE) comprises three entities with their own etiology, and therapy. The cubital tunnel syndrome represents the most common disorder. Its pathological basis is a nerve compression under the aponeurosis between the origins of the ulnar flexor muscle of the wrist (humeroulnar arcade). Correspondingly, ultrasound shows a flattening of the nerve under the arcade with a proximal swelling in the sulcus. Cross-sectional areas greater than 0.1 cm^2 accompanied by a hypoechoic appearance and loss of the honeycomb echotexture, are diagnostic for cubital tunnel syndrome. Another entity is caused by a repetitive subluxation or luxation of the nerve out of the sulcus leading to chronic pressure damage. A lacking or loose humeroulnar arcade is postulated as a reason for this. In the case of subluxation, the ulnar nerve is located at the tip of the medial epicondyle at maximum elbow flexion. In the case of luxation, it is dislocated volar to the medial epicondyle. The nerve dislocation is often accompanied by a nerve swelling [2].

Further, space-occupying lesions such as ganglia, lipomas, arthritic changes, accessory muscles, or a dislocation of the medial triceps head ("snapping triceps syndrome") can be reliably identified. In these cases, the compression is often located proximal to the cubital tunnel, which may result in atypical electrophysiological findings.

The diagnostic value of sonography is comparable with electrophysiological methods, in combination it improves the diagnostic yield. In addition, it provides prognostic information: the extent of swelling in the sulcus correlates negatively with clinical improvement after surgery [8].

Less common compression syndromes

Since the less common compression syndromes affect mostly smaller nerves, the sonographic depiction of a direct nerve compression is more difficult. Therefore, the main role of sonography lies in the recognition of neighborhood processes as compression factors. Thus, sonography can detect space-occupying lesions such as ganglia or lipomas affecting the ulnar nerve in Guyon's Loge, the median nerve at the proximal forearm, the interosseous posterior nerve in the supinator tunnel, the axillary nerve in the quadrilateral space as well as the suprascapular nerve. In the so-called algetic interosseus-posterior-syndrome an ultrasound-guided infiltration can be performed for diagnostic purposes. In thoracic-outlet-sydrome, sonography can reveal a compression of the spinal nerve C7 or C8 by a cervical rib. In the lower extremities, peroneal nerve at the fibular head and tibial nerve in the tarsal tunnel can be affected by different soft tissue masses (enlarged bursae, ganglia, heterotopic ossification after trauma). Especially the peroneal nerve can be affected by intraneural ganglia emerging from tibiofibular joint via the articular branch [9]. In Morton's metatarsalgia a "neuroma-like enlargment" of the second or third plantar interdigital nerve can be seen. Even in obese patients with meralgia paresthetica, a compression of the lateral femoral cutaneous nerve can be demonstrated and combined with an ultrasound-guided infiltration (personal experience).

Sonography of peripheral nerve tumors

The diagnosis of peripheral nerves with ultrasound was described in literature back in the 1980s. This was possible because large nerve tumors could be detected even with older transducers with a low scanning frequency (around 7 MHz). The two most common types of tumors are schwannomas (neurinoma) and neurofibromas. Sonographically, both appear as well-defined, round masses with a hyperechoic rim, which are localized in the course of a peripheral nerve. Schwannomas (Fig. 3) are mostly homogeneously hypoechoic and lie eccentric to the long nerve axis, in contrast to neurofibromas, which lie central. Neurofibroma's echogenicity is higher and distributed in the center of the mass (so called target sign) [10]. Schwannomas show often a hypervascularization in color coded examination, in neurofibromas no significant internal perfusion can be seen even in contrast enhanced ultrasound [11]. Plexiform neurofibromas, which occur typically in neurofibromatosis type 1 (von Recklinghausen's disease), spread over long segments of one or more nerves. The nerves are infiltrated with small nodules which form a dysmorph mass of heterogeneous echogenicity uplifting the inner nerve architecture ("sack full of worms") [12]. Perineuriomas are generally less well known. They

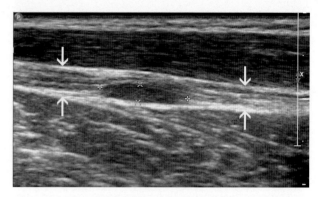

Figure 3 Longitudinal scan of a small ulnar nerve schwannoma (markers) in the forearm. Arrows = ulnar nerve.

appear often in young patients and present with painless progressive motor deficits. With NUS they appear as fusiform hypoechogenic structures without vascularization spreading over several centimeters.

A sonographic screening examination for the presence of nerve tumors should be performed in every etiologically unexplained neuropathy. The affected nerve has to be visualized in its entire course of the limb. This investigation is also possible without a high-quality technical equipment.

Generalized neuropathies (polyneuropathies)

In generalized neuropathies, ultrasonography is not routinely used yet. In a variety of diseases, however, NUS can demonstrate a generalized enlargement (edema) of the peripheral nerves, e.g. in acromegaly, or diabetes mellitus, which explains the frequent occurrence of entrapment syndromes. A generalized nerve hypertrophy is also found in hereditary neuropathies (e.g. HMSN 1) [13]. In immune-mediated inflammatory neuropathies (e.g. AIDP, CIDP, MMN), a so called hypertrophic remodeling of the peripheral nerves is present. It is characterized by nerve hypertrophy and a variation of individual fascicle thickness changing in the nerve course (personal experience). Focal nerve or fascicle thickening can also be found in painful mononeuropathies with a possibly immunologic etiology. Sonography can also differentiate nerve compression syndromes in polyneuropathies, which is particularly difficult with electrophysiological methods.

Sonography of traumatic nerve lesions

Sonography has an important role in the assessment of traumatic neuropathies. For the investigation is a high-quality equipment of great benefit, since it facilitates the presentation of changes in difficult conditions with tissue edema, hematomas, and scars. NUS can assess the continuity and integrity of the nerve, characterize the defect, and identify secondary nerve compression. Thereby, location, extent and type of damage are determined. This allows displaying a complete and partial nerve transection, the distance and condition of the stumps (formation of a neuroma) or a compression of the nerve, for example by scars, osteosynthetic material, callus formation, bone fragments, hematomas, or foreign bodies [2]. The most frequent

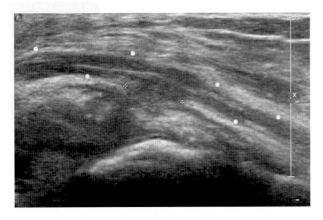

Figure 4 Longitudinal scan of an iatrogenic lesion of the ulnar nerve (points) after arthroscopy. Notice the partial nerve transection with discontinuous epifascicular epineurium (between markers).

alteration found in nerve trauma is axonal swelling. The nerve and its fascicles show a hypoechoic thickening over several centimeters, in proximal limb lesions sometimes affecting the whole extremity. In severe traumas, axonal swelling persists over several months and diminishes from proximal to distal with the forthcoming reinnervation (personal experience). Sonography allows differentiating major nerve trauma that requires surgical therapy, i.e. a complete and partial nerve neurotmesis. Since the degree of stump dehiscence determines the surgical procedure (neurorrhaphy in the case of a small defect, nerve transplant in the case of greater dehiscence), the distance of the nerve stumps should be measured. In longitudinal scans an amputation neuroma appears as a hypoechoic thickening or a bulbous mass where the nerve ends. In the case of a partial nerve transection, also intact parts of the nerve and its interfascicular epineurium can be seen (Fig. 4). This type of lesion is very difficult to diagnose with clinical and electrophysiological methods especially in the early post-traumatic period (within 3 months). Neuroma-in-continuity is represented by a fusiform hypoechoic thickened nerve with extincted nerve echotexture. Thus, NUS can facilitate the therapeutic decisions and initiate early surgical intervention using the appropriate method (neurorrhaphy, nerve grafting or neurolysis). Postoperative complications such as dehiscence of the nerve sutures or abnormal scarring can be identified, too.

Conclusion

The complete diagnosis of peripheral nerve damage includes not only the evaluation of nerve function with clinical and electrophysiological methods, but also the assessment of nerve morphology with imaging methods. Sonography allows not only to set the diagnosis, but also to reveal the etiology of the condition. Hence, early and appropriate therapeutic measures can be derived. Sonography can be used as the screening imaging tool for all disease categories of the peripheral nervous system.

References

[1] Fornage BD. Peripheral nerves of the extremities: imaging with US. Radiology 1988;167:179—82.
[2] Kopf H, Loizides A, Mostbeck GH, Gruber H. Diagnostic sonography of peripheral nerves: indications, examination technique and pathological findings. Ultraschall Med 2011;32:242—63.
[3] Martinoli C, Bianchi S, Derchi LE. Ultrasonography of peripheral nerves. Semin Ultrasound CT MRI 2000;21:205—13.
[4] Beekman R, Visser LH. High-resolution sonography of the peripheral nervous system—a review of the literature. Eur J Neurol 2004;11:305—14.
[5] Buchberger W, Schoen G, Strasser K, et al. High-resolution ultrasonography of the carpal tunnel. J Ultrasound Med 1991;10:531—7.
[6] Kele H, Verheggen R, Bittermann HJ, Reimers CD. The potential value of ultrasonography in the evaluation of carpal tunnel syndrome. Neurology 2003;61:389—92.
[7] Kele H, Verheggen R. Median nerve neurofibroma. J Neurol Neurosurg Psychiatry 2003;74:912.
[8] Beekman R, Schoemaker MC, van der Plas JP, et al. Diagnostic value of high-resolution sonography in ulnar neuropathy at the elbow. Neurology 2004;62:767—73.
[9] Visser LH. High-resolution sonography of the common peroneal nerve: detection of intraneural ganglia. Neurology 2007;67:1473—5.
[10] Lin J, Martel W. Cross-sectional imaging of peripheral nerve sheath tumors: characteristic signs on CT MR imaging, and sonography. AJR Am J Roentgenol 2001;176:75—82.
[11] Reynolds Jr DL, Jacobson JA, Inampudi P, Jamadar DA, Ebrahim FS, et al. Sonographic characteristics of peripheral nerve sheath tumors. Am J Roentgenol 2004;182:741—4.
[12] Bacigalupo L, Bianchi S, Valle M, et al. Ultrasonography of the peripheral nerves. Radiology 2003;43:841—9.
[13] Martinoli C, Schenone A, Bianchi S, Mandich P, Caponetto C, Abruzzese M, Derchi LE. Sonography of the median nerve in Charcot-Marie-tooth disease. Am J Roentgenol 2002;178:1553—6.

Ultrasonography of peripheral nerves — Clinical significance

Ulf Schminke*

Department of Neurology, Ernst Moritz Arndt University Greifswald, Ferdinand-Sauerbruch-Str, 17475 Greifswald, Germany

KEYWORDS
Ultrasonography;
Entrapment neuropathy;
Nerve sheath tumor;
Traumatic nerve lesion;
Polyneuropathy

Summary   Over the past two decades, high-resolution ultrasonography of peripheral nerves has been evolved as an adjunctive examination technique in clinical neurophysiology laboratories providing complementary information to electrodiagnostic studies. In addition to the information on nerve function, which are typically obtained by nerve conduction studies and electromyography, ultrasonography permits direct assessment of pathologic changes in nerve structure and/or in the adjacent tissue, as well. This article reviews the clinical significance of ultrasonography for the diagnostic evaluation of focal neuropathies, particularly entrapment neuropathies, traumatic nerve lesions, nerve sheath tumors, and several types of polyneuropathies. Ultrasonography offers neuromuscular clinicians a unique opportunity to conduct both complementary examination modalities by themselves without referring patients to another laboratory.
© 2012 Elsevier GmbH. All rights reserved.

Introduction

Since the first reports on sonographic evaluation of peripheral nerves [1,2], high-resolution ultrasound has evolved rapidly over the past two decades. The ability of ultrasonography to visualize even small structures like peripheral nerves makes ultrasonography complementary to electrodiagnostic studies. In addition to the information on nerve function, which is typically provided by nerve conduction studies (NCS) and electromyography (EMG), neuromuscular ultrasound permits direct assessment of pathologic changes in nerve structure and/or in the adjacent tissue, as well. Most commonly, ultrasonography has been studied for the diagnosis of focal neuropathies, specifically of entrapment neuropathies at various sites throughout the arm and leg. Furthermore, this technique has been proved valuable for the examination of traumatic nerve lesions, nerve sheath tumors and several types of polyneuropathies.

Entrapment neuropathies

The most common cause of focal neuropathies is entrapment of a nerve while passing through an osseo-fibrous tunnel, such as the carpal tunnel at the wrist and the cubital tunnel at the elbow. The pathophysiological feature of nerve compression comprises disturbed vascular microcirculation, impaired axonal transport, edema within the nerve, and thickening of perineurium resulting in an enlargement of the nerve diameter, which is typically located proximally to the entrapment site [3]. Consequently, changes in nerve cross-sectional area are the most relevant sonographic findings in entrapment neuropathies (Supplementary Fig. 1; to view the figure, please visit the online supplementary file in ScienceDirect). In patients with carpal tunnel syndrome (CTS), numerous studies demonstrated high accuracy for both, the

* Tel.: +49 3834 866819; fax: +49 3834 866806.
  E-mail address: ulf.schminke@uni-greifswald.de

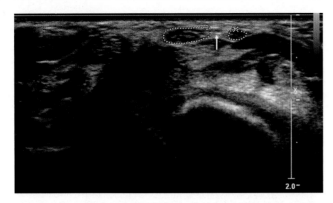

Figure 1 Cross-sectional view of the median nerve at the inlet of the carpal tunnel at the wrist showing a bifid median nerve (dotted line) and a small persistent median artery (arrow).

maximum cross-sectional area of the median nerve proximal to the entrance of the carpal tunnel and the ratio of the median nerve area at the wrist to the area of the nerve at the forearm [4—11]. For example, according to a cut-off value for the cross-sectional area of 10 mm², sensitivity and specificity were 82% and 87% in a study by Ziswiler et al. [6]. Increasing the cut-off value to 12 mm² resulted in a 100% specificity at the expense of a lower sensitivity of 44%. Secondary findings in patients with CTS are nerve flattening within the carpal tunnel and bowing of the flexor retinaculum [2]. In contrast to electrodiagnosis, ultrasonography has the capability to rule out secondary causes of CTS such as tenosynovitis, ganglion cysts, accessory muscles or tumors [4,5]. In case the nerve branches proximal to the carpal tunnel, ultrasonography can further demonstrate a bifid median nerve [11] or a persistent median artery (Fig. 1) [12]. If symptoms persist or worsen after surgery, ultrasonography may be valuable to assess incomplete splitting of the retinaculum or intra-operative injuries of the ulnar branch of the median nerve (Fig. 2). However, in contrast to NCS, ultrasonography is obviously not suitable for post-treatment follow-up of CTS since Lee et al. [13] pointed out

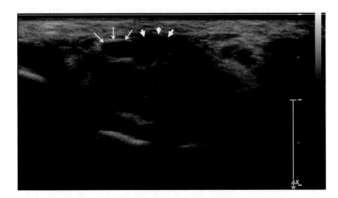

Figure 2 Cross-sectional view of the median nerve in the carpal tunnel in a patient who underwent surgery for carpal tunnel syndrome and complained about numbness of the ulnar portion of the middle finger and the radial portion of the ring finger. Nodular enlargement of the ulnar branch of the median nerve (arrowheads), probably, as consequence of nerve injury during surgery. (Long arrows indicate the not affected radial portion of the median nerve.)

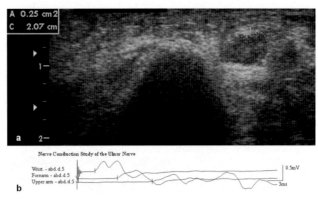

Figure 3 Cross-sectional view of the ulnar nerve (dotted line) in the ulnar groove between the medial epicondyle and the olecranon process. (a) Enlargement of the cross-sectional area to 25 mm² in a patient with ulnar neuropathy at the elbow. (b) Nerve conduction study of the ulnar nerve. Motor potentials are recorded from the abductor digiti minimi muscle after stimulation at the wrist (upper curve), below (middle curve) and above the elbow (bottom curve). Low amplitudes of compound motor potentials indicate severe Wallerian degeneration of axons, which makes it difficult to determine the exact site of nerve entrapment.

that the cross-sectional area of the median nerve remained unchanged 6 months after surgery.

Supplementary material related to this article can be found, in the online version, at http://dx.doi.org/10.1016/j.permed.2012.03.012.

As with carpal tunnel syndrome, several studies investigated the sensitivity and the specificity of ultrasonography for the diagnosis of ulnar neuropathy at the elbow in comparison to electrodiagnosis [14—19]. Specifically, if electrodiagnostic studies are inconclusive, which may occur in case of severe Wallerian degeneration of axons when conduction velocities are difficult to determine, ultrasonography helps either to localize the exact site of nerve entrapment around the elbow (Fig. 3) or to rule out ulnar neuropathy at sites different from the elbow segment [14,20]. Dynamic ultrasonography during flexion of the elbow may further demonstrate subluxation or dislocation of the ulnar nerve from its normal position in the ulnar groove, which may occur either isolated or in combination with the medial head of the triceps muscle [16,20].

In clinical practice, it is always recommended to track the entire course of each nerve from the wrist to the axilla for several reasons: Focal inflammatory neuropathy, which is frequently located at proximal sites of the upper extremities, or nerve tumors may be otherwise mistaken for entrapment syndromes. Demyelinating polyneuropathies such as Charcot—Marie—Tooth disease or chronic inflammatory demyelinating polyneuropathy (CIDP) showing a diffuse swelling of nerves may be missed if only a single measurement is performed at the wrist or at the ulnar groove between the medial epicondyle and the olecranon process. Further sites of entrapment that can be evaluated with ultrasound are the supraspinous notch (suprascapular nerve), the quadrilateral space (axillary nerve), the spiral groove of the humerus (radial nerve), the proximal edge of

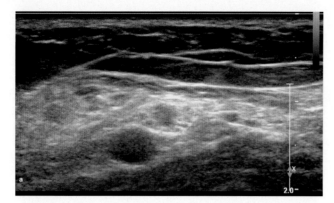

Figure 4 Cross-sectional view of the median nerve (dotted line) at the upper arm proximal to the cubital fossa in a patient with chronic inflammatory demyelinating polyneuropathy (CIDP). The cross-sectional area is enlarged and some fascicles are more swollen than others.

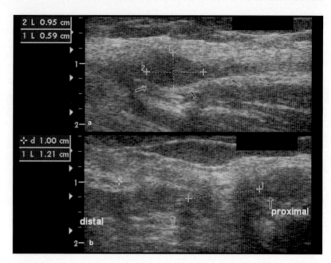

Figure 5 Longitudinal view of a completely transected ulnar nerve (arrows) at the upper arm. (a) Traumatic neuroma at the terminal end of a transected nerve with homogeneous texture and hypoechoic echogenicity. (b) Retraction of both nerve stumps after complete nerve transection with a gap of 12 mm.

the supinator muscle (posterior interosseus nerve), and the osseo-fibrous tunnel at the fibular head (peroneal nerve).

Polyneuropathies

As expected from histology and from magnetic resonance imaging (MRI) studies, patients with CIDP show diffuse enlargement of both, cervical nerve roots and peripheral nerves. Typically, some fascicles are more affected than others within a single nerve and additional areas of focal enlargement may occur (Fig. 4) [21–23]. These areas of focal enlargement, which have also been reported in patients with multifocal motor neuropathies [24], correlate well with nerve conduction blocks in electrodiagnostic studies [25]. This finding is clinically relevant because conduction blocks are sometimes difficult to assess in proximal portions of peripheral nerves [25]. Diffuse nerve enlargement is also a characteristic finding in patients with hereditary motor and sensory neuropathy (Charcot–Marie–Tooth disease) [26–28]. In contrast to CIDP, the enlargement involves uniformly all fascicles of an individual nerve with the result that the fascicular structure of the nerve is preserved (Supplementary Fig. 2; to view the figure, please visit the online supplementary file in ScienceDirect). Although diabetic neuropathy is the most common polyneuropathy, only a few studies have addressed this topic and findings are inconclusive, so far [23].

Supplementary material related to this article can be found, in the online version, at http://dx.doi.org/10.1016/j.permed.2012.03.012.

Traumatic nerve lesions

In patients with traumatic nerve lesions, adding ultrasonography to electrodiagnosis may provide a lot of important complementary information about the localization and the cause of impaired nerve function, both being essential for deciding upon surgical treatment. Ultrasonography not only allows one to precisely localize the site of nerve injury, it also indicates whether a nerve is completely transected or partially dissected or whether the nerve is displaced or even encased by surrounding scar formation or by a fibrous or bony callus after bone fracture [29–32]. Furthermore, ultrasonography may identify fracture fragments compressing nerves in close vicinity to bone fractures or may quantify the amount of nerve retraction after complete nerve transection (Fig. 5). Traumatic neuroma can occur at the site of either partial or complete dissection of the nerve. Neuroma appears as a bulbous concentric enlargement at the terminal end of a transected nerve with homogeneous texture and hypoechoic echogenicity. In case of only partial dissection, the continuity of the nerve is preserved and neuroma appears as nodular shaped broadening of the nerve contour (Supplementary Fig. 3; to view the figure, please visit the online supplementary file in ScienceDirect). Intraoperative ultrasonography is a promising new field enabling morphological examination of nerve lesions in continuity in order to assess the extent of nerve fibrosis and to discriminate between intraneural or perineural fibrosis. [33]. Both information are valuable to estimate the regenerative potential of a nerve lesion.

Supplementary material related to this article can be found, in the online version, at http://dx.doi.org/10.1016/j.permed.2012.03.012.

Tumors involving peripheral nerves

Schwannomas (neurilemmomas) and solitary neurofibromas are the most common benign nerve sheath tumors. Sonographically, they appear as well-defined hypoechoic masses with a fusiform shape and a normal-appearing nerve that enters and exits the tumor (Supplementary Fig. 4; to view the figure, please visit the online supplementary file in ScienceDirect) [34,35]. Because of their capsule, schwannoma are located more excentric, while not encapsulated neurofibroma are located more centrally compared to the course of the nerve. Since many nerve fascicles remain intact, benign nerve sheath tumors may be missed with electrodiagnostic studies alone. In contrast to benign tumors, malignant nerve

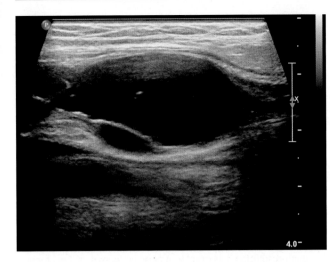

Figure 6 Longitudinal view of an intraneural ganglion of the tibial nerve/sciatic nerve at the level of the poplitea.

sheath tumors are characterized by rapid growth and progressive neurological symptoms. Their shape is ill-defined and their echotexture is more heterogeneous [35].

Supplementary material related to this article can be found, in the online version, at http://dx.doi.org/10.1016/j.permed.2012.03.012.

Leakage of joint fluid into the sheath of a joint nerve branch, which is subsequently pumped into the nerve sheath of a main nerve, is the pathophysiological substrate of intraneural ganglia [36,37]. Ultrasonography characteristically shows multiple well-defined anechoic cysts within the continuity of the nerve, which are filled with joint fluid and displace the nerve fascicles (Fig. 6). Most ganglia arise from the superior tibio-fibular joint involving either the common peroneal or the tibial nerve, but they may also affect the tibial nerve at the ankle or the ulnar nerve at the elbow. A recent study by Visser [36] has demonstrated that intraneural ganglia account for approximately 18% of peroneal mononeuropathies at the fibular head, which underlines that ultrasonography is a valuable examination technique that is complementary to electrodiagnostic studies in these patients.

Outlook

In summary, ultrasonography of peripheral nerves is a valuable adjunctive modality in the clinical neurophysiology laboratory. Information on pathologic changes in nerve structure and in the adjacent tissue in conjunction with information obtained by electrodiagnostic studies on the severity and chronicity of a disturbed nerve function and on the underlying demyelinating or axonal process may provide a more comprehensive picture of peripheral nerve diseases compared to what can be provided by each modality alone [38]. Furthermore, information on nerve structure are often indispensable for clinical decision making. With respect to that purpose, ultrasonography is superior to magnetic resonance imaging in several aspects including not only costs, accessibility, portability, speed of examination, and patient comfort, but also technical properties such as spatial resolution and the ability to perform dynamic examinations during limb movements. Ultrasonography offers neuromuscular clinicians a unique opportunity to conduct both complementary examination modalities by themselves without referring patients to another laboratory. Currently, however, only a few neuromuscular clinicians are familiar with neuromuscular ultrasound. More efforts are necessary toward establishing examination guidelines and launching educational programs with appropriate certification by relevant accrediting societies to achieve a more widespread use of ultrasonography in clinical neurophysiology laboratories.

Conflict of interest

The author declares that there is no actual or potential conflict of interest including any financial, personal or other relationships with other people or organizations within three years of beginning the submitted work that could inappropriately influence, or be perceived to influence, his work.

References

[1] Fornage BD. Peripheral nerves of the extremities: imaging with US. Radiology 1988;167:179—82.
[2] Buchberger W, Judmaier W, Birbamer G, Lener M, Schmidauer C. Carpal tunnel syndrome: diagnosis with high-resolution sonography. American Journal of Roentgenology 1992;159:793—8.
[3] Rempel D, Dahlin L, Lundborg G. Pathophysiology of nerve compression syndromes: response of peripheral nerves to loading. Journal of Bone and Joint Surgery 1999;81:1600—10.
[4] Nakamichi K, Tachibana S. Ultrasonographic measurement of median nerve cross-sectional area in idiopathic carpal tunnel syndrome: diagnostic accuracy. Muscle and Nerve 2002;26:798—803.
[5] Kele H, Verheggen R, Bittermann HJ, Reimers CD. The potential value of ultrasonography in the evaluation of carpal tunnel syndrome. Neurology 2003;61:389—91.
[6] Ziswiler HR, Reichenbach S, Vögelin E, Bachmann LM, Villiger PM, Jüni P. Diagnostic value of sonography in patients with suspected carpal tunnel syndrome: a prospective study. Arthritis and Rheumatism 2005;52:304—11.
[7] Hobson-Webb LD, Massey JM, Juel VC, Sanders DB. The ultrasonographic wrist-to-forearm median nerve area ratio in carpal tunnel syndrome. Clinical Neurophysiology 2008;119:1353—7.
[8] Visser LH, Smidt MH, Lee ML. High-resolution sonography versus EMG in the diagnosis of carpal tunnel syndrome. Journal of Neurology, Neurosurgery and Psychiatry 2008;79:63—7.
[9] Klauser AS, Halpern EJ, De Zordo T, Feuchtner GM, Arora R, Gruber J, et al. Carpal tunnel syndrome assessment with US: value of additional cross-sectional area measurements of the median nerve in patients versus healthy volunteers. Radiology 2009;250:171—7.
[10] Karadağ YS, Karadağ O, Ciçekli E, Oztürk S, Kiraz S, Ozbakir S, et al. Severity of Carpal tunnel syndrome assessed with high frequency ultrasonography. Rheumatology International 2010;30:761—5.
[11] Klauser AS, Halpern EJ, Faschingbauer R, Guerra F, Martinoli C, Gabl MF, et al. Bifid median nerve in carpal tunnel syndrome: assessment with US cross-sectional area measurement. Radiology 2011;259:808—15.
[12] Kele H, Verheggen R, Reimers CD. Carpal tunnel syndrome caused by thrombosis of the median artery: the importance of high-resolution ultrasonography for diagnosis. Case report. Journal of Neurosurgery 2002;97:471—3.

[13] Lee CH, Kim TK, Yoon ES, Dhong ES. Postoperative morphologic analysis of carpal tunnel syndrome using high-resolution ultrasonography. Annals of Plastic Surgery 2005;54:143−6.

[14] Beekman R, Schoemaker MC, Van Der Plas JP, Van Den Berg LH, Franssen H, Wokke JH, et al. Diagnostic value of high-resolution sonography in ulnar neuropathy at the elbow. Neurology 2004;62:767−73.

[15] Yoon JS, Walker FO, Cartwright MS. Ultrasonographic swelling ratio in the diagnosis of ulnar neuropathy at the elbow. Muscle and Nerve 2008;38:1231−5.

[16] Mondelli M, Filippou G, Frediani B, Aretini A. Ultrasonography in ulnar neuropathy at the elbow: relationships to clinical and electrophysiological findings. Neurophysiologie Clinique 2008;38:217−26.

[17] Volpe A, Rossato G, Bottanelli M, Marchetta A, Caramaschi P, Bambara LM, et al. Ultrasound evaluation of ulnar neuropathy at the elbow: correlation with electrophysiological studies. Rheumatology 2009;48:1098−101.

[18] Gruber H, Glodny B, Peer S. The validity of ultrasonographic assessment in cubital tunnel syndrome: the value of a cubital-to-humeral nerve area ratio (CHR) combined with morphologic features. Ultrasound in Medicine and Biology 2010;36:376−82.

[19] Bayrak AO, Bayrak IK, Turker H, Elmali M, Nural MS. Ultrasonography in patients with ulnar neuropathy at the elbow: comparison of cross-sectional area and swelling ratio with electrophysiological severity. Muscle and Nerve 2010;41:661−6.

[20] Beekman R, Visser LH, Verhagen WI. Ultrasonography in ulnar neuropathy at the elbow: a critical review. Muscle and Nerve 2011;43:627−35.

[21] Taniguchi N, Itoh K, Wang Y, Omoto K, Shigeta K, Fujii Y, et al. Sonographic detection of diffuse peripheral nerve hypertrophy in chronic inflammatory demyelinating polyradiculoneuropathy. Journal of Clinical Ultrasound 2000;28:488−91.

[22] Matsuoka N, Kohriyama T, Ochi K, Nishitani M, Sueda Y, Mimori Y, et al. Detection of cervical nerve root hypertrophy by ultrasonography in chronic inflammatory demyelinating polyradiculoneuropathy. Journal of the Neurological Sciences 2004;219:15−21.

[23] Zaidman CM, Al-Lozi M, Pestronk A. Peripheral nerve size in normals and patients with polyneuropathy: an ultrasound study. Muscle and Nerve 2009;40:960−6.

[24] Beekman R, van den Berg LH, Franssen H, Visser LH, van Asseldonk JT, Wokke JH. Ultrasonography shows extensive nerve enlargements in multifocal motor neuropathy. Neurology 2005;65:305−7.

[25] Granata G, Pazzaglia C, Calandro P, Luigetti M, Martinoli C, Sabatelli M, et al. Ultrasound visualization of nerve morphological alteration at the site of conduction block. Muscle and Nerve 2009;40:1068−70.

[26] Heinemeyer O, Reimers CD. Ultrasound of radial, ulnar, median, and sciatic nerves in healthy subjects and patients with hereditary motor and sensory neuropathies. Ultrasound in Medicine and Biology 1999;25:481−5.

[27] Martinoli C, Schenone A, Bianchi S, Mandich P, Caponetto C, Abbruzzese M, et al. Sonography of the median nerve in Charcot—Marie—Tooth disease. American Journal of Roentgenology 2002;178:1553−6.

[28] Cartwright MS, Brown ME, Eulitt P, Walker FO, Lawson VH, Caress JB. Diagnostic nerve ultrasound in Charcot—Marie—Tooth disease type 1B. Muscle and Nerve 2009;40:98−102.

[29] Bodner G, Buchberger W, Schocke M, Bale R, Huber B, Harpf C, et al. Radial nerve palsy associated with humeral shaft fracture: evaluation with US—initial experience. Radiology 2001;219:811−6.

[30] Peer S, Bodner G, Meirer R, Willeit J, Piza-Katzer H. Examination of postoperative peripheral nerve lesions with high-resolution sonography. American Journal of Roentgenology 2001;177:415−9.

[31] Gruber H, Peer S, Kovacs P, Marth R, Bodner G. The ultrasonographic appearance of the femoral nerve and cases of iatrogenic impairment. Journal of Ultrasound in Medicine 2003;22:163−72.

[32] Gruber H, Glodny B, Galiano K, Kamelger F, Bodner G, Hussl H, et al. High-resolution ultrasound of the supraclavicular brachial plexus—can it improve therapeutic decisions in patients with plexus trauma? European Radiology 2007;17:1611−20.

[33] Koenig RW, Schmidt TE, Heinen CP, Wirtz CR, Kretschmer T, Antoniadis G, et al. Intraoperative high-resolution ultrasound: a new technique in the management of peripheral nerve disorders. Journal of Neurosurgery 2011;114:514−21.

[34] Hughes DG, Wilson DJ. Ultrasound appearances of peripheral nerve tumours. British Journal of Radiology 1986;59:1041−3.

[35] Gruber H, Glodny B, Bendix N, Tzankov A, Peer S. High-resolution ultrasound of peripheral neurogenic tumors. European Radiology 2007;17:2880−8.

[36] Visser LH. High-resolution sonography of the common peroneal nerve: detection of intraneural ganglia. Neurology 2006;67:1473−5.

[37] Young NP, Sorenson EJ, Spinner RJ, Daube JR. Clinical and electrodiagnostic correlates of peroneal intraneural ganglia. Neurology 2009;72:447−52.

[38] Padua L, Aprile I, Pazzaglia C, Frasca G, Caliandro P, Tonali P, et al. Contribution of ultrasound in a neurophysiological lab in diagnosing nerve impairment: a one-year systematic assessment. Clinical Neurophysiology 2007;118:1410−6.

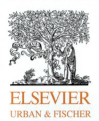
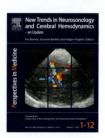

Bartels E, Bartels S, Poppert H (Editors):
New Trends in Neurosonology and Cerebral Hemodynamics — an Update.
Perspectives in Medicine (2012) 1, 427—430

journal homepage: www.elsevier.com/locate/permed

An overview of musculoskeletal ultrasound — A thirteen years experience in Pakistan

Syed Amir Gilani*

Department of Radiological Sciences and Medical Imaging (AISMI), The University of Lahore, Lahore, Pakistan

KEYWORDS
Ultrasound;
Musculoskeletal;
Shoulder;
Elbow;
Wrist;
Hand;
Hip;
Knee;
Ankle;
Foot;
Back;
Lumbosacral region;
Calf;
Thigh

Summary

Objective: (1) To provide an overview on 13 years experience on patients with musculoskeletal disorders in Pakistan. (2) To assess accuracy of ultrasound in musculoskeletal disorders. (3) To determine percentage of different regional pathologies referred for musculoskeletal ultrasound.

Material and methods: We scanned 25,437 patients coming from all over Pakistan including 18,715 males and 6722 females from 1 month to 85 years of age.

We used two ultrasound equipments with a multi-frequency (6—14 MHz) linear probe to perform studies in patients with possible musculoskeletal system problems.

Results: All patients with different joint or specific problems of musculoskeletal system were scanned, the total number of patients of any specific disorder was calculated and the accuracy of ultrasound was compared with MRI in a given percentage of patients.

Discussion: In all musculoskeletal disorders ultrasound was found to be accurate in about 84.8%. It was 83.5% accurate in the cases which went for MRI, its accuracy with other lab tests was 81.2% and that with surgery was 93.3%.

Conclusion: Musculoskeletal ultrasound is a very useful tool in almost all disorders of musculoskeletal system and shall be a necessary tool of a physicians, specially a family physician, orthopedic surgeon, physiotherapist and rheumatologist.
© 2012 Elsevier GmbH. All rights reserved.

Introduction

Musculoskeletal ultrasound has been used widely in many radiology services around the world. The use of this tool in the clinician setting is recent. We present our experience of 13 years in musculoskeletal ultrasound. We scanned about 25,437 patients, whereby most of them complained about different musculoskeletal acute and chronic problems.

Objective

(1) To provide an overview on 13 years experience on patients with musculoskeletal disorders in outdoor clinic of our department, Lahore, Pakistan.
(2) To assess accuracy of ultrasound in musculoskeletal disorders.
(3) To determine the percentage of different regional pathologies referred for musculoskeletal ultrasound.

* Tel.: +92 300 8460876; fax: +92 423 7521118.
E-mail address: profgilani@gmail.com

2211-968X/$ — see front matter © 2012 Elsevier GmbH. All rights reserved.
doi:10.1016/j.permed.2012.02.056

Material and methods

We scanned 25,437 symptomatic patients coming from all over Pakistan including 18,715 males and 6722 females from 1 month to 85 years of age.

We used two ultrasound equipments with a multi-frequency (6—14 MHz) linear probe to perform studies in patients with possible musculoskeletal system problems. Age, gender, previous diagnosis and morbidity were registered.

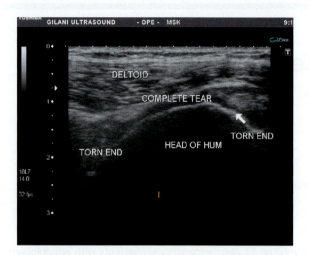

Figure 1 Complete tear of M. suprispinatous.

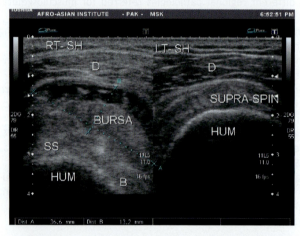

Figure 2 Right shoulder in chronic SASD-bursitis.

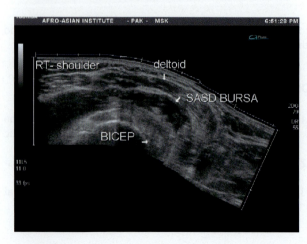

Figure 3 Panoramic view of right SASD bursitis.

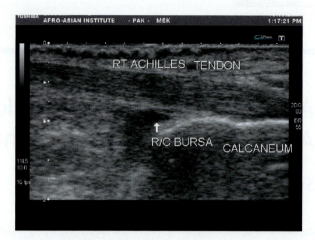

Figure 4 Right retrocalcaneal bursitis.

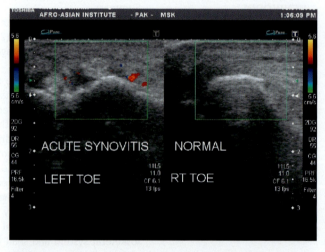

Figure 5 Left toe acute synovitis-Rheumatoid arthritis.

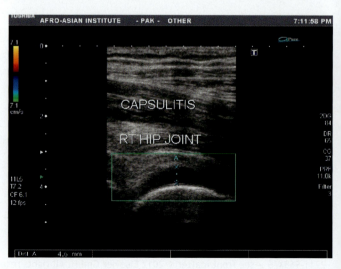

Figure 6 Right hip joint showing acute capsulitis.

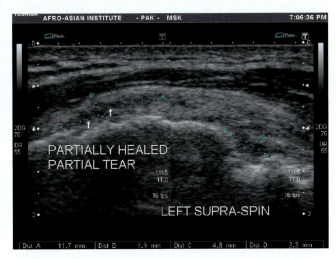

Figure 7 Shoulder: partially healed partial tear of left M. supraspinatous.

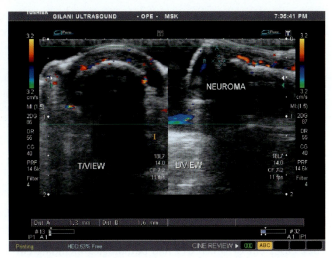

Figure 10 Nail bud with hyperechoic avascular neuroma.

Results

Our study included 12,072 patients with *shoulder* complaints, out of which 10,822 had some pathology whereas the remaining patients were normal. The main pathologies were bilateral supraspinatous complete tear, unilateral superspinatous complete tear (67% right, 33% left), maximum partial tear of supraspinatous, minimum partial tear of supraspinatous, partial tear of supraspinatous with subacromial impingment, subacromial impingment with tendonitis of supraspinatous, bilateral complete tear of subscapularis, unilateral complete tear of subscapularis, partial tear of subscapularis, bilateral complete tear of infraspinatous, unilateral complete tear of infraspinatous, partial tear of infraspinatous, tendonitis of infraspinatous, bilateral complete tear of long head of biceps, unilateral complete tear of long head of biceps, partial tear of long head of biceps, effusion around long head of biceps, subluxation of long head of biceps, dislocation of long head of biceps, teres minor complete tear, teres minor partial tear, acute subacromial-subdeltoid (SASD) bursitis, chronic SASD bursitis, AC joint pathologies, AC ligament pathologies, anterior labrum pathologies, posterior labrum pathologies, synovitis of rotator cuff tendons, tenosynovitis of rotator cuff tendons, partially healed tendons of rotator cuff, chronic tendonitis of rotator cuff, tendomuscular junctions, osteoarthritis, osteoporosis, osteomyelitis, transverse humeral ligament pathologies and soft tissue pathologies.

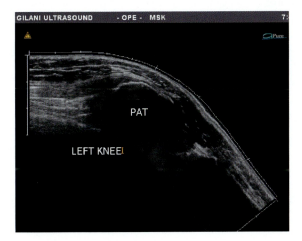

Figure 8 Normal panoramic view of left knee.

The total number of cases of *elbow* scanned were 2355, out of which 2198 had pathologies including tendon tear, tendonitis, tenosynovitis, bursal pathologies, ligament pathologies, soft tissue pathologies, and vascular pathologies whereas in wrist and hand we scanned 2136 patients out of which 2086 had pathologies of *wrist and hand* like soft tissues, synovitis, tenosynovitis, acute tendonitis, chronic tendonitis, hood injury, trigger finger, foreign bodies, nail bud pathologies, vascular pathologies.

We scanned 812 patients of *hip* and in 766 found pathologies like effusions, bursal pathologies, tendon pathologies, snapping hip, muscle pathologies, soft tissue lesions, sciatic nerve pathologies, and vascular pathologies.

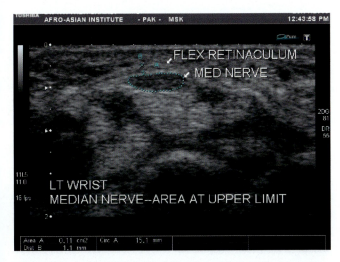

Figure 9 Left wrist showing flexor retinaculum and median nerve (circumference = 15 mm).

In *neonates* we scanned 603 cases for developmental dysplasia of the hip (DDH) and found DDH in 142 cases, 14 cases of effusion and 5 cases soft tissue pathologies.

In *groin and thigh* we scanned 256 cases and we found the pathologies in 217 of soft tissue, vascular pathologies, hernias, lymph node pathologies, tendonitis, tendon tear.

We scanned 4852 cases of *knee*, out of 4794 showed pathologies including fluid in suprapatellar recess, infrapatellar tendon pathologies, bursal pathologies, quadriceps tendon pathologies, PCL (Posterior Crutiate Ligament) pathologies, baker's cyst, popliteal vessels pathologies, MCL (Medial Collateral Ligament) pathologies, LCL (Lateral Collateral Ligament) pathologies, medial meniscal pathologies, lateral meniscal pathologies, soft tissue pathologies, (2 bilateral), osteomyelitis, osteoarthritis, rheumatoid arthritis, tendonitis, and muscle pathologies. In *calf* we scanned 622 cases out of which 619 had pathologies including cellulitis, soft tissue pathologies, muscle pathologies, vascular pathologies, osteomyelitis.

We also scanned 1290 cases of *ankle joint and foot* out of which 1252 showed pathologies including tendon tear, tendonitis, tenosynovitis, bural pathologies, ligament pathologies, soft tissue pathologies, foot pathologies, and fascial pathologies in foot.

In *lumbosacral region (back)* we scanned 74 cases out of which we had just 21 pathologies including intervertebral disc prolapse (posterior), vertebral pathologies, muscular tear, muscular spasm, and muscular sprains.

Chest wall was scanned anteriorly and posteriorly in 26 patients out of which 9 had pathologies including soft tissue pathologies, rib pathologies, intercostal muscle pathologies, and costochondral joint pathologies.

Conclusion

Musculoskeletal ultrasound is a very useful tool in almost all disorders of musculoskeletal system and shall be a necessary tool of a physicians, specially a family physician, orthopedic surgeon, physiotherapist and rheumatologist. This technique also allows to have a correct guidance for therapeutic procedures.

Four-dimensional ultrasound calf muscle imaging in patients with genetic types of distal myopathy

Ekaterina Titianova [a,b,*], Teodora Chamova [c], Velina Guergueltcheva [c], Ivailo Tournev [c,d]

[a] Clinic of Functional Diagnostics of Nervous System, Military Medical Academy, 3 Georgi Sofiiski Str., 1606 Sofia, Bulgaria
[b] Medical Faculty, Sofia University, 1 Koziak Str., 1407 Sofia, Bulgaria
[c] Clinic of Neurology, University Hospital "Alexandrovska", 1 Georgi Sofiiski Str., 1431 Sofia, Bulgaria
[d] Department of Cognitive Science and Psychology, New Bulgarian University, 21 Montevideo Str., 1618 Sofia, Bulgaria

KEYWORDS
Distal myopathies;
4D ultrasound imaging;
HIBM2;
Myosonology;
TMD;
VCPDM

Abstract

Purpose: To demonstrate the capabilities of 4D ultrasound calf muscle imaging in patients with genetic types of distal myopathies (DMs).

Methods: Three patients with DM were studied: a 58-year-old man with Vocal Cord and Pharyngeal Weakness Distal Myopathy (VCPDM), a 36-year-old woman with Tibial Muscular Dystrophy (TMD) and a 27-year-old woman with Hereditary Inclusion Body Myopathy Type 2 (HIBM2). Their calf muscles were evaluated in rest and during maximal plantar flexion using 3D/4D ultrasound imaging. The results were compared to myosonograms of healthy controls.

Results: All patients had myopathic syndrome due to advanced muscular dystrophy. In comparison to controls abnormal calf muscle architectonics, reduced muscle contractility and a combination of spot-like hypo- and hyperechoic areas were established on 4D ultrasound imaging. The changes were associated with the degree of muscle atrophy, fat and fibrous tissue infiltration.

Conclusions: Four-dimensional myosonology gives additional information for muscle architectonics in patients with genetic types of DM. Further studies are needed to evaluate if the described findings are typical for specific genetic types of myopathy.
© 2012 Elsevier GmbH. All rights reserved.

Introduction

The concept of space—time or a four-dimensional (4D) space, combines space and time to a single abstract "space" with three spatial (length, width and height), and one temporal (time) dimensions. Volume 3D/4D ultrasound is mainly used in obstetric sonology during pregnancy, providing space—time images of the fetus. Its application in adult neurology is limited and not well investigated [1,2]. The conventional ultrasound imaging, recently introduced for structural and functional evaluation of muscles and nerves in

Abbreviations: DM, distal myopathy; 4D, four-dimensional; HIBM2, Hereditary Inclusion Body Myopathy Type 2; PF, plantar flexion; TMD, Tibial Muscular Dystrophy; VCPDM, Vocal Cord and Pharyngeal Weakness Distal Myopathy.

* Corresponding author at: Clinic of Functional Diagnostics of Nervous System, Military Medical Academy, 3 Georgi Sofiiski Str., 1606 Sofia, Bulgaria. Tel.: +359 2 9225454.

E-mail addresses: titianova@yahoo.com (E. Titianova), teodoratch@abv.bg (T. Chamova), vguerbliz@abv.bg (V. Guergueltcheva), itournev@emhpf.org (I. Tournev).

Table 1	Patients' characteristics.		
Parameters	VCPDM	TMD	HIBM2
Gene locus	5q31	2q13—q33	9p1—q1
Protein	Matrin 3	Titin	UDP-N-acetylglucosamine 2 epimerase/N-acetyl mannosamine kinase
Age of onset/assessment	40/57	17/38	17/27
MRC scale (TS)	3—/5	4+/5	2—/5
Muscle histology	Advanced muscular dystrophy, fat and fibrous tissue	Muscle fibers are replaced by fat and fibrous tissue	Not performed

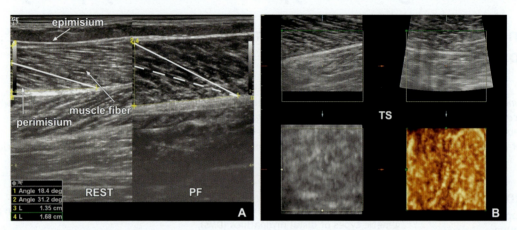

Figure 1 (A) B-mode image of TS muscle in rest and PF in a 27-year-old healthy woman. Dotted line presents the orientation of muscle fibers in rest. (B) 4D myosonogram with a reticular TS architectonics.

patients with neuromuscular disorders, is mainly of clinical use [3,4].

The aim of the present study was to demonstrate the capabilities of 4D ultrasound calf muscle imaging in 3 patients with genetically verified types of distal myopathy (DM).

Materials and methods

The study included 3 patients with genetically verified types of DM: a 58-year-old man with Vocal Cord and Pharyngeal Weakness Distal Myopathy (VCPDM) due to heterozygous mutation in exon 2 of the *MATR3* gene [5], a 36-year-old woman with Tibial Muscular Dystrophy (TMD), due to heterozygous mutation in exon 362 of TTN-gene and a 27-year-old woman with Hereditary Inclusion Body Myopathy Type 2 (HIBM2), due to double heterozygous mutation in the GNE-gene [6]. Neurological assessment (including MRC scale) at the time of myosonology showed clinical features of myopathic syndrome more pronounced for distal leg muscles in all patients. Normal conduction velocities of the fibular, tibial, median nerves and myogenic changes of distal calves and hand muscles were found by electromyography. An advanced muscular dystrophy was proved by muscle biopsy, performed in the patients with VCPDM and TMD (Table 1).

Triceps surae muscles were evaluated in a lying position by using a special probe for 3D/4D real time imaging (Logic 7, GE). The transverse diameter of both TS heads in longitudinal plan, the angle of inclination of the muscle fibers towards the surface of the aponeurosis and 3D/4D imaging of calf architectonics were evaluated in rest and during maximal plantar flexion (PF). The results were compared to myosonograms of 3 age- and sex-matched healthy controls.

Results

The normal TS myosonogram is demonstrated in Fig. 1. The whole muscle is enveloped by hyperechoic epimysium. The muscle fibers are hypoechoic and grouped in fascicles, divided by hyperechoic septs of fibrous and fat tissue of the perimysium. In a longitudinal B-mode image the perimysium is depicted as oblique parallel hyperechoic lines. The PF causes calf muscle contraction that increases the transverse muscle diameter and the angle of muscle fiber towards the aponeurosis. The 4D ultrasound imaging shows a reticular TS architectonics despite the muscle activity, age and sex of healthy controls. Its hypoechoic areas increase during PF, due to thickening of the contracted muscle fibers.

Compared to healthy controls all patients with DM had a reduced transverse TS diameter and decreased muscle contractility. The muscle fibers were inclined and their

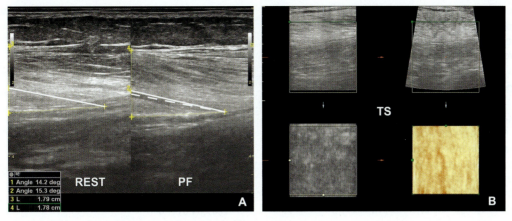

Figure 2 (A) B-mode image of TS muscle in rest and during PF in the woman with HIBM2. Dotted line presents the orientation of the muscle fibers in rest. (B) An abnormal 4D architectonics of the same muscle.

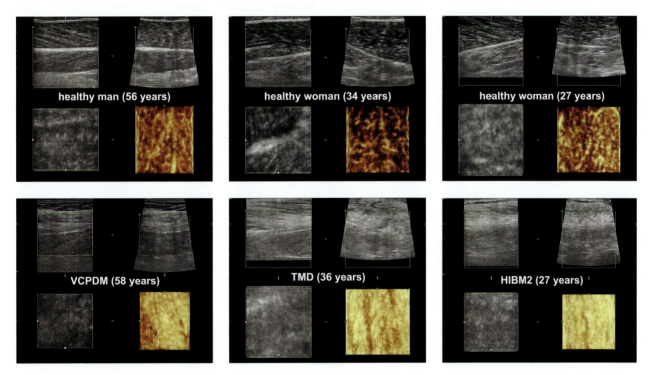

Figure 3 4D architectonics of TS muscles in patients with DM and age- and sex-matched controls.

orientation was under a smaller angle towards the aponeurosis during rest and PF (Fig. 2). The normal reticular muscle structure was replaced by granular myoarchitectonics — a combination of spot-like hypo- and hyperechoic areas on 4D ultrasound imaging was found in association with the degree of muscle atrophy, fat tissue infiltration and fibrosis. The hyperechoic areas had a tendency of fusing in the patient with HIBM2 (Fig. 3).

Discussion

Distal myopathies are a group of genetically and clinically heterogeneous disorders classified into one broad category, due to the presentation of weakness involving distal skeletal muscles of upper and lower limbs. The identified genes, whose mutations cause DM, encode different proteins: sarcomere proteins (titin, myosin); membrane proteins (dysferlin, caveolin); Z-disc proteins or proteins important for the Z-disc stability (ZASP; desmin; myotilin; filamin C; a-b crystalin) and cytosol proteins (GNE), nuclear matrix proteins (MATR 3). They are characterized by progressive muscular dystrophy, followed by replacement of the normal muscle fibers with fibrous and adipous tissue [7,8] that increases muscle echogenicity — the muscles become whiter in B-mode ultrasound imaging [9].

Our study confirms that in comparison to controls all patients with DM had reduced muscle fiber contractility and an abnormal TS architectonics with a combination of spot-like hyper- and hypoechoic areas on 4D ultrasound imaging. The changes in space—time myosonograms were associated with the degree of muscle atrophy, fat tissue infiltration and fibrosis. The presence of fusing hyperechoic zones in the patient with HIBM2 allows us to speculate that different DM could have different 4D ultrasound pattern. As there is no any available 4D myosonographic data in the literature except our publications [1,2], we could not make a comparative analysis of our findings with other studies.

Conclusions

The study shows that 4D myosonology is a safe noninvasive method for space—time imaging of the structural and functional changes in muscle architectonics in patients with genetic types of DM. It can be used for determining the most appropriate areas for muscle biopsy (not too destroyed and not too preserved). Further studies are needed to evaluate if the described findings are typical for specific genetic types of myopathy.

References

[1] Titianova E, Guergueltcheva V, Mihaylova V, Chamova T, Tournev I. Myosonography and clinical genetic studies in a patient with distal myopathy. Neurosonol Cereb Hemodyn 2010;6:87—94.

[2] Chamova T, Titianova E, Tournev I, Dimova R. Myosonographic assessment of triceps surae muscle in a patient with autosomal recessive hereditary inclusion body myopathy. Neurosonol Cereb Hemodyn 2011;7:93—9.

[3] Pillen S. Skeletal muscle ultrasound. Eur J Transl Myol 2010;1:145—55.

[4] Lee JC, Healy J. Sonography of lower limb muscle injury. AJR 2004;184:341—51.

[5] Malicdan MV, Nonaka I. Distal myopathies a review: highlights on distal myopathies with rimmed vacuoles. Neurol India 2008;56:314—24.

[6] Senderek J, Garvey SM, Krieger M, Guergueltcheva V, Urtizberea A, Roos A, et al. Autosomal-dominant distal myopathy associated with a recurrent missense mutation in the gene encoding the nuclear matrix protein, Matrin 3. Am J Hum Genet 2009;84:511—8.

[7] Nonaka I. Distal myopathies. Curr Opin Neurol 1999;2:493—9.

[8] Mastaglia FL, Lamont PJ, Laing NG. Distal myopathies. Curr Opin Neurol 2005;18:504—10.

[9] Pillen S, Tak R, Lammens M, Verrijp K, Arts I, Zwarts M, et al. Skeletal muscle ultrasound: correlation between fibrous tissue and echo intensity. Ultrasound Med Biol 2009;35:443—6.

12. Case Reports

"A horse, a horse, my kingdom for a horse" — Saddle thrombosis of carotid bifurcation in acute stroke

Edoardo B. Vicenzini [a,*], Maria Fabrizia Giannoni [b], Maria Chiara Ricciardi [a], Gaia Sirimarco [a], Massimiliano Toscano [a], Gian Luigi Lenzi [a], Vittorio Di Piero [a]

[a] *Stroke Unit — Neurosonology, Department of Neurology and Psychiatry, Sapienza University of Rome, Viale dell'Università 30, 00185 Rome, Italy*
[b] *Vascular Ultrasound Investigation, Department "Paride Stefanini", Sapienza University of Rome, Viale dell'Università 30, 00185 Rome, Italy*

KEYWORDS
Saddle thrombosis;
High-resolution ultrasound;
Acute stroke care;
Endarterectomy

Summary

Background: Saddle thrombosis is less frequently detected in carotid arteries than in peripheral arterial embolism. The clot and the distal vessel patency have to be promptly recognized in these cases, because if the carotid vessel is open distally, chances may arise for successful emergent surgical procedures to remove the thrombus. At conventional static imaging, mobile floating thrombi may be difficult to differentiate from thrombosis on carotid complicated lesions of atherosclerotic origin. High-resolution ultrasound (US), with its unique capability of real-time imaging, adds fundamental data for interpretation of the findings.
Methods: Carotid ultrasound has been performed in acute stroke patients with high-resolution probes. Real-time clips are analyzed and imaging is presented.
Results: Saddle carotid bifurcation thrombosis of cardiac origin has been identified in 2 patients with acute homolateral ischemic stroke, with prompt successful surgical removal in one case. Moreover, an example of a thrombus attached on the ruptured surface of a complicated atherosclerotic plaque in an acute symptomatic stroke patient that was successfully operated in emergency is presented.
Conclusions: Early high-resolution ultrasound with real-time imaging can easily identify peculiar characteristics of carotid vulnerable diseases in acute stroke phase. Different clinical implications result from the early identification of these different conditions, modifying the therapeutical strategies.
© 2012 Elsevier GmbH. All rights reserved.

Introduction

"Saddle" arterial thrombi, by definition, are clots located at the sites of vessels bifurcations, "riding" the tips of the flow dividers. The most common sites for the peripheral localization of the saddle emboli are the aortic-femoral artery bifurcation, in cases of distal limbs arterial embolism, the pulmonary artery and across a patent

* Corresponding author. Tel.: +39 06 49914705;
fax: +39 06 49914194.
E-mail address: edoardo.vicenzini@uniroma1.it (E.B. Vicenzini).

interatrial foramen ovale [1–6]. Saddle carotid bifurcation embolism due to cardiac thrombi — paradoxical or not — is uncommon to be displayed with conventional static imaging in clinical practice, but it is not so rare a condition that may be observed, especially with high-resolution, real-time ultrasound (US) imaging [7].

In respect to "static" imaging with the computerized tomography (CTA) and magnetic resonance angiographies (MRAs), high-resolution ultrasound have the unique possibility to study real-time pathophysiology, displaying the emboli floating in the carotid lumen during their way to the intracranial district, when they find adhesion to the carotid arteries wall. These aspects clearly differentiate these clots from those arising on complicated atherosclerotic plaques, with the consequent therapeutical implications [7]. The identification of these highly unstable conditions is indeed particularly important in the acute stroke phases, since emergency surgery procedures — such as thrombus mechanical retrieval or emergent carotid surgery — can be performed, in order to prevent further deterioration of neurological conditions [8–11]. This surgical approach is similar, but more risky, than well-established mechanical thrombus retrieval procedure commonly applied in peripheral arteries embolism [12].

We describe two cases of uncommon carotid bifurcation saddle thrombosis of cardiac origin and a case of local thrombosis on a complicated carotid plaque. All these features could be detected easily with ultrasound, leading to the following implicated therapeutical decisions.

Description of cases

Case 1

DR, male, 84 years old, hypertensive, affected by chronic atrial fibrillation, presented acute left hemiplegia. Cerebral CT scan showed an extensive ischemic damage in the right middle cerebral artery (MCA) territory, with CT hyperdense MCA sign, indicative of intracranial vessel M1 occlusion (Fig. 1A). Carotid duplex (Siemens S2000; 9, 14, 18 MHz linear probes) showed a saddle thrombus at the right carotid bifurcation: the head of the clot was floating in the internal carotid artery and only partially reducing the lumen, and the tail was mobile in the external carotid artery (Fig. 1 C and D, Clip 1). Flow in the distal internal carotid artery was preserved, with only slight increased resistive indices (Fig. 1D, Clip 2). Even though the mobile clot seemed to be very harmful for the possibility of further distal embolism, considering the MCA occlusion and the extensive ischemic cerebral damage, surgery was however considered not indicated and the patient underwent only medical treatment.

Case 2

FR, male, 47 years old, asymptomatic for relevant cardiovascular history, presented acute mental confusion and bilateral strength deficit at the lower limbs. Cerebral MRI scan showed an ischemic damage in both the anterior

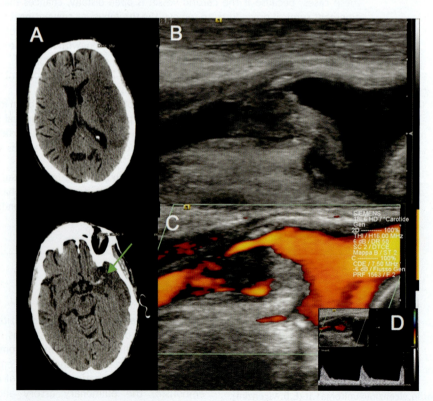

Figure 1 Case 1. Cerebral CT scan (A) with middle cerebral artery hyperdense occlusive sign (green arrow, below). Carotid ultrasonography: B-mode (B), power duplex (C) of a "horse riding" thrombus located at the carotid bifurcation. The distal tract of the internal carotid artery is patent, as revealed by both power Doppler (C) as well as by the pulsed wave Doppler (D).

cerebral arteries (ACA) territory. Both ACA were scarcely visible at magnetic resonance angiography while MCAs were patent and the related brain parenchyma spared from ischemic damage (Fig. 2A). Carotid duplex (Siemens S2000; 9, 14, 18 MHz linear probes) showed a clot in the left carotid bulb, adherent to the anterior vessel wall (Fig. 2 B–D, Clip 3). Considering the patency of both the MCAs and that the cerebral tissue was still normal in the left MCA territory, the patient was successfully operated in emergency, to prevent further embolism. A second MRA revealed that both ACAs were originating from the left side, thus explaining why embolism affected the ACA bilaterally from the left bifurcation. Further cardiovascular screening revealed multiple thromboses, at the pulmonary artery and at the saphenofemoral right junction and the patient was also positioned a caval filter. Blood coagulation tests revealed altered AT III, Prot C and Prot S levels. Patient was then treated with anticoagulants.

Case 3

MD, 63 years old, slight hypercholesterolemic, presented acute transient mild left hemiparesis, with rapid spontaneous recovery. Carotid duplex showed moderate, non-hemodynamic, internal carotid artery stenosis by a heterogeneous, partially hypoecoic plaque with a soft component. High-resolution B-mode imaging revealed that the plaque had a ruptured surface and a very soft and compressible area and with the superimposition of a mobile clot, the tail freely floating in the lumen of the internal carotid artery (Fig. 3A–C, Clips 6–7). Cerebral MRI showed a small ischemic lesion in the right deep MCA territory, in the internal capsule (Fig. 3D). Patient underwent successful early urgent endarterectomy and intraoperative findings (Fig. 3E) confirmed the presence of a complicated plaque with a thrombus attached to its surface

Discussion

Therapeutical decisions in acute stroke patients have to be taken in few minutes, due to the narrowness of the therapeutical window. The decisions depend not only from the characteristics of the patient (age, time, co-morbidity, clinical severity, etc.), but also from the results of the first instrumental evaluation performed such as CT, MR with diffusion/perfusion sequences, MRA and sonography. Cases addressed to acute surgery or acute cerebrovascular treatments are though not so frequent (almost 5—10% of all acute presentations), also due to the frequent lack of 24 h availability of diagnostic facilities and expert performers.

Characterizations of carotid plaque morphology and of internal carotid artery stenosis hemodynamics have become nowadays a fundamental step for the surgical management. In cases of tight, pre-occlusive proximal internal carotid artery stenosis inducing distal low-flow velocities a vessel ''occlusion'' may indeed be over diagnosed, if the vessel hemodynamics are not correctly evaluated. While the occlusion excludes further indications for surgical revascularization, this well-known misleading entity — the so-called ''pseudo-occlusion'' — may be a very high-risk condition, since further distal embolism may still occur thorough the patent vessel and, thus, the debate on the opportunity of a surgical approach [13,14]. The pseudo-occlusion diagnosis has then to be promptly done, because emergent surgery can still be indeed successful in selected cases [15]. In these regards, several are the factors that may concur for the decision to perform a surgical procedure. First, the lumen of the vessels distal to the stenosis has to be patent and without excessive distal extension of the atherosclerotic process, that could hamper the surgical approach. Second, in cases of stroke, cerebral parenchyma should not be severely compromised, for the negative effects exerted by revascularization when performed in an already cerebral necrotic tissue. Conventional imaging with CT and MR provides the information on the status of cerebral tissue, but, on the other hand, when the distal tract of the carotid artery is patent and with low flow velocities, they may misinterpret the vessel as occluded, because of the low signal relate to the low-flow velocities [7]. High-resolution ultrasound, with real-time imaging of the vessel wall and hemodynamics evaluation with Pulsed-Wave Doppler, can be of valuable help for the identification of distal vessel patency in such cases [7], even with the aid of ultrasound contrast agents [16,17].

Another point to be taken into account for the management of the patient is the comprehension of the local bifurcation disease causing the pseudo-occlusion: atherosclerotic processes usually involve longer tracts of the artery, limiting the possibilities of surgery when the stenosis extends too distally, while a migrating thrombus is usually of smaller size and induces damage of the vessel wall only at the site of adhesion. We have already described the advantages of US in respect to CT and MR to identify carotid occlusions due to cardiac embolism [7] and, in these new cases, US could easily identify uncommon carotid ''saddle'' thrombi attached to the vessel wall and leaving the distal tract of the vessel open and without wall disease. Even without strictly following stroke guidelines, surgery was performed successfully in one case. The identification with high-resolution US of the embolic source on the plaque surface in case 3 indicated that surgery had to be performed as soon as possible, and not on elective bases.

This small case series underline that high-resolution US, even with contrast agents, is a feasible and reliable technique, nowadays commonly diffused in clinical practice, with more and more detailed imaging quality. These better resolution pictures can be of help in reducing operator's dependency, usually claimed as a major limit of US investigations. The detection of dynamic, real-time, aspects ''in motion'' is a strong potentiality of this technique, to better understand vascular pathophysiology. Moreover, ultrasound can easily differentiated cardiac clots from local thrombosis on a complicated atherosclerotic plaque, with the related clinical implications. All these findings underline the role of early ultrasound in the management of acute stroke patients. In conclusion, the achievement of his ''kingdom'' for the patient is linked to the availability of an expert joker, able to obtain the best results from his horse, besides ... ''saddle problems''.

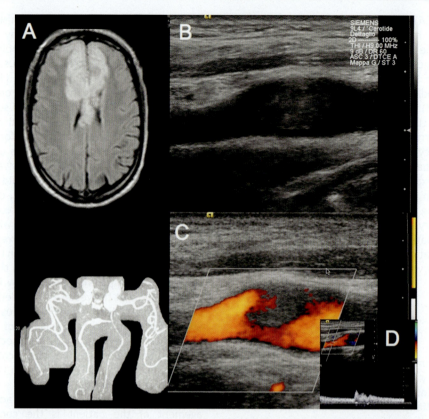

Figure 2 Case 2. Cerebral MR scan (A) with both anterior cerebral arteries ischemic lesions and normal middle cerebral arteries at MRA (below). Carotid utrasonography: B-mode (B), power mode (C) of a mobile clot adherent to the superior wall of the carotid bulb. Distally, the internal carotid artery is patent, as shown by the power Doppler (B) and pulsed wave Doppler (D).

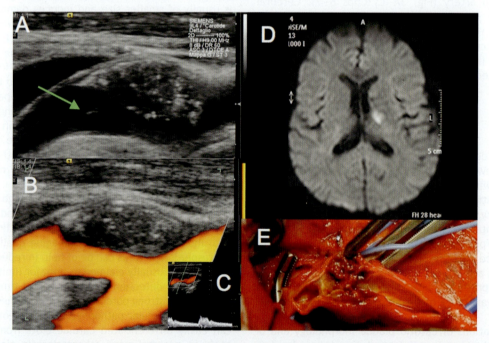

Figure 3 Case 3. Carotid ultrasonography: B-mode imaging (A) of the internal carotid stenosis with heterogeneous structure in a homolateral middle cerebral artery acute ischemic stroke patient. High-resolution images show a small thrombus with the head adhesion at the ruptured surface of the plaque, freely floating in the internal carotid lumen (green arrow). The distal tract of the artery is fully patent at the color Doppler (B), with normal blood flow velocities (C). Cerebral MRI scan shows a small lacuna in the homolateral internal capsule (D) and intraoperative findings (E) confirm the presence of a complicated plaque, with a thrombus attached to the surface of the plaque.

Appendix A. Supplementary data

Supplementary data associated with this article can be found, in the online version, at doi:10.1016/j.permed.2012.02.001.

References

[1] Musani MH. Asymptomatic saddle pulmonary embolism: case report and literature review. Clin Appl Thromb Hemost 2011;17(March):337—9.
[2] Kanjanauthai S, Couture LA, Fissha M, Gentry M, Sharma GK. Saddle pulmonary embolism visualized by transthoracic echocardiography. J Am Coll Cardiol 2010;56:e21.
[3] Chughtai H, Basora J, Khan K, Matta J. Massive pulmonary embolism and paradoxical migration during surgical embolectomy: role of transesophageal echocardiogram. Clin Cardiol 2010;33:E20—2.
[4] Shavit L, Appelbaum L, Grenader T. Atrial myxoma presenting with total occlusion of the abdominal aorta and multiple peripheral embolism. Eur J Intern Med 2007;18:74—5.
[5] Olearchyk AS. Saddle embolism of the aorta with sudden paraplegia. Can J Surg 2004;47:472—3.
[6] Kavanagh DO, Richards S, Barry MC, Sheehan S. Aortic saddle embolus causing paraplegia. Ir Med J 2004;97:117.
[7] Vicenzini E, Giannoni MF, Ricciardi MC, Toscano M, Sirimarco G, Di Piero V, et al. Noninvasive imaging of carotid arteries in stroke: emerging value of real-time high-resolution sonography in carotid occlusion due to cardiac embolism. J Ultrasound Med 2010;29:1635—41.
[8] Turnbull RG, Tsang VT, Teal PA, Salvian AJ. Successful innominate thromboembolectomy of a paradoxic embolus. J Vasc Surg 1998;28:742—5.
[9] McKinney WB, O'Hara W, Sreeram K, Hudson JA, Solis M. The successful surgical treatment of a paradoxical embolus to the carotid bifurcation. J Vasc Surg 2001;33:880—2.
[10] Smith WS, Sung G, Saver J, Budzik R, Duckwiler G, Liebeskind DS, et al. Mechanical thrombectomy for acute ischemic stroke: final results of the multi MERCI trial. Stroke 2008;39:1205—12.
[11] Ederle J, Bonati LH, Dobson J, Featherstone RL, Gaines PA, Beard JD, et al. Endovascular treatment with angioplasty or stenting versus endarterectomy in patients with carotid artery stenosis in the Carotid and Vertebral Artery Transluminal Angioplasty Study (CAVATAS): long-term follow-up of a randomised trial. Lancet Neurol 2009;8:898—907.
[12] Allaqaband S, Kirvaitis R, Jan F, Bajwa T. Endovascular treatment of peripheral vascular disease. Curr Probl Cardiol 2009;34:359—476.
[13] Garner C, Saver JL, Quiñones-Baldrich WJ. Pseudo-occlusion and/or pseudo-stenosis of the intracranial internal carotid artery. Ann Vasc Surg 1999;13:629—33.
[14] Fürst G, Saleh A, Wenserski F, Malms J, Cohnen M, Aulich A, et al. Reliability and validity of noninvasive imaging of internal carotid artery pseudo-occlusion. Stroke 1999;30:1444—9.
[15] Ringelstein EB, Zeumer H, Angelou D. The pathogenesis of strokes from internal carotid artery occlusion diagnostic and therapeutical implications. Stroke 1983;14:867—75.
[16] Ferrer JM, Samsó JJ, Serrando JR, Valenzuela VF, Montoya SB, Docampo MM. Use of ultrasound contrast in the diagnosis of carotid artery occlusion. J Vasc Surg 2000;31:736—41.
[17] Vicenzini E, Giannoni MF, Puccinelli F, Ricciardi MC, Altieri M, Di Piero V, et al. Detection of carotid adventitial vasa vasorum and plaque vascularization with ultrasound cadence contrast pulse sequencing technique and echo-contrast agent. Stroke 2007;38:2841—3.

Intravascular papillary endothelial hyperplasia at the origin of internal carotid artery: A rare cause of stroke

Nicola Carraro [a,*], Vittoria Maria Sarra [a], Airì Gorian [a], Francesco Pancrazio [b], Sergio Bucconi [c], Paola Martingano [d], Gilberto Pizzolato [a], Fabio Chiodo Grandi [a]

[a] DUC SMIT, UCO di Clinica Neurologica, AOTS, Trieste, Italy
[b] DUC ACADEM, UCO di Chirurgia Vascolare, AOTS, Trieste, Italy
[c] DUC ACADEM, UCO di Anatomia e Istologia Patologica, AOTS, Trieste, Italy
[d] DUC SMIT, UCO di Radiologia, AOTS, Trieste, Italy

KEYWORDS
Intravascular papillary endothelial hyperplasia;
IPEH;
Carotid artery;
Extracranial ultrasound examination

Summary Intravascular papillary endothelial hyperplasia (IPEH), also known as Masson's tumor, is a rare, generally considered a non neoplastic vascular lesion, caused by an abnormal endovascular proliferation of endothelial cells.
We describe, as far as we know, the first case of this lesion, localized at the origin of the internal carotid artery, which was responsible for an ischemic stroke. Although this entity is very rare, it is important for the clinician to become familiar with this lesion, since the complete removal of the lesion is the only treatment of choice. A partial removal may lead to further clinical events.
© 2012 Elsevier GmbH. All rights reserved.

Introduction

Intravascular papillary endothelial hyperplasia (IPEH) is a relatively uncommon benign and non-neoplastic vascular lesion [1–4]. Firstly described by Masson in 1923, as an endothelial proliferation associated with thrombosis and fibrin deposition, leading to obliteration of the vascular lumen [1–4]. Histologically it is characterized by the presence of endothelium-lined papillary structures composed by a single layer of plump cells around a fibrin core that sometimes forms irregular anatomizing clefts, simulating an angiosarcoma [5–8]. However, the absence of cellular polymorphism, mitotic activity and necrosis represent a differential feature of IPEH [5]. The prognosis of this lesion is excellent, and recurrence is an unusual finding. It is cured by simple excision in primary forms, and by treating the underlying condition in the secondary ones [6,8]. Its pathogenesis is believed to be associated with trauma, but it has also been reported as an unusual form of organized thrombus [6–9].

Case report

A 43 years old female with neither previous history of neurological diseases nor vascular risk factors other

* Corresponding author. Tel.: +39 040 421712; fax: +39 040 910861.
E-mail address: n.carraro@fmc.units.it (N. Carraro).

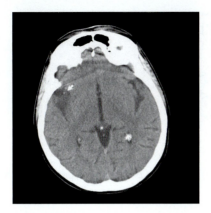

Figure 1 Brain CT: the "dot sign" (arrow) is visible in a M_2 branch of the right middle cerebral artery.

than smoking custom, was admitted to our Neurological Department — Stroke Unit, because of a left hemiparesis. She had felt her left arm somehow weak, strangely "cold", in the previous afternoon, but believing that this was related to fatigue she went to sleep. On admission a mild left sided sensorimotor hemiparesis was found with a NIHSS of 8.

The brain CT scan performed at the admission showed a "dot sign" in a M_2 branch of the right Middle Cerebral Artery (MCA) (Fig. 1) and a right fronto-parietal ischemic stroke (PACI) (Fig. 2). The EC US revealed at the origin of the internal carotid artery, an hyperechogenic lesion (Figs. S1 and S2). It was somehow different from an atherosclerotic plaque and more similar to a soft tissue mass. Its echogenicity was homogenous and, in its distal portion, it was partially separated from the arterial wall, but no flapping movement was evident (video). The lesion occupied more than 75% of the cross sectional area of the vessel, but no increased velocity was present (Figs. S3, and 3). At TCCD all the major intracranial arteries were insonated; an asymmetry of the MCA velocities (R < L), with a Zanette index of 26.39 suspicious for a right MCA distal occlusion, was found (Figs. S4 and S5). The Angio-CT confirmed these features (Figs. 4 and 5). The patient was evaluated for vascular risk factors, dietary

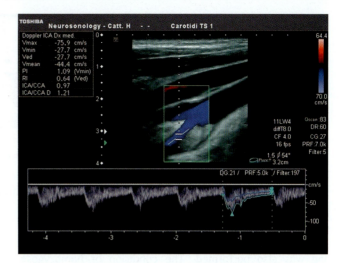

Figure 3 Extracranial carotid ultrsound examination. Right internal carotid artery and the flow waveform.

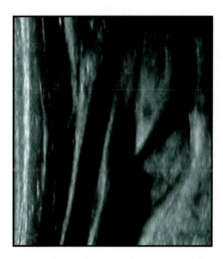

Figure 4 Internal carotid artery by extracranial carotid ultrsound examination.

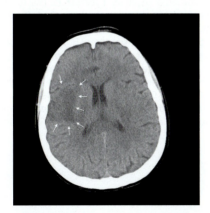

Figure 2 Brain CT: the right sided hypodense ischemic lesion is clearly detectable (arrows).

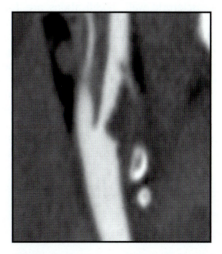

Figure 5 Internal carotid artery by Angio-CT performed the same day of ECUS.

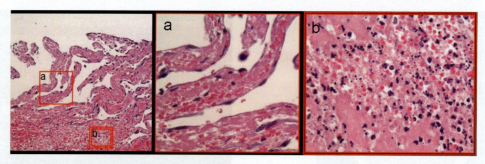

Figure 6 Histological specimens (EE stain) at different magnifications (a and b) showing an endothelial hyperplasia with a papillary distribution, surrounding a fibrin core with leucocytes and erythrocytes.

factors (Folate, B12), and methylene tetra hydro folate reductase (MTHFR) polymorphism; a thrombophilic screening was also performed. The condition of homozygosis for MTHFR was present. The histological diagnosis was consistent with a diagnosis of IPEH (Fig. 6): a marginal endothelial papillary hyperplasia, surrounding a fibrous and hematic material like an organized thrombotic formation, was described.

From the therapeutical point of view an antiplatelet therapy was started at the admission and the following days the clinical condition progressively improved. The vascular surgeon was then consulted and a surgical procedure was performed to remove the lesion.

When dismissed the patient was asymptomatic, the NIHSS equal to 0 and she did not suffer from any other symptom during the following 2 years. The EC US (Figs. S6 and S7), 2 years later, revealed some hyperplasia at the origin of the ICA possibly representing the over-expression of the post-CEA neoendothelial growth or the evolution of the incompletely removed lesion and showed that a longer follow-up is necessary.

Discussion

This pathology is quite rare compared with the common atherosclerotic lesions located at the carotid bifurcation; nevertheless the ultrasonographer may suspect it if no other atherosclerotic wall modifications are found elsewhere at the extracranial level, when the lesion is partly separated from the arterial wall in its distal portion and when no flow modification is found despite the huge lesion's dimensions. Moreover it is relevant to make the diagnosis for the clinician, since this lesion is highly prone to induce thrombus formation on its surface, with the possibility of embolic events. Early CEA is recommended and it is again relevant for the surgeon to suspect this diagnosis since, if the lesion is not completely removed, it can grow back again, with the risk of further embolic events.

Appendix A. Supplementary data

Supplementary data associated with this article can be found, in the online version, at http://dx.doi.org/10.1016/j.permed.2012.04.006.

References

[1] De Courten A, Küffer R, Samson J, Lombardi T. Intravascular papillary endothelial hyperplasia of the mouth: report of six cases and literature review. Oral Diseases 1999;5:175—8.

[2] Matsuzaka K, Koike Y, Yakushiji T, Shimono M, Inoue T. Intravascular papillary endothelial hyperplasia arising from the upper lip. Bulletin of Tokyo Dental College 2003;44:55—9.

[3] Devi M, Nalin Kumar S, Ranganathan K, Saraswathi TR. Oral intra vascular papillary endothelial hyperplasia in the floor of the mouth. Indian Journal of Dental Research 2004;15:149—51.

[4] Wang XY, Namiq A, Fan F. A 55-year-old woman with a buccal mass intravascular papillary endothelial hyperplasia. Archives of Pathology and Laboratory Medicine 2006;130:877—8.

[5] Inalöz HS, Patel G, Knight AG. Recurrent intravascular papillary endothelial hyperplasia developing from a pyogenic granuloma. Journal of the European Academy of Dermatology and Venereology 2001;15:156—8.

[6] Kim D, Israel H, Friedman M, Kuhel W, Langevin CJ, Plansky T. Intravascular papillary endothelial hyperplasia manifesting as a submandibular mass: an unusual presentation in an uncommon location. Journal of Oral and Maxillofacial Surgery 2007;65:786—90.

[7] Santonja C, De Sus J, Moragón M. Extramedullary hematopoiesis within endothelial papillary hyperplasia (Masson's pseudoangiosarcoma) of the tongue. Medicina Oral Patologia Oral y Cirugia Bucal 2007;12:E556—9.

[8] Anthony SG, Mudgal CS, DeLaney TF, Shin RD, Raskin KA, Ring DC. Recurrent intravascular papillary endothelial hyperplasia of the right middle finger treated with radiation therapy. Journal of Bone and Joint Surgery (British Volume) 2008;90:95—7.

[9] Cagli S, Oktar n, Dalbasti T, Islekel S, Demirtas E, Ozdamar N. Intravascular papillary endothelial hyperplasia of the cental nervous system. Neurologia Medico-Chirurgica 2004;44:302—10.

Reversible cerebral vasoconstriction syndrome after preeclampsia

Robert Müller*, Oliver Meier, Roman L. Haberl

Städtisches Klinikum München, Klinik für Neurologie und Neurologische Intensivmedizin Sanatoriumsplatz 2, 81545 München, Germany

KEYWORDS
Transcranial color coded ultrasound;
Reversible cerebral vasoconstriction syndrome

Summary Reversible cerebral vasoconstriction is a syndrome characterized by typical clinical manifestation and by the detection of vasoconstriction in cerebral arteries. Clinical symptoms are thunderclap headache, nausea, vomiting, confusion and seizures. Stenosis and dilatation of the cerebral arteries can be detected. Ultrasound as a non-invasive examination can also detect and control the findings. We describe the syndrome by reporting the case of a 32 year old primipara with vasoconstriction syndrome after preeclampsia.
© 2012 Published by Elsevier GmbH.

Background

Since the work of Call and Fleming in 1988 [1] a variety of similar syndromes with reversible cerebral vasoconstriction were published. Today these syndromes are unified in the term reversible cerebral vasoconstriction syndrome [2]. According to literature the reversible cerebral vasoconstriction syndrome is characterized by the following facts.

The mean age of onset is 42 years. Women are affected 2—3 times more often than men [5]. The syndrome is associated with pregnancy and puerperium, drugs such as cocaine, cannabis, LSD, ergotamine or selective serotonin reuptake inhibitors, different types of headache such as migraine, primary thunderclap headache, primary headache associated with sexual activity and other conditions such as porphyria, pheochromocytoma, craniocerebral injury [3,4].

According to the work of Ducros et al. the main clinical manifestation in 94% of 67 patients were thunderclap headache recurring over a mean period of one week. Other symptoms were nausea, vomiting, confusion and blurred vision. 3% of the patients in this review showed seizures [5].

Several vascular complications are reported. According to the work of Ducros 22% of the patients developed subarachnoidal hemorrhage, 6% intracerebral hemorrhage, 14% showed transient ischemic symptoms and 4% developed cerebral infarction in the course of disease [5].

Neuroimaging shows diffuse, multiple stenosis and dilatation of the cerebral vessels (string and beads) which resolve spontaneously in 1—3 months. There are no common transcranial color coded ultrasound criteria for diagnosis. Therefore common criteria for intracerebral stenosis or vasospamus are used. Ultrasound is shown to be safe in diagnosing and in controlling the course of disease [6].

There is no standard treatment. Due to literature mainly the calcium antagonist nimodipine in systemic application or in some case reports in local application is used.

The disease is self-limiting and has a low incidence of recurrence. But for prolonged vasoconstriction a higher risk of posterior leukencephalopathy and strokes is reported [6].

Case report

We report the case of a 32 year old primipara. The patient was admitted to an academical hospital with maximum medical care. The cause of admission was preeclampsia. For

* Corresponding author.
 E-mail address: Mueller_Rob@web.de (R. Müller).

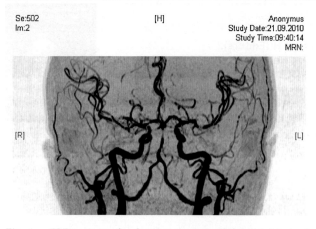

Fig. 1 TOF angiography showing stenosis of the distal A. basilaris, of the left A. cerebri media in the distal M1 section. *Abbreviations*: TOF MRA = Time-of-flight magnetic resonance angiography.

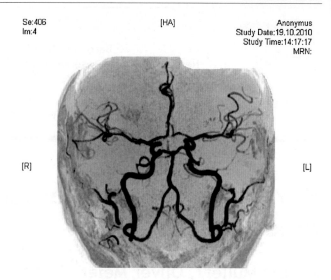

Fig. 2 1 month later no stenosis could be found.

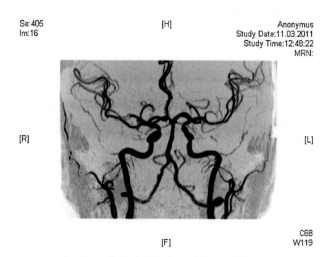

Fig. 3 6 months later no stenosis could be found.

gynecological reasons a Ceasarean section (C-section) was necessary.

There were several complications: Before C-Section the patient had a generalised tonic—clonic seizure, after the C-Section there was an atonic bleeding of the uterus with hemorragic shock with the need of erythrocyte concentrate transfusion. Four days after C-Section the patient complained about dyspnoea, CT-scan of the thorax and ultrasound of the deep veins of the leg showed pulmonal artery embolism after deep vein thrombosis. Hematological testing showed no dysfunction of the blood clotting or vasculitis associated antibodies. Anticoagulation was immediately initiated with i.v. heparin. Overlapping oral anticoagulation with phenoprocuomon was started.

Due to the generalised tonic—clonic seizure a neurologist was consulted. Physical examination showed no deficit of the cranial nerve function, the motor function, the sensibility, the coordination or the reflexes. No headache was reported. A MRI scan of the brain was done with a TOF angiography. The angiography showed stenosis of the distal A. basilaris and of the left A. cerebri media and stenosis with lower degree of the right A. cerebri media and of the left A. cerebri anterior. There was also a small infarction in the left A. cerebri anterior territory and no signs for sinus thrombosis or cerebral edema (Fig. 1). One month later the MRI-angiography showed no stenosis of the cerebral vessels (Fig. 2), another MRI 6 months after the onset also showed no stenosis of the cerebral vessels (Fig. 3).

Transcranial ultrasound showed decreasing peak systolic flow over the time (Table 1).

Retrospectively, with the findings from the MRI-scans and the ultrasound examination diagnosis of reversible cerebral vasoconstriction syndrome was verified.

Due to the benign course of disease we did not start any specific medical treatment.

Table 1 Transcranial Doppler findings over the time.

	28.09.			15.12.			18.04.		
	Depth (cm)	PSF (cm/s)	Mean (cm/s)	Depth (cm)	PSF (cm/s)	Mean (cm/s)	Depth (cm)	PSF (cm/s)	Mean (cm/s)
ACM left	5.0	150	125	5.0	84	55	5.0	93	64
ACA left	6.5	143	108	6.5	91	54	6.5	93	47
A. basilaris	10.0	140	100	10.0	82	58	10.0	95	62

Abbreviations: ACM = middle cerebral artery, ACA = anterior cerebral artery, PSF = peak systolic flow velocity (cm/s).

Discussion

Transcranial color coded ultrasound is a good and safe technique in diagnosing reversible vasoconstriction syndrome and in monitoring the course of disease. The main difficulty in this disease is to distinguish between reversible vasoconstriction syndrome and other vascular diseases of the central nerve system especially cerebral angiitis. Of course vascular imaging, e.g. with MRI is necessary.

Cerebral reversible vasoconstriction syndrome seems to be diagnosed insufficiently. On the other hand the more frequent use of non invasive cerebral vascular imaging as well as the more frequent use of vasoactive drugs may increase the number seen in daily practice.

Although in our reported case no headache was reported, thunderclap headache is one of the typical symptoms. Therefore the reversible vasoconstriction syndrome should be considered in differential diagnosis of thunderclap headache.

Women with an acute neurological deficit after birth or a Ceasarean section need a transcranial color-coded duplex sonography to detect cerebral vasoconstriction syndrome as soon as possible.

References

[1] Call GK, Fleming MC, Sealfon S, Levine H, Kistler JP, Fisher CM. Reversible cerebral segmental vasoconstriction. Stroke 1988;19:1159—70.

[2] Sattar A, Manousakis G, Jensen MB. Systematic review or reversible cerebral vasoconstriction syndrome. Expert Rev Cardiovasc Ther 2010;8(10):1417—21.

[3] Calabrese LH, Dodick DW, Schwedt TJ, et al. Narrative review: reversible cerebral vasoconstriction syndromes. Ann Intern Med 2007;146:34—44.

[4] Krämer M, Berlit P. Reversibles cerebrales Vasokonstriktions syndrom versus zerebrale Vaskulitis. Der Nervenarzt 2011;82:500—5.

[5] Ducros A, Boukobza M, Porcher R, Sarov M, Valade D, Bousser MD. The clinical and radiological spectrum of reversible cerebral vasoconstriction syndrome. A prospective series of 67 patients. Brain 2007;130:3091—101.

[6] Chen SP, Fuh JL, Chang FC, Lirng JF, Shia BC, Wang SJ. Reversible vasoconstriction syndrome. Ann Neurol 2008;63:751—7.

Transcranial and cervical duplex: A feasible approach to the diagnosis of pulsatile tinnitus

Pedro Cardona [a,*], Helena Quesada [a], Luis Cano [a], Jaume Campdelacreu [a], Anna Escrig [b], Paloma Mora [c], Francisco Rubio [a]

[a] Department of Neurology, Bellvitge University Hospital, Barcelona, Spain
[b] Department of Neurology, Sant Boi Hospital, Spain
[c] Department of Neuroradiology, Bellvitge University Hospital, Barcelona, Spain

KEYWORDS
Fistula;
Transcranial Doppler;
Duplex;
Tinnitus;
Pulsatile;
Dissection

Summary Pulsatile tinnitus is an uncommon form of tinnitus. Several vascular causes, such as carotid dissection and arteriovenous fistulae, have been associated to pulsatile tinnitus.
Methods: We present two patients who complained of pulsatile tinnitus and headache in the last 2 weeks.
Results: Transcranial Doppler demonstrated disturbances in systolic blood flow consisting of turbulences in the middle cerebral artery in one patient and disturbances in a vertebral artery in the other. MR and CT angiography confirmed the diagnosis of vertebrobasilar arteriovenous fistula. Daily compression maneuvers reduced the flow and bruit of both fistulas.
Conclusions: Hemodynamic changes in cerebral flow through a non-invasive and feasible test such as TCD or duplex can be very useful for the etiological diagnosis of pulsatile tinnitus.
© 2012 Elsevier GmbH. All rights reserved.

Introduction

Pulsatile tinnitus is an uncommon form of tinnitus. It has some well-known causes including hypertension, heart murmur or Eustachian tube dysfunction.

Pulsatile tinnitus could be a non-specific sign of cerebral blood flow disturbances, or a disturbance of a cervical vein or artery. Turbulent blood flow occurs when the wall of a blood vessel becomes irregular or stenotic.

Several vascular causes, such as carotid dissection and arteriovenous fistulae, have been associated to pulsatile tinnitus [1,2].

Methods

We present two patients, a 27-year-old woman and a 43-year-old man, who complained of pulsatile tinnitus and headache in the last 2 weeks. Neurological examination was normal in both cases. The tinnitus was not associated with dizziness or vertigo and neither were there any related drugs. CT scan and MR showed normal brain structures. In the following weeks the patients explained that they were obtaining a transient relief of tinnitus through compression maneuvers on the neck.

Results

Transcranial Doppler demonstrated disturbances in systolic blood flow consisting of turbulences in the middle cerebral

* Corresponding author. Tel.: +34 932607919; fax: +34 932607882.
E-mail address: pcardonap@bellvitgehospital.cat (P. Cardona).

2211-968X/$ — see front matter © 2012 Elsevier GmbH. All rights reserved.
doi:10.1016/j.permed.2012.02.062

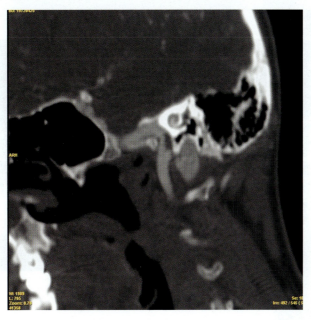

Figure 1   CT angiography: intracranial carotid stenosis next to cochlea.

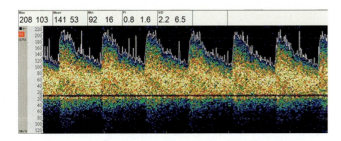

Figure 2   Turbulences in TCD test during left MCA and carotid insonation (M1 segment left MCA).

artery in one patient and disturbances in a vertebral artery in the other. Intracranial carotid dissection next to the temporal bone and cochlea was diagnosed by CT angiography in one patient. In the other patient, duplex of the extracranial vertebral artery showed a dampened pulse wave and turbulence with audible bruit. Duplex through the cervical-occipital window showed an oscillating vascular flow related to ipsilateral cervical compression maneuvers. MR and CT angiography confirmed the diagnosis of vertebrobasilar arteriovenous fistula [3]. Daily compression maneuvers reduced the flow and bruit of both the carotid artery and the arteriovenous fistula as visualized by transcranial Doppler (TCD) and duplex. Two months later the carotid artery recovered its normal flow pattern in TCD and CT angiography, allowing treatment with aspirin to be discontinued (Figs. 1—3).

Discussion

Two types of blood flow disturbances are associated with pulsatile tinnitus: a generalized increased flow, which can occur in conditions like severe anemia, hyperthyroidism or thyrotoxicosis and in the context of punishing exercise or pregnancy; and a localized increased flow. Vascular causes of tinnitus have been well described and include arteriovenous malformations, arteriovenous fistula, carotid artery-cavernous sinus fistula, vascular tumors in the middle ear, intracranial vascular stenosis usually from atheroma plaques and moya-moya syndrome. We present a patient with an uncommon cause of stroke such as an isolated intracranial carotid artery dissection. Vascular examination through magnetic resonance or CT is mandatory for the diagnosis of pulsatile tinnitus because it is sometimes very difficult to determine the cause and location of these bruits [4]. TCD or carotid-intracranial duplex can help us determine whether there is a disturbance flow with high sensitivity. However, a CT or MR angiography is necessary to increase specificity for the diagnosis [5]. At first, patients with pulsatile tinnitus should be investigated with noninvasive techniques like ultrasounds. If these tests fail to identify abnormal findings, selective angiography can help us to the diagnosis and management [6,7].

The most common ultrasound findings in carotid artery dissection are an absence of flow signal in the internal carotid artery, a biphasic (stump) flow in its bulb and a high-resistance flow pattern of the ipsilateral common carotid artery. Pulsatile tinnitus can occur in up to 25% of patients with dissection of the internal carotid artery.

An arteriovenous fistula is an abnormal connection or passageway between an artery and a vein, what causes hemodynamic changes that can give rise to audible bruits. Trancranial color-coded sonography (TCCS) is a good screening technique for the diagnosis of fistulae and contrast-enhancement could be a good test to monitor complete embolization of dural arteriovenous fistulae.

Treatment of vascular pulsatile tinnitus generally involves a multi-disciplinary approach and includes a variety of symptom management methods. A possible endovascular or surgical treatment should be considered in selected cases of vascular etiology [8,9].

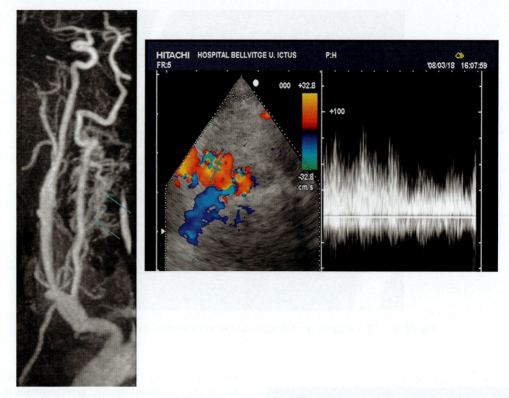

Figure 3 MR angiography shows several venous vessels next to left vertebral artery. Duplex through cervical/occipital window shows a vascular flow that oscillates with ipsilateral cervical compression maneuvers.

Conclusion

The finding of direct or indirect hemodynamic changes in cerebral flow through a non-invasive and feasible test such as TCD or duplex can be very useful for the etiological diagnosis of pulsatile tinnitus. MR and CT angiography are needed to confirm the diagnosis and for treatment planning [10].

References

[1] Mattox DE, Hudgins P. Algorithm for evaluation of pulsatile tinnitus. Acta Otolaryngol 2008;128(April (4)):427—31.
[2] Sonmez G, Basekim CC, Ozturk E, Gungor A, Kizilkaya E. Imaging of pulsatile tinnitus: a review of 74 patients. Clin Imaging 2007;31(March—April (2)):102—8.
[3] Corr P, Tsheole-Marishane L. Pulsatile tinnitus. Br J Radiol 2001;74(July (883)):669—70.
[4] Weissman JL, Hirsch BE. Imaging of tinnitus: a review. Radiology 2000;216(August (2)):3429.
[5] Mehanna R, Shaltoni H, Morsi H, Mawad M. Endovascular treatment of sigmoid sinus aneurysm presenting as devastating pulsatile tinnitus. A case report and review of literature. Interv Neuroradiol 2010;16(December (4)):451—4.
[6] De Candia A, Como G, Passon P, Pedace E, Bazzocchi M. Sonographic findings in glomus tympanicum tumor. J Clin Ultrasound 2002;30(May (4)):236—40.
[7] Narvid J, Do HM, Blevins NH, Fischbein NJ. CT angiography as a screening tool for dural arteriovenous fistula in patients with pulsatile tinnitus: feasibility and test characteristics. AJNR Am J Neuroradiol 2011;32(March (3)):446—53.
[8] Singh DP, Forte AJ, Brewer MB, Nowygrod R. Bilateral carotid endarterectomy as treatment of vascular pulsatile tinnitus. J Vasc Surg 2009;50(July (1)):183—5.
[9] Baumgartner RW, Arnold M, Baumgartner I, Mosso M, Gönner F, Studer A, et al. Carotid dissection with and without ischemic events: local symptoms and cerebral artery findings. Neurology 2001;57(September (5)):827—32.
[10] Harrer JU, Popescu O, Henkes HH, Klötzsch C. Assessment of dural arteriovenous fistulae by transcranial color-coded duplex sonography. Stroke 2005;36(May (5)):976—9.

Pitfall of vertebral artery insonation: Bidirectional flow without subclavian artery pathology

Susanne Johnsen [a,*], Stephan J. Schreiber [b], Florian Connolly [b], Karsten Schepelmann [a], Jose M. Valdueza [c]

[a] Department of Neurology, Schlei-Klinikum, Schleswig, Germany
[b] Department of Neurology, University Hospital Charité, Berlin, Germany
[c] Neurological Centre, Segeberger Kliniken, Bad Segeberg, Germany

KEYWORDS
Vertebral artery;
Pitfall;
Alternating flow;
Bidirectional flow;
Duplex sonography;
Subclavian steal syndrom

Summary

Background: A bidirectional flow pattern within the intracranial segment of the vertebral artery (V4—VA) should be indicative of a proximal steno-occlusive disorder of the ipsilateral subclavian artery (SA). Here we present two patients revealing this ultrasound finding without evidence of a specific SA pathology.

Methods/case reports: In case 1 duplex sonography revealed a diameter of the left V2—VA of 3.3 mm and 2.7 mm on the right side. Normal flow signals were detected in the left V2—VA, a systolic flow deceleration was seen on the right side. Intracranially, a biphasic flow pattern was observed in the right V4—VA. The left V4—VA, the basilar artery and the brachial arteries (BrA) as well as the cuff-test were normal. Conventional angiography ruled out a SA or VA pathology. A bilateral fetal-type posterior cerebral artery (FT-PCA) was seen. CT angiography demonstrated a small diameter of the right intracranial V4—VA close to the basilar confluens.

In case 2 VA diameter of the left and right V2—VA was 3.3 and 2.3 mm, respectively. Flow signals, similar to case 1 were observed in the non-dominant V2—VA and V4—VA segment. The remaining vessels and the cuff-test were normal. MR angiography demonstrated a FT-PCA and an incomplete posterior inferior cerebellar artery (PICA)-ending VA on the right side.

Conclusions: A bidirectional flow in V4—VA can not prove a subclavian steal phenomenon. A normal triphasic flow signal of the brachial artery excludes a relevant proximal obstruction of the SA. Also, diameter measurements of the VA are mandatory.

It seems that physiological variants of the vertebrobasilar circulation like a VA hypoplasia, PICA-ending VA or FT-PCA might also cause the above type of VA flow pattern.
© 2012 Elsevier GmbH. All rights reserved.

Introduction

A bidirectional flow pattern within the intracraniel segment of the vertebral artery (V4—VA) normally indicates a proximal steno-occlusive disorder of the ipsilateral subclavian artery. Depending on the grade of the SA stenosis a reduced systolic flow (systolic deceleration) may be observed within

* Corresponding author. Tel.: +49 431802149.
E-mail address: sjohnsen@ki.tng.de (S. Johnsen).

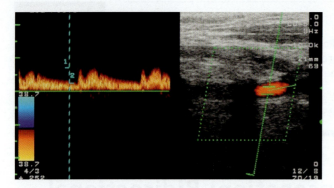

Figure 1 Right V2—VA with assumed systolic deceleration.

the ipsilateral VA in grade 1, an alternating flow in grade 2 or even a retrograde flow in grade 3 (Fig. S1). Indirect hemodynamic signs of obstruction of the SA can be seen in the distal depending vessels, e.g. in the ipsilateral brachial artery. In this case an attenuated flow pattern usually with a bi- or monophasic flow signal instead of the typical triphasic flow profile will be observed.

Here we present two patients revealing an alternating flow pattern in the intracranial segment of a vertebral artery without indication of subclavian artery pathology. There was also no evidence for a stenoocclusive disorder in the ipsilateral brachiocephalic trunc or the proximal segment of the vertebral artery.

Case reports

Case 1

A 69-year-old man was admitted after an episode of severe headache. Duplex sonography revealed mild atherosclerotic plaques. V2—VA diameter was 3.3 mm on the left, 2.7 mm on the right side. Normal flow signals were detected in the left V2—VA (Fig. S2), a flow pattern considered as a systolic flow deceleration was seen on the right side (Fig. 1). Intracranially, a biphasic flow pattern was observed in the right V4—VA distal the posterior inferior cerebellar artery (PICA) (Fig. 2). A normal flow pattern was seen in the right V4—VA proximal PICA (Fig. 3). The left V4—VA, the basilar artery and the brachial arteries (BrA) as well as the cuff-test were normal. Conventional angiography ruled out a SA or VA pathology (Fig. 4). A bilateral fetal-type posterior cerebral

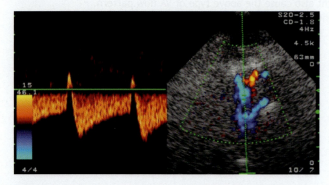

Figure 2 Right V4—VA distal PICA with bidirectional flow pattern.

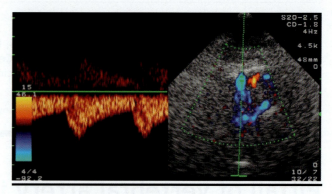

Figure 3 Right V4—VA proximal PICA with normal flow pattern.

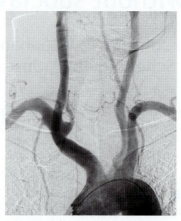

Figure 4 Conventional angiography without SA stenosis.

artery (FT-PCA) was seen (Fig. 5). CT angiography demonstrated a small diameter of the right intracranial V4—VA close to the basilar confluens.

Case 2

This 79-year-old lady was seen after carotid surgery of a symptomatic right-sided internal carotid artery stenosis. Duplexsonography revealed a moderate left ICA stenosis. V2—VA diameter measurement showed a hypoplasia of the right side (2.3 mm) and a normal caliber on the left side (3.3 mm). Flow signals, similar to case 1 were observed in the non-dominant right V2—VA (Fig. 6) and V4—VA (Fig. S3). The brachial arteries (Fig. S4), the left-sided

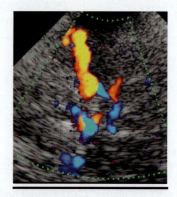

Figure 5 Circle of Willis with bilateral fetal type PCA.

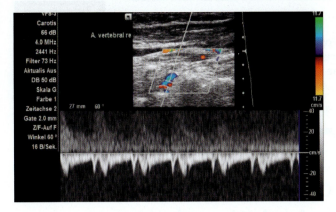

Figure 6 Right V2—VA with assumed systolic deceleration.

V2—VA (Fig. S5), and the cuff-test were normal. MR angiography demonstrated a FT-PCA and an incomplete posterior inferior cerebellar artery (PICA)-ending VA on the right side.

Results

In these two cases we saw a bidirectional flow pattern in the intracranial V3- and/or V4-segment of the vertebral artery. In both cases a systolic deceleration was seen in the V2-segment of the ipsilateral vertebral artery. None of them had an obstruction of the subclavian artery, the brachiocephalic trunc or the proximal vertebral artery. In both cases we found variations of the vertebrobasilar circulation with a bilateral incomplete fetal type PCA, a PICA-ending vertebral artery and a hypoplasia of the ipsilateral vertebral artery.

Discussion

In both cases we assumed that the bidirectional flow in the V4-segment of the vertebral artery might derive from the V4-segment distal of the PICA origin. In such condition the main blood flow from the right vertebral artery takes the way through the right posterior inferior cerebellar artery. In case 1 this was seen in CT angiography, in case 2 in MR angiography. Due to a lower blood stream with less pressure for the flow through the very thin ipsilateral V4-segment and the normal flow in the contralateral vertebral artery this bidirectional flow pattern may arise. The situation may be intensified by difficult outflow conditions via the basilar artery and the incomplete fetal type of the posterior cerebral arteries.

Conclusion

A bidirectional flow in the V4-segment of the vertebral artery cannot prove a subclavian steal syndrome. It may occur in normal subjects without evidence for an obstruction of the brachiocephalic trunc or of the ipsilateral proximal vertebral artery. To avoid such a pitfall the flow pattern of the brachial artery should be part of the examination. A normal triphasic flow pattern excludes a relevant obstruction of the proximal subclavian artery. Also diameter measurements of the VA are mandatory. It seems that variations of the vertebrobasilar circulation like PICA-ending vertebral artery, hypoplasia of the vertebral artery and fetal-type PCA might also cause a biphasic intracranial flow pattern. Regional different pressure ratios witch are caused by individual in- and outflow conditions might be a main cause. Larger series are required to confirm these preliminary observations.

Appendix A. Supplementary data

Supplementary data associated with this article can be found, in the online version, at http://dx.doi.org/10.1016/j.permed.2012.04.003.

Migraine-like presentation of vertebral artery dissection after cervical manipulative therapy

Dalius Jatuzis*, Jurgita Valaikiene

Vilnius University, Neurology and Neurosurgery Clinic, Centre of Neurology, Vilnius, Lithuania

KEYWORDS
Vertebral artery dissection;
Cervical manipulative therapy;
Headache;
Migraine

Summary Headache is the common symptom in patients with cervical artery dissection. However, it rarely occurs in isolation, without focal neurological signs, and even more rarely mimics migraine. We present a clinical case of young woman with new severe throbbing unilateral headache which started one week after cervical manipulative therapy. No history of migraine was present. Vertebral artery dissection was diagnosed after duplex ultrasound and CT angiography. Local symptoms and signs were absent, and diffusion-weighted MRI did not show any acute brain ischemic lesions. Throbbing headache gradually resolved in 10 days. Follow-up 5 months later showed near-complete normalization of lumen and flow of dissected vertebral artery. The possibility of extracranial dissection should be considered in patients with first attack of migraine-like hemicrania, especially if cervical manipulations or trauma occurred recently.
© 2012 Elsevier GmbH. All rights reserved.

Introduction

Headache is the common symptom in patients with cervical artery dissection (CAD). However, it rarely occurs in isolation, without focal neurological signs, and even more rarely mimics migraine. Spontaneous CAD can be associated with minor traumas of various origin, including stretches, sudden neck movements, and chiropractic manipulation [1,2]. We present a clinical case of patient with new severe migraine-like hemicrania after cervical manipulative therapy (CMT) in whom dissection of vertebral artery (VA) was diagnosed after ultrasound and neuroimaging assessment.

Case report

A 26 years old woman arrived to our out-patient neurological department due to persistent severe throbbing unilateral left-side headache, predominantly in the temporal region, which started 1 week ago. Nausea, photophobia, intolerance of physical activity was also present. Her clinical history revealed that three weeks ago cervical manipulations were applied for recurrent right-side neck pain which exacerbated episodically during the last few years. No other minor trauma or severe coughing was reported by patient. Dull cervical pain alleviated after CMT and resolved 1 week before the onset of pulsating hemicrania. The patient did not have attacks of episodic hemicrania or symptoms compatible with migraine aura never before.

General examination was unremarkable. Height of the patient was 160 cm, weight 48 kg (patient had intense training in gymnastics during adolescence). *Neurological examination* revealed no focal signs and was normal. *Extracranial color duplex ultrasound* showed typical direct signs of right VA dissection (dilation of V1 before the

* Corresponding author at: Department of Neurology, Vilnius University Hospital, Santariskiu Klinikos, Santariskiu Str. 2, Vilnius LT-08661, Lithuania. Tel.: +370 686 89795; fax: +370 523 65165.
E-mail address: dalius.jatuzis@santa.lt (D. Jatuzis).

entrance into C6 vertebra (Fig. 1a), double lumen of V2 segment and narrowing of true lumen (Fig. 1b) (video supplement)) and abnormal extracranial flow (decreased flow velocities and high resistance index) in right VA (Fig. 1c). It has never been performed before. *Transcranial color coded sonography* confirmed normal flow within Willis circle (the circle of Willis), however, flow within the intracranial segment of the right VA was not detected. The *CT angiography* confirmed a long dissection of the right VA, with a large intramural hematoma and a string-like true lumen (Fig. 2). *Diffusion-weighted MRI* did not show any acute brain ischemic lesions.

Antithrombotic treatment (aspirin) was given for prevention of cerebral embolism. The possibility of endovascular stenting of the right VA was considered, however, it was not performed because of own risks of stenting related to long dissected segment and needs for multiple stents.

Hemicrania lasted for approximately 10 days and gradually resolved. Follow-up 1 and 5 months later showed near-complete normalization of lumen and flow of the right VA (Fig. S1 (A) and (B)). Migraine-like hemicrania did not appear again.

Discussion

The characteristics of pain associated with CAD are not specific and can sometimes resemble migraine or even cluster headache [3]. CAD with isolated pain might be more common than expected and is more often caused by extracranial VA dissection [4]. Recently a clinical case of VA dissection presenting with isolated occipital headache was published [5]. In a large series of CAD patients in whom pain was the only symptom, the pain was continuous in most cases, and headaches were mostly of a severe intensity and throbbing quality, whereas neck pain was more commonly constrictive and of moderate intensity [4]. The onset type ranged from thunderclap headache to progressive pain. In our case pain was intensive, throbbing, started gradually and mimicked migraine, however, it lasted much more than typical migraine attack. Interestingly, hemicranial left-sided pain started on the contralateral side to the dissection of right VA. No local symptoms and signs or ischemic manifestations occurred.

The cause of cervical artery dissection remains disputed. The most likely pathological mechanism is the trauma (torsional or stretching) of the arterial wall causing a tear in the intima that separates the intima from the tunica media. The mechanism and the severity of external trauma sufficient to cause dissection varies from blunt and penetrating external to trivial trauma such as coughing, or torsion of the neck as in forced head rotation on chiropractic manipulation or sporting injuries [6].

Though recognized as therapy for spinal pain for thousands of years, manipulation of the spine has been performed since the 18th century to treat, or even prevent, symptoms of neck pain, muscle tension and migraine without any medical or scientific background. There has been significant discussion and debate about the possible association between VA dissection and CMT. The first recorded case of fatal brain stem infarction due to vertebrobasilar vessel injury after neck manipulation was in 1947 [7].

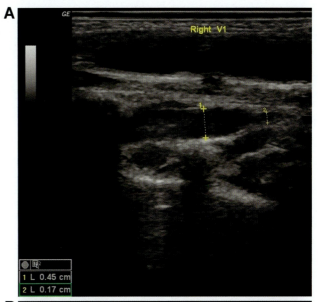
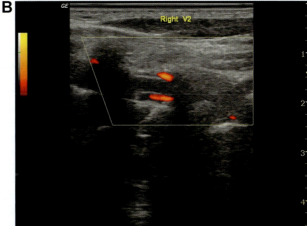
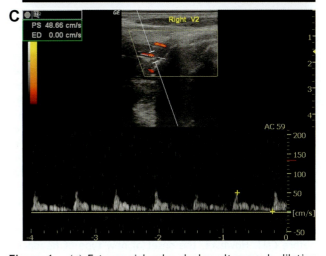

Figure 1 (a) Extracranial color duplex ultrasound: dilation of V1 before the entrance into C6 vertebra. (b) Extracranial color duplex ultrasound: double lumen of V2 segment and narrowing of true lumen. (c) Extracranial color duplex ultrasound: abnormal extracranial flow (decreased flow velocities and high resistance index).

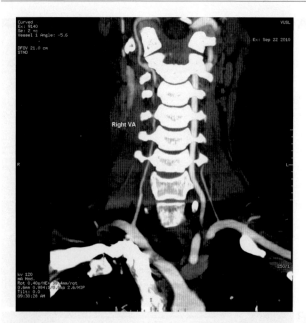

Figure 2 CT angiography: dissection of right vertebral artery.

More than one-quarter of cases of stroke from VA dissection were attributed to neck manipulation in one published case series [8]. However, a clear causal relationship has not yet been established, therefore, the role of CMT in VA dissection remains a controversy that sparks debate and disagreement between neurologists and chiropractors. For example, a recent paper in *Chiropractic & Osteopathy* came to conclusions that the relationship is not causal—patients with VA dissection already present prior to the manipulation often have initial symptoms which cause them to seek care from a chiropractic physician and have a stroke some time after, independent of the chiropractic visit [9]. A cause-and-effect relationship is even less convincing when the delay between manipulation and symptoms is hours or even days [6]. The question "Does CMT cause VA dissection and subsequent ischemic stroke?" was addressed with a structured evidence-based clinical neurologic practice review [10]. Authors found burden of evidence to support a cause-and-effect relationship between CMT with VA dissection. Young vertebrobasilar artery territory stroke patients were 5 times more likely than controls to have had CMT within 1 week of the event date. The best available estimate of incidence was approximately 1.3 cases of VA dissection or occlusion attributable to CMT for every 100,000 persons <45 years of age receiving CMT within 1 week of manipulative therapy [10].

In our case we are also not able to prove a causal relationship between CMT and VA dissection, as ultrasound examination of extracranial arteries has not been performed before CMT. However, the onset of new type of headache (different from common neck pain) weeks after CMT and confirmed new VA dissection make this relationship plausible.

Conclusions

Causative relationship between CMT and VA dissection remains unproven. However, the possibility of extracranial dissection should be considered in patients with first attack of migraine-like hemicrania, especially if cervical manipulations or trauma were present recently. CMT should not be started without ultrasound screening of extracranial arteries in cases of atypical neck pain.

Acknowledgements

We thank Dr. Mindaugas Mataciunas and Jurate Dementaviciene for radiological tests and comments.

Appendix A. Supplementary data

Supplementary data associated with this article can be found, in the online version, at http://dx.doi.org/10.1016/j.permed.2012.03.010.

References

[1] Debette S, Leys D. Cervical-artery dissections: predisposing factors, diagnosis, and outcome. The Lancet Neurology 2009;8:668—78.
[2] Ernst E. Adverse effects of spinal manipulation: a systematic review. Journal of the Royal Society of Medicine 2007;100:330—8.
[3] Morelli N, Mancuso M, Gori S, Maluccio MR, Cafforio G, Chiti A, et al. Vertebral artery dissection onset mimics migraine with aura in a graphic designer. Headache 2008;48: 621—4.
[4] Arnold M, Cumurciuc R, Stapf C, Favrole P, Berthet K, Bousser MG. Pain as the only symptom of cervical artery dissection. Journal of Neurology, Neurosurgery and Psychiatry 2006;77:1021—4.
[5] Luigetti M, Profice P, Pilato F, Della Marca G, Broccolini A, Morosetti R, et al. Vertebral artery dissection presenting with isolated occipital headache. Headache 2010;50: 1378—80.
[6] Menon RK, Norris JW. Cervical arterial dissection: current concepts. Annals of the New York Academy of Sciences 2008;1142:200—17.
[7] Pratt-Thomas HR, Berger KE. Cerebellar and spinal injuries after chiropractic manipulation. The Journal of the American Medical Association 1947;133:600—3.
[8] Norris JW, Beletsky V, Nadareishvili ZG. Sudden neck movement and cervical artery dissection. The Canadian Stroke Consortium. Canadian Medical Association Journal 2000;163:38—40.
[9] Murphy DR. Current understanding of the relationship between cervical manipulation and stroke: what does it mean for the chiropractic profession? Chiropractic & Osteopathy 2010;18:22.
[10] Miley ML, Wellik KE, Wingerchuk DM, Demaerschalk BM. Does cervical manipulative therapy cause vertebral artery dissection and stroke. The Neurologist 2008;14:66—73.

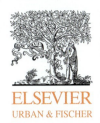

**Bartels E, Bartels S, Poppert H (Editors):
New Trends in Neurosonology and Cerebral Hemodynamics — an Update.**

The impact of recanalization on ischemic stroke outcome: A clinical case presentation

Silva Andonova[a,*], Filip Kirov[a], Chavdar Bachvarov[b]

[a] Second Clinic of Neurology, St. Marina University Hospital, Varna, Bulgaria
[b] Centre of Radiology, St. Marina University Hospital, Varna, Bulgaria

KEYWORDS
Ischemic stroke;
Recanalization;
Intravenous thrombolysis

Summary

Background and purpose: Stroke remains the third most common cause of death in industrialized nations, and the single most common reason for permanent disability. Intravenous thrombolysis (IVT) with recombinant tissue plasminogen activator (rtPA, Alteplase) for the treatment of acute ischemic stroke within 4.5 h of onset is becoming a worldwide conventional standard of care. Thrombolytic stroke therapy is based on the ''recanalization hypothesis'' that reopening of occluded vessels improves clinical outcome in acute ischemic stroke through regional reperfusion and salvage of threatened tissues. However, intravenous thrombolysis is successful in approximately one-third of patients. Thrombaspiration through either a microcatheter, or a guiding catheter may be an option for a fresh nonadhesive clot. The use of mechanical thrombectomy devices in patients experiencing ischemic stroke and reocclusion after intravenous thrombolysis can now gain approval on the basis of recanalization, demonstrating better recanalization rates.

Case description: We present a clinical case of IVT followed by re-occlusion, and intra-arterial thrombaspiration and stenting.

Results: After IVT was started, a significant improvement of the neurological deficit was observed. After the end of the fibrinolysis, the patient had severe deterioration of the symptoms. The patient underwent control CT of the head to exclude intracerebral hemorrhage — the CT was normal. Through a guiding catheter thrombaspiration and stenting was performed with effective reperfusion with reversal of the neurological deficits.

Conclusions: Revascularization remains the most intuitive strategy to reverse ischemic injury associated with arterial occlusion in acute strokes. This case represents a valuable example of two recanalization therapies in acute ischemic stroke to improve clinical outcome by restoring anterograde perfusion and salvaging the ischemic brain.
© 2012 Elsevier GmbH. All rights reserved.

Background and purpose

Despite the substantial advances in preventive and treatment strategies, stroke still remains the third most common cause of death in industrialized nations, and the single most common reason for permanent disability [1,14]. Bulgaria is

* Corresponding author at: Department of Neurology, St. Marina University Hospital, 1 HristoSmirnenski St., Varna 9010, Bulgaria. Tel.: +359 52 978236.
E-mail address: drsilva@abv.bg (S. Andonova).

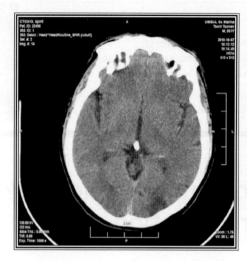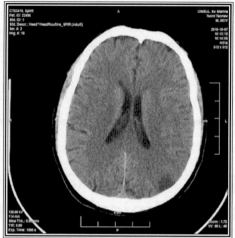

Figure 1 Brain CT.

the worst example in the European Union, by heading the list of stroke mortality [13].

Intravenous thrombolysis (IVT) with recombinant tissue plasminogen activator (rtPA, Alteplase) within 4.5 h of stroke onset is now the worldwide standard of care [7].

However, the cumulated experience from IVT reveals some substantial drawbacks: short time window, long list of exclusion criteria, and more importantly — a not negligible rate of no treatment effect or re-occlusion [5]. The only possible solution in the latter case is an attempt for rapid intra-arterial recanalization [3,4,9,11,14].

Case description

We present a clinical case of IVT followed by re-occlusion, and intra-arterial thrombaspiration and stenting.

A 51 years old male was admitted in the emergency department at 07:50 with dextral hemiparesis and speech difficulties. The patient has had diabetes mellitus type II for 5 years with good control without treatment, and arterial hypertension treated with ACE-inhibitor. His wife reported the symptoms appeared at 06:50 when preparing to leave for work. Brain CT (at 08:30) revealed a hypodense area in the left occipital region. The color-coded duplex sonography revealed this as high grade stenosis of the left internal carotid artery (Fig. 1).

He was transferred to the Neuro-Critical Care Unit for IVT. At the start of the infusion — an intravenous rt-Pa by protocol: body weight × 0.9 mg/kg rt-PA — with 10% bolus and i.v. infusion for 60 min, (on 08:39) his NIHSS was 8 points. At 09:10 the patient showed clinical improvement with NIHSS = 5 p., but at 09:40, at the end of the rt-Pa infusion, the patient became suddenly hemiplegic and aphasic. His NIHSS was 15. The second brain CT did not show any differences from the previous one (Fig. 2).

A decision was made for an immediate attempt for intra-arterial recanalization, after obtaining a written informed consent from his wife. Cerebral angiography with right-sided femoral access was started at 10:36, revealing an occlusion of the left internal carotid artery. A mechanical thrombaspiration with 20 cc syringe was successfully performed leading to recanalization at 11:32. As there was a significant stenosis on the place of the occlusion a self-expandable stent was placed at 11:45. The patient's improvement started a few minutes later with NIHSS — 12 at 11:45, and 6 at 12:00.

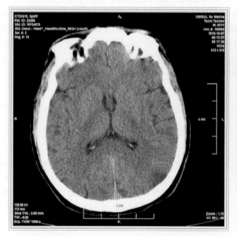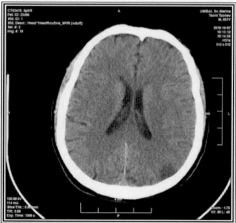

Figure 2 Control CT (10.15 h) to exclude intracerebral hemorrhage NIHSS = 15.

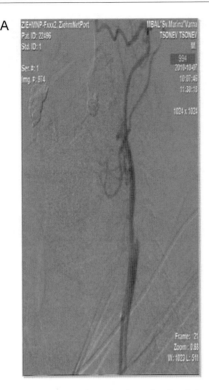 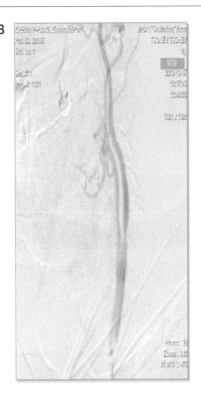

Figure 3 Digital subtraction angiography: (A) thrombosis of the left internal carotid artery; (B) after thrombaspiration and stent with effective reperfusion.

Brain CT showed small hemorrhagic infarction in the left hemisphere. The patient was discharged after five days with motor dysphasia and NIHSS of 3. Three months later he had recovered completely (Figs. 3—5).

Figure 4 Intracranial image of left carotid artery after fibrinolysis, thrombaspiration and stenting.

Revascularization remains the most intuitive strategy to reverse ischemic injury associated with arterial occlusion in acute strokes. Revascularization may lead to opening of an occluded artery, or recanalization, yet restoration of downstream flow, or reperfusion, may not ensue.

This case represents a valuable example of two recanalization therapies in acute ischemic stroke to improve clinical outcome by restoring anterograde perfusion and salvaging the ischemic brain.

Discussion

The potential role of intravenous thrombolysis for recanalization of various occlusion sites has also been examined in depth [6]. In the Echoplanar Imaging Thrombolytic Evaluation Trial, intravenous tissue plasminogen activator administered in the 3—6-h time window showed poor recanalization of intracranial carotid artery (ICA) lesions and far better results with middle cerebral artery (MCA) occlusions [6]. Intra-arterial recanalization in acute ischemic stroke is nowadays the second option for saving the ischemic brain after the officially recognized IVT, and is a landmark for experienced and advanced acute stroke centers worldwide [2,10,12]. Several methods and a substantial arsenal of devices and systems are currently in use routinely or under investigation in different trials [9,14]. Mechanical thrombaspiration with a syringe in acute stroke is today more likely a topic from the history of endovascular treatment [8,11]. Most case series have been published in the last 15 years with promising results, but so far there is no data from clinical trials [12]. For Bulgaria this is one of the few known clinical cases of successful recanalization in acute stroke.

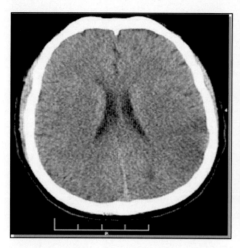 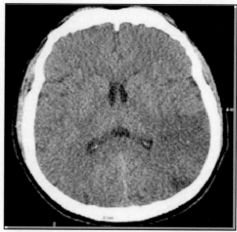

Figure 5 Second control CT (24h after the onset) — ischemic zone in left parietal lobe; with reversal of neurological deficits — NIHSS 3 points.

References

[1] Adams HP, del Zoppo G, Alberts MJ. ASA recommendations. Circulation 1996;94:1167—74.
[2] Alexandrov AV. Current and future recanalization strategies for acute ischemic stroke. Journal of Internal Medicine 2010;267:209—19.
[3] Brekenfeld C, Remonda L, Nedeltchev K, Bredow F, Ozdoba C, Wiest R, et al. Endovascular neuroradiological treatment of acute ischemic stroke: techniques and results in 350 patients. Neurological Research 2005;27(1):29—35.
[4] Chapot R, Houdart E, Rogopoulos A, Wessel M, Bisdorff A, Merland J. Thromboaspiration in the basilar artery: report of two cases. American Journal of Neuroradiology 2002;23:282—4.
[5] Clark WM, Wissman S, Albers G. Intravenous rt-PA for acute ischemic stroke beyond 3-hours (ATLANTIS). Journal of American Medical Association 1999;282:2019—26.
[6] De Silva DA, Brekenfeld C, Ebinger M, Christensen S, Barber PA, Butcher KS, et al. The benefits of intravenous thrombolysis relate to the site of baseline arterial occlusion in the Echoplanar Imaging Thrombolytic Evaluation Trial (EPITHET). Stroke 2010;41:295—9.
[7] European Stroke Organization (ESO) Executive Committee and the ESO Writing Committee. Guidelines for Management of Ischemic Stroke and Transient Ischemic Attack; 2008.
[8] Fisher M. Characterizing the target of acute stroke treatment. Stroke 1997;28:866—72.
[9] Hussein HM, Georgiadis AL, Vazquez G, Miley JT, Memon MZ, Mohammad YM, et al. Occurrence and predictors of futile recanalization following endovascular treatment among patients with acute ischemic stroke: a multicenter study. American Journal of Neuroradiology 2010;31:454—8.
[10] Menon BK, Hill MD, Eesa M, Modi J, Bhatia R, Wong J, et al. Initial experience with the Penumbra Stroke System for recanalization of large vessel occlusions in acute ischemic stroke. Neuroradiology 2011;53:261—6.
[11] Loh Y, Jahan R, McArthur DL, Shi ZS, Gonzalez NR, Duckwiler GR, et al. Recanalization rates decrease with increasing thrombectomy attempts. American Journal of Neuroradiology 2010;31:935—9.
[12] Lutsep HL, Clark WM, Nesbit GM, Berlis A, Barnwell S, Norbash A, et al. Intraarterial suction thrombectomy in acute stroke. American Journal of Neuroradiology 2002;23:783—6.
[13] Titianova E, Velcheva I, Stamenov B. Treatment of acute ischemic stroke with thrombolysis in Bulgaria. Neurosonography and Cerebral Hemodynamic 2010;1(6):9—14.
[14] Tomsick TA, Khatri P, Jovin T, Demaerschalk B, Malisch T, Demchuk A, et al. Equipoise among recanalization strategies. Neurology 2010;74:1069—76.

Semantic aphasia in a sonothrombolysed patient. A treatment without use of rt-PA

Marko Klissurski*, Evgenii Vavrek, Nelly Nicheva-Vavrek

Clinic of Neurology, University Hospital "Tzaritza Ioanna-ISUL", Sofia, Bulgaria

KEYWORDS
Sonothrombolysis;
Semantic aphasia

Summary The objectives were to describe a case of a patient with acute ischemic stroke who achieved recanalization of the occluded middle cerebral artery and a good clinical improvement after immediate application of standard medical treatment (including aspirin) plus sonothrombolysis for 2 h without use of rt-PA. After the first 24 h, a rare form of aphasia, a semantic type of aphasia was described. On day 5, the NIHSS score of the patient was 2, on day 30, his NIHSS and modified Rankin score was 0. The main factors influencing favorable outcome were discussed. Despite controversial evidence, it is worth studying the efficacy and safety of sonothrombolysis without rt-PA, but with commonly used drugs. This approach could be easily applied in eligible patients almost in every stroke unit worldwide.
© 2012 Published by Elsevier GmbH.

Introduction

The ultrasound energy could increase the intrinsic fibrinolysis in occluded vessels even in the absence of thrombolytic agents, such as alteplase (rt-PA) [1—5]. The results of CLOTBUST clinical trials showed that the sonothrombolysis (STL) or the combination of rt-PA plus 2 h of continuous transcranial Doppler (TCD) was able to increase recanalization rates in acute ischemic stroke (AIS), with a trend toward better functional outcomes compared to rt-PA alone [6]. Spontaneous recanalization of the middle cerebral artery (MCA) in AIS was observed despite a poor initial thrombolysis in Brain Ischemia (TIBI) score in some patients who were not eligible for (or not treated with) thrombolysis (TL) using rt-PA [2,7—10]. The factors leading to spontaneous recanalization, its natural rate, and whether STL without rt-PA should be worth doing in large clinical series or is potentially ineffective, are still unresolved questions.

The objectives of the current report were to describe a case of a patient who suffered AIS and achieved good clinical improvement after immediate application of standard medical treatment plus STL for 2 h (transcranial color-coded duplex sonography) without use of rt-PA.

Abbreviations: rt-PA, recombinant tissue plasminogen activator; STL, sonothrombolysis; TCD, transcranial Doppler; AIS, acute ischemic stroke; MCA, middle cerebral artery; TIBI, thrombolysis in brain ischemia; TL, thrombolysis; TCCDS, transcranial color-coded duplex sonography; PSV/EDV, peak systolic/end diastolic velocity.
* Corresponding author at: Clinic of Neurology, University Hospital "Tzaritza Ioanna-ISUL", 8 Bialo more str., 1527 Sofia, Bulgaria. Tel.: +359 885 630 610; fax: +359 2 9432 109/160.
E-mail address: mklissurski@yahoo.com (M. Klissurski).

Materials and methods

A 59-year old patient presented in the emergency room with right hemiplegia and complete motor aphasia 1.5 h after he was found earlier in the morning. The exact time of his stroke onset was not known, but according to his wife, it was definitely between 2 and 6 h before the admission.

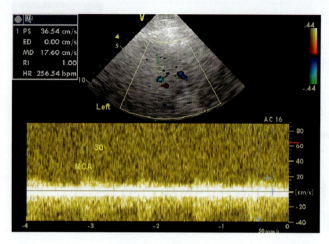 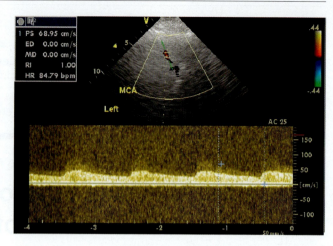

Figure 1   Minute 30.   Figure 2   Day 1.

On admission, the patient had a NIHSS score of 10, and blood pressure of 150/80 mm Hg. From the past medical history, he had only mild arterial hypertension, treated with beta-blocker. The routine blood tests, ECG, and conventional computed tomography (CT) of the head were carried out (according to the Bulgarian AIS guideline). When the diagnosis of AIS was accepted after CT, the patient was given immediately aspirin 300 mg, bisoprolol 5 mg, atorvastatin 10 mg orally; normal saline 0.9% 1.5 L, pyracetam (Nootropil) 3.0 g intravenously; and fraxiparine 0.4 mL subcutaneously. The values of his complete blood count, biochemistry and lipids panel were within normal limits, except for the leucocytes count of $13.3 \times 10^9/l$ and hematocrit of 0.54.

The extracranial and transcranial color-coded duplex sonography (TCCDS) was performed after admission in the stroke unit. The exact vessel pathology and hemodynamic status were defined in accordance to TIBI and COGIF criteria [7,11—14] using General Electric Vivid 7 Pro diagnostic TCCDS device. The extracranial ultrasound showed mild atheromatous carotid changes with higher intima—media thickness complex values bilaterally and several small hypoechogenic nonstenotic plaques around the bifurcations. On TCCDS, there was evidence of occlusion in the left MCA, its proximal M1 segment. Signals from corresponding A1, P1 and C1 segments of the basal cerebral arteries were recorded as needed [13]. The monitoring of intracranial velocities and STL of the left MCA were done by manually holding a 2-MHz transducer for 2 h via transtemporal window (sample volume 5 mm, low velocity scale; broad color duplex window to be able to see A1, C1, P1 arteries; mild oscillations and adjustments along the course of affected M1 segment). The neurologic and hemodynamic status of the patient was assessed after 3, 6, and 12 h, as well as on the 1st, 3rd, 5th, 30th, and 90th day by a neurologist, speech therapist and neurosonologist.

Results

On starting TCCDS monitoring (minute 0), there was not any detectable signal from the initial M1 segment of MCA, TIBI scale score 0. From minute 30 (Fig. 1) until minute 120, a minimal, spike-like MCA flow occurred, with peak systolic/end diastolic velocity (PSV/EDV) 20/5 cm/s, and TIBI score was between 1 and 2. Respectively, TIBI 3 was detected on the sixth hour with a dampened MCA flow pattern and PSV/EDV 50/24 cm/s. On the first day, MCA PSV/EDV were 68/26 cm/s (Fig. 2). On the third day, there was no significant asymmetry between the two MCA arteries, with PSV/EDV of 76/40 cm/s, TIBI 5 score. On day 30, blood flow velocities of both MCAs were within normal range (Figs. 3—7).

The patient's neurological status improved on the first day after admission. His NIHSS score changed from 10 to 5, and his complete motor aphasia resolved to a semantic one. This particular and rare type of aphasia was characterized by impaired simultant gnosis, comprehension of time relations, and constructions of affiliations, such as ''my father's brother is my...''. This rare type of aphasia (described first by Russian neuropsychologist A.R. Luria) is not included in all modern classifications. It is thought to be a part of the sensory aphasia [15].

On discharge at day 5, the NIHSS score of the patient was 2. On the follow-up at the first month the patient achieved complete neurological recovery. At the third month his modified Rankin Scale was 0.

Discussion and conclusion

The acute occlusion of the proximal MCA segment is a dangerous event that could lead to a large brain infarct, severe disability, and poor functional outcome in cases with no recanalization [9,10]. That is why we applied STL 3.5—6 h after the onset of AIS. We observed the evolution of recanalization in the occluded MCA within the first 6—12 h after the procedure [8,16]. In the presented case, two rare clinical situations deserve attention. First, the favorable outcome was achieved using simple and non-expensive treatment including STL without rt-PA. Second, there was a quick resolution of an almost complete motor aphasia to a specific semantic type that was connected to the location of the brain ischemic changes in MCA territory and their functional compensation.

The quick clinical improvement of our patient could be a result of mere chance for spontaneous recanalization [9,10]. We believe that early aspirin administration (immediately after CT, and approximately 3.5 h after the stroke onset) was an important factor for the disease evolution and long-term prognosis [17]. Based only on a single observation, it would be a speculative suggestion to accept that 2 h of STL combined with 300 mg aspirin given orally contributed to the mechanical breakdown of thrombus and recanalization in the left MCA. The data from a clinical study showed evidence toward better recanalization rate in patients not eligible for IV rt-PA [2,8]. However, the role of other medications given to those patients, their dosages and time of administration along with the STL was not clear as a contributing factor.

In some acute clinical presentations with unknown time of stroke onset, still there are no reliable criteria to distinguish who would benefit from TL and who would benefit from STL. Perhaps, younger age, lower initial NIHSS score, MRI mismatch and TIBI scale or COGIF grade improvements could be used as favorable prognostic parameters [4,11–13,16,18].

Despite controversial evidence in literature [1,2,5,10–12], we think that it is worth studying the efficacy and safety of this simple method, TCCDS STL without TL agent, but with aspirin or other commonly used drugs. This approach could be easily applied in eligible patients almost in every stroke unit facility worldwide.

Appendix A. Supplementary data

Supplementary data associated with this article can be found, in the online version, at http://dx.doi.org/10.1016/j.permed.2012.03.018.

References

[1] Alexandrov AV, Mikulik R, Ribo M, Sharma VK, Lao AY, Tsivgoulis G, et al. A pilot randomized clinical safety study of sonothrombolysis augmentation with ultrasound-activated perflutren-lipid microspheres for acute ischemic stroke. Stroke 2008;39(5):1464–9.

[2] Eggers J, Koch B, Meyer K, Konig I, Seidel G. Effect of ultrasound on thrombolysis of middle cerebral artery occlusion. Annals of Neurology 2003;53(6):797–800.

[3] Pfaffenberger S, Devcic-Kuhar B, Kollmann C, Kastl SP, Kaun C, Speidl WS, et al. Can a commercial diagnostic ultrasound device accelerate thrombolysis? An in vitro skull model. Stroke 2005;36(1):124–8.

[4] Polak JF. Ultrasound energy and the dissolution of thrombus. New England Journal of Medicine 2004;351(21):2154–5.

[5] Rubiera M, Alexandrov AV. Sonothrombolysis in the management of acute ischemic stroke. Posted: 03/03/2010. American Journal of Cardiovascular Drugs 2010;10(1):5–10.

[6] Alexandrov AV, Molina CA, Grotta JC, Garami Z, Ford SR, Alvares-Sabin J, et al. Ultrasound-enhanced systemic thrombolysis for acute ischemic stroke. New England Journal of Medicine 2004;351(21):2170–8.

[7] Demchuk AM, Burgin WS, Christou I, Felberg RA, Barber PA, Hill MD, et al. Thrombolysis in brain ischemia (TIBI) transcranial Doppler flow grades predict clinical severity, early recovery and mortality in intravenous TPA treated patients. Stroke 2001;32:89–93.

[8] Eggers J, Seidel G, Koch B, Konig I. Sonothrombolysis in acute ischemic stroke for patients ineligible for rt-PA. Neurology 2005;64(6):1052–4.

[9] Hacke W, Donnan G, Fieschi C, Kaste M, von Kummer R, Broderick JP, et al. Association of outcome with early stroke treatment: pooled analysis of ATLANTIS, ECASS, and NINDS rt-PA stroke trials. Lancet 2004;363:768–74.

[10] Wardlaw JM, Marray V, Berge E, del Zoppo GJ. Thrombolysis in acute ischemic stroke. Part 1. Thrombolysis versus control. Cochrane Database of Systematic Reviews 2009;4: CD000213.

[11] Alexandrov AV, Grotta JC. Arterial re-occlusion in stroke patients treated with intravenous tissue plasminogen activator. Neurology 2002;59:862–7.

[12] Alexandrov AV, Labiche LA, Wojner AW. Ultra-early prediction of stroke outcome in patients treated with 0.9 mg/kg IV tPA. Stroke 2002;33:342.

[13] Kaps M, Damian MS, Teschendorf U, Dorndorf W. Transcranial Doppler ultrasound findings in the middle cerebral artery occlusion. Stroke 1990;21:532–7;
Ley-Pozo J, Ringelstein EB. Noninvasive detection of occlusive disease of the carotid siphon and middle cerebral artery. Annals of Neurology 1990;28:640–7.

[14] Nedelmann M, Stolz E, Gerriets T, Baumgartner RW, Malferrari G, Seidel G, et al. Consensus recommendations for transcranial color-coded duplex sonography for the assessment of intracranial arteries in clinical trials on acute stroke. Stroke 2009;40:3238–44.

[15] Мавлов Л. Фундаментална неврология, Бойко Стаменов, София; 2000.

[16] Alexandrov AV, Burgin WS, Demchuk AM, El-Mitwalli A, Grotta JC. Speed of intracranial clot lysis with intravenous tPA therapy: sonographic classification and short-term improvement. Circulation 2001;103:2897–902.

[17] Chen ZM, Sandercock P, Pan HC, Counsell C, Collins R, Liu LS, et al. Indication for early aspirin use in acute ischemic stroke. A combined analysis of 40 000 randomized patients from the Chinese acute stroke trial and the International stroke trial. Stroke 2000;31:1240–9.

[18] Brown DL, Johnston KC, Wagner DP, Haley Jr EC. Predicting major neurological improvement with intravenous recombinant tissue plasminogen activator treatment of stroke. Stroke 2004;35(1):147–50.

My worst case with sonothrombolysis

Evgenii Vladislav Vavrek*

Emergency Neurological Unit, University Hospital "Tzaritza Ioanna-ISUL", 8 Bialo More Str., Sofia, Bulgaria

KEYWORDS
TCCS;
Sonothrombolysis;
Asymptomatic hemorrhage

Summary This article presents the case of a 63-year-old man with an acute ischemic stroke due to extracranial thrombosis of the left internal carotid artery, associated with about 70% stenoses of the right common and internal carotid arteries. The patient was treated with rtPA associated with a temporal transcranial ultrasound examination (TCCS) for an hour during a rtPA infusion. During the transcranial monitoring the left middle cerebral artery (LMCA) was rated between 2 and 3 on the TIBI scale. At the 24th hour two small ischemic zones and two intracranial hematomas were detected. No new symptoms were added. There are data showing that transcranial ultrasound monitoring (TCD and TCCS) and microbubble administration in acute ischemic stroke patients are associated with an early recanalization and a high rate of hemorrhagic transformation but do not seem to increase the risk of a symptomatic intracranial hemorrhage. According to CLOTBUST TCD alone is safe in acute ischemic stroke patients. TCCS alone is also tested in a smaller study. In the presented case report an association between the transtemporal insonation and the hematomas is possible but not probable.
© 2012 Elsevier GmbH. All rights reserved.

Introduction

Sonothrombolysis is still a new branch in the thrombolytic treatment of the acute ischemic stroke. Sonothrombolysis in neurology is usually a combination between thrombolysis (in most cases with r-TPA) augmented with ultrasound. There are many parameters which have to be defined, such as frequencies, position, time for insonation, inclusion and exclusion criteria (time window, etc.), type and dosis of microbubbles [1]. There is data for some parameters, for example low frequencies showed to induce bleeding [2]. The trials use two types of ultrasound — transcranial Doppler (TCD) and transcranial color-coded sonography (TCCS) [2—9]. There are a few proposed theories for the action of the sonothrombolysis — mechanical, temperature, through NO [1,10—14].

Usually the focus of the insonation is the place with the worst Thrombolysis In Brain Ischemia (TIBI) score and the trials include patients with a middle cerebral artery (MCA) occlusion [3—9].

The main positive results include an earlier and better recanalization rate and clinical outcome and the main problem is the hemorrhage. The hemorrhage is mostly asymptomatic [3—9]. TCCS was associated 18% symptomatic hemorrhage in a recent study with a MCA occlusion and insonation on the M1 segment of MCA [4].

In a very small group of patients treated with sonothrombolyis versus thrombolysis alone we published a better clinical improvement in a sonothrombolytic arm, but with one death, due to a malignant stroke. We had no hemorrhage in the sonothrombolytic arm [15].

Abbreviations: TCD, transcranial Doppler; TCCS, transcranial color-coded sonography; ICA, internal carotid artery; MCA, middle cerebral artery; TEICA, thrombosis of extracranial segment of ICA; TIBI, thrombolysis in Brain Ischemia; r-TPA, recombinant Tissue Plasminogen Activator.

* Tel.: +359 888981403; fax: +359 29432109.
E-mail address: evavrek@hotmail.com

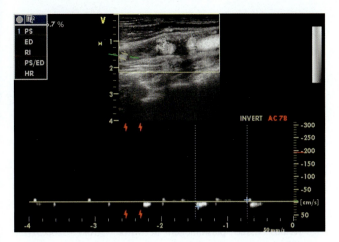

Figure 1 Thrombosis of the left ICA after the bifurcation.

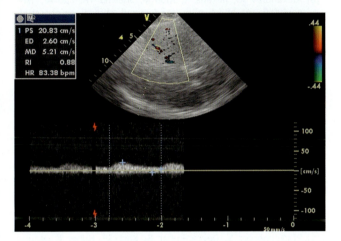

Figure 2 Left MCA.

Materials and methods

A 63-year-old man with a sudden onset of right paresis, lesion of the right facial nerve and aphasia, NIHSS 10, thrombosis of the left ICA after the bifurcation (Fig. 1), stenosis of the right ICA, left MCA — TIBI 2 (Fig. 2), with a history of essential hypertension, dyslipidemia and TIA with dysarthria

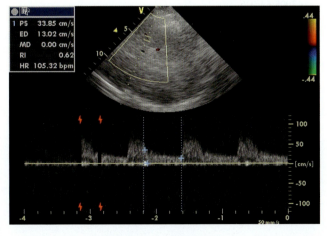

Figure 3 Right MCA.

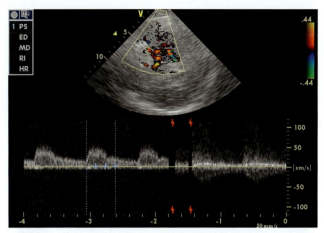

Figure 4 Transient improvement of the bloodstream in the left MCA.

and right paresthesia was admitted to our hospital. Blood tests on admission were normal. He was treated with r-TPA associated with temporal transcranial ultrasound (hand helped TCCS using *General Electric* Vivid 7 Pro device.) for an hour during standard r-TPA infusion. The insonation was focused on M1 segment of the left MCA. The start time since the onset of the stroke was 3 h 15 min (see Fig. 3).

Results

During the insonation, at the 30the min a transient improvement was achieved with TIBI 3—4 (Fig. 4), NIHSS 5—6. At the 120th min NIHSS was 11. At the 24th hour an asymptomatic hemorrhage was detected (Fig. 5). On the 4th day NIHSS was 4 and on discharge (day 9) NIHSS was 3 points. On the 30th day a complete resorption of the hemorrhage was achieved and no neurological deficit was detected (Fig. 6).

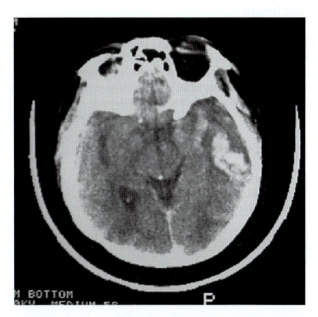

Figure 5 Day 1.

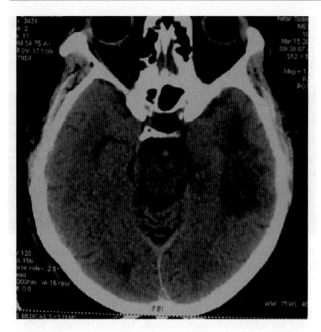

Figure 6 Day 30.

Discussion

The recanalization of thrombosis of the extracranial segment of ICA (TEICA) is rare. The thrombolysed patients with TEICA usually improve after thrombolysis. After TEICA secondary thromboses are detected, including the MCA area. Our patient was relatively young and he suffered a big stroke — we can speculate that the patient was at risk of a malignant stroke; none of the criteria for DESTINY — one of the biggest trials including patients at risk of a malignant stroke — was met [16]. The focus of the TCCS was chosen to prevent secondary thrombosis. It can be assumed that the patient received benefit from the treatment, because of the good clinical recovery.

Conclusion

The proper decision in patients with TEICA is not clear yet. In this case a connection between the TCCS and the hemorrhagic transformation is possible, but cannot be proven. The good clinical outcome in this case gives an argument in favor of the application of sonothrombolysis in patients with TEICA.

References

[1] Vavrek E. Acute ischemic stroke. A therapeutic application of the Doppler sonography with(out) thrombolysis — oral presentation. Krems, Austria: Danube University; 2008.

[2] Daffertshofer M, Gass A, Ringleb P, Sitzer M, Sliwka U, Els T, et al. Transcranial low-frequency ultrasound-mediated thrombolysis in brain ischemia: increased risk of hemorrhage with combined ultrasound and tissue plasminogen activator: results of a phase II clinical trial. Stroke 2005;36(7):1441—6.

[3] Alexandrov AV, Molina CA, Grotta JC, Garami Z, Ford SR, Alvarez-Sabin J, et al. Ultrasound-enhanced systemic thrombolysis for acute ischemic stroke. N Engl J Med 2004;351(21):2170—8.

[4] Eggers J, Koch B, Meyer K, König I, Seidel G. Effect of ultrasound on thrombolysis of middle cerebral artery occlusion. Ann Neurol 2003;53(6):797—800.

[5] Molina CA, Ribo M, Rubiera M, Montaner J, Santamarina E, Delgado-Mederos R, et al. Microbubble administration accelerates clot lysis during continuous 2-MHz ultrasound monitoring in stroke patients treated with intravenous tissue plasminogen activator. Stroke 2006;37(2):425—9.

[6] Alexandrov AV, Mikulik R, Ribo M, Sharma VK, Lao AY, Tsivgoulis G, et al. A pilot randomized clinical safety study of sonothrombolysis augmentation with ultrasound-activated perflutren-lipid microspheres for acute ischemic stroke. Stroke 2008;39(5):1464—9.

[7] IMARx. TUCSON trial [online]. Available from URL: http://www.imarx.com/ImaRx/clinical_trials5_0 [accessed 28.09.09].

[8] Larrue AV, Arnaud C. Trancranial ultrasound combined with intravenous microbubbles and tissue plasminogen activator for acute ischemic stroke: a randomized controlled study. Stroke 2007;38:472 [abstract].

[9] Perren F, Loulidi J, Poglia D, Landis T, Sztajzel R. Microbubble potentiated transcranial duplex ultrasound enhances IV thrombolysis in acute stroke. J Thromb Thrombolysis 2008;25:219—23.

[10] Klisurski M. Sonotromboliza. Neurosonol Cerebral Hemodynam 2006;2:61—6.

[11] Pfaffenberger S, Devcic-Kuhar B, Kast SP, Huber K, Maurer G, Wojta J, et al. Ultrasound thrombolysis. Thromb Haemost 2005;94:26—36.

[12] Slikkerveer J, Dijkmans PA, Sieswerda GT, Doevendans PA, van Dijk AP, Verheugt FW, et al. Ultrasound enhanced prehospital thrombolysis using microbubbles infusion in patients with acute ST elevation myocardial infarction: rationale and design of the sonolysis study. Trials 2008;9:72.

[13] Suchkova VN, Baggs RB, Sahni SK, Francis CW. Ultrasound improves tissue perfusion in ischemic tissue through a nitric oxide dependent mechanism. Thromb Haemost 2002;88(5):865—70.

[14] Francis C. Therapeutic effects of ultrasound. Neurology 2005;64:935.

[15] Klissurski M, Vavrek E. Sonothrombolysis in Bulgaria — poster. Madrid, Spain: ESNCH; 2010.

[16] Juttler E, Schwab S, Schmiedek P, Unterberg A, Hennerici M, Woitzik J, et al. Decompressive surgery for the treatment of malignant infarction of the middle cerebral artery (DESTINY). Stroke 2007;38:2518.

Transient brainstem ischemia and dural arteriovenous malformation

Jurgita Valaikiene [a,*], Jurate Dementaviciene [b], Dalius Jatuzis [a], Loreta Cimbalistiene [c]

[a] Vilnius University, Medical Faculty, Neurology and Neurosurgery Clinic, Centre of Neurology, Vilnius, Lithuania
[b] Vilnius University, Medical Faculty, Department of Radiology, Nuclear Medicine and Medical Physics, Vilnius, Lithuania
[c] Vilnius University, Medical Faculty, Department of Human and Medical Genetics, Vilnius, Lithuania

KEYWORDS
Arteriovenous malformation;
Transient ischemic attack;
Hereditary hemorrhagic telangiectasia;
Transcranial color-coded duplex sonography

Summary

Background: Hereditary hemorrhagic telangiectasia (HHT), is a very rare vascular disorder, characterized by arteriovenous malformations of various types. High cervical dural arteriovenous fistulas are extremely rare and usually manifestate with progressive myelopathy.

Case presentation: We present neurovascular imaging in a patient suffering from a cervical intradural extramedullar and intracranial arteriovenous malformation who presented with repeated transient ischemic brainstem attacks. This case illustrates the hemodynamic and anatomical information derived from multimodal neuroimaging procedures. The chest CT detected a pulmonary AVM.

Conclusion: Evaluating younger patients with acute brain ischemia, HHT has to be kept in mind. Pulmonary AVM often leads to TIA or stroke due to paradoxical embolization.
© 2012 Elsevier GmbH. All rights reserved.

Introduction

Hereditary hemorrhagic telangiectasia (HHT) or Osler—Weber—Rendu disease, is an extremely rare (1:5000) disorder of the vascular system. The disease is characterized by various vascular malformations: small arteriovenous junctions are called telangiectasia, and large — arteriovenous malformation (AVM). Clinical disease expression depends on the AVM location and extent. Cerebral AVM occurs in about 10%, spinal AVM less than 1% of all HHT cases [1]. Multimodal neuroimaging of patient suffering from brainstem ischemic attacks revealed extremely rare cervical intradural extramedullar and intracranial arteriovenous malformation. According to guidelines for the diagnosis of HHT [2] thoracic CT was done and pulmonary AVM was found, which, potentially, can cause transient ischemic attack (TIA) or a stroke.

A clinical case

A 40 year old woman was urgently admitted for the first time to the hospital with sudden onset speech disorder and left limb weakness. Until then, in the patient's own estimation, she had been healthy. After hospitalization in the district hospital, neurological examination revealed dysarthria, horizontal nystagmus and left hemiparesis. An urgent brain computed tomography (CT) excluded ischemia or hemorrhagia, but there was suspicion of aneurysm of basilar artery

* Corresponding author. Tel.: +370 65682642; fax: +3705365221.
E-mail address: jurgita.valaikiene@santa.lt (J. Valaikiene).

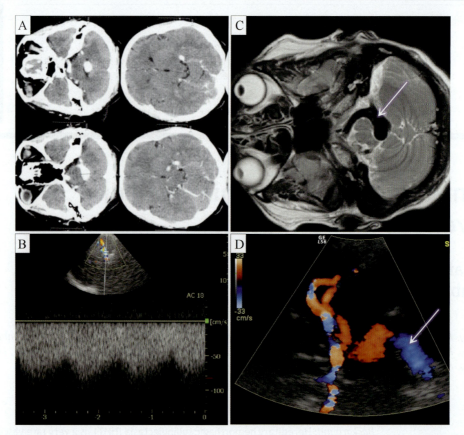

Figure 1 (A) Cerebral CT, contrast enhanced: enlarged vessel at the mesencephalic brainstem level. (B) TCCS, transtemporal: pathologically increased venous flow. (C) Cerebral MRT, T2W sequence: enlarged vessel at the mesencephalic brainstem level (arrow). (D) TCCS, transtemporal: enlarged Rosenthal vein (arrow).

(BA) and left middle cerebral artery (MCA) (Fig. 1A). The patient was quickly transported to the Vilnius University Hospital. Neurological examination revealed no focal neurological symptoms.

Laboratory and instrumental investigations

Patient's blood test revealed no clinical and biochemical abnormalities. Electrocardiogram showed sinus heart rhythm. Echocardioscopy revealed good function of left ventricle, and normal heart chambers. An urgent extracranial color-coded sonography (ECCS) was unremarkable. Transcranial color-coded sonography (TCCS) showed normal basal arteries, but detected an enlarged vein of Rosenthal and deep middle cerebral vein with pathologically increased blood flow velocities (Fig. 1B and D). In addition a large vein found at the mesencephalic brainstem level adjacent to the BA. Transforaminal examination revealed increased blood flow velocity of anterior spinal artery in conjunction with venous enlargement (Fig. 2A and B). Brain and spinal magnetic resonance imaging (MRI) disclosed a large intradural extramedullar cervical and intracranial arteriovenous malformation (Figs. 1 and 2C). The cervical spinal cord was deformed by the enlarged draining vein running cranially into posterior fossa draining into the straight sinus. Digital subtraction angiography (DSA), revealed multiple arteriovenous junctions with feeding arteries arising from V2 to V3 segments of both vertebral arteries (Fig. 3A and C).

The chest CT detected an 18 mm pulmonary AVM (Fig. 4).

Discussion

Transcranial color-coded duplexsonography plays an important role in the urgent diagnostic of neurovascular diseases, especially in younger people with stroke. Noninvasive, bed side performed TCCS helps quickly differentiate arterial and venous pathological changes, and diagnose AVM [3,4]. In this case the brain CT showed possible BA and MCA aneurysm, TCCS method showed not arterial, but venous dilatation at the mesencephalic brainstem level, passing down through the *foramen magnum* (Fig. 2A). The data were confirmed performing brain and spinal MRI (Figs. 1 and 2C) and DSA (Fig. 3). Extremely rare cervical/upper thoracic part AVM with high-pressure, fast flow and feeding from the vertebral arteries, especially the left side, was found. High cervical dural arteriovenous fistulas usually manifest with progressive myelopathy. In this case no symptoms of myelopathy had been observed. Despite impressive venous congestion within the cervical spinal canal, no congestive edema of the spinal cord was seen, indicated that venous overflow was well compensated. Explaining the genesis of recurrent TIA was thought to be related to the steal mechanism. Radiologists analyzing brain CT and MRI images also observed

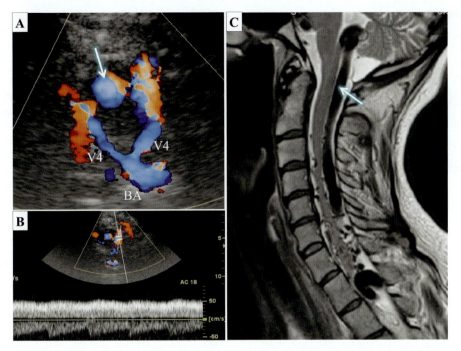

Figure 2 (A) TCCS, transforaminal: venous enlargement in conjunction with anterior spinal artery (arrow) and adjacent to vertebral artery. (B) TCCS, transforaminal: an enlarged vein adjacent to vertebral artery with pathologically increased blood flow velocities. (C) Spinal MRT, T2W: a large intradural extramedullar cervical/upper thoracic and intracranial AVM (arrow).

telangiectasia in the nose, small AVM in left side of the forehead — the image is characterized by HHT. Asked about bleeding from the nose, the patient responded positively. Constant light bleeding from the nose starting from age 10 had become normal condition, the patient claimed to have been completely healthy. The patient was consulted by clinical geneticist (LC) and was diagnosed definite HHT according to all four Curaçao diagnostic criteria (Table 1)

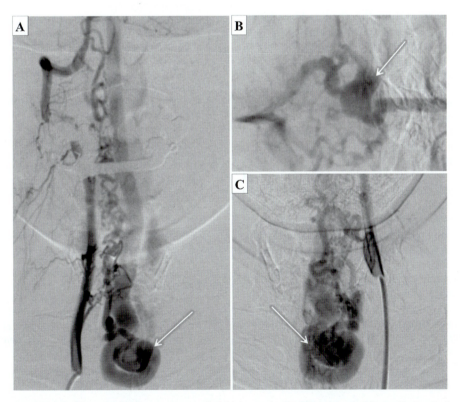

Figure 3 (A) Selective DSA of right vertebral artery: spinal AVM (arrow). (B) DSA: enlarged Rosenthal vein (arrow). (C) Selective DSA of left vertebral artery: spinal AVM (arrow).

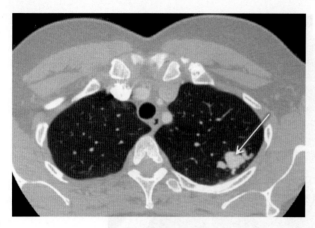

Figure 4   Chest CT: pulmonary AVM (arrow).

Table 1   Clinical HHT diagnostic criteria and their frequence [1,5].

I	Recurrent spontaneous epistaxis because of nasal telangiectasia (~90%)
II	Mucocutaneous telangiactasia on the face, nose, fingertips and mouth mucosa (~80%)
III	Internal organ damage — gastrointestinal telangiectasia (~20%), lungs (~50%), liver (~30%), brain (~10%), spinal cord (~1%) AVM
IV	Family anamnesis first degree relatives have following criterias

At least three criteria confirm diagnosis, if two criterias — possible HHT and one criteria — HHT is doubtfull.

[5]: epistaxis, telangiectasia on the cheeks, lips, hands, fingers, spinal, cerebral and pulmonary AVM, a positive family anamnesis (patient's father, brother, two children have signs of HHT). An autosomal dominant inheritance type was found. Blood was taken for DNA genetic testing. It should be noted that pulmonary AVM often leads to neurological complications. Often the patient has a TIA/stroke due to paradoxical embolization, the patient may develop a brain abscess due to septic embolus [6—8]. According to International guidelines for the diagnosis and management of HHT, if pulmonary AVM diameter is >3 mm, it is recommended to perform transcatheter embolotherapy in an HHT center of excellence (level of evidence II, strong recommendation) [2]. Management tactics of cervical, thoracic intradural extramedullar and intracranial arteriovenous malformations (the endovascular embolization, surgery) are uncertain. Therapy for these AVM with multiple feeders is preferingly using interventional closure of the primary fistula. There are no ongoing intervention procedures, since the patient is currently neurologically asymptomatic. In a past year the patient experienced two episodes of TIA with transient left arm numbness and weakness. Often high cervical AVM treatment even in highly experienced centers may end in serious neurological complications. The patient is monitored periodically giving neurological examination and TCCS.

Summary

Urgent TCCS is a very useful diagnostic tool, obtaining unique information about real time arteriovenous cerebral status in case of acute brain ischemia. It helps to plan further diagnostic procedures. HHT has to be in mind evaluating younger patient with acute brain ischemia. Despite the rarity of the disease, HHT is often accompanied with TIA/stroke due to pulmonary AVM. Multidisciplinary approach in management of HHT is required.

Consent

The patient has given permission to publish her medical history, clinical data and findings.

Acknowledgements

We thank professor Rüdiger von Kummer for radiological test and comments, PD Dr. Felix Schlachetzki for scientifical advices.

The clinical case was presented at the 16th ESNCH Meeting in Munich, Germany, May 2011.

References

[1] Govani FS, Shovlin CL. Hereditary hemorrhagic telangiectasia: a clinical and scientific review. Eur J Hum Genet 2009;17(7):860—71.
[2] Faughnan ME, Palda VA, Garcia-Tsao G, Geisthoff UW, McDonald J, Proctor DD, et al. International guidelines for the diagnosis and management of hereditary hemorrhagic telangiectasia. J Med Genet 2011;48(2):73—87.
[3] Bartels E. Intrakranielle Gefäßmalformationen. In: Bogdahn U, Becker G, Schlachetzki, editors. Echosignalverstärker und transkranielle Farbduplex-Sonographie. Berlin: Blackwell Wiss-Verl; 1998. p. 276—97.
[4] Harrer JU, Popescu O, Henkes HH, Klötzsch C. Assessment of dural arteriovenous fistulae by transcranial color-coded duplex sonography. Stroke 2005;36(5):976—9.
[5] Shovlin CL, Guttmacher AE, Buscarini E, Faughnan ME, Hyland RH, Westermann CJ, et al. Diagnostic criteria for hereditary hemorrhagic telangiectasia (Rendu—Osler—Weber syndrome). Am J Med Genet 2000;91(1):66—7.
[6] Gallitelli M, Pasculli G, Fiore T, Carella A, Sabbà C. Emergencies in hereditary hemorrhagic telangiectasia. QJM 2006;99(1):15—22.
[7] Manawadu D, Vethanayagam D, Ahmed SN. Hereditary hemorrhagic telangiectasia:. transient ischemic attacks. CMAJ 2009;180(8):836—7.
[8] Ribeiro E, Cogez J, Babin E, Viader F, Defer G. Stroke in hereditary hemorrhagic telangiectasia patients. New evidence for repeated screening and early treatment of pulmonary vascular malformations: two case reports. BMC Neurol 2011;11:84.

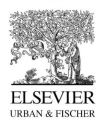
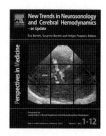

Bartels E, Bartels S, Poppert H (Editors):
New Trends in Neurosonology and Cerebral Hemodynamics — an Update.
Perspectives in Medicine (2012) 1, 1—12

journal homepage: www.elsevier.com/locate/permed

List of Contributors

Foad **Abd-Allah**, Department of Neurology, Cairo University, Cairo, Egypt
Noha **Abo-Krysha**, Department of Neurology, Cairo University, Cairo, Egypt
Marina **Abramova**, Russian National Research, Medical University, Laboratory of Child Cerebrovascular Disorders, Moscow, Russia
Rob G. **Ackerstaff**, Department of Clinical Neurophysiology, St. Antonius Hospital, Utrecht, The Netherlands
Andrei V. **Alexandrov**, Comprehensive Stroke Center, University of Alabama Hospital, Birmingham, Al, USA
Vugar **Aliev**, Russian Polenov Neurosurgical Institute, St. Petersburg, Russia
Angelika **Alonso**, Department of Neurology, UniversitätsMedizin Mannheim, University of Heidelberg, Mannheim, Germany
Mathias **Altmann**, Department of Opthalmology, University of Regensburg, Regensburg, Germany
Grethe **Andersen**, The Department of Neurology, Aarhus Hospital, Aarhus University Hospital, Aarhus, Denmark
Silva **Andonova**, Second Clinic of Neurology, St. Marina University Hospital, Varna, Bulgaria
Gian Paolo **Anzola**, Ospedale S. Orsola, Unita' Operativa di Cardiologia — Fatebenefratelli, Service of Neurology, Brescia, Italy
Nicole **Apostolidou**, Department of Neurology, Democritus University of Alexandroupolis School of Medicine, Alexandroupolis, Greece
Rocco A. **Armonda**, Walter Reed National Military Medical Center, Bethesda, MD, USA
Dimitrios **Artemis**, Department of Neurology, UniversitätsMedizin Mannheim, University of Heidelberg, Mannheim, Germany
Rei **Asami**, Life Science Research Center, Central Research Laboratory, Tokyo, Japan
Elsa **Azevedo**, Department Neurology, Hospital São João, Faculty of Medicine of University of Porto, Porto, Portugal
Chavdar **Bachvarov**, Centre of Radiology, St. Marina University Hospital, Varna, Bulgaria
Mathias **Bähr**, Department of Neurology, University of Göttingen, Göttingen, Germany
Andrea **Balasso**, Interdisciplinary Research Laboratory of the Klinikum rechts der Isar der TU München, München, München
Essam **Baligh**, Department of Cardiovascular Medicine, Cairo University, Cairo, Egypt
Galina **Baltgaile**, Riga Stradina University, Neurological Department, Riga, Latvia
Caroline **Banahan**, Medical Physics Department, University Hospitals of Leicester NHS Trust, Leicester, UK
Claudio **Baracchini**, Department of Neuroscience, University of Padua, Padua, Italy
Eva **Bartels**, Center for Neurological Vascular Diagnostics, München, Technische Universität München, Germany
Susanne **Bartels**, Department of Psychiatry and Psychotherapy, Albert-Ludwigs-University Freiburg, Freiburg, Germany
Vanja **Bašič Kes**, University Department of Neurology, University Hospital Center Sestre Milosrdnice, Zagreb, Croatia
Poorang **Bassir**, Student Scientific Research Committee (SSRC), Tehran University of Medical Sciences, Tehran, Iran
Jochen **Bäuerle**, Department of Neurology, Justus-Liebig-University, Giessen, Germany
Randy S. **Bell**, Walter Reed National Military Medical Center, Bethesda, MD, USA
Hermann **Berger**, Interdisciplinary Research Laboratory of the Klinikum rechts der Isar der TU München, München, München
Valery **Bersnev**, Russian Polenov Neurosurgical Institute, St. Petersburg, Russia
Daniela **Bertens**, Department of Neurology, VU University Medical Center, Amsterdam, The Netherlands
Angelo **Bignamini**, School of Specialization in Hospital Pharmacy, University of Milan, Milan, Italy
Yana **Bocheva**, Central Clinical Laboratory, St. Marina University Hospital, Varna, Bulgaria
Eduard H. **Boezeman**, Department of Clinical Neurophysiology, St. Antonius Hospital, Utrecht, The Netherlands
Ulrich **Bogdahn**, Department of Neurology, University of Regensburg, Bezirksklinikum Regensburg, Regensburg, Germany
Manuel **Bolognese**, Department of Neurology, UniversitätsMedizin Mannheim, University of Heidelberg, Mannheim, Germany
Mikhail A. **Bolotnov**, Moscow Clinical Hospital 13, Moscow, Russia
Marijana **Bosnar Puretic**, University Department of Neurology, University Hospital Center "Sisters of Mercy", Zagreb, Croatia
Michiel L. **Bots**, Department of Primary Care, University Medical Center Utrecht, Utrecht, The Netherlands
Sandra **Boy**, Department of Neurology, University of Regensburg, Bezirksklinikum Regensburg, Regensburg, Germany
Biljana **Bozic**, Institute for Physiology and Biochemistry, University of Belgrade, Belgrade, Serbia
Bogdan **Brodacki**, Clinic of Neurology, Military Medical Institute, Warsaw, Poland
Sergio **Bucconi**, DUC ACADEM, UCO di Anatomia e Istologia Patologica, AOTS, Trieste, Italy
Wolfgang F. **Buhre**, Department of Anesthesiology, University Medical Center Utrecht, Utrecht, The Netherlands
Gianfranco **Butera**, Policlinico San Donato, San Donato Milanese, Italy

Jaume **Campelacreu**, Department of Neurology, Bellvitge University Hospital, Barcelona, Spain
Luis **Cano**, Department of Neurology, Bellvitge University Hospital, Barcelona, Spain
Luigi **Caputi**, Fondazione IRCCS Neurological Institute C. Besta. Department of Cerebrovascular Diseases, Milan, Italy
Pedro **Cardona**, Department of Neurology, Bellvitge University Hospital, Barcelona, Spain
Mario **Carminati**, Policlinico San Donato, San Donato Milanese, Italy
Nicola **Carraro**, DUC SMIT, UCO di Clinica Neurologica, AOTS, Trieste, Italy
Pedro **Castro**, Department Neurology, Hospital São João, Faculty of Medicine of University of Porto, Porto, Portugal
Teodora **Chamova**, Clinic of Neurology, University Hospital "Alexandrovska", Sofia, Bulgaria
Sylvia **Cherninkova**, Clinic of Neurology, University Hospital "Alexandrovska, Sofia, Bulgaria
Massimo **Chessa**, Policlinico San Donato, San Donato Milanese, Italy
Vladislav Y. **Chirkin**, Russian Polenov Neurosurgical Institute, St. Petersburg, Russia
Emma M.L. **Chung**, Department of Cardiovascular Sciences, University of Leicester, Leicester, UK
Loreta **Cimbalistiene**, Vilnius University, Medical Faculty, Department of Human and Medical Genetics, Vilnius, Lithuania
Raffaella **Colombatti**, Department of Pediatrics, University of Padua, Padua, Italy
Florian **Connolly**, Department of Neurology, University Hospital Charité, Berlin, Germany
Lejla **Ćorić**, University Department of Neurology, University Hospital Center Sestre Milosrdnice, Zagreb, Croatia
László **Csiba**, Department of Neurology, University of Debrecen Medical and Health Science Center, Debrecen, Hungary
Daniel **Czerný**, Department of Radiology, University Hospital, Ostrava, Czech Republic
Marek **Czosnyka**, Academic Neurosurgical Unit, Addenbrooke's Hospital, Cambridge, UK
Gianni **De Berti**, Neuroradiology Unit, Department of Radiology, Azienda Ospedaliera ASMN, Istituto di Ricovero e Cura a Carattere Scientifico, Reggio Emilia, Italy
Gert J. **de Borst**, Department of Vascular Surgery, University Medical Center Utrecht, Utrecht, The Netherlands
S.F.T.M. **de Bruijn**, Department of Neurology and Clinical Neurophysiology, Haga Teaching Hospitals, The Hague, The Netherlands
Jelle R. **de Kruijk**, Department of Neurology, Tergooiziekenhuizen, Blaricum, The Netherlands
Jean-Paul P. **de Vries**, Department of Vascular Surgery, St. Antonius Hospital, Utrecht, The Netherlands
Massimo **Del Sette**, Neurology Unit, Ospedale Sant'Andrea, La Spezia, Italy
Vida **Demarin**, University Department of Neurology, University Hospital Center Sestre Milosrdnice, Zagreb, Croatia
Jurate **Dementaviciene**, Vilnius University, Medical Faculty, Department of Radiology, Nuclear Medicine and Medical Physics, Vilnius, Lithuania
Vittorio **Di Piero**, Stroke Unit – Neurosonology, Department of Neurology and Psychiatry, Sapienza University of Rome, Rome, Italy
Orlando **Diaz-Daza**, The Methodist Hospital Neurological Institute, Houston, TX, USA
Ralf **Dittrich**, Department of Neurology, University of Münster, Münster, Germany
Banafsheh **Dormanesh**, AJA University of Medical Sciences, Tehran, Iran
Robert **Ecker**, Maine Medical Cente, Portland, ME, USA
Hans-Henning **Eckstein**, Interdisciplinary Research Laboratory of the Klinikum rechts der Isar der TU München, München, München
Jürgen **Eggers**, Neurology, University Hospital Schleswig-Holstein, Lübeck, Germany
Reiko **Endoh**, Medical Engineering Laboratory, Research Center for Medical Sciences, Jikei University School of Medicine, Tokyo, Japan
Mario **Ermani**, Department of Neuroscience, University of Padua, Padua, Italy
Michael **Ertl**, Department of Neurology, University of Regensburg, Bezirksklinikum Regensburg, Regensburg, Germany
Anna **Escrig**, Department of Neurology, Sant Boi Hospital, Barcelona, Spain
David H. **Evans**, Department of Cardiovascular Sciences, University of Leicester, Leicester, UK
Táňa **Fadrná**, Department of Neurology, University Hospital and Ostrava University Medical School, Ostrava, Czech Republic
Filippo Maria **Farina**, Department of Neuroscience, University of Padua, Padua, Italy
Szabolcs **Farkas**, Department of Neurology, University of Debrecen Medical and Health Science Center, Debrecen, Hungary
Franz **Fazekas**, Department of Neurology, Medical University of Graz, Graz, Austria
Seyed-Mohammad **Fereshtehnejad**, Firoozgar Clinical Research Development Center (FCRDC), Tehran University of Medical Sciences, Tehran, Iran
Michael **Frank**, Intensive Care, Haga Teaching Hospitals, The Hague, The Netherlands
João **Freitas**, Autonomic Unit, Hospital São João, Faculty of Medicine of University of Porto, Porto, Portugal
Takahiro **Fukuda**, Division of Neuropathology, Department of Neuroscience, Research Center for Medical Sciences, Jikei University School of Medicine, Tokyo, Japan
Hiroshi **Furuhata**, Medical Engineering Laboratory, Research Center for Medical Sciences, Jikei University School of Medicine, Tokyo, Japan
Paolo **Gallo**, Department of Neuroscience, University of Padua, Padua, Italy
Anreea **Gamulescu**, Department of Opthalmology, University of Regensburg, Regensburg, Germany
Zsolt **Garami**, The Methodist Hospital Research Institute, Houston, TX, USA
Maria Fabrizia **Giannoni**, Vascular Ultrasound Investigation, Department "Paride Stefanini", Sapienza University of Rome, Rome, Italy
Sotirios **Giannopoulos**, Department of Neurology, University of Ioannina School of Medicine, Ioannina, Greece
Syed Amir **Gilani**, Department of Radiological Sciences and Medical Imaging (AISMI), The University of Lahore, Lahore, Pakistan
Aleksandar **Gopcevic**, Department of Anesthesiology, University Hospital Center "Sisters of Mercy", Zagreb, Croatia
Airì **Gorian**, DUC SMIT, UCO di Clinica Neurologica, AOTS, Trieste, Italy
Jan **Gralla**, Institute of Diagnostic and Interventional Neuroradiology, Inselspital, University of Bern, Bern, Switzerland
Fabio Chiodo **Grandi**, DUC SMIT, UCO di Clinica Neurologica, AOTS, Trieste, Italy
Sonja **Gröschel**, Department of Neurology, University of Göttingen, Göttingen, Germany

List of Contributors

Klaus **Gröschel**, Department of Neurology, University of Mainz, Mainz, Germany
Velina **Guergueltcheva**, Clinic of Neurology, University Hospital "Alexandrovska", Sofia, Bulgaria
Roman L. **Haberl**, Städtisches Klinikum München, Klinik für Neurologie und Neurologische Intensivmedizin, München, Germany
James P. **Hague**, Department of Physical Sciences, Open University, Milton Keynes, UK
Hiroshi **Hano**, Department of Pathology, Jikei University School of Medicine, Tokyo, Japan
Andreas **Harloff**, Department of Neurology, University of Freiburg, Freiburg, Germany
Salim **Harris**, Neurovascular and Neurosonology Division, Neurology Department, Medical Faculty, University of Indonesia, Jakarta, Indonesia
H.S. Moeniralam **Hazra**, Intensive Care, St. Antonius Hospital, Utrecht, The Netherlands
Horst **Helbig**, Department of Opthalmology, University of Regensburg, Regensburg, Germany
Michael G. **Hennerici**, Department of Neurology, UniversitätsMedizin Mannheim, University of Heidelberg, Mannheim, Germany
Roman **Herzig**, Department of Neurology, Faculty of Medicine and Dentistry, Palacký University and University Hospital Olomouc, Olomouc, Czech Republic
Andreas **Hetzel**, Department of Neurology, University of Freiburg, Freiburg, Germany
Sven M. **Hochheimer**, Walter Reed National Military Medical Center, Bethesda, MD, USA
Bernd M. **Hofmann**, Siemens AG, Healthcare Sector, Erlangen, Germany
Remco **Hoogenboezem**, Department of Neurology and Clinical Neurophysiology, Haga Teaching Hospitals, The Hague, The Netherlands
Susanna **Horner**, Department of Neurology, Medical University of Graz, Graz, Austria
Tibor **Hortobágyi**, Department of Neurology, University of Debrecen Medical and Health Science Center, Debrecen, Hungary
Maayke **Hunfeld**, Department of Neurology and Clinical Neurophysiology, Haga Teaching Hospitals, The Hague, The Netherlands
Rogier V. **Immink**, Department of Anesthesiology, University Medical Center Utrecht, Utrecht, The Netherlands
Takuya **Inagaki**, Department of Pathology, Jikei University School of Medicine, Tokyo, Japan
Dalius **Jatuzis**, Vilnius University, Medical Faculty, Neurology and Neurosurgery Clinic, Centre of Neurology, Vilnius, Lithuania
Marek **Jauss**, Department of Neurology, Oekumenisches Hainich Klinikum, Muehlhausen, Mühlhausen, Germany
Vikram **Jeyagopal**, Department of Cardiovascular Sciences, University of Leicester, Leicester, UK
Soeren Paaske **Johnsen**, The Department of Clinical Epidemiology, Aarhus University Hospital, Aarhus, Denmark
Susanne **Johnsen**, Department of Neurology, Schlei-Klinikum, Schleswig, Germany
Tomáš **Jonszta**, Department of Radiology, University Hospital, Ostrava, Czech Republic
Rasadul **Kabir**, The Methodist Hospital Neurological Institute, Houston, TX, USA
Jaap **Kappelle**, Department of Neurology and Julius Center for Health Sciences, University Medical Center Utrecht, Utrecht, The Netherlands
Sonja **Karakaneva**, Clinic of Functional Diagnostics of Nervous System, Military Medical Academy, Sofia, Bulgaria
László **Kardos**, Kenézy Hospital and Outpatient Services, Infection Control Unit, Debrecen, Hungary
Alexey V. **Kascheev**, Moscow State University for Medicine and Dentistry, Department of Neurology, Moscow, Russia
Ken-ichi **Kawabata**, Life Science Research Center, Central Research Laboratory, Tokyo, Japan
Jesada **Keandaoungchan**, Division of Neurology, Department of Medicine, Faculty of Medicine Ramathibodi Hospital, Mahidol University, Bangkok, Thailand
Henrich **Kele**, Neurologie Neuer Wall, Hamburg, Germany
Pawel **Kermer**, Department of Neurology, Nordwestkrankenhaus Sanderbusch GmbH, Sande, Germany
R. Rolf **Kern**, Department of Neurology, UniversitätsMedizin Mannheim, University of Heidelberg, Mannheim, Germany
Ruud W.M. **Keunen**, Department of Neurology and Clinical Neurophysiology, Haga Teaching Hospitals, The Hague, The Netherlands
Filip **Kirov**, Second Clinic of Neurology, St. Marina University Hospital, Varna, Bulgaria
Jürgen **Klingelhöfer**, Department of Neurology, Medical Center Chemnitz, Chemnitz, Germany
Marko **Klissurski**, Clinic of Neurology, University Hospital "Tzaritza Ioanna-ISUL", Sofia, Bulgaria
Richard **Klucznik**, The Methodist Hospital Neurological Institute, Houston, TX, USA
Réka Katalin **Kovács**, Department of Neurology, University of Debrecen Medical and Health Science Center, Debrecen, Hungary
Michiyo **Koyama**, Department of Clinical Neurosciences, Kyoto Takeda Hospital, Kyoto, Japan
Alexandr **Kozlov**, Russian Polenov Neurosurgical Institute, St. Petersburg, Russia
Jan **Krajča**, Department of Radiology, University Hospital, Ostrava, Czech Republic
Sandro M. **Krieg**, Department of Neurosurgery, Klinikum rechts der Isar, Technische Universität München, München, Germany
Zeljko **Krsmanovic**, Department of Neurology, Military Medical Academy, Belgrade, Serbia
Martin **Kuliha**, Department of Neurology, University Hospital and Ostrava University Medical School, Ostrava, Czech Republic
Boban **Labovic**, Department of Neurology, Military Medical Academy, Belgrade, Serbia
Gian Luigi **Lenzi**, Stroke Unit – Neurosonology, Department of Neurology and Psychiatry, Sapienza University of Rome, Rome, Italy
Toplica **Lepic**, Department of Neurology, Military Medical Academy, Belgrade, Serbia
Milan **Lepic**, Department of Neurology, Military Medical Academy, Belgrade, Serbia
Brigitta **Léránt**, Department of Neurology, University of Debrecen Medical and Health Science Center, Debrecen, Hungary
Christopher **Levi**, Centre for Translational Neuroscience & Mental Health Research, University of Newcastle & Hunter Medical Research Institute, Newcastle, NSW, Australia
Dieter **Liepsch**, Insitut f. Biotechnik e.V., University of Applied Sciences, München, München
Jan **Liman**, Department of Neurology, University of Göttingen, Göttingen, Germany
Luca **Lodigiani**, Ultrasound Operational Marketing, ESAOTE SpA, Genova, Italy
Goran **Loncar**, Department of Cardiology, Clinical Center Zvezdara, Belgrade, Serbia
Arijana **Lovrencic-Huzjan**, University Department of Neurology, University Hospital Center "Sisters of Mercy", Zagreb, Croatia

Massimo **Maggi**, Neuroradiology Unit, Department of Radiology, Azienda Ospedaliera ASMN, Istituto di Ricovero e Cura a Carattere Scientifico, Reggio Emilia, Italy

Seyed Mohammad Hossein **Mahmoodi**, Student Scientific Research Committee (SSRC), Tehran University of Medical Sciences, Tehran, Iran

Giovanni **Malferrari**, Neurology Unit, Department of Neuromotor Physiology, Azienda Ospedaliera ASMN, Istituto di Ricovero e Cura a Carattere Scientifico, Reggio Emilia, Italy

Renzo **Manara**, Institute of Neuroradiology, University of Padua, Padua, Italy

Marcello **Mancini**, Consiglio Nazionale delle Ricerche, Istituto di Biostrutture␣Bioimmagini, University Federico II, Napoli, Italy

Norina **Marcello**, Neurology Unit, Department of Neuromotor Physiology, Azienda Ospedaliera ASMN, Istituto di Ricovero e Cura a Carattere Scientifico, Reggio Emilia, Italy

Michael **Markl**, Departments of Radiology and Biomedical Engineering, Northwestern University, Chicago, IL, USA

Scott A. **Marshall**, Department of Neurology, Uniformed Services University of the Health Sciences, Bethesda, MD, USA

Paola **Martingano**, DUC SMIT, UCO di Radiologia, AOTS, Trieste, Italy

Irena **Martinic Popovic**, University Department of Neurology, University Hospital Center "Sisters of Mercy", Zagreb, Croatia

Stephan **Meairs**, Department of Neurology, UniversitätsMedizin Mannheim, University of Heidelberg, Mannheim, Germany

Oriano **Mecarelli**, Stroke Unit – Neurosonology, Department of Neurology and Psychiatry, Sapienza University of Rome, Rome, Italy

Masoud **Mehrpour**, Firoozgar Clinical Research Development Center (FCRDC), Neurology Department, Tehran University of Medical Sciences, Tehran, Iran

Oliver **Meier**, Städtisches Klinikum München, Klinik für Neurologie und Neurologische Intensivmedizin, München, Germany

Giorgio **Meneghetti**, Department of Neuroscience, University of Padua, Padua, Italy

Bernhard **Meyer**, Department of Neurosurgery, Klinikum rechts der Isar, Technische Universität München, München, Germany

Milija D. **Mijajlovic**, Neurology Clinic, Clinical Center of Serbia, School of Medicine University of Belgrade, Belgrade, Serbia

Samira **Mirzaeizadeh**, Student Scientific Research Center (SSRC), Tehran University of Medical Sciences, Tehran, Iran

Amit **Mistri**, Medical Physics Department, University Hospitals of Leicester NHS Trust, Leicester, UK

Hidetaka **Mitsumura**, The Jikei University School of Medicine, Department of Neurology, Tokyo, Japan

Takayuki **Mizuno**, Department of Neurology, Kyoto Prefectural University of Medicine, Kyoto, Japan

Alexandr O. **Mnushkin**, Moscow State University for Medicine and Dentistry, Department of Neurology, Moscow, Russia

Soichiro **Mochio**, The Jikei University School of Medicine, Department of Neurology, Tokyo, Japan

Carlos A. **Molina**, Vall d'Hebron Stroke Unit, Department of Neurosciences, Hospital Universitari Vall d'Hebron, Barcelona, Spain

Frans L. **Moll**, Department of Vascular Surgery, University Medical Center Utrecht, Utrecht, The Netherlands

Sándor **Molnár**, Department of Neurology, Sopron Elizabeth Hospital, Sopron, Hungary

Maria **Montanaro**, Department of Pediatrics, University of Padua, Padua, Italy

Paloma **Mora**, Department of Neuroradiology, Bellvitge University Hospital, Barcelona, Spain

Pasquale **Mordasini**, Institute of Diagnostic and Interventional Neuroradiology, Inselspital, University of Bern, Bern, Switzerland

A. **Mosch**, Department of Neurology and Clinical Neurophysiology, Haga Teaching Hospitals, The Hague, The Netherlands

Mohammad Reza **Motamed**, Firoozgar Clinical Research Development Center (FCRDC), Neurology Department, Tehran University of Medical Sciences, Tehran, Iran

Robert **Müller**, Städtisches Klinikum München, Klinik für Neurologie und Neurologische Intensivmedizin, München, Germany

Rashid S. **Musin**, Moscow State University for Medicine and Dentistry, Department of Neurology, Moscow, Russia

Masoud **Nabavi**, Neurology Department, Shahed University of Medical Sciences, Tehran, Iran

Katalin **Nagy**, Department of Neurology, University of Debrecen Medical and Health Science Center, Debrecen, Hungary

Neda **Najimi**, Firoozgar Clinical Research Development Center (FCRDC), Tehran University of Medical Sciences, Tehran, Iran

Masanori **Nakagawa**, Department of Neurology, Kyoto Prefectural University of Medicine, Kyoto, Japan

Max **Nedelmann**, Department of Neurology, Justus-Liebig-University, Giessen, Germany

Pamela **New**, The Methodist Hospital Neurological Institute, Houston, TX, USA

Nelly **Nicheva-Vavrek**, Clinic of Neurology, University Hospital "Tzaritza Ioanna-ISUL", Sofia, Bulgaria

Kurt **Niederkorn**, Department of Neurology, Medical University of Graz, Graz, Austria

László **Oláh**, Department of Neurology, University of Debrecen Medical and Health Science Center, Debrecen, Hungary

Viktor E. **Olyushin**, Russian Polenov Neurosurgical Institute, St. Petersburg, Russia

Angelo **Onofri**, Department of Neuroscience, University of Padua, Padua, Italy

Eustaquio **Onorato**, Ospedale S. Orsola, Unita' Operativa di Cardiologia – Fatebenefratelli, Service of Neurology, Brescia, Italy

Stephen M. **Oppenheimer**, Maine Medical Cente, Portland, ME, USA

Francesco **Pancrazio**, DUC ACADEM, UCO di Chirurgia Vascolare, AOT, Trieste, Italy

Ronney **Panerai**, Department of Cardiovascular Sciences, University of Leicester, Leicester, UK

G.K. **Panuntsev**, Russian Polenov Neurosurgical Institute, St. Petersburg, Russia

Eugenio **Parati**, Fondazione IRCCS Neurological Institute C. Besta. Department of Cerebrovascular Diseases, Milan, Italy

Mark **Parsons**, Centre for Translational Neuroscience & Mental Health Research, University of Newcastle & Hunter Medical Research Institute, Newcastle, NSW, Australia

Rizwan **Patel**, Department of Cardiovascular Sciences, University of Leicester, Leicester, UK

Andreas **Patzak**, University Hospital Charite, Humboldt-University of Berlin, Johannes-Mueller Institute of Physiology, Berlin, Germany

Dmitriy A. **Pechiborsch**, Russian Polenov Neurosurgical Institute, St. Petersburg, Russia

Claire W. **Pennekamp**, Department of Vascular Surgery, University Medical Center Utrecht, Utrecht, The Netherlands

Denis **Perko**, University Medical Centre Ljubljana, Department of Neurology, Ljubljana, Slovenia,

Diana **Petkova**, Clinic of Pneumology and Physiology, St. Marina University Hospital, Varna, Bulgaria

Renata Anna **Piusińska-Macoch**, Clinic of Neurology, Military Medical Institute, Warsaw, Poland

List of Contributors

Gilberto **Pizzolato**, DUC SMIT, UCO di Clinica Neurologica, AOTS, Trieste, Italy
Z. **Podgajny**, Clinic of Endocrinology, Military Medical Institute, Warsaw, Poland
Holger **Poppert**, Klinikum rechts der Isar, Universität München, Department of Neurology, München, Germany
Janja **Pretnar-Oblak**, University Medical Centre Ljubljana, Department of Neurology, Ljubljana, Slovenia,
Stefano **Pro**, Stroke Unit – Neurosonology, Department of Neurology and Psychiatry, Sapienza University of Rome, Rome, Italy
Václav **Procházka**, Department of Radiology, University Hospital, Ostrava, Czech Republic
Patrizia **Pulitano**, Stroke Unit – Neurosonology, Department of Neurology and Psychiatry, Sapienza University of Rome, Rome, Italy
Helena **Quesada**, Department of Neurology, Bellvitge University Hospital, Barcelona, Spain
Ranko **Raicevic**, Department of Neurology, Military Medical Academy, Belgrade, Serbia
Shakhob **Ramazanov**, Russian Polenov Neurosurgical Institute, St. Petersburg, Russia
Patrizia **Rampazzo**, Department of Neuroscience, University of Padua, Padua, Italy
Disya **Ratanakorn**, Division of Neurology, Department of Medicine, Faculty of Medicine Ramathibodi Hospital, Mahidol University, Bangkok, Thailand
Alexander **Razumovsky**, Sentient NeuroCare Services, Hunt Valley, MD, USA
Matthias **Reinhard**, Department of Neurology, University of Freiburg, Freiburg, Germany
Michael **Remmers**, Department of Neurology, Amphia Hospital, Breda, The Netherlands
Maria Chiara **Ricciardi**, Stroke Unit – Neurosonology, Department of Neurology and Psychiatry, Sapienza University of Rome, Rome, Italy
Florian **Ringel**, Department of Neurosurgery, Klinikum rechts der Isar, Technische Universität München, München, Germany
Erich B. **Ringelstein**, Department of Neurology, University of Münster, Münster, Germany
Martin A. **Ritter**, Department of Neurology, University of Münster, Münster, Germany
Bojan **Rode**, Department of Anesthesiology, University Hospital Center "Sisters of Mercy", Zagreb, Croatia
Bernhard **Rosengarten**, Department of Neurology, Justus-Liebig-University, Giessen, Germany
Martin **Roubec**, Department of Neurology, University Hospital and Ostrava University Medical School, Ostrava, Czech Republic
Larisa **Rozhchenko**, Russian Polenov Neurosurgical Institute, St. Petersburg, Russia
Francisco **Rubio**, Department of Neurology, Bellvitge University Hospital, Barcelona, Spain
Angelica **Ruiz Franco**, The Instituto Nacional de Neurología y Neurocirugía Manuel Velasco, Suárez, México City, Mexico
Tatjana **Rundek**, Department of Neurology, Miller School of Medicine, University of Miami,, Miami, FL, USA
David **Russell**, Department of Neurology, Oslo University Hospital, Oslo, Norway
Sebastian **Rutsch**, Department of Neurology, University of Freiburg, Freiburg, Germany
Fatemeh Naderi **Safa**, Student Scientific Research Center (SSRC), Tehran University of Medical Sciences, Tehran, Iran
Mohammad Ali **Sahraeian**, Neurology Department, Tehran University of Medical Sciences, Tehran, Iran
Laura **Sainati**, Department of Pediatrics, University of Padua, Padua, Italy
Daniel **Šaňák**, Department of Neurology, Faculty of Medicine and Dentistry, Palacký University and University Hospital Olomouc, Olomouc, Czech Republic
Dirk **Sander**, Department of Neurology, Benedictus Krankenhaus Tutzing, Technische Universität München, München, Germany
Giuseppe **Sangiorgi**, Modena University, Modena, Italy
Sandro **Sanguigni**, Neurology Unit, Ospedale Madonna del Soccorso, San Benedetto del Tronto, Italy
Gennaro **Santoro**, S.O.D. "Diagnostica ed Interventistica Cardiovascolare, AOU Careggi, Florence, Italy
Rosa **Santos**, Department Neurology, Hospital São João, Faculty of Medicine of University of Porto, Porto, Portugal
Vittoria Maria **Sarra**, DUC SMIT, UCO di Clinica Neurologica, AOTS, Trieste, Italy
Leonid A. **Savin**, Moscow State University for Medicine and Dentistry, Department of Neurology, Moscow, Russia
Enrico **Sbarigia**, Vascular Ultrasound Investigation, Department "Paride Stefanini", Sapienza University of Rome, Rome, Italy
Peter D. **Schellinger**, Departments of Neurology and Geriatry, Johannes Wesling Klinikum Minden, Minden, Germany
Karsten **Schepelmann**, Department of Neurology, Schlei-Klinikum, Schleswig, Germany
Felix **Schlachetzki**, Department of Neurology, University of Regensburg, Bezirksklinikum Regensburg, Regensburg, Germany
Bernhard **Schmidt**, Department of Neurology, Medical Center Chemnitz, Chemnitz, Germany
Ulf **Schminke**, Department of Neurology, Ernst Moritz Arndt University Greifswald, Greifswald, Germany
Stephan J. **Schreiber**, Department of Neurology, University Hospital Charité, Berlin, Germany
Gerhard **Schroth**, Institute of Diagnostic and Interventional Neuroradiology, Inselspital, University of Bern, Bern, Switzerland
Günter **Seidel**, Department of Neurology, Asklepios Klinik Hamburg Nord, Hamburg, Germany
Vladimir **Semenyutin**, Russian Polenov Neurosurgical Institute, St. Petersburg, Russia
Renpei **Sengoku**, The Jikei University School of Medicine, Department of Neurology, Tokyo, Japan
Giovanna **Servillo**, DUC SMIT, UCO di Clinica Neurologica, AOTS, Trieste, Italy
Meryl A. **Severson**, Walter Reed National Military Medical Center, Bethesda, MD, USA
Vijay K. **Sharma**, Division of Neurology, National University Hospital, Singapore, Singapore
Svetlana **Shayunova**, Russian National Research, Medical University, Laboratory of Child Cerebrovascular Disorders, Moscow, Russia
Jun **Shimizu**, Medical Engineering Laboratory, Research Center for Medical Sciences, Jikei University School of Medicine, Tokyo, Japan
Toshiyuki **Shiogai**, Department of Clinical Neurosciences, Kyoto Takeda Hospital, Kyoto, Japan
Mikhail V. **Sinkin**, Moscow Clinical Hospital 11, Moscow, Russia
Gaia **Sirimarco**, Stroke Unit – Neurosonology, Department of Neurology and Psychiatry, Sapienza University of Rome, Rome, Italy
David **Skoloudík**, Department of Neurology, University Hospital and Ostrava University Medical School, Ostrava, Czech Republic
Andrea **Skultéty Szárazová**, University Hospital of Bratislava, 1st Neurological Clinic, Bratislava, Slovakia
P. **Smużyński**, Clinic of Cardiology, Military Medical Institute, Warsaw, Poland

Darja **Sodec Simicevic**, University Department of Neurology, University Hospital Center "Sisters of Mercy", Zagreb, Croatia

Denis S. **Solonskiy**, Moscow State University for Medicine and Dentistry, Department of Neurology, Moscow, Russia

Isabella **Spadoni**, Ospedale "G: Pasquinucci" U.O. Cardiologia Pediatrica e GUCH, Montepepe, Massa, Italy

Francesco **Speziale**, Vascular Ultrasound Investigation, Department "Paride Stefanini", Sapienza University of Rome, Rome, Italy

Wilco **Spiering**, Department of Vascular Medicine, University Medical Center Utrecht, Utrecht, The Netherlands

Boyko **Stamenov**, Department of Neurology, Pleven Medical University, Pleven, Bulgaria

Jacek **Staszewski**, Clinic of Neurology, Military Medical Institute, Warsaw, Poland

Irina **Stepanova**, Russian National Research, Medical University Named After N.I. Pirogov, Pediatric Faculty, Neurology, Neurosurgery and Medical Genetics Department, Laboratory of Child Cerebrovascular Disorders, Moscow, Russia

Fred L. **Stephens**, Walter Reed National Military Medical Center, Bethesda, MD, USA

Adam **Stępień**, Clinic of Neurology, Military Medical Institute, Warsaw, Poland

Konrad **Stock**, Klinikum rechts der Isar, Universität München, Department of Nephrolog, München, Germany

Jeffrey **Stoll**, Siemens Ultrasound, Mountain View, CA, USA

Erwin **Stolz**, Department of Neurology, CaritasKlinikum Saarbruecken, Saarbrücken, Germany

Zlatka **Stoyneva**, St. Ivan Rilsky University Hospital, Sofia,, Bulgaria

Christina **Straesser**, Department of Neurology, University of Debrecen Medical and Health Science Center, Debrecen, Hungary

Igor D. **Stulin**, Moscow State University for Medicine and Dentistry, Department of Neurology, Moscow, Russia

Denes L. **Tavy**, Department of Neurology and Clinical Neurophysiology, Haga Teaching Hospitals, The Hague, The Netherlands

Teodoro A. **Tigno**, The University of Texas Medical Branch, Galveston, TX, USA

Ekaterina **Titianova**, Clinic of Functional Diagnostics of Nervous System, Military Medical Academy, Sofia, Bulgaria

Kazimierz **Tomczykiewicz**, Clinic of Neurology, Military Medical Institute, Warsaw, Poland

Elisabeth **Torka**, Department of Neurology, University of Regensburg, Bezirksklinikum Regensburg, Regensburg, Germany

Massimiliano **Toscano**, Stroke Unit – Neurosonology, Department of Neurology and Psychiatry, Sapienza University of Rome, Rome, Italy

Ivailo **Tournev**, Department of Cognitive Science and Psychology, New Bulgarian University, Sofia, Bulgaria

Selma C. **Tromp**, Department of Clinical Neurophysiology, St. Antonius Hospital, Utrecht, The Netherlands

Georgios **Tsivgoulis**, Department of Neurology, Democritus University of Alexandroupolis School of Medicine, Alexandroupolis, Greece

Peter **Turčáni**, University Hospital of Bratislava, 1st Neurological Clinic, Bratislava, Slovakia

Gian Paolo **Ussia**, Ospedale Ferrarotto, Laboratorio di Emodinamica Divisione Clinicizzata di Cardiologia, Azienda Policlinico Vittorio Emanuele, Catania, Italy

Jurgita **Valaikiene**, Vilnius University, Medical Faculty, Neurology and Neurosurgery Clinic, Centre of Neurology, Vilnius, Lithuania

Jose M. **Valdueza**, Neurological Centre, Segeberger Kliniken, Bad Segeberg, Germany

Michael **Valet**, Department of Neurology, Benedictus Krankenhaus Tutzing, Technische Universität München, München, Germany

Marianne **van der Mee**, Department of Clinical Neurophysiology, St. Antonius Hospital, Utrecht, The Netherlands

Agnes **van Sonderen**, Department of Neurology and Clinical Neurophysiology, Haga Teaching Hospitals, The Hague, The Netherlands

Evgenii Vladislav **Vavrek**, Emergency Neurological Unit, University Hospital "Tzaritza Ioanna-ISUL", Sofia, Bulgaria

Dragana **Veljancic**, Department of Neurology, Military Medical Academy, Belgrade, Serbia

Narayanaswamy **Venketasubramanian**, Division of Neurology, University Medicine Cluster, Singapore, Singapore

Federica **Viaro**, Department of Neuroscience, University of Padua, Padua, Italy

Edoardo B. **Vicenzini**, Stroke Unit – Neurosonology, Department of Neurology and Psychiatry, Sapienza University of Rome, Rome, Italy

Alexander H. **Vo**, The University of Texas Medical Branch, Galveston, TX, USA

John J. **Volpi**, The Methodist Hospital Neurological Institute, Houston, TX, USA

Gerhard-Michael **von Reutern**, Ambulantes Kardiologisches Zentrum, Neurologische Praxis, Bad Nauheim, Germany

Paul **von Weitzel-Mudersbach**, The Department of Neurology, Aarhus Hospital, Aarhus University Hospital, Aarhus, Denmark

Marinko **Vucic**, Department of Anesthesiology, University Hospital Center "Sisters of Mercy", Zagreb, Croatia

Vlasta **Vukovic Cvetkovic**, University Department of Neurology, University Hospital Center "Sisters of Mercy", Zagreb, Croatia

Uwe **Walter**, Department of Neurology, University of Rostock, Rostock, Germany

Katrin **Wasser**, Department of Neurology, University of Göttingen, Göttingen, Germany

Janin **Wohlfahrt**, Department of Neurology, University of Göttingen, Göttingen, Germany

Masakazu **Yamamoto**, Department of Clinical Neurosciences, Kyoto Takeda Hospital, Kyoto, Japan

Makiko **Yogo**, The Jikei University School of Medicine, Department of Neurology, Tokyo, Japan

Masayuki **Yokoyama**, Medical Engineering Laboratory, Research Center for Medical Sciences, Jikei University School of Medicine, Tokyo, Japan

Kenjiro **Yoshikawa**, Department of Stroke Medicine, Hoshigaoka Kouseinenkin Hospital, Osaka, Japan

Marjan **Zaletel**, University Medical Centre Ljubljana, Department of Neurology, Ljubljana, Slovenia,

Maciej **Zarębiński**, Department of Invasive Cardiology, SPS Szpital Zachodni, Grodzisk Mazowiecki, Poland

Hossein **Zareie**, Centre for Translational Neuroscience & Mental Health Research, University of Newcastle & Hunter Medical Research Institute, Newcastle, NSW, Australia

Iris **Zavoreo**, University Department of Neurology, University Hospital Center Sestre Milosrdnice, Zagreb, Croatia

Marialuisa **Zedde**, Neurology Unit, Department of Neuromotor Physiology, Azienda Ospedaliera ASMN, Istituto di Ricovero e Cura a Carattere Scientifico, Reggio Emilia, Italy

Viviane Flumignan **Zétola**, Hospital de Clínicas, Rua General Carneiro 181, Serviço de Neurologia, Curitiba, Brazil

Udo **Zikeli**, Siemens AG, Healthcare Sector, Erlangen, Germany

Sanne M. **Zinkstok**, Department of Neurology, Academic Medical Center, University of Amsterdam, Amsterdam, The Netherlands

Marino **Zorzon**, DUC SMIT, UCO di Clinica Neurologica, AOTS, Trieste, Italy

Bojana **Žvan**, University Medical Centre Ljubljana, Department of Neurology, Ljubljana, Slovenia

Subject index of volume 1

Acetazolamide vasoreactivity
   Brain tissue perfusion monitoring using Sonopod for transcranial color duplex sonography, 34
Acute cerebral ischemia
   Early ultrasound imaging of carotid arteries in the acute ischemic cerebrovascular patients, 108
   Cerebral autoregulation in acute ischemic stroke, 194
Acute ischemic stroke
   Sonothrombolysis for treatment of acute ischemic stroke: Current evidence and new developments, 14
   Hemodynamic causes of deterioration in acute ischemic stroke, 177
   Transcranial Doppler in acute stroke management – A "real-time" bed-side guide to reperfusion and collateral flow, 185
   Evaluation of very early recanalization after tPA administration monitoring by transcranial color-coded sonography, 331
Acute stroke
   Imaging of plaque perfusion using contrast-enhanced ultrasound – Clinical significance, 44
Acute stroke care
   "A horse, a horse, my kingdom for a horse" – Saddle thrombosis of carotid bifurcation in acute stroke, 435
Acute stroke treatment
   Mechanical recanalization in acute stroke treatment, 54
Alternating flow
   Pitfall of vertebral artery insonation: Bidirectional flow without subclavian artery pathology, 449
Angiogenesis
   Imaging of plaque perfusion using contrast-enhanced ultrasound – Clinical significance, 44
Angioplasty
   Predictors of carotid artery in-stent restenosis, 122
Angle-independent Doppler technique by QuantixND system
   Volume flow rate, 203
Ankle
   An overview of musculoskeletal ultrasound – A thirteen years experience in Pakistan, 427
Ankle-brachial index
   Optimized prevention of stroke: What is the role of ultrasound?, 100
Aortitis
   Diagnosis and management of Takayasu arteritis, 255
Arterial occlusion
   Endovascular sono-lysis using EKOS system in acute stroke patients with a main cerebral artery occlusion – A pilot study, 65
Arterial stiffness
   Breath holding index and arterial stiffness in evaluation of stroke risk in diabetic patients, 156
Arterial wall stiffness
   Arterial wall dynamics, 146
Arteriovenous malformation
   Transcranial color-coded duplex ultrasonography in routine cerebrovascular diagnostics, 325
   Transient brainstem ischemia and dural arteriovenous malformation, 465

Arteritis
   Diagnosis and management of Takayasu arteritis, 255
Artery
   Exploration of a zero-tolerance regime on cerebral embolism in symptomatic carotid artery disease, 218
Association
   Are impaired endothelial function in the posterior cerebral circulation and intact endothelial function in the anterior cerebral and systemic circulation associated with migraine: A post hoc study, 297
Asymptomatic
   Medical management of asymptomatic carotid stenosis, 116
   Moyamoya like arteriopathy: Neurosonological suspicion and prognosis in adult asymptomatic patients, 257
Asymptomatic carotid stenosis
   How to treat an asymptomatic carotid stenosis? The view of the neurologist, 112
Asymptomatic hemorrhage
   My worst case with sonothrombolysis, 462
Atherosclerosis
   Symptomatic intracranial stenosis: A university hospital-based ultrasound study, 211
Atherosclerotic plaques
   Plaque angiogenesis identification with Contrast Enhanced Carotid Ultrasonography: Statement of the Consensus after the 16th ESNCH Meeting – Munich, 20-23 May 2011, 51
Atrial fibrillation
   The contribution of microembolic signals (MES) detection in cardioembolic stroke, 214

Basal ganglia
   Transcranial sonography of the cerebral parenchyma: Update on clinically relevant applications, 334
   Transcranial sonography in psychiatric diseases, 357
Bidirectional flow
   Pitfall of vertebral artery insonation: Bidirectional flow without subclavian artery pathology, 449
Bifurcation
   In vivo wall shear stress patterns in carotid bifurcations assessed by 4D MRI, 137
Biopsy
   Ultrasound fusion imaging, 80
Blindness
   The retrobulbar spot sign in sudden blindness – Sufficient to rule out vasculitis?, 408
Blood-brain barrier (BBB)
   Advances in neurosonology – Brain perfusion, sonothrombolysis and CNS drug delivery, 5
Blood flow velocity
   The long-term effects of hypobaric and hyperbaric conditions on brain hemodynamic: A transcranial Doppler ultrasonography of blood flow velocity of middle cerebral and basilar arteries in pilots and divers, 316
B-mode
   Arterial wall dynamics, 146

Brain activation studies
Adaptation of cerebral pressure-velocity hemodynamic changes of neurovascular coupling to orthostatic challenge, 290

Brain death
Oscillating transcranial Doppler patterns of brain death associated with therapeutic maneuvers, 321
The role of color duplex sonography in the brain death diagnostics, 362
Ultrasonography of the optic nerve sheath in brain death, 414

Brain hemodynamic
The long-term effects of hypobaric and hyperbaric conditions on brain hemodynamic: A transcranial Doppler ultrasonography of blood flow velocity of middle cerebral and basilar arteries in pilots and divers, 316

Brain perfusion
Update on ultrasound brain perfusion imaging, 30

Brain tissue perfusion
Brain tissue perfusion monitoring using Sonopod for transcranial color duplex sonography, 34

Brainstem raphe
Transcranial sonography in psychiatric diseases, 357

Brasilian Guideline
Role of TCD in sickle cell disease: A review, 265

Breath holding index
Breath holding index and arterial stiffness in evaluation of stroke risk in diabetic patients, 156

Calf
An overview of musculoskeletal ultrasound – A thirteen years experience in Pakistan, 427

Cardioembolic stroke
The contribution of microembolic signals (MES) detection in cardioembolic stroke, 214

Carotid
Exploration of a zero-tolerance regime on cerebral embolism in symptomatic carotid artery disease, 218

Carotid arteries imaging
Threedimensional imaging of carotid arteries: Advantages and pitfalls of ultrasound investigations, 82

Carotid artery
In vivo wall shear stress patterns in carotid bifurcations assessed by 4D MRI, 137
Carotid intima-media thickness (cIMT) and plaque from risk assessment and clinical use to genetic discoveries, 139
Intravascular papillary endothelial hyperplasia at the origin of internal carotid artery: A rare cause of stroke, 440

Carotid artery models
How local hemodynamics at the carotid bifurcation influence the development of carotid plaques, 132

Carotid artery stenosis
Plaque angiogenesis identification with Contrast Enhanced Carotid Ultrasonography: Statement of the Consensus after the 16th ESNCH Meeting – Munich, 20-23 May 2011, 51
Predictors of carotid artery in-stent restenosis, 122

Carotid atherosclerosis
Carotid atherosclerosis: Socio-demographic issues, the hidden dimensions, 167

Carotid Doppler
Cerebral blood flow in the chronic heart failure patients, 304

Carotid endarterectomy
How to treat an asymptomatic carotid stenosis? The view of the neurologist, 112
When to perform transcranial Doppler to predict cerebral hyperper-fusion after carotid endarterectomy?, 119

Carotid IMT/cIMT
Carotid intima-media thickness (cIMT) and plaque from risk assessment and clinical use to genetic discoveries, 139
The association of carotid intima-media thickness (cIMT) and stroke: A cross sectional study, 164

Carotid stenosis
Imaging of plaque perfusion using contrast-enhanced ultrasound – Clinical significance, 44
The role of extracranial ultrasound in the prevention of stroke based on the new guidelines, 94
Optimized prevention of stroke: What is the role of ultrasound?, 100
Measuring the degree of internal carotid artery stenosis, 104
Threedimensional imaging of carotid arteries: Advantages and pitfalls of ultrasound investigations, 82
Medical management of asymptomatic carotid stenosis, 116

Carotid stenting
How to treat an asymptomatic carotid stenosis? The view of the neurologist, 112
Post-carotid stent ultrasound provides critical data to avoid rare but serious complications, 129

Carotid surgery
Early ultrasound imaging of carotid arteries in the acute ischemic cerebrovascular patients, 108

Carotid ultrasound
Predictors of carotid artery in-stent restenosis, 122
Post-carotid stent ultrasound provides critical data to avoid rare but serious complications, 129

CBF velocity during normal sleep and sleep disorders
Cerebral blood flow velocity in sleep, 275

CCSVI
Fact or fiction: Chronic cerebro-spinal insufficiency, 371
Italian multicenter study on venous hemodynamics in multiple sclerosis: Advanced Sonological Protocol, 399

Central retinal artery occlusion
The retrobulbar spot sign in sudden blindness – Sufficient to rule out vasculitis?, 408

Cerebral autoregulation
Cerebral autoregulation in acute ischemic stroke, 194
Asymmetry of cerebral autoregulation does not correspond to asymmetry of cerebrovascular pressure reactivity, 285
Adaptation of cerebral pressure-velocity hemodynamic changes of neurovascular coupling to orthostatic challenge, 290
Informativity of pulsatility index and cerebral autoregulation in hydrocephalus, 311

Cerebral blood arrest
The role of color duplex sonography in the brain death diagnostics, 362

Cerebral blood flow
Cerebral blood flow in the chronic heart failure patients, 304
Asymmetry of cerebral autoregulation does not correspond to asymmetry of cerebrovascular pressure reactivity, 285

Cerebral blood flow velocity
Posttraumatic vasospasm and intracranial hypertension after wartime traumatic brain injury, 261

Cerebral electrical activity
Cerebral blood flow velocity in sleep, 275

Cerebral hemodynamics
Adaptation of cerebral pressure-velocity hemodynamic changes of neurovascular coupling to orthostatic challenge, 290

Cerebral hyperperfusion syndrome
When to perform transcranial Doppler to predict cerebral hyperper-fusion after carotid endarterectomy?, 119

Cerebral perfusion pressure
Asymmetry of cerebral autoregulation does not correspond to asymmetry of cerebrovascular pressure reactivity, 285

Cerebral veins
Virtual Navigator study: Subset of preliminary data about cerebral venous circulation, 385
Ipsilateral evaluation of the transverse sinus: Transcranial color-coded sonography approach in comparison with magnetic resonance venography, 390

Cerebral venous hemodynamics
Possibilities of transcranial color-coded sonography in pathology of deep brain veins in children, 353
Italian multicenter study on venous hemodynamics in multiple sclerosis: Advanced Sonological Protocol, 399

Cerebrospinal fluid
Informativity of pulsatility index and cerebral autoregulation in hydrocephalus, 311

Cerebrovascular reactivity
Asymmetry of cerebral autoregulation does not correspond to asymmetry of cerebrovascular pressure reactivity, 285

Cervical artery dissection
Ultrasound in spontaneous cervical artery dissection, 250

Cervical manipulative therapy
Migraine-like presentation of vertebral artery dissection after cervical manipulative therapy, 452

Subject index of volume 1

Chiari abnormalities
    Possibilities of transcranial color-coded sonography in pathology of deep brain veins in children, 353

Child/Children
    Transcranial ultrasound in adults and children with movement disorders, 349
    Possibilities of transcranial color-coded sonography in pathology of deep brain veins in children, 353

Chronic cerebrospinal venous insufficiency (CCSVI)
    Chronic cerebrospinal venous insufficiency in patients with multiple sclerosis: A case-control study from Iran, 375

Chronic heart failure
    Cerebral blood flow in the chronic heart failure patients, 304

Chronic hyperventilation syndrome
    An increased frequency of right-to-left shunt in patients with chronic hyperventilation syndrome, 241

Clinical application
    Clinical application of laser Doppler flowmetry in neurology, 89

Cognitive impairment
    Intellectual impairment and TCD evaluation in children with sickle cell disease and silent stroke, 272

Collateral flow
    Transcranial Doppler in acute stroke management – A "real-time" bed-side guide to reperfusion and collateral flow, 185

Color Doppler imaging
    Diagnosis of non-atherosclerotic carotid disease, 244

Color velocity imaging quantification
    Volume flow rate, 203

Combat associated wartime traumatic brain injury
    Posttraumatic vasospasm and intracranial hypertension after wartime traumatic brain injury, 261

Common carotid artery
    Comparative in vivo and in vitro postmortem ultrasound assessment of intima-media thickness with additional histological analysis in human carotid arteries, 170

Comparative analysis
    Comparative in vivo and in vitro postmortem ultrasound assessment of intima-media thickness with additional histological analysis in human carotid arteries, 170

Compliance
    Arterial wall dynamics, 146

Compression
    Ultrasonography of the peripheral nervous system, 417

Computed tomography angiography (CTA)
    Vertebral artery hypoplasia and the posterior circulation stroke, 198

Confirmatory test
    The role of color duplex sonography in the brain death diagnostics, 362

Consensus conference
    Plaque angiogenesis identification with Contrast Enhanced Carotid Ultrasonography: Statement of the Consensus after the 16th ESNCH Meeting – Munich, 20-23 May 2011, 51

Contrast agents
    Plaque angiogenesis identification with Contrast Enhanced Carotid Ultrasonography: Statement of the Consensus after the 16th ESNCH Meeting – Munich, 20-23 May 2011, 51

Contrast carotid ultrasound
    Imaging of plaque perfusion using contrast-enhanced ultrasound – Clinical significance, 44

Contrast enhanced ultrasound
    Early ultrasound imaging of carotid arteries in the acute ischemic cerebrovascular patients, 108

Critical closing pressure
    Adaptation of cerebral pressure-velocity hemodynamic changes of neurovascular coupling to orthostatic challenge, 290

Cryptogenic stroke
    Patent foramen ovale, 228

Computed tomographie (CT)
    Ultrasound fusion imaging, 80

Deep brain stimulation
    Intra- and post-operative monitoring of deep brain implants using transcranial ultrasound, 344

Degree of stenosis
    Measuring the degree of internal carotid artery stenosis, 104

Diabetes mellitus
    Breath holding index and arterial stiffness in evaluation of stroke risk in diabetic patients, 156

Diagnostic ultrasound
    The retrobulbar spot sign in sudden blindness – Sufficient to rule out vasculitis?, 408

Dissection
    Diagnosis of non-atherosclerotic carotid disease, 244
    Transcranial and cervical duplex: A feasible approach to the diagnosis of pulsatile tinnitus, 446

Distal myopathies
    Four-dimensional ultrasound calf muscle imaging in patients with genetic types of distal myopathy, 431

Distensibility
    Arterial wall dynamics, 146

Doppler method
    Volume flow rate, 203

Doppler ultrasound
    Measuring the degree of internal carotid artery stenosis, 104

Doppler ultrasound imaging
    Ultrasound findings of the optic nerve and its arterial venous system in multiple sclerosis patients with and without optic neuritis vs. healthy controls, 381

Drug delivery
    Advances in neurosonology – Brain perfusion, sonothrombolysis and CNS drug delivery, 5

Duplex
    The association of carotid intima-media thickness (cIMT) and stroke: A cross sectional study, 164
    Transcranial and cervical duplex: A feasible approach to the diagnosis of pulsatile tinnitus, 446

Duplex scanning
    Intima-media thickness of the carotid artery in OSAS patients, 160

Duplex sonography
    Measuring the degree of internal carotid artery stenosis, 104
    Ultrasound examination techniques of extra- and intracranial veins, 366
    Pitfall of vertebral artery insonation: Bidirectional flow without subclavian artery pathology, 449

Duplex ultrasonography
    Vertebral artery hypoplasia and the posterior circulation stroke, 198

Dural sinus
    Ultrasound examination techniques of extra- and intracranial veins, 366

Dysfunction
    Are impaired endothelial function in the posterior cerebral circulation and intact endothelial function in the anterior cerebral and systemic circulation associated with migraine: A post hoc study, 297

Early neurological deterioration
    Hemodynamic causes of deterioration in acute ischemic stroke, 177

Echocardiography
    Italian patent foramen ovale survey (I.P.O.S.): Early results, 236

Egyptian population
    Carotid atherosclerosis: Socio-demographic issues, the hidden dimensions, 167

Elbow
    An overview of musculoskeletal ultrasound – A thirteen years experience in Pakistan, 427

Electrode position control
    Transcranial sonography of the cerebral parenchyma: Update on clinically relevant applications, 334
    Intra- and post-operative monitoring of deep brain implants using transcranial ultrasound, 344

Embolus
    Late septic encephalopathy and septic shock are not associated with ongoing cerebral embolism, 224
    Exploration of a zero-tolerance regime on cerebral embolism in symptomatic carotid artery disease, 218

Embolus detection
   Microbubble signal properties from PFO tests using transcranial Doppler ultrasound, 232
Encephalopathy
   Late septic encephalopathy and septic shock are not associated with ongoing cerebral embolism, 224
Endarterectomy
   "A horse, a horse, my kingdom for a horse" - Saddle thrombosis of carotid bifurcation in acute stroke, 435
Endothelium
   Are impaired endothelial function in the posterior cerebral circulation and intact endothelial function in the anterior cerebral and systemic circulation associated with migraine: A post hoc study, 297
Endovascular stroke treatment
   Mechanical recanalization in acute stroke treatment, 54
Entrapment neuropathy
   Ultrasonography of peripheral nerves - Clinical significance, 422
Extracranial carotid arteries tortuosity and kinking
   Threedimensional imaging of carotid arteries: Advantages and pitfalls of ultrasound investigations, 82
Extracranial ultrasound examination
   Intravascular papillary endothelial hyperplasia at the origin of internal carotid artery: A rare cause of stroke, 440

Fistula
   Transcranial and cervical duplex: A feasible approach to the diagnosis of pulsatile tinnitus, 446
4D flow MRI
   In vivo wall shear stress patterns in carotid bifurcations assessed by 4D MRI, 137
Flow mediated dilatation
   Are impaired endothelial function in the posterior cerebral circulation and intact endothelial function in the anterior cerebral and systemic circulation associated with migraine: A post hoc study, 297
Flow visualization
   How local hemodynamics at the carotid bifurcation influence the development of carotid plaques, 132
Flow-sensitive MRI
   In vivo wall shear stress patterns in carotid bifurcations assessed by 4D MRI, 137
Foot
   An overview of musculoskeletal ultrasound - A thirteen years experience in Pakistan, 427
Functional TCD
   Withdraw of statin improves cerebrovascular reserve in radiation vasculopathy, 309
Fusion
   Ultrasound fusion imaging, 80
Fusion imaging
   Virtual Navigator study: Subset of preliminary data about cerebral venous circulation, 385

Gaseous emboli
   Microbubble signal properties from PFO tests using transcranial Doppler ultrasound, 232
Guideline
   The role of extracranial ultrasound in the prevention of stroke based on the new guidelines, 94

Hand
   An overview of musculoskeletal ultrasound - A thirteen years experience in Pakistan, 427
Headache
   Migraine-like presentation of vertebral artery dissection after cervical manipulative therapy, 452
Heliox
   Effect of helium on cerebral blood flow: A $n = 1$ trial in a healthy young person, 301
Helium
   Effect of helium on cerebral blood flow: A $n = 1$ trial in a healthy young person, 301
Hemodynamic
   Hemodynamic causes of deterioration in acute ischemic stroke, 177

Hereditary hemorrhagic telangiectasia
   Transient brainstem ischemia and dural arteriovenous malformation, 465
HIBM2
   Four-dimensional ultrasound calf muscle imaging in patients with genetic types of distal myopathy, 431
High-resolution ultrasound
   "A horse, a horse, my kingdom for a horse" - Saddle thrombosis of carotid bifurcation in acute stroke, 435
Hip
   An overview of musculoskeletal ultrasound - A thirteen years experience in Pakistan, 427
Hydrocephalus
   Informativity of pulsatility index and cerebral autoregulation in hydrocephalus, 311
Hyperbaric condition
   The long-term effects of hypobaric and hyperbaric conditions on brain hemodynamic: A transcranial Doppler ultrasonography of blood flow velocity of middle cerebral and basilar arteries in pilots and divers, 316
Hypobaric condition
   The long-term effects of hypobaric and hyperbaric conditions on brain hemodynamic: A transcranial Doppler ultrasonography of blood flow velocity of middle cerebral and basilar arteries in pilots and divers, 316
Hypoplasia of cerebral venous sinuses
   Possibilities of transcranial color-coded sonography in pathology of deep brain veins in children, 353

Idiopathic intracranial hypertension
   B-mode sonography of the optic nerve in neurological disorders with altered intracranial pressure, 404
In vitro ultrasonography
   Comparative in vivo and in vitro postmortem ultrasound assessment of intima-media thickness with additional histological analysis in human carotid arteries, 170
In vivo ultrasonography
   Comparative in vivo and in vitro postmortem ultrasound assessment of intima-media thickness with additional histological analysis in human carotid arteries, 170
Insonation rate
   Ipsilateral evaluation of the transverse sinus: Transcranial color-coded sonography approach in comparison with magnetic resonance venography, 390
Internal cerebral vein
   Chronic cerebrospinal venous insufficiency in patients with multiple sclerosis: A case-control study from Iran, 375
Internal jugular vein
   Ultrasound examination techniques of extra- and intracranial veins, 366
   Chronic cerebrospinal venous insufficiency in patients with multiple sclerosis: A case-control study from Iran, 375
   Italian multicenter study on venous hemodynamics in multiple sclerosis: Advanced Sonological Protocol, 399
Intima-media thickness (IMT)
   Arterial wall dynamics, 146
   Morphological, hemodynamic and stiffness changes in arteries of young smokers, 152
   Intima-media thickness of the carotid artery in OSAS patients, 160
   Comparative in vivo and in vitro postmortem ultrasound assessment of intima-media thickness with additional histological analysis in human carotid arteries, 170
Intracranial atherosclerosis
   Intra- and extracranial stenoses in TIA - Findings from the Aarhus TIA-study: A prospective population-based study, 207
Intracranial pressure
   Posttraumatic vasospasm and intracranial hypertension after wartime traumatic brain injury, 261
   Informativity of pulsatility index and cerebral autoregulation in hydrocephalus, 311
   Ultrasonography of the optic nerve sheath in brain death, 414
Intracranial pressure (ICP)
   Oscillating transcranial Doppler patterns of brain death associated with therapeutic maneuvers, 321

Subject index of volume 1

Intracranial stenosis
    Symptomatic intracranial stenosis: A university hospital-based ultrasound study, 211
    Moyamoya like arteriopathy: Neurosonological suspicion and prognosis in adult asymptomatic patients, 257

Intracranial veins
    Ultrasound examination techniques of extra- and intracranial veins, 366

Intraoperative
    Intraoperative color-coded duplex sonography of the superior sagittal sinus in parasagittal meningiomas, 395

Intravascular papillary endothelial hyperplasia (IPEH)
    Intravascular papillary endothelial hyperplasia at the origin of internal carotid artery: A rare cause of stroke, 440

Intravenous thrombolysis
    The impact of recanalization on ischemic stroke outcome: A clinical case presentation, 455

Ischemic stroke
    Update on ultrasound brain perfusion imaging, 30
    Relationship between refill-kinetics of ultrasound perfusion imaging and vascular obstruction in acute middle cerebral artery stroke, 39
    Symptomatic intracranial stenosis: A university hospital-based ultrasound study, 211
    The impact of recanalization on ischemic stroke outcome: A clinical case presentation, 455

Knee
    An overview of musculoskeletal ultrasound – A thirteen years experience in Pakistan, 427

Laser Doppler flowmetry
    Clinical application of laser Doppler flowmetry in neurology, 89

Left ventricular assist devices
    The contribution of microembolic signals (MES) detection in cardioembolic stroke, 214

Left ventricle ejection fraction
    Cerebral blood flow in the chronic heart failure patients, 304

Lumbosacral region
    An overview of musculoskeletal ultrasound – A thirteen years experience in Pakistan, 427

Macular degeneration
    Four-dimensional ultrasound imaging in neuro-ophthalmology, 86

Magnetic resonance angiography (MRA)
    Vertebral artery hypoplasia and the posterior circulation stroke, 198
    Evaluation of very early recanalization after tPA administration monitoring by transcranial color-coded sonography, 331

Magnetic resonance imagine (MRI)
    Ultrasound fusion imaging, 80

Magnetic resonance venography
    Intraoperative color-coded duplex sonography of the superior sagittal sinus in parasagittal meningiomas, 395

Management
    Diagnosis and management of Takayasu arteritis, 255

Mechanical recanalization
    Mechanical recanalization in acute stroke treatment, 54

Mechanical thrombectomy
    Mechanical recanalization in acute stroke treatment, 54

Medical treatment
    How to treat an asymptomatic carotid stenosis? The view of the neurologist, 112
    Medical management of asymptomatic carotid stenosis, 116

Microbubbles
    Advances in neurosonology – Brain perfusion, sonothrombolysis and CNS drug delivery, 5
    Sonothrombolysis: Current status, 11
    Safety evaluation of superheated perfluorocarbon nanodroplets for novel phase change type neurological therapeutic agents, 25
    Relationship between refill-kinetics of ultrasound perfusion imaging and vascular obstruction in acute middle cerebral artery stroke, 39

Microembolic signals
    Transcranial Doppler in acute stroke management – A "real-time" bed-side guide to reperfusion and collateral flow, 185
    The contribution of microembolic signals (MES) detection in cardioembolic stroke, 214

Middle cerebral artery (MCA)
    Moyamoya like arteriopathy: Neurosonological suspicion and prognosis in adult asymptomatic patients, 257
    Transcranial color-coded duplex ultrasonography in routine cerebrovascular diagnostics, 325

Migraine
    Are impaired endothelial function in the posterior cerebral circulation and intact endothelial function in the anterior cerebral and systemic circulation associated with migraine: A post hoc study, 297
    Migraine-like presentation of vertebral artery dissection after cervical manipulative therapy, 452

M-mode ultrasound
    Arterial wall dynamics, 146

Movement disorder
    Transcranial ultrasound in adults and children with movement disorders, 349

Moyamoya
    Moyamoya like arteriopathy: Neurosonological suspicion and prognosis in adult asymptomatic patients, 257

Multiple sclerosis (MS)
    Fact or fiction: Chronic cerebro-spinal insufficiency, 371
    Chronic cerebrospinal venous insufficiency in patients with multiple sclerosis: A case-control study from Iran, 375
    Italian multicenter study on venous hemodynamics in multiple sclerosis: Advanced Sonological Protocol, 399

Musculoskeletal
    An overview of musculoskeletal ultrasound – A thirteen years experience in Pakistan, 427

Myosonology
    Four-dimensional ultrasound calf muscle imaging in patients with genetic types of distal myopathy, 431

Nanodroplets
    Safety evaluation of superheated perfluorocarbon nanodroplets for novel phase change type neurological therapeutic agents, 25

Navigated brain stimulation
    Functional guidance in intracranial tumor surgery, 59

Nerve
    Ultrasonography of the peripheral nervous system, 417

Nerve sheath tumor
    Ultrasonography of peripheral nerves – Clinical significance, 422

Neurovascular coupling
    Adaptation of cerebral pressure-velocity hemodynamic changes of neurovascular coupling to orthostatic challenge, 290

Non-atherosclerotic
    Diagnosis of non-atherosclerotic carotid disease, 244

Obstructive sleep apnea
    Intima-media thickness of the carotid artery in OSAS patients, 160

Occlusion
    Transcranial color-coded duplex ultrasonography in routine cerebrovascular diagnostics, 325

Ophthalmic venous flow
    Ultrasound findings of the optic nerve and its arterial venous system in multiple sclerosis patients with and without optic neuritis vs. healthy controls, 381

Optic disc swelling
    Four-dimensional ultrasound imaging in neuro-ophthalmology, 86

Optic Nerve atrophy
    Ultrasound findings of the optic nerve and its arterial venous system in multiple sclerosis patients with and without optic neuritis vs. healthy controls, 381

Optic nerve edema
    Four-dimensional ultrasound imaging in neuro-ophthalmology, 86

Optic nerve sheath diameter
    Ultrasonography of the optic nerve sheath in brain death, 414

B-mode sonography of the optic nerve in neurological disorders with altered intracranial pressure, 404
Optic nerve sonography
B-mode sonography of the optic nerve in neurological disorders with altered intracranial pressure, 404
Optic neuritis
Ultrasound findings of the optic nerve and its arterial venous system in multiple sclerosis patients with and without optic neuritis vs. healthy controls, 381
Oscillating flow
Oscillating transcranial Doppler patterns of brain death associated with therapeutic maneuvers, 321
Outcome
Current trends in sonothrombolysis for acute ischemic stroke, 21
Act on Stroke – Optimization of clinical processes and workflow for stroke diagnosis and treatment, 73

Parasagittal meningioma
Intraoperative color-coded duplex sonography of the superior sagittal sinus in parasagittal meningiomas, 395
Parkinsonism
Transcranial sonography of the cerebral parenchyma: Update on clinically relevant applications, 334
Patch plastic
How local hemodynamics at the carotid bifurcation influence the development of carotid plaques, 132
Patent foramen ovale
Patent foramen ovale, 228
Italian patent foramen ovale survey (I.P.O.S.): Early results, 236
An increased frequency of right-to-left shunt in patients with chronic hyperventilation syndrome, 241
Peak systolic velocity
Measuring the degree of internal carotid artery stenosis, 104
Pediatric
Transcranial ultrasound in adults and children with movement disorders, 349
Percutaneous PFO closure
Italian patent foramen ovale survey (I.P.O.S.): Early results, 236
Perfluorocarbon
Safety evaluation of superheated perfluorocarbon nanodroplets for novel phase change type neurological therapeutic agents, 25
Perfusion
Advances in neurosonology – Brain perfusion, sonothrombolysis and CNS drug delivery, 5
Pitfall
Pitfall of vertebral artery insonation: Bidirectional flow without subclavian artery pathology, 449
Plaque
Carotid intima-media thickness (cIMT) and plaque from risk assessment and clinical use to genetic discoveries, 139
Polyneuropathy
Ultrasonography of the peripheral nervous system, 417
Ultrasonography of peripheral nerves – Clinical significance, 422
Posterior circulation stroke
Vertebral artery hypoplasia and the posterior circulation stroke, 198
Post-operative monitoring
Intra- and post-operative monitoring of deep brain implants using transcranial ultrasound, 344
Power modulation imaging
Brain tissue perfusion monitoring using Sonopod for transcranial color duplex sonography, 34
Preoperative mapping
Functional guidance in intracranial tumor surgery, 59
Prevalence
Intra- and extracranial stenoses in TIA – Findings from the Aarhus TIA-study: A prospective population-based study, 207
Prevention
The role of extracranial ultrasound in the prevention of stroke based on the new guidelines, 94
Primary prevention
Medical management of asymptomatic carotid stenosis, 116

Process optimization
Act on Stroke – Optimization of clinical processes and workflow for stroke diagnosis and treatment, 73
Psychiatric diseases
Transcranial sonography in psychiatric diseases, 357
Pulsatile
Transcranial and cervical duplex: A feasible approach to the diagnosis of pulsatile tinnitus, 446

Quality of care
Act on Stroke – Optimization of clinical processes and workflow for stroke diagnosis and treatment, 73
Quantitative flow measurement system
Volume flow rate, 203

Radiation vasculopathy
Withdraw of statin improves cerebrovascular reserve in radiation vasculopathy, 309
Recanalization
Current trends in sonothrombolysis for acute ischemic stroke, 21
Endovascular sono-lysis using EKOS system in acute stroke patients with a main cerebral artery occlusion – A pilot study, 65
Transcranial Doppler in acute stroke management – A "real-time" bed-side guide to reperfusion and collateral flow, 185
Evaluation of very early recanalization after tPA administration monitoring by transcranial color-coded sonography, 331
The impact of recanalization on ischemic stroke outcome: A clinical case presentation, 455
Refill kinetics
Relationship between refill-kinetics of ultrasound perfusion imaging and vascular obstruction in acute middle cerebral artery stroke, 39
Reocclusion
Hemodynamic causes of deterioration in acute ischemic stroke, 177
Restenosis
Predictors of carotid artery in-stent restenosis, 122
Retinal detachment
Four-dimensional ultrasound imaging in neuro-ophthalmology, 86
Reversible cerebral vasoconstriction syndrome
Reversible cerebral vasoconstriction syndrome after preeclampsia, 443
Right to left shunt
Patent foramen ovale, 228
An increased frequency of right-to-left shunt in patients with chronic hyperventilation syndrome, 241
Risk factors
Carotid intima-media thickness (cIMT) and plaque from risk assessment and clinical use to genetic discoveries, 139
Rolandic region
Functional guidance in intracranial tumor surgery, 59
rt-PA
Sonothrombolysis: Current status, 11

Saddle thrombosis
"A horse, a horse, my kingdom for a horse" – Saddle thrombosis of carotid bifurcation in acute stroke, 435
Safety
Safety evaluation of superheated perfluorocarbon nanodroplets for novel phase change type neurological therapeutic agents, 25
Second harmonic imaging
Brain tissue perfusion monitoring using Sonopod for transcranial color duplex sonography, 34
Semantic aphasia
Semantic aphasia in a sonothrombolysed patient. A treatment without use of rt-PA, 459
Sepsis
Late septic encephalopathy and septic shock are not associated with ongoing cerebral embolism, 224
Septic
Late septic encephalopathy and septic shock are not associated with ongoing cerebral embolism, 224

Subject index of volume 1

Shock
  Late septic encephalopathy and septic shock are not associated with ongoing cerebral embolism, 224
Shoulder
  An overview of musculoskeletal ultrasound – A thirteen years experience in Pakistan, 427
Sickle cell disease
  Role of TCD in sickle cell disease: A review, 265
  Transcranial Doppler sonography in children with sickle cell disease and silent ischemic lesions, 269
  Intellectual impairment and TCD evaluation in children with sickle cell disease and silent stroke, 272
Silent strokes
  Transcranial Doppler sonography in children with sickle cell disease and silent ischemic lesions, 269
  Intellectual impairment and TCD evaluation in children with sickle cell disease and silent stroke, 272
Sinus cavernous
  Possibilities of transcranial color-coded sonography in pathology of deep brain veins in children, 353
Sleep apnea syndrome
  Cerebral blood flow velocity in sleep, 275
Smoking
  Morphological, hemodynamic and stiffness changes in arteries of young smokers, 152
Snap freezing
  Comparative in vivo and in vitro postmortem ultrasound assessment of intima-media thickness with additional histological analysis in human carotid arteries, 170
Socio-demographic
  Carotid atherosclerosis: Socio-demographic issues, the hidden dimensions, 167
Sonography
  Intraoperative color-coded duplex sonography of the superior sagittal sinus in parasagittal meningiomas, 395
  Ultrasonography of the peripheral nervous system, 417
Sono-lysis
  Endovascular sono-lysis using EKOS system in acute stroke patients with a main cerebral artery occlusion – A pilot study, 65
Sonothrombolysis
  Advances in neurosonology – Brain perfusion, sonothrombolysis and CNS drug delivery, 5
  Sonothrombolysis: Current status, 11
  Sonothrombolysis for treatment of acute ischemic stroke: Current evidence and new developments, 14
  Safety evaluation of superheated perfluorocarbon nanodroplets for novel phase change type neurological therapeutic agents, 25
  Endovascular sono-lysis using EKOS system in acute stroke patients with a main cerebral artery occlusion – A pilot study, 65
  Semantic aphasia in a sonothrombolysed patient. A treatment without use of rt-PA, 459
  My worst case with sonothrombolysis, 462
Spasmophilia
  An increased frequency of right-to-left shunt in patients with chronic hyperventilation syndrome, 241
Spikes
  Oscillating transcranial Doppler patterns of brain death associated with therapeutic maneuvers, 321
Spontaneous
  Ultrasound in spontaneous cervical artery dissection, 250
Spontaneous intracranial hypotension
  B-mode sonography of the optic nerve in neurological disorders with altered intracranial pressure, 404
Statin
  Withdraw of statin improves cerebrovascular reserve in radiation vasculopathy, 309
Stenosis
  Transcranial color-coded duplex ultrasonography in routine cerebrovascular diagnostics, 325
Stent/Stents
  Predictors of carotid artery in-stent restenosis, 122
  How local hemodynamics at the carotid bifurcation influence the development of carotid plaques, 132

Stiffness
  Morphological, hemodynamic and stiffness changes in arteries of young smokers, 152
Stroke
  Advances in neurosonology – Brain perfusion, sonothrombolysis and CNS drug delivery, 5
  Current trends in sonothrombolysis for acute ischemic stroke, 21
  Endovascular sono-lysis using EKOS system in acute stroke patients with a main cerebral artery occlusion – A pilot study, 65
  Act on Stroke – Optimization of clinical processes and workflow for stroke diagnosis and treatment, 73
  Telestroke – How does that work?, 77
  The role of extracranial ultrasound in the prevention of stroke based on the new guidelines, 94
  Predictors of carotid artery in-stent restenosis, 122
  Post-carotid stent ultrasound provides critical data to avoid rare but serious complications, 129
  The association of carotid intima-media thickness (cIMT) and stroke: A cross sectional study, 164
  Exploration of a zero-tolerance regime on cerebral embolism in symptomatic carotid artery disease, 218
  Italian patent foramen ovale survey (I.P.O.S.): Early results, 236
  Diagnosis of non-atherosclerotic carotid disease, 244
  Role of TCD in sickle cell disease: A review, 265
  Transcranial color-coded duplex ultrasonography in routine cerebrovascular diagnostics, 325
  Transcranial sonography of the cerebral parenchyma: Update on clinically relevant applications, 334
  The retrobulbar spot sign in sudden blindness – Sufficient to rule out vasculitis?, 408
Stroke prevention
  Optimized prevention of stroke: What is the role of ultrasound?, 100
  How to treat an asymptomatic carotid stenosis? The view of the neurologist, 112
Subclavian steal syndrom
  Pitfall of vertebral artery insonation: Bidirectional flow without subclavian artery pathology, 449
Substantia nigra
  Transcranial sonography of the cerebral parenchyma: Update on clinically relevant applications, 334
Superior sagittal sinus
  Intraoperative color-coded duplex sonography of the superior sagittal sinus in parasagittal meningiomas, 395
Surrogate markers
  Carotid intima-media thickness (cIMT) and plaque from risk assessment and clinical use to genetic discoveries, 139
Survey
  Italian patent foramen ovale survey (I.P.O.S.): Early results, 236

Takayasu
  Diagnosis and management of Takayasu arteritis, 255
Telemedicine
  Telestroke – How does that work?, 77
TEMPiS network
  Telestroke – How does that work?, 77
Tetania
  An increased frequency of right-to-left shunt in patients with chronic hyperventilation syndrome, 241
Therapy
  Advances in neurosonology – Brain perfusion, sonothrombolysis and CNS drug delivery, 5
  Sonothrombolysis for treatment of acute ischemic stroke: Current evidence and new developments, 14
  Endovascular sono-lysis using EKOS system in acute stroke patients with a main cerebral artery occlusion – A pilot study, 65
Thigh
  An overview of musculoskeletal ultrasound – A thirteen years experience in Pakistan, 427
Thrombolysis
  Sonothrombolysis for treatment of acute ischemic stroke: Current evidence and new developments, 14

Current trends in sonothrombolysis for acute ischemic stroke, 21

TIA
Exploration of a zero-tolerance regime on cerebral embolism in symptomatic carotid artery disease, 218

Timing of carotid surgery
Early ultrasound imaging of carotid arteries in the acute ischemic cerebrovascular patients, 108

Tinnitus
Transcranial and cervical duplex: A feasible approach to the diagnosis of pulsatile tinnitus, 446

Tissue plasminogen activator
Evaluation of very early recanalization after tPA administration monitoring by transcranial color-coded sonography, 331

TMD
Four-dimensional ultrasound calf muscle imaging in patients with genetic types of distal myopathy, 431

Transcranial
Moyamoya like arteriopathy: Neurosonological suspicion and prognosis in adult asymptomatic patients, 257
Virtual Navigator study: Subset of preliminary data about cerebral venous circulation, 385
Ipsilateral evaluation of the transverse sinus: Transcranial color-coded sonography approach in comparison with magnetic resonance venography, 390
Italian multicenter study on venous hemodynamics in multiple sclerosis: Advanced Sonological Protocol, 399

Transcranial color-coded duplex ultrasonography (TCCS)
Brain tissue perfusion monitoring using Sonopod for transcranial color duplex sonography, 34
Moyamoya like arteriopathy: Neurosonological suspicion and prognosis in adult asymptomatic patients, 257
Transcranial color-coded duplex ultrasonography in routine cerebrovascular diagnostics, 325
Possibilities of transcranial color-coded sonography in pathology of deep brain veins in children, 353
Virtual Navigator study: Subset of preliminary data about cerebral venous circulation, 385
Ipsilateral evaluation of the transverse sinus: Transcranial color-coded sonography approach in comparison with magnetic resonance venography, 390
Reversible cerebral vasoconstriction syndrome after preeclampsia, 443
My worst case with sonothrombolysis, 462
Transient brainstem ischemia and dural arteriovenous malformation, 465

Transcranial Doppler sonography (TCD)
When to perform transcranial Doppler to predict cerebral hyperperfusion after carotid endarterectomy?, 119
Hemodynamic causes of deterioration in acute ischemic stroke, 177
Transcranial Doppler in acute stroke management – A "real-time" bed-side guide to reperfusion and collateral flow, 185
Cerebral autoregulation in acute ischemic stroke, 194
Intra- and extracranial stenoses in TIA – Findings from the Aarhus TIA-study: A prospective population-based study, 207
Exploration of a zero-tolerance regime on cerebral embolism in symptomatic carotid artery disease, 218
Patent foramen ovale, 228
Late septic encephalopathy and septic shock are not associated with ongoing cerebral embolism, 224
Microbubble signal properties from PFO tests using transcranial Doppler ultrasound, 232
Italian patent foramen ovale survey (I.P.O.S.): Early results, 236
An increased frequency of right-to-left shunt in patients with chronic hyperventilation syndrome, 241
Diagnosis of non-atherosclerotic carotid disease, 244
Posttraumatic vasospasm and intracranial hypertension after wartime traumatic brain injury, 261
Role of TCD in sickle cell disease: A review, 265
Transcranial Doppler sonography in children with sickle cell disease and silent ischemic lesions, 269
Intellectual impairment and TCD evaluation in children with sickle cell disease and silent stroke, 272
Cerebral blood flow velocity in sleep, 275
Asymmetry of cerebral autoregulation does not correspond to asymmetry of cerebrovascular pressure reactivity, 285
Adaptation of cerebral pressure-velocity hemodynamic changes of neurovascular coupling to orthostatic challenge, 290
Are impaired endothelial function in the posterior cerebral circulation and intact endothelial function in the anterior cerebral and systemic circulation associated with migraine: A post hoc study, 297
Effect of helium on cerebral blood flow: A $n = 1$ trial in a healthy young person, 301
Informativity of pulsatility index and cerebral autoregulation in hydrocephalus, 311
The long-term effects of hypobaric and hyperbaric conditions on brain hemodynamic: A transcranial Doppler ultrasonography of blood flow velocity of middle cerebral and basilar arteries in pilots and divers, 316
Oscillating transcranial Doppler patterns of brain death associated with therapeutic maneuvers, 321
The role of color duplex sonography in the brain death diagnostics, 362
Transcranial and cervical duplex: A feasible approach to the diagnosis of pulsatile tinnitus, 446

Transcranial magnetic stimulation
Functional guidance in intracranial tumor surgery, 59

Transcranial sonography
Transcranial sonography of the cerebral parenchyma: Update on clinically relevant applications, 334
Intra- and post-operative monitoring of deep brain implants using transcranial ultrasound, 344
Transcranial sonography in psychiatric diseases, 357

Transcranial ultrasound
Sonothrombolysis for treatment of acute ischemic stroke: Current evidence and new developments, 14
Evaluation of very early recanalization after tPA administration monitoring by transcranial color-coded sonography, 331
Transcranial ultrasound in adults and children with movement disorders, 349

Transducer holder (Sonopod)
Brain tissue perfusion monitoring using Sonopod for transcranial color duplex sonography, 34

Transesophageal echocardiography
Patent foramen ovale, 228

Transient global amnesia
Italian multicenter study on venous hemodynamics in multiple sclerosis: Advanced Sonological Protocol, 399

Transient ischemic attack
Intra- and extracranial stenoses in TIA – Findings from the Aarhus TIA-study: A prospective population-based study, 207
Transient brainstem ischemia and dural arteriovenous malformation, 465

Transverse sinus
Virtual Navigator study: Subset of preliminary data about cerebral venous circulation, 385
Ipsilateral evaluation of the transverse sinus: Transcranial color-coded sonography approach in comparison with magnetic resonance venography, 390

Trauma
Ultrasonography of the peripheral nervous system, 417

Traumatic brain injury
B-mode sonography of the optic nerve in neurological disorders with altered intracranial pressure, 404

Traumatic nerve lesion
Ultrasonography of peripheral nerves – Clinical significance, 422

Tumor
Functional guidance in intracranial tumor surgery, 59
Ultrasonography of the peripheral nervous system, 417

Ultrasonography
Advances in neurosonology – Brain perfusion, sonothrombolysis and CNS drug delivery, 5
The role of extracranial ultrasound in the prevention of stroke based on the new guidelines, 94

Optimized prevention of stroke: What is the role of ultrasound?, 100
Early ultrasound imaging of carotid arteries in the acute ischemic cerebrovascular patients, 108
Carotid intima-media thickness (cIMT) and plaque from risk assessment and clinical use to genetic discoveries, 139
Vertebral artery hypoplasia and the posterior circulation stroke, 198
Ultrasound in spontaneous cervical artery dissection, 250
Diagnosis and management of Takayasu arteritis, 255
Transcranial ultrasound in adults and children with movement disorders, 349
Fact or fiction: Chronic cerebro-spinal insufficiency, 371
Ultrasonography of the optic nerve sheath in brain death, 414
Ultrasonography of peripheral nerves – Clinical significance, 422
An overview of musculoskeletal ultrasound – A thirteen years experience in Pakistan, 427

3D ultrasound
Threedimensional imaging of carotid arteries: Advantages and pitfalls of ultrasound investigations, 82

4D ultrasound imaging
Four-dimensional ultrasound imaging in neuro-ophthalmology, 86
Four-dimensional ultrasound calf muscle imaging in patients with genetic types of distal myopathy, 431

Ultrasound contrast agent
Update on ultrasound brain perfusion imaging, 30
Patent foramen ovale, 228

Ultrasound perfusion imaging
Relationship between refill-kinetics of ultrasound perfusion imaging and vascular obstruction in acute middle cerebral artery stroke, 39

Ultrasound-guided procedure
Intra- and post-operative monitoring of deep brain implants using transcranial ultrasound, 344

Unstable carotid plaques
Early ultrasound imaging of carotid arteries in the acute ischemic cerebrovascular patients, 108

Unstable plaque
Imaging of plaque perfusion using contrast-enhanced ultrasound – Clinical significance, 44

Vasculitis
The retrobulbar spot sign in sudden blindness – Sufficient to rule out vasculitis?, 408

Vasomotor reactivity
Withdraw of statin improves cerebrovascular reserve in radiation vasculopathy, 309

Vasospasm
Posttraumatic vasospasm and intracranial hypertension after wartime traumatic brain injury, 261

VCPDM
Four-dimensional ultrasound calf muscle imaging in patients with genetic types of distal myopathy, 431

Velocity measurement
How local hemodynamics at the carotid bifurcation influence the development of carotid plaques, 132

Vertebral artery
Pitfall of vertebral artery insonation: Bidirectional flow without subclavian artery pathology, 449

Vertebral artery dissection
Migraine-like presentation of vertebral artery dissection after cervical manipulative therapy, 452

Vertebral artery hypoplasia (VAH)
Vertebral artery hypoplasia and the posterior circulation stroke, 198

Virtual Navigator
Virtual Navigator study: Subset of preliminary data about cerebral venous circulation, 385
Ipsilateral evaluation of the transverse sinus: Transcranial color-coded sonography approach in comparison with magnetic resonance venography, 390

Volume flow rate
Volume flow rate, 203

Wall shear stress
In vivo wall shear stress patterns in carotid bifurcations assessed by 4D MRI, 137

Wartime traumatic brain injury
Posttraumatic vasospasm and intracranial hypertension after wartime traumatic brain injury, 261

Wrist
An overview of musculoskeletal ultrasound – A thirteen years experience in Pakistan, 427

Acknowledgments

The editors wish to express their gratitude to the following companies who have helped to make the production of this book possible with their support:

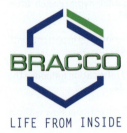
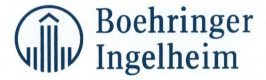
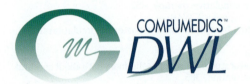
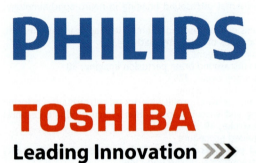
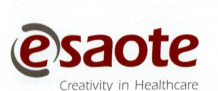